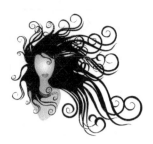

Book I
Dr. Julie Jackson

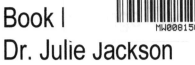

# Using the Rorschach Performance Assessment System® (R-PAS®)

# Using the
# Rorschach Performance
# Assessment System®
# (R-PAS®)

Edited by

## Joni L. Mihura
## Gregory J. Meyer

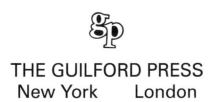

THE GUILFORD PRESS
New York     London

Copyright © 2018 The Guilford Press
A Division of Guilford Publications, Inc.
370 Seventh Avenue, Suite 1200, New York, NY 10001
www.guilford.com

Printed in the United States of America

This book is printed on acid-free paper.

Last digit is print number:  9  8  7  6  5  4  3  2  1

The authors have checked with sources believed to be reliable in their efforts to provide
information that is complete and generally in accord with the standards of practice that are
accepted at the time of publication. However, in view of the possibility of human error or
changes in behavioral, mental health, or medical sciences, neither the authors, nor the editors
and publisher, nor any other party who has been involved in the preparation or publication of
this work warrants that the information contained herein is in every respect accurate or complete,
and they are not responsible for any errors or omissions or the results obtained from the use of
such information. Readers are encouraged to confirm the information contained in this book
with other sources.

Library of Congress Cataloging-in-Publication Data is available from the publisher.

ISBN 978-1-4625-3253-7 (hardcover)

Rorschach Performance Assessment System® and R-PAS® are registered trademarks
of Rorschach Performance Assessment System, LLC.

Rorschach® is a registered trademark of Hogrefe. Hogrefe has not participated in the preparation
of this book.

# About the Editors

**Joni L. Mihura, PhD,** is Professor of Psychology at the University of Toledo, where she teaches personality assessment, advanced assessment, and psychodynamic/integrative psychotherapy. She received early career awards from the American Psychoanalytic Association and the Society for Personality Assessment (SPA), as well as the Walter G. Klopfer Award for Distinguished Contribution to the Literature from SPA, and is a Fellow and past board member of SPA. Dr. Mihura serves on the editorial boards of the *Journal of Personality Assessment* and *Rorschachiana,* has published many articles and chapters on psychological assessment, and is coeditor of the *Handbook of Gender and Sexuality in Psychological Assessment.* She is a codeveloper of R-PAS (*www.r-pas.org*) and presents invited lectures and trainings internationally.

**Gregory J. Meyer, PhD,** is Professor of Psychology at the University of Toledo. His research focuses on psychological assessment, with an emphasis on the integration of assessment methods. He is a four-time recipient of the Walter G. Klopfer Award for Distinguished Contribution to the Literature from SPA. Dr. Meyer also received the Award for Distinguished Contributions to Assessment Psychology from Section IX (Assessment Psychology) of the Society of Clinical Psychology, Division 12 of the American Psychological Association (APA), and is a Fellow of Division 5 (Quantitative and Qualitative Methods) of APA, as well as of SPA. With more than 75 peer-reviewed publications, he is a past editor of the *Journal of Personality Assessment.* He is a codeveloper of R-PAS and presents invited lectures and trainings internationally.

# Contributors

**Marvin W. Acklin, PhD, ABAP, ABPP,** Department of Psychiatry,
John A. Burns School of Medicine, University of Hawaii at Manoa, Honolulu, Hawaii

**Filippo Aschieri, PhD,** European Center for Therapeutic Assessment,
Università Cattolica del Sacro Cuore, Milan, Italy

**Ety Berant, PhD,** Baruch Ivcher School of Psychology, Interdisciplinary Center,
Herzliya, Israel

**Cassandra Berbary, PhD,** College of Health Sciences and Technology,
Rochester Institute of Technology, Rochester, New York

**Anthony Bram, PhD, ABAP,** Boston Psychoanalytic Society and Institute,
Newton Centre, Massachusetts; Cambridge Health Alliance/Harvard Medical School,
Cambridge, Massachusetts; and private practice, Lexington, Massachusetts

**Alessandra Chinaglia, MS,** Department of Psychology, Università Cattolica del Sacro Cuore,
Milan, Italy

**Hilde De Saeger, MA,** De Viersprong, Halsteren, The Netherlands

**Nicolae Dumitrascu, PhD,** Danielsen Institute at Boston University, Boston, Massachusetts

**Philip Erdberg, PhD, ABPP,** Department of Psychiatry, University of California
San Francisco School of Medicine, Greenbrae, California, and private practice,
Corte Madera, California

**Jack Fahy, PhD,** Masonic Center for Youth and Families, San Francisco, California

**Francesca Fantini, PhD,** European Center for Therapeutic Assessment and EDUCatt
(Ente per il Diritto allo studio dell'Università Cattolica), Università Cattolica
del Sacro Cuore, Milan, Italy

**Ellen J. Hartmann, CandPsychol,** Department of Psychology, University of Oslo,
Oslo, Norway

**Tammy L. Hughes, PhD,** Department of Counseling, Psychology, and Special Education, Duquesne University, Pittsburgh, Pennsylvania

**Saara Kaakinen, MA,** Department of Psychiatry, Unit of Forensic Psychiatry, Oulu University Hospital, Oulu, Finland

**Jan H. Kamphuis, PhD,** Department of Psychology, University of Amsterdam, Amsterdam, The Netherlands

**Nancy Kaser-Boyd, PhD, ABAP,** Department of Psychiatry and Biobehavioral Sciences, Geffen School of Medicine at the University of California, Los Angeles, and Semel Institute for Neuroscience and Human Behavior, Los Angeles, California

**Philip Keddy, PhD,** private practice, Oakland, California, and Wright Institute, Berkeley, California

**Reneau Kennedy, EdD,** Clinical and Forensic Psychology, Honolulu, Hawaii

**Ali Khadivi, PhD,** Department of Psychiatry, Bronx Lebanon Hospital Center, and Department of Psychiatry and Behavioral Sciences, Albert Einstein College of Medicine, Bronx, New York

**Andrea B. Kiss, MS,** Department of Psychology, University of Toledo, Toledo, Ohio

**James H. Kleiger, PsyD, ABPP, ABAP,** private practice, Bethesda, Maryland

**S. Margaret Lee, PhD,** private practice, Mill Valley, California

**Jessica Lipkind, PsyD,** WestCoast Children's Clinic, and private practice, Oakland, California

**Gregory J. Meyer, PhD,** Department of Psychology, University of Toledo, Toledo, Ohio

**Joni L. Mihura, PhD,** Department of Psychology, University of Toledo, Toledo, Ohio

**Emiliano Muzio, PhD,** private practice, Helsinki, Finland

**Peder Chr. B. Nørbech, MS, CandPsychol,** Department of Psychology, University of Oslo, Oslo, Norway

**Kate Piselli, PhD,** Department of Counseling, Psychology, and Special Education, Duquesne University, Pittsburgh, Pennsylvania

**Hannu Säävälä, MD, PhD,** Department of Psychiatry, Unit of Forensic Psychiatry, Oulu University Hospital, Oulu, Finland

**Justin D. Smith, PhD,** Department of Psychiatry and Behavioral Sciences, Northwestern University Feinberg School of Medicine, Chicago, Illinois

# Preface

While this book was being written, rumors existed that the Rorschach was never, or very rarely, used in clinical practice. However, recent surveys of clinicians and clinical training programs show that the Rorschach continues to be taught and used in practice at a high frequency (Mihura, Roy, & Graceffo, 2017; Wright et al., 2017). Most importantly, recent research has addressed the primary criticisms leveled against the previous, most commonly used Rorschach system, Exner's Comprehensive System (CS). This research culminated in the development of a new, empirically sound Rorschach system—the Rorschach Performance Assessment System (R-PAS; Meyer, Viglione, Mihura, Erard, & Erdberg, 2011)—and the self-proclaimed "Rorschach critics" lifting their call for an all-out moratorium on the use of the Rorschach in clinical and forensic settings (see Mihura & Meyer, Chapter 1, this volume).

## Why Use the Rorschach at All?

As described further in Chapter 1, there are several essential reasons for using the Rorschach:

1. To date, the Rorschach has, by far, the most published meta-analyses of validity for its clinical scales of any psychological test—over 50 published validity meta-analyses of Rorschach scales compared to only two Minnesota Multiphasic Personality Inventory–2 (MMPI-2) clinical scales.
2. The Rorschach provides incremental validity over self-report scales.
3. The Rorschach is the best psychological test for assessing psychosis, particularly when using R-PAS scales.
4. The Rorschach, using R-PAS, provides a valid behavioral assessment of psychological characteristics not available through any other normed test. These characteristics include reality testing and thought disturbance; preoccupations

and intrusions of mental imagery like those seen in posttraumatic stress disorder, obsessive–compulsive disorder, or major depression; and self and other
mental representations. It also provides a typical performance measure of
cognitive complexity and coded behaviors when interacting with the examiner to compare to norms.

## Why Was R-PAS Developed?

After Exner's death in 2006, the CS needed revisions to implement the changes on
which his Rorschach Research Council had been working. Exner had revised the CS
test manuals for administration, scoring, and interpretation every 2–5 years, starting
with the original manual in 1974 and culminating with his final manual in 2005.
However, Exner did not provide an avenue for the Research Council to continue
his work, and problems with the CS needed to be fixed. For example, the editors of
this casebook (Joni L. Mihura and Gregory J. Meyer) had been working on extensive systematic reviews of the CS validity literature to address the major concerns
that had been raised by critics of the Rorschach method, and that had led one of
those critics (Howard Garb) to call for a moratorium on the use of the Rorschach in
clinical and forensic practice in 1999. As members of Exner's Research Council, the
R-PAS developers were in a unique position to be aware of existing problems and
to be working toward solutions. Therefore, after 2 years of encouraging the Exner
family to continue making CS revisions and the family's ultimate decision to leave
the CS as it was, Meyer, Viglione, Mihura, Erard, and Erdberg decided to develop a
replacement system, implementing changes based on their research, which was substantially derived from the numerous Research Council projects endorsed by Exner
(see Exner, 2000). The R-PAS manual and online scoring program became available
in August 2011.

## Why Is This Book Essential for Using R-PAS?

Providing psychologists with clinical examples to assist in the application of different assessment and treatment methods is common practice. For example, there are a
number of casebooks available (e.g., Barnhill, 2014) for the *Diagnostic and Statistical Manual of Mental Disorders, Fifth Edition* (DSM-5; American Psychiatric Association, 2013). After the Rorschach CS was first published in 1974, several casebooks
followed. Exner wrote three, the most recent (and last) published in 2005 (Exner &
Erdberg, 2005). Other psychologists have also written or edited CS casebooks, such
as *Rorschach Assessment of the Personality Disorders* (Huprich, 2006), *Principles of
Rorschach Interpretation* (Weiner, 2004), and *Contemporary Rorschach Interpretation* (Meloy, Acklin, Gacono, Murray, & Peterson, 1997).
    However, at the time of this writing, there are no books that thoroughly demon-
strate or illustrate how R-PAS is implemented and interpreted. The existing CS casebooks cannot be used for R-PAS interpretation. The R-PAS results pages are entirely
different from those of the CS (e.g., R-PAS reports results using standard scores),
its variables have different names, it has variables not included in the CS, and the

interpretations for most R-PAS variables are different from those in the CS. For this reason, we created this volume.

The book's format is most similar to *Contemporary Rorschach Interpretation* (Meloy et al., 1997) in that it contains chapters written by experts on various topics, such as psychopathy, psychosis, and use of the Rorschach with children. However, our book differs in two important ways. First, it is edited by two of the R-PAS developers (Mihura and Meyer), which helps ensure fidelity to the system. Second, both editors reviewed the administration, scoring, and interpretation of every case and worked with the authors on revisions to maintain fidelity to R-PAS. Therefore, the examples in this book are valuable resources with which to see how administration is conducted and documented, to learn accurate coding, and to understand the process of interpretation.

## REFERENCES

American Psychiatric Association. (2013). *Diagnostic and statistical manual of mental disorders* (5th ed.). Arlington, VA: Author.

Barnhill, J. W. (2014). *DSM-5 clinical cases.* Arlington, VA: American Psychiatric Association.

Exner, J. E. (2000). *2000 alumni newsletter.* Asheville, NC: Rorschach Workshops.

Exner, J. E., & Erdberg, P. (2005). *The Rorschach: A comprehensive system: Vol. 2. Advanced interpretation* (3rd ed.). New York: Wiley.

Huprich, S. K. (Ed.). (2006). *Rorschach assessment of the personality disorders.* Mahwah, NJ: Erlbaum.

Meloy, J. R., Acklin, M. W., Gacono, C. B., Murray, J. F., & Peterson, C. A. (1997). *Contemporary Rorschach interpretation.* Mahwah, NJ: Erlbaum.

Meyer, G. J., Viglione, D. J., Mihura, J. L., Erard, R. E., & Erdberg, P. (2011). *Rorschach Performance Assessment System: Administration, coding, interpretation, and technical manual.* Toledo, OH: Rorschach Performance Assessment System.

Mihura, J. L., Roy, M., & Graceffo, R. A. (2017). Psychological assessment training in clinical psychology doctoral programs. *Journal of Personality Assessment, 99,* 153–164.

Weiner, I. B. (2003). *Principles of Rorschach interpretation* (2nd ed.). Mahwah, NJ: Erlbaum.

Wright, C. V., Beattie, S. G., Galper, D. I., Church, A. S., Bufka, L. F., Brabender, V. M., & Smith, B. L. (2017). Assessment practices of professional psychologists: Results of a national survey. *Professional Psychology: Research and Practice, 48,* 73–78.

# Contents

## PART III.  USING R-PAS IN FORENSIC EVALUATIONS

## PART IV.  USING R-PAS IN PRE-EMPLOYMENT, NEUROPSYCHOLOGICAL, AND EDUCATIONAL EVALUATIONS

# PART I

## The Basics of R-PAS and Its Interpretation

# CHAPTER 1

# Introduction to R-PAS

Joni L. Mihura
Gregory J. Meyer

The purpose of this book is to illustrate how to use and interpret the Rorschach Performance Assessment System (R-PAS; Meyer, Viglione, Mihura, Erard, & Erdberg, 2011) in a wide variety of situations. Through a presentation of illustrative cases, the book focuses on the ways in which the Rorschach is often used and can be helpful—thus, the title *Using the Rorschach Performance Assessment System® (R-PAS®)*. We designed the chapters to serve as exemplars for students and psychologists working in particular settings or situations (e.g., child custody, violence risk assessments, criminal responsibility evaluations), with certain populations (e.g., couples, female psychopaths, inpatients with a recent suicide attempt), and answering certain referral questions (e.g., detecting psychosis).

This volume should be considered essential for everyone who uses R-PAS, including practitioners, instructors, supervisors, and students. Its individual chapters, each of which has been thoroughly reviewed and vetted by the editors for administration, coding, and interpretation, can also be used as exemplars for students or psychologists who are using, or are considering using, R-PAS in any of these situations. There are many other audiences for this book as well. Psychologists whose expertise is not the Rorschach but who work in settings in which the Rorschach is used can read examples of its potential application. Judges or attorneys can use the book as a resource for relevant information on the Rorschach and the ways it is being used (or can or should be used) in legal settings.

## What Is R-PAS?

R-PAS (Meyer et al., 2011) is a Rorschach system that vastly improves upon the most commonly used previous system, the Comprehensive System (CS; Exner,

2003), by addressing its major criticisms (Meyer, Viglione, & Mihura, 2017; Mihura, Meyer, Bombel, & Dumitrascu, 2015; Mihura, Meyer, Dumitrascu, & Bombel, 2013; Wood, Garb, Nezworski, Lilienfeld, & Duke, 2015). R-PAS was designed as a replacement for the CS by members of Exner's Rorschach Research Council (Gregory J. Meyer, Donald J. Viglione, Joni L. Mihura, and Philip Erdberg) and a prominent forensic psychologist (Robert E. Erard). The council viewed this replacement as a necessary step following Exner's death in 2006 and the decision by his heirs, about 2 years later, not to further develop the CS. The CS itself was first published in 1974 (Exner, 1974), designed as a replacement for five previous competing Rorschach systems that were popular in the United States at the time (i.e., Beck, Beck, Levitt, & Molish, 1961; Hertz, 1970; Klopfer & Davidson, 1967; Piotrowski, 1957; Rapaport, Gill, & Schafer, 1968), which themselves were designed as extensions of and replacements for Hermann Rorschach's original test approach (Rorschach, 1921/1942).

## What Are the Essential Components of R-PAS?

An R-PAS assessment starts with a standardized administration of the test stimuli (i.e., the 10 inkblots) by an examiner, who asks the respondent to look at each card and answer the question "What might this be?" and then records the respondent's responses verbatim along with any relevant nonverbal expressions (Meyer et al., 2011). All Rorschach systems use the same 10 inkblots,[1] which were originally designed by Hermann Rorschach (1921/1942) after pilot-testing various iterations of the inkblots and refining them to improve their evocative features. After administering the test, the examiner codes the responses according to R-PAS guidelines and enters these codes into the online scoring and interpretation program (*www.r-pas.org*). This secure online program calculates the scores to be interpreted and plots them on a graph using standardized scores—similar to those used by other popular tests, such as intelligence tests—to compare the examinee's scores to norms. Next, the examiner interprets the test results using the R-PAS interpretive guidelines provided in the test manual or the editable case-based interpretive guidelines that are available from the online program. The R-PAS results are interpreted in the context of other assessment data, taking into account the method by which all of the information was obtained (e.g., clients' performance behavior on the Rorschach vs. self-report of their personality on questionnaires).

Table 1.1, "Brief Guide to Variables on the R-PAS Profile Pages," provides the names and a brief description of each scale and its basic interpretation. Figure 1.1 provides an image of the R-PAS Page 1 Profile to illustrate the results printout.[2] These resources are provided for readers who are encountering R-PAS for the first time, in order to give them a basic idea of its components. The table and figure are not sufficient for using and interpreting the system, however. Instead, the full manual is needed.

---

[1] Other inkblot tests have been developed, but they are rarely used.

[2] The R-PAS variables and results pages are updated with the emerging research.

**TABLE 1.1. Brief Guide to Variables on the R-PAS Profile Pages**

| Term | Description |
| --- | --- |

Page 1

*Administration Behaviors and Observations*

| | |
| --- | --- |
| Pr | Prompt; used to encourage the respondent to give an additional response when only one is given to a card. Giving only one response is a concrete instance of underproductive behavior that does not meet the situational demands of the environment. |
| Pu | Pull; when four responses are given to a card, the examiner asks for the card back and reminds the participant of the desired number of responses. Giving four responses is a concrete instance of overproductive behavior that does not meet environmentally set demands. |
| CT | Card Turns; total number of responses in which the card was turned, regardless of final orientation for the response. Depending on how it is contextually expressed, card turning may be linked to intellectual curiosity, flexibility, compulsivity, hostility or defiance, anxiety, authoritarianism, or suspiciousness. |

*Engagement and Cognitive Processing*

| | |
| --- | --- |
| Complexity | A composite variable that quantifies the amount of differentiation and integration involved in a protocol based on Location, Space, and Object Qualities; Contents; and Determinants summed across all responses. |
| R | Number of Responses; R is associated with both ability and motivation, and the latter may be due to intrinsic factors or situational factors. |
| F% | Form Percent, computed as F/R (replaces the CS score Lambda). F is Form without other determinants, also referred to as Pure F, *"the shape of a head."* Determinants are perceptual dimensions that *"determine"* a response. They are coded for the characteristics of the inkblot or characteristics attributed to the inkblot, including movement, color (either chromatic or achromatic), shading, dimensionality, symmetrical reflection, and the form, shape, or outline of a blot region. F% is inversely related to noticing, reacting to, and articulating subtleties and nuances in the inkblot environment, which suggests similar processes when the person is attending to his or her inner life and external world. |
| Blend | Blend response; a response with two or more determinants other than F; the determinants are separated by a comma (e.g., Mp,FC). See F% for a description of F and determinants. Blend is like the inverse of F%, but related more specifically to the ability to identify and articulate multiple features of one's experiential environment. |
| Sy | A Synthesis response; two objects meaningfully related, *"two birds sitting on branch"* (equal to the CS codes DQ+ and DQv/+). Sy is a measure of complex and sophisticated processing and coping, which involve integrative cognitive activity or relational thinking. |
| MC | Sum of M and WSumC. (Replaces the CS term EA.) M is the Human Movement determinant, *"people dancing."* WSumC is the Weighted Sum of Color determinants: $(C\times1.5)+CF+(FC\times0.5)$. C is the Color determinant without form, also referred to as Pure C, *"this blue stuff is water."* CF is the Color-Dominated determinant with form secondary, *"pink cotton candy; sort of curved."* FC is the Form-Dominated Color determinant, *"an airplane with a red wing."* MC is a measure of psychological activity and processing that is considered an index of psychological resources and adaptive capacity, based on the ability and propensity to populate, animate, and color one's experiential world. |

*(continued)*

**TABLE 1.1.** *(continued)*

| Term | Description |
| --- | --- |
| MC –PPD | The MC to PPD Difference Score; subtract PPD from MC (replaces the CS D-score and in CS terms is equivalent to EA – es). MC is as defined above. PPD refers to the Potentially Problematic Determinants, which are the sum of FM+m+Y+T+V+C′ (replaces the CS acronym, es, for Experienced Stimulation). FM is the Animal Movement determinant, *"a bear eating a fish."* The variables m, Y, T, V, and C′ are described below. MC – PPD is obtained by contrasting codes that suggest resources (MC) associated with ideational elaboration (Human Movement) and lively responsiveness to the world (chromatic color) to codes that suggest potential liabilities (PPD). |
| M | Human Movement determinant, *"people dancing."* Movement is not an actual attribute of the inkblot; it is a mental embellishment that requires some capacity to envision or imagine. M reflects the ability to use one's imagination to elaborate human experiences or activities; it represents a type of mentalization process that contributes to the capacity for empathy, a sense of active personal agency, a capacity to reflect on events and experiences, and a degree of developmental maturity. |
| M/MC | Human Movement Proportion, M divided by the sum of M and WSumC (replaces the CS EB ratio or M:WSumC). M is as defined above. WSumC is defined above with MC. M/MC assesses the degree to which decisions and actions are influenced by thoughtful deliberation and mentalization (M) versus spontaneous reactivity, vitality, and emotional expressiveness (WSumC). |
| (CF+C)/ SumC | The CF+C Proportion or Color Dominance Proportion, CF+C divided by SumC (replaces the FC:CF+C ratio in the CS). FC, CF, and C are described under MC. SumC is the sum of all the Color determinants, FC+CF+C. The CF+C Proportion is a rough measure of the relative absence, or relaxation, of cognitive control and modulation in one's reactions to the environment, especially when there is emotional provocation. |

*Perception and Thinking Problems*

| Term | Description |
| --- | --- |
| EII-3 | Ego Impairment Index—3rd version; a broadband, composite measure of thinking disturbance and severity of psychopathology. Its components include poor reality testing (FQ–), thought disturbance (WSumCog), crude and disturbing thought content (Critical Contents), and measures of interpersonal misunderstanding and disturbance (M–, PHR vs. GHR). As it increases, there is greater likelihood of difficulty accomplishing day-to-day tasks effectively. |
| TP-Comp | Thought and Perception Composite; assesses reality testing (via FQ variables) and thought disorganization (via Cognitive Codes), making it a broadband composite measure of psychopathology severity. (TP-Comp is a fully dimensional replacement for the CS PTI.) |
| WSumCog | Weighted Sum of Cognitive Codes; a measure of disturbed and disordered thought. Two groups of Cognitive Codes may characterize a person's responses: those that are visual and involve illogical or implausible relationships in the inkblot stimuli (i.e., INC, FAB, CON) and those that are linguistic and involve illogical reasoning or difficulties with effective communication (e.g., DV, DR, PEC). INC, FAB, DV, and DR are weighted for severity (Level 1 or 2). |
| SevCog | Sum of Severe Cognitive Codes, that is, DV2+INC2+DR2+FAB2+PEC+CON. SevCog captures significant or severe disruptions in thought processes. At least among adults and adolescents, these kinds of disruptions are typically most indicative of psychotic-level lapses in conceptualization, reasoning, communication, or thought organization. |
| FQ–% | "FQ Minus Percent"; percentage of all responses that are distorted—that is, FQ–/R (equal to X–% in the CS). FQ–% is a measure of distortion, misinterpretation, or mistaken perception, often leading to poor judgments, odd behavior, or poor adaptation. Internal imagery and concerns may interfere with the person's ability to process and interpret external reality, and the person may see and describe things in a mistaken, distorted, personalized way that others will not see or understand. |

*(continued)*

**TABLE 1.1.** *(continued)*

| Term | Description |
|------|-------------|
| WD−% | "WD Minus Percent," computed as WD−/WD. WD−% is similar to FQ−%, but it more specifically indicates whether distortions occur even in perceptual situations that are more common and conventional and tied to familiarly identified objects. Distortions in this context may be considered more atypical and problematic. |
| FQo% | "F-Q-O Percent"; percentage of all responses that are common, easy to see, and accurate—that is, FQo/R (equal to X+% in the CS). FQo% is a measure of conventional judgment, good reality testing, and seeing the world the way most other people do. Like FQ−, FQo is a product of developmental maturation, such that FQo% increases progressively from childhood to adolescence to young adulthood to adulthood (and FQ− decreases). |
| P | Popular response, *"a bat"* (Card I). Popular objects are relatively obvious perceptions that are seen by a large proportion of people taking the test. Thus, P is a measure of highly conventional interpretations of the environment and sensitivity to obvious external cues. |

*Stress and Distress*

| Term | Description |
|------|-------------|
| YTVC' | "Y-T-V-C-Prime," or Sum of Shading and Achromatic Color; Total number of shading (Y, T, V) and achromatic color (C') determinants (equal to SumShading in the CS). YTVC' is a rough measure of being drawn to inconsistencies, uncertainties, and nuances in the environment, which extends to real and imagined interactions with others. In terms of response process, incorporating these features into response descriptions adds inconsistencies and nuances to the task, while also distracting the respondent from focusing on the shape of the inkblot to answer the question of what it might be. |
| m and Y | m = Inanimate Movement determinant, sometimes referred to as "little m," *"a falling rock."* Y = Diffuse Shading determinant, *"the shading makes it look camouflaged"* (equal to the CS score SumY). Both m and Y have shown a relationship to moderate to severe stressors. The m code involves mechanical or nonsentient activity that lacks volitional control and is typically characterized by external forces acting on an object. Y indicates sensitivity to nuance, minor gradations, and inconsistencies in the inkblot, as well as an effort to make sense of, or account for, these features. Y is thought to indicate a helpless feeling in the face of the stressors, whereas m is related to an anxious kind of ideation that is outside of one's control or possibly impinging on oneself from external forces. |
| MOR | Morbid Content Thematic Code; a response incorporating a damaged, dead, or depressive quality, *"a broken branch,"* or a *"sad person crying."* MOR responses indicate morbid, pessimistic, injured, damaged, or sad ideational themes. |
| SC-Comp | Suicide Concern Composite (a fully dimensional replacement for the CS S-CON). SC-Comp is an implicit measure of risk for suicide or serious self-destructive behavior with many false-positives (elevated score but person does not engage in actual self-harm). |

*Self and Other Representation*

| Term | Description |
|------|-------------|
| ODL% | Oral Dependent Language, *"Fried shrimp on a plate,"* divided by R. (ODL was formerly abbreviated ROD for Rorschach Oral Dependency; Food content [Fd] in the CS is included in ODL.) ODL codes the words that suggest or images that convey themes of nurturance, needed support or help, oral activity, food and eating, or birth and fragility. Elevations identify respondents who are implicitly motivated by dependent needs, related to an underlying dependent trait or a state. |
| SR | Space Reversal; the object seen resides within and is defined by the white space contours so that the typical perspective of seeing ink on a white background is perceptually reversed. The response may or may not include inked areas, *"A (white) lamp in the center"* (the CS had combined Space Integration, described below, and SR into one code, S). SR is an implicit behavioral measure of independence strivings, inventive or creative perspective taking, and oppositionality. |

*(continued)*

**TABLE 1.1.** *(continued)*

| Term | Description |
|---|---|
| MAP/<br>MAHP | The Mutuality of Autonomy Pathology Proportion, MAP divided by MAHP. MAP is the Mutuality of Autonomy–Pathology Thematic Code, *"some sort of organism swallowing up that bird."* MAHP is the total number of Mutuality of Autonomy Health (MAH) and MAP codes. MAH is defined below. MAP/MAHP assesses the extent to which relationships are viewed as destructive or harmful. |
| PHR/<br>GPHR | The Poor Human Representation Proportion; the sum of Poor Human Representation (PHR) codes divided by the sum of Good and Poor Human Representation codes (GPHR; replaces the GHR:PHR ratio from the CS and their difference score, the HRV). GHR suggests an ability to envision the self and relationships with others in an adaptive or positive way. PHR suggests a propensity to misunderstand others, relationships, and/or the self, or to imbue relationships with themes of damage or aggression. |
| M– | "M Minus"; Human Movement determinant with FQ–. M– is a rough measure of significant misunderstanding or misperceptions of people that can result in disturbed interpersonal relations. |
| AGC | Aggressive Content, *"a weapon."* Regularly seeing aggressive, powerful, dangerous, predatory, or threatening images is a behavioral indication that these themes are on the person's mind. |
| H | Whole Human content, *"a person,"* also referred to as Pure H. Reporting images of whole human beings is associated with the ability to envision people in complete, intact, multifaceted, and integrated ways. |
| COP | Cooperative Movement; cooperative, positive, or pleasant interactions between objects, *"two people dancing."* COP reflects a generally positive template for envisioning relationships. |
| MAH | Mutuality of Autonomy–Health, *"two women leaning in on a table between them, talking."* Like COP but more restricted, MAH suggests the potential for mature and healthy interpersonal relationships. |

Page 2

*Engagement and Cognitive Processing*

| Term | Description |
|---|---|
| W% | Whole Percent, W/R. W% reflects a capacity for generalization and abstraction—subsuming various facts under a larger concept, the big picture. |
| Dd% | Unusual Detail Percent; Dd/R. Dd% reflects a tendency to focus on rare, small, or idiosyncratic details in the experiential environment. |
| SI | Space Integration; background space is used in a response along with an inked blot area, *"A dark face, the white is eyes"* (the CS combined SI and SR into one code, S). SI is typically indicative of cognitive effort, motivation, complex integration, and possibly creative thinking. |
| IntCont | Intellectualized Content, (2×ABS)+Art+Ay. ABS is Abstract Representation, *"the swirling represents fear"* (AB in the CS). Art is Art content, *"a painting."* Ay is Anthropology content; content with particular cultural, historical, or ethnographic significance, *"a Greek temple."* IntCont reflects an abstract or symbolic, intellectualized style of information processing. |
| Vg% | Vague percent; Vg/R. Vg is Vagueness, *"some haze"* (corresponds to the CS codes DQv and DQv/+). Vg% reflects a vague, impressionistic, and relatively ineffective processing style. |

*(continued)*

**TABLE 1.1.** *(continued)*

| Term | Description |
|---|---|
| V | Vista determinant, where shading creates a sense of dimensionality, *"a deep cave, it's darker in the back"* (equal to the CS score SumV). V reflects using nuance and subtleties as a basis for taking perspective, gaining distance, or seeing through things. It can be a cognitive resource. |
| FD | Form Dimension determinant, for dimensional responses based on form, *"a road; the end looks far off the way it gets narrower at the top."* FD suggests a general evaluative perspective or capacity for taking a distancing perspective. |
| R8910% | "R-8-9-10 Percent," R8910/R (replaces the Afr from the CS). R8910 is the total number of responses on Cards VIII, IX, and X. R8910% taps a general responsiveness to compelling or vibrant stimuli, which may include emotional situations with other people. |
| WSumC | Weighted Sum of Color determinants; (C×1.5)+CF+(FC×0.5). C, CF, and FC are described under MC, above. WSumC is related to an interest in and awareness of stimulating, compelling features of the environment, which may include one's emotional reactions to them. |
| C | Color determinant without form, also referred to as Pure C, *"this blue stuff is water."* C suggests a cognitively passive or even helpless receptivity to activating or compelling experiences. |
| Mp/ (Ma+Mp) | The Passive Human Movement Proportion, Mp/(Ma+Mp) (replaces the CS Ma:Mp ratio). Mp is the sum of Passive Human Movement determinants, *"a woman looking down,"* and Ma is the sum of Active Human Movement determinants, *"two men wrestling."* Mp/(Ma+Mp) indicates a propensity for passive (versus active) fantasy and ideation. |

*Perception and Thinking Problems*

| Term | Description |
|---|---|
| FQu% | "F-Q-U Percent"; percentage of all responses that are relatively uncommon but reasonably accurate, FQu/R (equal to Xu% in the CS). FQu responses are midrange in terms of frequency and accuracy between FQo and FQ–. FQu% is associated with unconventional and individualistic ways of interpreting experiences. |

*Stress and Distress*

| Term | Description |
|---|---|
| PPD | Potentially Problematic Determinants; FM+m+Y+T+V+C' (replaces the CS acronym, es, for Experienced Stimulation). PPD is related to an environmental sensitivity or attunement because it reflects the capacity to animate percepts, to envision static objects in motion, and to use and describe the saturation of ink or its achromatic colors when generating images. However, this kind of sensitivity or attunement can be a liability because these codes also can be indicative of stressors that are outside one's control in terms of impulses, needs, or feelings that are stimulating, irritating, upsetting, or pressing. |
| CBlend | Color Blend, in which a color (FC, CF, C) determinant is blended with a shading (Y, T, V) or achromatic color (C') determinant in one response; for example, CF,T (equal to Col-Shd in the CS). CBlend suggests emotional or environmental sensitivity in which emotionally spontaneous reactions (Color) can be compromised by concerns with inconsistencies, indefiniteness, and nuances (Shading) or gloomy darkness and deadening numbness (C'), thus suggesting that one is vulnerable to mixed affective experiences. |
| C' | Any achromatic color determinant using black, gray, or white, *"a black coat"* (equal to the CS score SumC'). C' suggests being drawn to dreary, dark, and gloomy stimuli. |

*(continued)*

**TABLE 1.1.** *(continued)*

| Term | Description |
|---|---|
| V | Vista determinant, as defined above. V involves perspective taking or an evaluative attitude and may be associated with some discomfort or dissatisfaction when directed against the self or others. |
| CritCont% | Critical Contents divided by R. Critical Contents is an EII-3 subcomponent, equal to An+Bl+Ex+Fi+Sx+AGM+MOR. Bl is Blood content. Ex is Explosion content, *"an atomic bomb going off."* Fi is Fire or smoke content, *"a candle flame."* Sx is Sexual content, *"a nude guy."* MOR is described above; An and AGM are described below. CritCont% may be elevated from traumatic experiences, primitive thinking, or exaggeration and malingering. |

*Self and Other Representation*

| Term | Description |
|---|---|
| SumH | Sum of all Human content codes, H+(H)+Hd+(Hd). SumH reflects an awareness of, or interest in, other people. |
| NPH/ SumH | The Non-Pure Human Proportion, NPH/SumH (replaces the CS H:(H)+Hd+(Hd) ratio). NPH is the sum of Non-Pure Human content, that is, the total number of human-like or human detail contents, (H)+Hd+(Hd). NPH/SumH indicates the tendency to mentally represent human objects in incomplete, unrealistic, or fanciful ways. |
| V-Comp | Vigilance Composite (a fully dimensional replacement for the CS HVI). V-Comp assesses guardedness, effortful and focused cognition, sensitivity to cues of danger, tense affective constriction, interpersonal wariness, and distancing. |
| r | Reflection determinant, *"a parrot looking in the mirror"* (equal to the CS variable Fr+rF). r may reflect a need for mirroring support, experiencing oneself as reflected in the world in a self-centered way, and/or a propensity to use the self as a frame of reference when processing information. |
| p/(a+p) | The Passive Movement Proportion, p/(a+p) (replaces the a:p ratio from the CS). p is the sum of Passive Movement determinants, *"sitting."* p/(p+a) is a rough measure of passive versus active inclinations in a person's behaviors or attitudes. |
| AGM | Aggressive Movement, *"men fighting"* (AG in the CS). AGM indicates that the person has imagined, and, at some level, probably identified with, aggressive activity, but it does not indicate the person's attitude toward this aggressive activity. |
| T | Texture determinant, where shading designates a tactile sensation, *"the coloration makes it seem furry"* (equal to the CS score SumT). T suggests that the person is attuned to touch and to tactile experiences in his or her environment, which may reflect an implicit desire for interpersonal closeness. |
| PER | Personal Knowledge Justification, the use of personal experience to justify a response, *"it's a fancy bicycle; I've seen one just like that."* PER suggests a tendency to justify one's views and positions based on private, personal knowledge or authority. |
| An | Anatomy content, *"a heart,"* which includes medical imaging content, *"an X-ray of a chest"* (equal to the CS An+Xy). An suggests that a person is concerned about bodily, physical, or medical issues. |

## R-PAS Summary Scores and Profiles – Page 1

C-ID: Mr. J - Applications of R-PAS    P-ID: 50    Age: 19    Gender: Male    Education: 12

| Domain/Variables | Raw Scores | Raw %ile | Raw SS | Cplx. Adj. %ile | Cplx. Adj. SS | Standard Score Profile R-Optimized | Abbr. |
|---|---|---|---|---|---|---|---|
| **Admin. Behaviors and Obs.** | | | | | | | |
| Pr | 1 | 62 | 104 | | | | Pr |
| Pu | 0 | 40 | 96 | | | | Pu |
| CT (Card Turning) | 1 | 38 | 95 | | | | CT |
| **Engagement and Cog. Processing** | | | | | | | |
| Complexity | 89 | 76 | 110 | | | | Cmplx |
| R (Responses) | 20 | 21 | 88 | 4 | 73 | | R |
| F% [Lambda=0.18] (Simplicity) | 15% | 5 | 75 | 12 | 83 | | F% |
| Blend | 8 | 88 | 118 | 76 | 110 | | Bln |
| Sy | 11 | 87 | 117 | 72 | 109 | | Sy |
| MC | 9.5 | 75 | 110 | 54 | 102 | | MC |
| MC - PPD | -6.5 | 17 | 85 | 20 | 87 | | MC-PPD |
| M | 7 | 88 | 118 | 74 | 110 | | M |
| M/MC [7/9.5] | 74% | 84 | 115 | 83 | 114 | | M Prp |
| (CF+C)/SumC [2/2] | NA | | | | | | CFC Prp |
| **Perception and Thinking Problems** | | | | | | | |
| EII-3 | 1.5 | 97 | 127 | 97 | 127 | | EII |
| TP-Comp (Thought & Percept. Com...) | 2.5 | 97 | 128 | 96 | 127 | | TP-C |
| WSumCog | 27 | 98 | 131 | 98 | 130 | | WCog |
| SevCog | 4 | 99 | 138 | 99 | 138 | | Sev |
| FQ-% | 20% | 93 | 122 | 92 | 121 | | FQ-% |
| WD-% | 24% | 98 | 132 | 96 | 126 | | WD-% |
| FQo% | 30% | 2 | 71 | 2 | 70 | | FQo% |
| P | 4 | 22 | 88 | 25 | 89 | | P |
| **Stress and Distress** | | | | | | | |
| YTVC' | 10 | 92 | 122 | 88 | 117 | | YTVC' |
| m | 4 | 90 | 119 | 80 | 112 | | m |
| Y | 0 | 17 | 85 | 17 | 85 | | Y |
| MOR | 1 | 51 | 100 | 41 | 96 | | MOR |
| SC-Comp (Suicide Concern Comp.) | 5.0 | 65 | 106 | 53 | 101 | | SC-C |
| **Self and Other Representation** | | | | | | | |
| ODL% | 40% | 98 | 133 | 98 | 131 | | ODL% |
| SR (Space Reversal) | 0 | 19 | 87 | 19 | 87 | | SR |
| MAP/MAHP [1/2] | NA | | | | | | MAP Prp |
| PHR/GPHR [7/11] | 64% | 91 | 120 | 91 | 120 | | PHR Prp |
| M- | 0 | 36 | 95 | 36 | 95 | | M- |
| AGC | 5 | 85 | 116 | 80 | 113 | | AGC |
| H | 6 | 94 | 123 | 89 | 119 | | H |
| COP | 1 | 54 | 102 | 45 | 98 | | COP |
| MAH | 1 | 64 | 105 | 34 | 93 | | MAH |

© 2010-2016 R-PAS

**FIGURE 1.1.** R-PAS results: Page 1 Profile. Reproduced from the Rorschach Performance Assessment System® (R-PAS®) Scoring Program (© 2010–2016) and excerpted from the *Rorschach Performance Assessment System: Administration, Coding, Interpretation, and Technical Manual* (© 2011) with copyrights by Rorschach Performance Assessment System, LLC. All rights reserved. Used by permission of Rorschach Performance Assessment System, LLC. Further reproduction is prohibited without written permission from R-PAS.

## How Is R-PAS an Improvement Over the CS?

R-PAS addresses many problems with the CS that have been expressed by different constituents: the self-proclaimed "Rorschach critics" (Wood, Nezworski, Garb, & Lilienfeld, 2006), psychologists who research and use the Rorschach in practice (Meyer & Archer, 2001; Meyer, Hsiao, Viglione, Mihura, & Abraham, 2013), and students learning to use the task for the first time (Viglione, Meyer, Resende, & Pignolo, 2017). The following sections briefly summarize these improvements. See Meyer et al. (2017) for more detail.

### Validity Meta-Analyses for Individual Scores

Although many narrative reviews of the Rorschach validity literature exist, including Exner's research reviews in the CS test manuals (Exner, 2003), meta-analyses based on systematic reviews of the literature have become the expected norm in psychology to summarize the existing research on a topic. Because the Rorschach has always been somewhat controversial, by 2001, three independent meta-analyses had been conducted on the *general* validity of the Rorschach (Atkinson, 1986; Hiller, Rosenthal, Bornstein, Berry, & Brunell-Neuleib, 1999; Parker, Hanson, & Hunsley, 1988). In each case, the authors compared the general validity of Rorschach to the general validity of the Minnesota Multiphasic Personality Inventory (MMPI). Meyer and Archer (2001) greatly expanded one of those meta-analyses (Parker et al.) and then statistically summarized the results across all three meta-analyses. They showed that, on average, Rorschach scores were as valid as MMPI scores, both when considering all hypothesized effects ($r = .32$ for both, using 523 effect sizes for the Rorschach and 533 effect sizes for the MMPI) and when considering all studies examining heteromethod validity ($r = .29$ for both, using 73 studies for the Rorschach with $N = 6,520$, and 85 studies for the MMPI with $N = 15,985$).

However, much less systematic work had been done on the validity of individual Rorschach variables. Until 2011, validity meta-analyses for six Rorschach scores had been published. Four of these were not CS scores, and validity support was found for all four scores (Bornstein, 1999; Diener, Hilsenroth, Shaffer, & Sexton, 2011; Meyer & Handler, 1997; Romney, 1990). For the two CS scores, support was found for the Schizophrenia Index but not the Depression Index (Jørgensen, Andersen, & Dam, 2000, 2001).[3] However, over 60 Rorschach variables are interpreted in the CS, leaving the great majority of variables unaccounted for by meta-analyses.

In 2012, the online version of Mihura and colleagues' (2013) systematic meta-analytic reviews of 65 CS variables was published in the top scientific review journal in psychology (*Psychological Bulletin*). This extensive project was started in 2005 in response to the critics' call for meta-analyses on all CS scales, and eventually took over 6 years and thousands of hours to complete. Although this project was originally planned as a contribution to the CS, after Exner's death, the prepublication versions of the meta-analyses eventually formed the backbone of the revised system, R-PAS.

---

[3]Three of the five Rorschach scores with meta-analytic validity support are now included in R-PAS (the Schizophrenia Index, which has been renamed the Thought and Perception Composite, the Ego Impairment Index–3, and the Oral Dependent Language Scale).

In a momentous event, in response to these meta-analyses, the most vocal critics of the Rorschach lifted their call for a global moratorium on the use of the Rorschach in clinical and forensic settings (see Wood et al., 2015; and our response, Mihura et al., 2015). Because the CS is frozen in time without the possibility of updating, it cannot incorporate any of these meta-analytic findings.

In addition to their importance for the Rorschach, Mihura and colleagues' (2013) large-scale meta-analyses were notable for any multiscale psychological test. As of this writing, compared to the Rorschach, no other psychological tests have so many published meta-analyses addressing the construct validity of their individual scales. Mihura et al. systematically reviewed the published validity literature for 65 Rorschach scales; enough data existed to perform meta-analyses on 53 of these scales.[4] R-PAS included seven other non-CS variables that have published validity meta-analyses (Bornstein, 1999; Diener et al., 2011; Graceffo, Mihura, & Meyer, 2014), systematic reviews (Mihura, Dumitrascu, Roy, & Meyer, 2017), and meta-analyses in progress (Kiss, Mihura, & Meyer, 2017). In contrast, meta-analyses on the popular MMPI-2 have mainly been conducted on the scales designed to detect faking (e.g., Rogers, Sewell, Martin, & Vitacco, 2003). The MMPI-2 has published validity meta-analyses for only 2 of its 112 clinical and treatment scales, supporting the relationship between two depression scales and the diagnosis of depression (Gross, Keyes, & Greene, 2000).

## More Accurate Norms Than the CS

The CS norms have been an area of contention. Wood and his colleagues published research suggesting that many of the CS normative values were inaccurate, in the direction of overpathologizing clients (Wood, Nezworski, Garb, & Lilienfeld, 2001a, 2001b). At first, Exner and members of his Rorschach Research Council thought this criticism was largely in error (Exner, 2001; Meyer, 2001), but research they conducted on their own showed that the CS norms were substantially different for many important scores (e.g., those assessing psychosis; Meyer, Erdberg, & Shaffer, 2007; Viglione & Giromini, 2016). Subsequently, new international norms were published the year after Exner's death (Meyer et al., 2007), which R-PAS adopted with some modifications (see Chapter 16, "Generating Normative Reference Data," in the R-PAS manual; Meyer et al., 2011, pp. 469–484; Meyer, Shaffer, Erdberg, & Horn, 2015; Viglione & Giromini, 2016). The R-PAS developers are currently collecting new norms.

## Less Variable Number of Responses Than the CS

The Rorschach in general (Cronbach, 1949) and the CS in particular (Meyer, 1992, 1993) have been criticized for using a method of administration that results in a widely varying number of responses, depending on the respondent and the examiner. Practically, this varying number of responses also makes it difficult for examiners to allot time for an administration. In addition, examiners using the CS are often faced with the need to readminister the task due to an insufficient number of responses,

---

[4]R-PAS relies on CS research as part of its evidence base. Throughout the history of the CS, it also relied on research from previous ways of scoring and administering the Rorschach.

resulting in frustration for the respondent and in confusion and scheduling complications for the examiner. Therefore, R-PAS instituted new administration guidelines that were first reviewed, vetted, and tested in an early form by the Research Council before Exner's death (Dean, 2005; Dean, Viglione, Perry, & Meyer, 2007, 2008). These guidelines were revised several times until they resulted in significantly reduced variability in the number of responses and virtually eliminated the need to readminister the task (Hosseininasab et al., in press; Reese, Viglione, & Giromini, 2014; Viglione et al., 2015). The latter is an improvement that is especially important in forensic settings where the client might be resistant to engage in an assessment.

### Reduces Examiner Differences Compared to the CS

Different examiner styles can significantly affect important Rorschach variables when using CS administration and coding guidelines—particularly the complexity of a person's responses and the degree to which the objects he or she sees fit the blot contours, which is used as a measure of reality testing (see Exner, 2007, Table 1). To address this problem, R-PAS made numerous improvements to reduce ambiguities in administration and coding and to ensure that both steps are undertaken with more consistency and reliability across examiners (Meyer et al., 2011, 2017). R-PAS also provides many online resources to help clinicians and students practice and calibrate to R-PAS standards for administration and coding (*www.r-pas.org*). These resources include administration videos; practice protocols for role-playing the examiner and respondent, along with one for a "coach"; administration checklists; and several R-PAS cases coded by its developers.

### Interpretation Is More Efficient and Credible Than in the CS

Two changes from the CS to R-PAS—(1) using standardized scores instead of raw scores and (2) basing interpretations on the response process—make interpretation notably more efficient and credible. These improvements are especially important for students who are learning the test for the first time, although making Rorschach interpretation more credible and plausible is important for many constituents: the general public; psychologists who doubt the Rorschach simply based on its association with psychoanalytic theory; and judges, attorneys, and juries.

#### *Standardized Score Printout*

The R-PAS scoring program provides test results that compare the client's data to norms using standardized scores like those used on self-report tests (e.g., MMPI-2, MMPI-2-RF, and Personality Assessment Inventory [PAI]) and intelligence tests (e.g., Wechsler Adult Intelligence Scale—Fourth Edition [WAIS-IV]). In contrast, the CS uses raw score results, requiring users to memorize or look up the normative values for over 60 scores each time they interpret the test. CS interpretation presents an overwhelming situation for students who are first learning the test. To illustrate the difference, compare the R-PAS Page 1 results presented in Figure 1.1 to the bottom third of the CS Structural Summary, which contains the main CS results, presented in Figure 1.2. Instructors switching from CS to R-PAS say that the standardized

**RATIOS, PERCENTAGES, AND DERIVATIONS**

| | AFFECT | INTERPERSONAL |

| R = 16 | L = 0.33 |
|---|---|

| EB | = | 6 : 5.0 | EA | = 11.0 | EBPer | = N/A |
|---|---|---|---|---|---|---|
| eb | = | 2 : 2 | es | = 4 | D | = +2 |
| | | | Adj es | = 4 | Adj D | = +2 |

| FM | = | 1 | SumC' | = 1 | SumT | = 0 |
|---|---|---|---|---|---|---|
| m | = | 1 | SumV | = 1 | SumY | = 0 |

**AFFECT**

| FC:CF+C | = 0 : 4 |
|---|---|
| Pure C | = 2 |
| SumC' : WSumC | = 1 : 5.0 |
| Afr | = 0.33 |
| S | = 2 |
| Blends:R | = 4 : 16 |
| CP | = 0 |

**INTERPERSONAL**

| COP | = 1 | AG | = 3 |
|---|---|---|---|
| GHR:PHR | = 1 : 6 | | |
| a:p | = 5 : 3 | | |
| Food | = 1 | | |
| SumT | = 0 | | |
| Human Content | = 7 | | |
| Pure H | = 3 | | |
| PER | = 4 | | |
| Isolation Index | = 0.19 | | |

**IDEATION**

| a:p | = 5 : 3 | Sum6 | = 10 |
|---|---|---|---|
| Ma:Mp | = 4 : 2 | Lvl-2 | = 3 |
| 2AB+(Art+Ay) | = 2 | WSum6 | = 34 |
| MOR | = 2 | M- | = 3 |
| | | M none | = 0 |

**MEDIATION**

| XA% | = 0.56 |
|---|---|
| WDA% | = 0.54 |
| X-% | = 0.31 |
| S- | = 1 |
| P | = 2 |
| X+% | = 0.38 |
| Xu% | = 0.19 |

**PROCESSING**

| Zf | = 9 |
|---|---|
| W:D:Dd | = 8:5:3 |
| W : M | = 8 : 6 |
| Zd | = +4.5 |
| PSV | = 0 |
| DQ+ | = 6 |
| DQv | = 2 |

**SELF-PERCEPTION**

| 3r+(2)/R | = 0.25 |
|---|---|
| Fr+rF | = 0 |
| SumV | = 1 |
| FD | = 2 |
| An+Xy | = 1 |
| MOR | = 2 |
| H:(H)+Hd+(Hd) | = 3 : 4 |

| PTI = 5 | ☐ DEPI = 4 | ☐ CDI = 2 | ☐ S-CON = 7 | ☑ HVI = Yes | ☐ OBS = No |
|---|---|---|---|---|---|

**FIGURE 1.2.** Rorschach Comprehensive System (CS) Structural Summary: Main results section. Reproduced by special permission of the Publisher, Psychological Assessment Resource, Inc. (PAR), 16204 North Florida Avenue, Lutz, Florida 33549, from the Rorschach Interpretation Assistance Program: Version 5 by John E. Exner, Jr., PhD, Irving B. Weiner, PhD, and PAR Staff. Copyright 1976, 1985, 1990, 1994, 1995, 1999, 2001, 2003 by PAR. Further reproduction is prohibited without permission of PAR.

score results and response process foundation for interpretation significantly improve students' learning experiences. R-PAS users report that being able to view all of the main results at a glance is helpful, and they are less likely to lose track of important results. The main R-PAS results pages are described further in Chapters 2 and 3 and are illustrated in every case chapter (Chapters 4–19).

## Response Process-Based Interpretations

The *response process* refers to the psychological operations that occur in the process of generating a response to a task. As described further in Chapter 2, basing Rorschach interpretations on the response process is similar to interpreting cognitive performance tasks like those on the WAIS-IV. For example, on the WAIS-IV Block Design subtest, clinicians do not interpret the person's ability to put together blocks in everyday life; they generalize the psychological operations that occur in the process of generating a response (e.g., visual analysis and synthesis in the case of Block Design) to similar operations in everyday life. For CS interpretations, the lack of a clear link between the respondent's Rorschach response and the clinician's interpretation of that response has resulted in a sense of hiddenness and mystery around the

Rorschach that has surely led to an inherent doubting and discounting of the test. Therefore, R-PAS highlights the link between the coded behavior and its interpretation, and removes the mystery.

As a broader context, for many years, the Rorschach was associated with psychoanalytic theory (even though Hermann Rorschach did not describe it that way; Rorschach, 1921/1942; Searls, 2017). When psychoanalysis came under attack (Crews, 1996), the Rorschach did too. Exner (1974) tried to remove the stigma from the Rorschach by presenting his system as atheoretical and empirical, but for the vast majority of variables, he did not explain the link between the coding of the response and the resultant interpretation. In contrast, similar to Schachtel's (1966) phenomenological approach to understanding the Rorschach, R-PAS focuses strongly on the response process when interpreting the test results (see also Mihura et al., 2017). Response process-based interpretation makes Rorschach interpretation more credible, understandable, and easier for students to learn. We also expect that this strong link between response process and interpretation will lead clinicians to more accurately see examples of the associated attitudes and behaviors in their client's everyday life.

## Culture and Gender

The last improvement over the CS that we mention is R-PAS's nongendered international norms. In addition to being more accurate than Exner's CS norms (as previously noted), the R-PAS normative sample includes protocols from non-American countries (i.e., Argentina, Belgium, Brazil, Denmark, Finland, France, Greece, Israel, Italy, Portugal, Romania, and Spain), whereas Exner's (2003) norms, collected in the 1970s and early 1980s (Exner, 1986; Exner & Weiner, 1982), were entirely from the United States. There is no reliable evidence to date that the basic cognitive and perceptual task of the Rorschach results in cultural and gender differences (e.g., Meyer et al., 2007; Meyer, Giromini, Viglione, Reese, & Mihura, 2015; Meyer, Shaffer, et al., 2015). The main differences across countries occur with some salient cultural images—such as the "Christmas elves" in Scandinavian countries reported in response to Card II and totem poles in the U.S. Southwest reported in response to Card VI—but not, for example, how well the image fits the blot, the perceptual features that are described, or the base rates of thought disturbance. Six of the 16 case chapters in this book focus on cases from countries other than the United States (i.e., Finland, Israel, Italy, the Netherlands, and Norway).

## What Are Key Strengths and Applications of R-PAS?

### More Construct Validity Meta-Analyses Than Any Other Test

As previously noted, a significant strength of the Rorschach is that it has, by far, the most published construct validity meta-analyses for its clinical scales than any other psychological test—over 50 Rorschach scales compared to only two MMPI-2 clinical scales (Bornstein, 1999; Diener et al., 2011; Graceffo et al., 2014; Gross et al., 2000; Meyer, 2000; Mihura et al., 2013). The development of R-PAS was guided by these meta-analyses—which is not the case for any other existing Rorschach system.

## Incremental Validity Over Self-Report Measures

In clinical and forensic practice, the Rorschach offers a different method of assessment that provides incremental validity over self-report measures (for a discussion, see Meyer, 1996, 1997; Mihura, 2012; Mihura et al., 2013). There is strong support in the literature for valid Rorschach scores to add incremental validity over self-report measures, including Mihura et al.'s (2013) meta-analyses and a number of other studies (Blasczyk-Schiep, Kazén, Kuhl, & Grygielski, 2011; Dao, Prevatt, & Horne, 2008; Fowler, Piers, Hilsenroth, Holdwick, & Padawer, 2001; Hartmann & Grønnerød, 2009; Hartmann, Sunde, Kristensen, & Martinussen, 2003; Meyer, 2000; Ritsher, 2004; Viglione & Hilsenroth, 2001). This finding is not surprising, given that a substantial body of literature shows only small to moderate relationships between what people say about themselves and what they do (e.g., Mihura & Graceffo, 2014; Wilson & Dunn, 2004).

## The Best Normed Measure to Assess Psychosis

Especially strong and robust evidence exists regarding the Rorschach's ability to detect psychosis and psychotic symptoms (Jørgensen et al., 2000, 2001; Mihura et al., 2013, Table 4), something that even the Rorschach's staunchest critics do not contest (Garb, Wood, Lilienfeld, & Nezworski, 2005). Our recent, but as yet unpublished, systematic review of the literature on the ability of all versions of the MMPI to detect psychosis in clinical and forensic settings suggests that it is a less valid measure for this purpose than the Rorschach (Mihura, Ales, et al., 2017). This finding is consistent with published studies showing that the Rorschach provides incremental validity over self-report measures in detecting psychosis but not the other way around (e.g., Dao et al., 2008). In Chapters 4, 5, 6, 10, 11, 12, and 16, we provide case examples of using R-PAS when the referral question targets psychosis, as well as when the diagnosis of psychosis emerges as a possibility only after R-PAS is administered.

## Valid, Normed Behavioral Assessment of Psychological Characteristics Not Available on Other Tests

In addition to the general ability to detect psychosis, R-PAS also offers valid, normed behavioral assessment of psychological characteristics that are not available through other tests (for more discussion of this topic, see Mihura, 2012; Mihura & Graceffo, 2014). For example, reality testing and thought disturbance are components of psychosis, but they are also characteristics of other disorders and of personality in general. They run along a continuum that is not limited to psychosis or schizophrenia. Reality testing problems result in misinterpretations of the environment that can make successful treatment and healthy adaptation very challenging, even among patients who do not have psychotic-spectrum difficulties (e.g., Opaas, Hartmann, Wentzel-Larsen, & Varvin, 2016). R-PAS also provides a typical performance measure of cognitive complexity, in contrast to the maximal performance measures of cognitive complexity that are obtained by cognitive ability tests (e.g., intelligence, memory). There is empirical evidence that a client who scores low on these Rorschach measures of cognitive complexity is significantly more likely to report symptoms of alexithymia (the inability to notice and describe one's emotions; Porcelli & Mihura, 2010) and to have problems engaging in and benefiting from psychotherapy (Mihura et al., 2013; see the "Strongly Supported Variables" section in the Discussion).

The Rorschach also is the only performance test with norms to assess mental imagery—norms that can provide helpful information about preoccupations in general, as well as for disorders in which intrusive imagery is a symptom, such as PTSD (with traumatic images) and OCD (with obsessive images). Finally, relevant for all clinicians but especially those who integrate relational or psychodynamic components in their case conceptualizations, R-PAS provides (1) valid, normed measures of self and other representations and (2) coded behaviors with the examiner to compare to norms (e.g., Card Turning; evidence of not "following the rules," as in high number of Prompts and Pulls) that can be generalized to everyday life and to interpersonal dynamics that can be expected with the client's therapist.

## Orientation to This Book

This book contains three introductory chapters written by R-PAS developers: (1) the present introductory chapter by Mihura and Meyer; (2) a basic chapter on interpretation, by Mihura and Meyer (Chapter 2), that summarizes and extends the interpretive guidelines found in the R-PAS manual; and (3) a chapter on norms, by Meyer and Erdberg (Chapter 3), with a particular focus on using R-PAS with children and adolescents. For readers unfamiliar with R-PAS, Table 1.1 lists the variable names and a concise description of how they are coded and interpreted. The subsequent chapters (Chapters 4–19) illustrate R-PAS cases from various settings—clinical and forensic as well as also medical, pre-employment, neuropsychological, and educational. The chapter topics were chosen to represent referral questions that R-PAS can help answer. In all cases, client names and identifying information have been carefully altered to protect their anonymity. The chapters are written by international assessment experts; about two-thirds are United States authors, and the others represent the countries of Finland, Israel, Italy, the Netherlands, and Norway.

By design, the chapters have similar sections: (1) a brief introduction to the case, (2) the referral question(s), (3) a summary of other assessment data, (4) relevant research or legal matters, (5) reasons why R-PAS was chosen to help address the referral questions, (6) the experience of the R-PAS administration, (7) the deidentified Results (Responses, Code Sequence, and Profile Pages 1 and 2), and (8) a discussion of the results as applied to the case(s). The chapters are concise and tightly packed with information. To assist the chapter authors with their case interpretation, an early version of the R-PAS Case-Based Interpretive Guide was prepared for each of their cases. Depending on the particular assessment setting and situation, the chapters conclude with a summary about the impact that the R-PAS experience had on the person being assessed and/or the importance of the R-PAS data for understanding the person and answering the referral questions.

## REFERENCES

Atkinson, L. (1986). The comparative validities of the Rorschach and MMPI: A meta-analysis. *Canadian Psychology, 27,* 238–247.

Beck, S. J., Beck, A. G., Levitt, E. E., & Molish, H. B. (1961). *Rorschach's test: Vol. I. Basic processes* (3rd ed.). Oxford, UK: Grune & Stratton.

Blasczyk-Schiep, S., Kazén, M., Kuhl, J., & Grygielski, M. (2011). Appraisal of suicide risk among adolescents and young adults through the Rorschach test. *Journal of Personality Assessment, 93,* 518–526.

Bornstein, R. F. (1999). Criterion validity of objective and projective dependency tests: A meta-analytic assessment of behavioral prediction. *Psychological Assessment, 11,* 48–57.

Crews, F. (1996). The verdict on Freud. *Psychological Science, 7,* 63–67.

Cronbach, L. J. (1949). Statistical methods applied to Rorschach scores: A review. *Psychological Bulletin, 46,* 393–429.

Dao, T. K., Prevatt, F., & Horne, H. L. (2008). Differentiating psychotic patients from nonpsychotic patients with the MMPI-2 and Rorschach. *Journal of Personality Assessment, 90,* 93–101.

Dean, K. L. (2005). A method to increase Rorschach response productivity while maintaining comprehensive system validity. *Dissertation Abstracts International, 65,* 4280.

Dean, K. L., Viglione, D. J., Perry, W., & Meyer, G. J. (2007). A method to optimize the response range while maintaining Rorschach comprehensive system validity. *Journal of Personality Assessment, 89,* 149–161.

Dean, K. L., Viglione, D. J., Perry, W., & Meyer, G. J. (2008). Correction to: "A method to optimize the response range while maintaining Rorschach comprehensive system validity." *Journal of Personality Assessment, 90,* 204.

Diener, M. J., Hilsenroth, M. J., Shaffer, S. A., & Sexton, J. E. (2011). A meta-analysis of the relationship between the Rorschach Ego Impairment Index (EII) and psychiatric severity. *Clinical Psychology & Psychotherapy, 18,* 464–485.

Exner, J. E. (1974). *The Rorschach: A comprehensive system.* New York: Wiley.

Exner, J. E. (1986). *The Rorschach: A comprehensive system. Vol. 1: Basic foundations* (2nd ed.). New York: Wiley.

Exner, J. E. (2001). A comment on "The misperception of psychopathology: Problems with norms of the Comprehensive System for the Rorschach." *Clinical Psychology: Science and Practice, 8,* 386–396.

Exner, J. E. (2003). *The Rorschach: A comprehensive system* (4th ed.). New York Wiley.

Exner, J. E. (2007). A new U.S. adult nonpatient sample. *Journal of Personality Assessment, 89*(Suppl.), S154–S158.

Exner, J. E., & Weiner, I. B. (1982). *The Rorschach: A comprehensive system: Vol. 3. Assessment of children and adolescents.* New York: Wiley.

Fowler, J. C., Piers, C., Hilsenroth, M. J., Holdwick, D. J., & Padawer, J. R. (2001). The Rorschach Suicide Constellation: Assessing various degrees of lethality. *Journal of Personality Assessment, 76,* 333–351.

Garb, H. N., Wood, J. M., Lilienfeld, S. O., & Nezworski, M. T. (2005). Roots of the Rorschach controversy. *Clinical Psychology Review, 25,* 97–118.

Graceffo, R. A., Mihura, J. L, & Meyer, G. J. (2014). A meta-analysis of an implicit measure of personality functioning: The Mutuality of Autonomy Scale. *Journal of Personality Assessment, 96,* 581–595.

Gross, K., Keyes, M. D., & Greene, R. L. (2000). Assessing depression with the MMPI and MMPI-2. *Journal of Personality Assessment, 75,* 464–477.

Hartmann, E., & Grønnerød, C. (2009). Rorschach variables and Big Five scales as predictors of military training completion: A replication study of the selection of candidates to the Naval Special Forces in Norway. *Journal of Personality Assessment, 91,* 254–264.

Hartmann, E., Sunde, T., Kristensen, W., & Martinussen, M. (2003). Psychological measures as predictors of military training performance. *Journal of Personality Assessment, 80,* 87–98.

Hertz, M. R. (1970). *Frequency tables for scoring Rorschach responses* (5th ed.). Cleveland, OH: Case Western Reserve University.

Hiller, J. B., Rosenthal, R., Bornstein, R. F., Berry, D. T. R., & Brunell-Neuleib, S. (1999). A comparative meta-analysis of Rorschach and MMPI validity. *Psychological Assessment, 11,* 278–296.

Hosseininasab, A., Meyer, G. J., Viglione, D. J., Mihura, J. L., Berant, E., Resende, A. C., . . . Mohammadi, M. R. (in press). The effect of receiving CS administration or an R-optimized alternative on R-PAS variables: A meta-analysis of findings from six studies. *Journal of Personality Assessment.*

Jørgensen, K., Andersen, T. J., & Dam, H. (2000). The diagnostic efficiency of the Rorschach Depression Index and the Schizophrenia Index: A review. *Assessment, 7,* 259–280.

Jørgensen, K., Andersen, T. J., & Dam, H. (2001). "The diagnostic efficiency of the Rorschach Depression Index and the Schizophrenia Index: A review": Erratum. *Assessment, 8,* 355.

Kiss, A. B., Mihura, J. L., & Meyer, G. J. (2017). *A meta-analytic review of the AGC score and its relationship to real life violence.* Manuscript in preparation.

Klopfer, B., & Davidson, H. H. (1967). *The Rorschach procedure: An introduction.* New York: Harcourt, Brace & World.

Meyer, G. J. (1992). Response frequency problems in the Rorschach: Clinical and research implications with suggestions for the future. *Journal of Personality Assessment, 58,* 231–244.

Meyer, G. J. (1993). The impact of response frequency on Rorschach constellation indices and on their validity with diagnostic and MMPI-2 criteria. *Journal of Personality Assessment, 60,* 153–180.

Meyer, G. J. (1996). The Rorschach and MMPI: Toward a more scientifically differentiated understanding of cross-method assessment. *Journal of Personality Assessment, 67,* 558–578.

Meyer, G. J. (1997). On the integration of personality assessment methods: The Rorschach and MMPI. *Journal of Personality Assessment, 68,* 297–330.

Meyer, G. J. (2000). The incremental validity of the Rorschach Prognostic Rating Scale over the MMPI Ego Strength Scale and IQ. *Journal of Personality Assessment, 74,* 356–370.

Meyer, G. J. (2001). Evidence to correct misperceptions about Rorschach norms. *Clinical Psychology: Science and Practice, 8,* 389–396.

Meyer, G. J., & Archer, R. P. (2001). The hard science of Rorschach research: What do we know and where do we go? *Psychological Assessment, 13,* 486–502.

Meyer, G. J., Erdberg, P., & Shaffer, T. W. (2007). Toward international normative reference data for the Comprehensive System. *Journal of Personality Assessment, 89*(Suppl.), S201–S216.

Meyer, G. J., Giromini, L., Viglione, D. J., Reese, J. B., & Mihura, J. L. (2015). The association of gender, ethnicity, age, and education with Rorschach scores. *Assessment, 22,* 46–64.

Meyer, G. J., & Handler, L. (1997). The ability of the Rorschach to predict subsequent outcome: A meta-analysis of the Rorschach Prognostic Rating Scale. *Journal of Personality Assessment, 69,* 1–38.

Meyer, G. J., Hsiao, W.-C., Viglione, D. J., Mihura, J. L., & Abraham, L. M. (2013). Rorschach scores in applied clinical practice: A survey of perceived validity by experienced clinicians. *Journal of Personality Assessment, 95,* 351–365.

Meyer, G. J., Shaffer, T. W., Erdberg, P., & Horn, S. L. (2015). Addressing issues in the development and use of the Composite International Reference Values as Rorschach norms for adults. *Journal of Personality Assessment, 97,* 330–347.

Meyer, G. J., Viglione, D. J., & Mihura, J. L. (2017). Psychometric foundations of the Rorschach Performance Assessment System (R-PAS). In R. E. Erard & F. B. Evans (Eds.), *The Rorschach in multimethod forensic practice* (pp. 23–91). New York: Routledge.

Meyer, G. J., Viglione, D. J., Mihura, J. L., Erard, R. E., & Erdberg, P. (2011). *Rorschach Performance Assessment System: Administration, coding, interpretation, and technical manual.* Toledo, OH: Rorschach Performance Assessment System.

Mihura, J. L. (2012). The necessity of multiple test methods in conducting assessments: The role of the Rorschach and self-report. *Psychological Injury and Law, 5,* 97–106.

Mihura, J. L., Dumitrascu, N., Roy, M., & Meyer, G. J. (2017). The centrality of the response process in construct validity: An illustration via the Rorschach space response. *Journal of Personality Assessment.* [Epub ahead of print]

Mihura, J. L., & Graceffo, R. A. (2014). Multimethod assessment and treatment planning. In C. J. Hopwood & R. F. Bornstein (Eds.), *Multimethod clinical assessment* (pp. 285–318). New York: Guilford Press.

Mihura, J. L., Meyer, G. J., Bombel, G., & Dumitrascu, N. (2015). Standards, accuracy, and questions of bias in Rorschach meta-analyses: Reply to Wood, Garb, Nezworski, Lilienfeld, and Duke (2015). *Psychological Bulletin, 141,* 250–260.

Mihura, J. L., Meyer, G. J., Dumitrascu, N., & Bombel, G. (2013). The validity of individual Rorschach variables: Systematic reviews and meta-analyses of the comprehensive system. *Psychological Bulletin, 139,* 548–605.

Mihura, J. L., Ales, F., Meyer, G. J., Meadows, E. A., Roy, M., & Dumitrascu, N. (2017). *A meta-analytic review of the MMPI's (all versions) ability to detect psychosis in clinical and forensic settings.* Manuscript in progress.

Opaas, M., Hartmann, E., Wentzel-Larsen, T., & Varvin, S. (2016). Relationship of pretreatment Rorschach factors to symptoms, quality of life, and real-life functioning in a 3-year follow-up of traumatized refugee patients. *Journal of Personality Assessment, 98,* 247–260.

Parker, K. C., Hanson, R. K., & Hunsley, J. (1988). MMPI, Rorschach, and WAIS: A meta-analytic comparison of reliability, stability, and validity. *Psychological Bulletin, 103,* 367–373.

Piotrowski, Z. A. (1957). *Perceptanalysis.* New York: Macmillan.

Porcelli, P., & Mihura, J. L. (2010). Assessment of alexithymia with the Rorschach Comprehensive System: The Rorschach Alexithymia Scale (RAS). *Journal of Personality Assessment, 92,* 128–136.

Rapaport, D., Gill, M. M., & Schafer, R. (1968). *Diagnostic psychological testing* (rev. ed., R. Holt, Ed.). New York: International Universities Press.

Reese, J. B., Viglione, D. J., & Giromini, L. (2014). A comparison between Comprehensive System and an early version of the Rorschach Performance Assessment System administration with outpatient children and adolescents. *Journal of Personality Assessment, 96,* 515–522.

Ritsher, J. B. (2004). Association of Rorschach and MMPI psychosis indicators and schizophrenia spectrum diagnoses in a Russian clinical sample. *Journal of Personality Assessment, 83,* 46–63.

Rogers, R., Sewell, K. W., Martin, M. A., & Vitacco, M. J. (2003). Detection of feigned mental disorders: A meta-analysis of the MMPI-2 and malingering. *Assessment, 10,* 160–177.

Romney, D. M. (1990). Thought disorder in the relatives of schizophrenics: A meta-analytic review of selected published studies. *Journal of Nervous and Mental Disease, 178,* 481–486.

Rorschach, H. (1942). *Psychodiagnostik* [Psychodiagnostics]. Bern, Switzerland: Bircher. (Original work published 1921)

Schachtel, E. G. (1966). *Experiential foundations of Rorschach's test.* Hillsdale, NJ: Analytic Press.

Searls, D. (2017). *The inkblots: Hermann Rorschach, his iconic test, and the power of seeing.* New York: Crown.

Viglione, D. J., & Giromini, L. (2016). The effects of using the international versus Comprehensive System Rorschach norms for children, adolescents, and adults. *Journal of Personality Assessment, 98,* 391–397.

Viglione, D. J., & Hilsenroth, M. J. (2001). The Rorschach: Facts, fictions, and future. *Psychological Assessment, 13,* 452–471.

Viglione, D. J., Meyer, G. J., Jordan, R. J., Converse, G. L., Evans, J., MacDermott, D., & Moore, R. C. (2015). Developing an alternative Rorschach administration method to optimize the number of responses and enhance clinical inferences. *Clinical Psychology & Psychotherapy, 22,* 546–558.

Viglione, D. J., Meyer, G. J., Resende, A. C., & Pignolo, C. (2017). A survey of challenges experienced by new learners coding the Rorschach. *Journal of Personality Assessment, 99,* 315–323.

Wilson, T. D., & Dunn, E. W. (2004). Self-knowledge: Its limits, value, and potential for improvement. *Annual Review of Psychology, 55,* 493–518.

Wood, J. M., Garb, H. N., Nezworski, M. T., Lilienfeld, S. O., & Duke, M. C. (2015). A second look at the validity of widely used Rorschach indices: Comment on Mihura, Meyer, Dumitrascu, and Bombel (2013). *Psychological Bulletin, 141,* 236–249.

Wood, J. M., Nezworski, M. T., Garb, H. N., & Lilienfeld, S. O. (2001a). Problems with the norms of the Comprehensive System for the Rorschach: Methodological and conceptual considerations. *Clinical Psychology: Science and Practice, 8,* 397–402.

Wood, J. M., Nezworski, M. T., Garb, H. N., & Lilienfeld, S. O. (2001b). The misperception of psychopathology: Problems with norms of the Comprehensive System for the Rorschach. *Clinical Psychology: Science and Practice, 8,* 350–373.

Wood, J. M., Nezworski, M. T., Garb, H. N., & Lilienfeld, S. O. (2006). The controversy over Exner's Comprehensive System for the Rorschach: The critics speak. *Independent Practitioner, 26,* 73–82.

CHAPTER 2

# Principles of R-PAS Interpretation

## Joni L. Mihura
## Gregory J. Meyer

This chapter provides an overview of interpreting the Rorschach using the Rorschach Performance Assessment System (R-PAS). The chapter summarizes and extends the interpretive guidelines provided in the R-PAS test manual (Meyer, Viglione, Mihura, Erard, & Erdberg, 2011) using illustrative examples from the cases in this book.

## Initial Considerations for R-PAS Interpretation

### For Readers Transitioning from the CS to R-PAS

As we noted in our Introduction, R-PAS is different enough from the Comprehensive System (CS), the previous most commonly used Rorschach system (Exner, 2003), that it is necessary to learn how to interpret it in its own right; however, the learning transfer from knowing the CS will be significant, making the transition fairly easy to master. For example, many R-PAS variables are the same as variables in the CS, although some have different names, and results are interpreted using standardized scores. At the same time, R-PAS includes several empirically supported Rorschach variables that are not in the CS. Also, R-PAS interpretation differs from CS interpretation in that (1) R-PAS interpretation is directly shaped by the response process (i.e., the behaviors and psychological operations that occur when the examinee responds to the task in a way to warrant a particular code), which can result in different interpretations than the CS for the same variables; and (2) R-PAS does not use the CS interpretive search strategy. With respect to the latter, there is a sort of folklore that the steps in the CS search strategy were grounded in research, but this is not correct.

## Some Corrections for Common Misconceptions about the Rorschach

For several decades, psychology has classified and viewed the Rorschach as a "projective test," in contrast to an "objective test," which was the term used to characterize self-report inventories such as the Minnesota Multiphasic Personality Inventory–2 (MMPI-2). These classifications are unfortunate misnomers for several reasons. First, the Rorschach is a problem-solving task, and its response process is not truly, or even largely, projective in nature (e.g., there is considerable structure built into the inkblot images, and clients certainly can be aware of their Rorschach-assessed characteristics). Second, the term *objective* implicitly suggests a contrast with the antonym *subjective,* implying that tasks such as the Rorschach are influenced by personal, subjective feelings and opinions and that self-report tests are not. However, a person's self-report is inherently subjective. Third, projection is a concept tied to psychoanalytic theory, and critiques of that theory have been wrongly generalized to tasks with no direct links to it. Finally, tests referred to as *projective* (e.g., Rorschach, Thematic Apperception Test [TAT], sentence completion, drawings) have been viewed as using the same method of assessment, which is not the case. This grouping of tests uses different assessment methods (e.g., TAT interpretations are based on narrative themes; drawings are based on imaginal constructions). The Rorschach also does not use just one method of assessment. For example, in R-PAS, there are scores based on the accuracy and conventionality of one's perceptions (FQ), the coherence and plausibility of one's communication (Cognitive Codes), the nature of one's thematic imagery (e.g., Morbid) or language-based representations (Oral Dependent Language [ODL]), and the propensity to be attentive to subtle nuances of one's experiential environment (e.g., Shading).

Therefore, the contemporary assessment literature has moved beyond the outdated objective–projective classifications of psychological tests and, instead, aims to describe tests based on the nature of the test stimuli and the behaviors and psychological operations involved in responding to the task. Broadly speaking, the old objective versus projective classifications have been respectively referred to as *self-report* versus *performance tests* (Meyer & Kurtz, 2006; Meyer et al., 2017) or *self-attributed* versus *implicit methods* of assessment (McClelland, Koestner, & Weinberger, 1989). Yet keep in mind that the dichotomous nature of these classifications is a carryover from the objective–projective divide; there are actually many different assessment methods, each with unique implications for interpretation and treatment planning (see Hopwood & Bornstein, 2014).

Externally assessed data, such as observer ratings or laboratory behaviors, are typically more strongly associated with each other than with introspectively assessed (self-reported) characteristics (Mihura, 2012). As an external assessment measure, the Rorschach is no different. Research shows that the Rorschach has medium effect size relationships[1] with other externally assessed criteria but small associations with self-reported information (Mihura, Meyer, Dumitrascu, & Bombel, 2013). This finding means that, in an assessment, one would expect Rorschach data to converge more closely with assessment data obtained from a source external to the respon-

---

[1]This is the expected magnitude of cross-method association for valid scales (Hemphill, 2003; based on Meyer et al., 2001).

dent than with the respondent's own self-report. At the same time, research suggests that when people know themselves well and are open to disclosing personal information, their Rorschach scores will correspond more closely to scores derived from their self-reported characteristics (Berant, Newborn, & Orgler, 2008; Meyer, 1997, 1999). Therefore, some clients' R-PAS results will more closely converge with their self-reported characteristics (i.e., based on an interview or responses to a questionnaire) than will other clients' results.

## Basic Orientation to R-PAS Interpretation

After administering the 10 inkblots to the examinee and recording his or her verbal responses and relevant nonverbal communications, the examiner codes the responses using the guidelines in the R-PAS manual (Meyer et al., 2011) and enters these codes into the scoring and interpretation program (located at *www.r-pas.org*). The scoring output provides the Code Sequence (i.e., the codes for each of the examinee's responses) and the main test results, which, like cognitive performance tests such as the Wechsler Adult Intelligence Scale—Fourth Edition (WAIS-IV), are plotted using standard scores (SSs) that have a mean of 100 and a standard deviation (*SD*) of 15. The main results are on the "Page 1" and "Page 2" Profile Pages, with supplemental output containing the results for all of the individual components of the scores. Page 1 results have the strongest validity support and should be reviewed before the Page 2 variables.[2]

Although all variables occur along an underlying continuum, the examiner should interpret the SS results as higher or lower than average when the SS is above or below the mean of 100 by more than 10 SS for adults and more than 15 SS for children and adolescents. The scoring program has two ways in which the user can easily determine the interpretive range for the results: one with chromatic colors denoting the interpretive ranges, and another for users who wish to print achromatic results. To interpret chromatic results output, a green icon indicates the Average range (for adults, SS 90–110; for children and adolescents, SS 85–115). Successive interpretive bands extend beyond the Average range endpoints by 10 SS for adults and 15 for children and adolescents.[3] Low Average and High Average are indicated by yellow icons, Low and High are indicated by red icons, and Very Low and Very High are indicated by black icons. Chromatic color was not used in the printing of this book; therefore, Figure 2.1 uses an achromatic printout to illustrate the icons' interpretive ranges. For Average scores, the icon circles are open; for Low Average and High Average scores, the circles contain one vertical line; for Low and High scores, the circles

---

[2]The rationale for placing variables on Page 1 or 2 is described in the R-PAS manual (Meyer et al., 2011; pp. 459–464). The factors considered included (1) their support in Rorschach construct validity meta-analyses (e.g., Bornstein, 1999; Diener, Hilsenroth, Shaffer, & Sexton, 2011; Graceffo, Mihura, & Meyer, 2014; Mihura et al., 2013); (2) their support in a large clinician survey (Meyer, Hsiao, Viglione, Mihura, & Abraham, 2013); (3) the close link between the coded variable's response process and its interpretation; and (4) reducing redundancies in coding and interpretation by dropping scores that did not provide unique interpretive value. The R-PAS authors have the goal of moving all variables to Page 1 or out of the system altogether, depending on how the evidence develops.

[3]See Chapter 3 for more information about using R-PAS norms with children and adolescents.

| Perception and Thinking Problems | | | | | | 60 | 70 | 80 | 90 | 100 | 110 | 120 | 130 | 140 | |
|---|---|---|---|---|---|---|---|---|---|---|---|---|---|---|---|
| EII-3 | 1.1 | 92 | 121 | 93 | 123 | | | | | | | | | | EII |
| TP-Comp (Thought & Percept. Com...) | 2.1 | 95 | 124 | 95 | 124 | | | | | | | | | | TP-C |
| WSumCog | 34 | 99 | 136 | 99 | 135 | | | | | | | | | | WCog |
| SevCog | 3 | 98 | 131 | 98 | 131 | | | | | | | | | | Sev |
| FQ-% | 16% | 79 | 112 | 81 | 113 | | | | | | | | | | FQ-% |
| WD-% | 16% | 85 | 115 | 83 | 114 | | | | | | | | | | WD-% |
| FQo% | 40% | 7 | 78 | 5 | 75 | | | | | | | | | | FQo% |
| P | | 5 | 39 | 96 | 46 | 98 | | | | | | | | | P |

**FIGURE 2.1.** Example of R-PAS standard score results and their differentiated icons. Reproduced from the Rorschach Performance Assessment System® (R-PAS®) Scoring Program (© 2010–2016) and excerpted from the *Rorschach Performance Assessment System: Administration, Coding, Interpretation, and Technical Manual* (© 2011) with copyrights by Rorschach Performance Assessment System, LLC. All rights reserved. Used by permission of Rorschach Performance Assessment System, LLC. Further reproduction is prohibited without written permission from R-PAS.

contain two vertical lines; and for Very Low and Very High scores, the circles are completely filled.

## Applying the R-PAS Interpretive Guidelines

Before interpreting the results, the clinician should review assessment questions generated by the referral source and the client and develop hypotheses for the results, keeping in mind the unique methods of assessment the Rorschach task provides. The required materials are (1) the verbatim Responses and the Location Sheets, (2) the Code Sequence and the Results pages, and (3) behavioral observations recorded during the test administration.

The basic interpretive steps, as described in the manual (Meyer et al., 2011, pp. 321–328), use what are called the "four S's" (which works in the English language): *Scan, Sift, Synthesize*, and *Summarize*. The first interpretive step is to quickly *Scan* the Profile Pages. The goal is to become globally familiar with the results before starting the detailed interpretive process. To do so, scan Pages 1 and 2 for notably high or low scores, as indicated by the red icons with two vertical lines and the black icons that are completely filled (denoting extreme scores). The point is simply to register these scores in memory, so as you complete the other steps, these will be in mind, influencing your sifting and synthesizing. Ultimately, the scan should take less than a minute, although it will require a bit more time when one is initially becoming acquainted with the variables and Profile Pages.

After conducting the Scan, the next step is to sequentially consider each variable and *Sift* through the different interpretive possibilities for each one. Variables at a particular level of elevation produce a fan-like array of possible inferences, and the goal of this step is to narrow the possibilities to the one or two that are most likely correct for the client. While sifting, you will also be *Synthesizing* information across all other data sources (e.g., clinical interview, behavioral observations, other assessment results). Sifting and synthesizing are reciprocal processes, differentiated by their focus on a refined understanding of one variable via consideration of all other relevant data, respectively. The Sift and Synthesize steps include "burrowing into the data," which means that after you review the plotted results for each variable, you step down one level to that variable's subcomponents to further flesh out the meaning of the results. For example, when encountering an elevation on the Ego Impairment Index–3 (EII-3), burrow down one level and review its subcomponent parts to see if a particular type of impairment contributed to the elevation. Possibilities include thought disorder (WSumCog), reality testing (FQ–), disturbed object relations (PHR Proportion), misinterpretations of human actions (M–), and primitive thinking (Critical Contents). When a variable does not have subcomponent scores, stepping down one level would entail reading the original response, which is particularly helpful for Thematic codes (to review for salient themes) and poor Form Quality codes (to see if particular personally salient images are overwhelming the person's ability to respond to the inkblot contours). When the Complexity SS is less than 85 or more than 115, the interpreter should consider whether to plot and interpret Complexity Adjusted scores, discussed further in subsequent sections. Finally, *Summarize* what has been learned about the person from R-PAS, integrate that summary with conclusions from other test results taking into consideration the methods by which the information was acquired, and formulate answers to the referral questions.

## The Centrality of the Response Process in R-PAS Interpretation

The Rorschach task has been conceptualized in a variety of ways. For example, Leichtman (1996) focused on the creation of a Rorschach response as communication within an interpersonal field. Exner (2003) focused on the respondent's scanning of the inkblots and the decision-making processes involved in choosing a response. However, Exner's approach to interpreting the Rorschach task does not inform interpretation as directly and as all-encompassingly as R-PAS's focus on the response process. Our views are similar to Schachtel's (1966) experiential and phenomenological approach to interpreting the Rorschach. As Schachtel said, "No amount of validation of Rorschach-test-score meanings can substitute for the understanding of what goes on in the test and in its interpretation" (p. 2). Whatever broader theories one uses to conceptualize people and their psychological operations, one must ground R-PAS interpretation in an understanding of its basic response process.

### *What Is the "Response Process"?*

The *response process* refers to the psychological operations that occur in the process of generating a response to the task whose elements are coded or classified in a particular way (Meyer et al., 2011; Mihura, Dumitrascu, Roy, & Meyer, 2017). At its very core, R-PAS data comprise coded behaviors. For performance tests like the Rorschach and intelligence tests, the response process is the behavioral representation of the test's scores. For example, to "pass" the items in the Block Design subtest on the Wechsler intelligence tests, respondents must mentally represent the design they are asked to reproduce in an accurate fashion and then analyze the design components to ensure the faces of their blocks accurately match those components. Accomplishing this task requires the ability to analyze and synthesize abstract visual information, nonverbal concept formation and reasoning, fluid intelligence, visual perception and organization, and visual–motor coordination. In addition, respondents might mentally analyze and synthesize the components of the design before they start manipulating the blocks to create the design, or they might use physical trial-and-error manipulation of the blocks until the design looks like that in the figure. All of these elements are response process components that can be considered in interpretation, focusing not only on the mental analysis and synthesis but also on respondents' ability to physically manipulate the blocks.

In R-PAS, somewhat similarly, a Synthesis code indicates that the respondent has analyzed and synthesized distinct components of the inkblot to create a meaningful interrelationship of the parts. In contrast to Block Design, however, no physical manipulation is required, and the respondent is free to create his or her own mental designs to map onto the inkblot components. In addition, IQ tests are "maximal performance" tests with right and wrong answers on which people are asked to perform to their best ability, whereas R-PAS is a "typical performance" task that assesses what a person typically "will do" when left to his or her own predilections, not what the person "can do" when asked to perform optimally in response to clear guidelines. Engaging in the mental and physical operations that result in a Block Design score is a requirement of the task; in contrast, R-PAS instructions do not ask the respondent to perform the mental operations involved in the Synthesis response process. The respondent may explicitly or implicitly believe that this achievement is expected, but it is not part of the task instructions. Therefore, the mental and behavioral operations that result in a Synthesis code—as well as all other R-PAS coding (except, to some degree, R)—are almost entirely about the psychology of the person producing the response rather than the demands of the situation.

Because the response process of an R-PAS score is at the core of its interpretation, the R-PAS manual (Meyer et al., 2011) provides interpretation at the response level (pp. 330–346) prior to interpretation at the broader protocol level (pp. 347–376). Rorschach scores that are based on single codes, such as Human Movement (M), have the same interpretation at the response level as they do at the protocol level. On the other hand, for Rorschach scores that are derived from an amalgamation of different codes (e.g., M + Weighted Sum of Color [WSumC]), the interpreter must first understand the response process of the individual codes (e.g., M and WSumC) in order to understand the combination of these codes at the protocol level. Therefore, the interpreter should become familiar with the response process foundation for all of the individual R-PAS variables. This explicit response process approach to interpretation is a distinguishing feature of R-PAS compared to the CS.

## Enriching Formal Score Interpretation with Idiographic Interpretations

R-PAS strongly supports idiographic interpretations, using a disciplined approach grounded in principles described in the manual (Meyer et al., 2011, pp. 326–328). Similar to the TAT, it is important to know the *card pull* for common and uncommon reactions and elaborations to cards and their features. For instance, it is fairly common to identify breasts or penises as the rationale for assigning male or female sex to humans seen in the D9 areas on Card III; however, it is uncommon to identify both. As another example of card pull, most people experience Card VIII—the first completely colorful card—as having cheerful, pleasant colors. Therefore, when respondents have a negative reaction to Card VIII, it can be helpful to review the response to see what is obstructing or ruining their pleasant experience. Chapter case examples of such responses to Card VIII include Khadivi's (Chapter 6) case of attempted suicide; "Mary," who said, "Reminds me of a leaf in the fall losing its color"; Aschieri, Chinaglia, and Kiss's (Chapter 9) assessment of "Nora," a woman in couple therapy who said, "A beautiful color! An ugly flower drawn in a very inaccurate way"; and Bram's (Chapter 7) client, "Heidi," in a therapeutic impasse with negative reactions to her treatment providers: "Too happy! Too colorful! . . . All the colors are so bright. Like *too* happy. Every animal is smiling in happy land, *not my happy land.*"

Responses with personal significance (also called "projected" material; Exner, 1989) are more likely to contain codes of (1) movement (M, FM, m); (2) FQu or FQ–; and (3) Cognitive, Thematic Codes, or Critical Contents (see also Pianowski, Meyer, & de Villemor-Amaral, 2016). Conceptually, FQ– responses would be more likely to contain projected material, whereas FQu responses would be more idiographic or personalized. Case examples that fit these criteria include Lee's child custody case (Chapter 13), in which the father accused his ex-wife of being aggressive toward their child; the father provided the following response to Card X: "Angry mouse soldier . . . half-open eyes make it look angry, and nose with frowning mouth, ready to bite . . . a steel helmet because the color is metallic" (relevant codes: FQ– Ma,FC,C′ INC2 AGM,AGC). To Card VII, Kleiger and Khadivi's (Chapter 5) female adolescent, "Chandra," who was being assessed for emerging psychosis and who had been abusing her sister, who was also diagnosed with psychosis, said, "Looks like two girls that are looking at each other intensely. Looks like they are surprised. Looks like they have worms coming out of their heads . . . like they're gonna start a fight or something. . . . These look like worms, like they were rotting. It looks like their eyes were wide open like 'Oh!'" (relevant codes: FQu Ma,mp FAB2 AGM,MOR,MAP). One could hypothesize that this response represents the adolescent's experience of the emergent psychosis and her conflict with her sister, who has also been diagnosed with psychosis.

The idiographic response features aligning with the standard interpretation of the R-PAS code should give the clinician greater confidence in the code's interpretation and lend idiographic richness to it. Using the Achromatic Color (C′) code, the following responses are examples. In Acklin's (Chapter 10) evaluation of a client's criminal responsibility and competency to stand trial, he referred to the client as a "depressed and reluctant messiah"; he reported a countertransference experience of "almost complete absence" and described the client as having "extremely flat rapport." His client's C′ response was, " . . . somebody that has been squashed, flat, dead looking. (Examiner: Dead looking?) The color is dark, lifeless." Bram (Chapter 7) described his client, Heidi, as "feeling overwhelmed, depressed, and preoccupied with death and suicide"; her C′ response was, "It looks like depression. (Examiner: Why depression?) Because it's all black." For Dumitrascu's (Chapter 16) neuropsychological assessment of "Lisa," a young adult with a history of relational trauma who was currently feeling overwhelmed at school, her C′ response was "A person trapped in something . . . like a black sludge, I guess; like being trapped in something."

The examinee's behavior during the assessment is also a good source of idiographic information. For example, compare and contrast the level of self-awareness shown in responses for the following two cases. The last response of "Nora," Aschieri et al.'s (Chapter 9) client, was, "A woman wearing a coat, bra, legs, breast, head, and fur coat. It's very colored, very beautiful, but I'm disturbed by these four insects that are attacking the woman from every side. She is surrounded by the insects, but the coat protects her because it is thick. She is protected except from the insect that is attacking her at the head. *Wow, what am I saying!*" Nora's level of self-awareness is quite different than that of Nørbech et al.'s (Chapter 12) client, "Toni," a psychopathic female with trauma intrusions and thought disturbance, who responded to Card II: "A snake with an open mouth and long neck. *Why are you showing me these pictures?*" and to Card III, "Two birds or humans holding onto something. *Sick paintings.* . . . And you see an animal head sticking out of their chest here." And to Card IV, "Big animal. Legs, head. Two snakes here. The animal is spitting out something. *I can't stand looking at this picture.*"

We can also use Toni's response sequence to illustrate "sequence analysis," an advanced idiographic approach in which one attends to the scores and idiographic features of consecutive responses (see Peebles-Kleiger, 2002). As illustrated in the previous paragraph, in several responses in a row, Toni was disturbed by what she was seeing, and the responses themselves contained thought disturbance (R7 INC1; R8 INC1,FAB2; R9 DR1,FAB2). Toni seemed to try to get rid of these mental images by refusing to give another response, even though prompted to do so on Cards III and IV. Toni's response patterns demonstrate a unique benefit of performance-based personality tests: the ability to see "how it all fits together."

## Contending with Non-Normal Distributions and Low Base-Rate Scores

To contend with the non-normal distributions that characterize many Rorschach scores, the percentiles associated with every raw score were obtained and converted to their normal SS equivalent (see Meyer & Erdberg, Chapter 3, this volume, and Appendix E in the R-PAS manual). Therefore, the percentiles are organized for interpretation as if they belonged to the regular bell-shaped normal curve, which slightly accentuates differences in the more extreme ends and minimizes them in the middle of the distribution where the more common scores are (see Meyer et al., 2011, p. 480, for specifics). Understanding the implications of the non-normal distribution and low base rates or frequencies of many Rorschach scores (e.g., T, M−) is vital when interpreting R-PAS results. Low base rate scores can be defined as those that occur 5 times or less in every 100 responses. Because R-PAS protocols have about 24 responses, on average, low base-rate scores are those with means of 1.20 and below. These variables have limited distributions in normative data, with many people having scores of 0, some with scores of 1, a smaller number with scores of 2, and so on, up to the maximum value observed in the norms, which often is just a value of 4 or 5. With limited distributions like these, each score value encompasses a range of percentile values. For instance, 55% of the people in the R-PAS norms have Texture (T) values of 0, which encompasses the range from the very smallest percentile up through the 55th percentile. When computing the R-PAS norms, as is conventional in statistical analyses, every score value that encompassed multiple percentiles was assigned the percentile for its midpoint. Thus, in the case of T, a value of 0 was assigned a percentile of 27.5 (i.e., 55/2 = 27.5) as the best value to represent the score, even though the score actually encompassed a larger range on the percentile distribution.

## *Interpretation with Low Base-Rate Scores*

Using Space Reversal (SR) as an example of a low base-rate score for adults, as you can see in Figure 2.2, a raw score of 0 is plotted at an SS of 87. Although it may be difficult to see in the figure, there is a thin light-gray line superimposed on the dashed line at an SS of 95. That is called a *hash mark,* and it indicates the dividing line between the range encompassed by one score value and the range encompassed by the adjacent score value. In this case, that dividing line is between a score of 0 and a score of 1. There is another hash mark at an SS of 110, which is the dividing line between a score of 1 and a score of 2, and a third one that is more readily visible at an SS of 118, which is the dividing line between a score of 2 and a score of 3. These dividing lines are important to keep in mind during interpretation. Returning to the SR score of 0, the figure shows its range extends up to and encompasses an SS of 95. Therefore, even though a raw score of 0 is plotted at an SS of 87 in the interpretable Low Average range, the actual range of a raw score of 0 for SR extends to the right up to an SS of 95 and also encompasses the low end of the Average range. Consequently, only cautious interpretations can be made about low scores for low base-rate variables.

In fact, some variables have such a low base rate that a raw score of 0 is plotted in the Average range. For adults, Page 1 contains four such variables (i.e., Pu, SevCog, M–, and MAH); the current Page 2 contains seven such variables (i.e., V, Pure C, CBlend, r, AGM, T, and PER). Because one cannot have a negative number for these count variables, they have no "Low" interpretation.[4]

## Understanding and Using the Underlying Units

By selecting "Units" when looking at the profiled results output in a browser, the examiner accesses the R-PAS software option to view the underlying units for each test variable. In practical terms, choosing the option to plot the underlying units provides the ability to see the variables with low base rates and to take into consideration the caveats previously discussed. Viewing the underlying units also provides the ability to consider the impact of scoring uncertainties. For example, if someone

| Self and Other Representation | | | | | | 60 | 70 | 80 | 90 | 100 | 110 | 120 | 130 | 140 | |
|---|---|---|---|---|---|---|---|---|---|---|---|---|---|---|---|
| ODL% | 40% | 98 | 133 | 98 | 131 | | | | | | | | | | ODL% |
| SR (Space Reversal) | 0 | 19 | 87 | 19 | 87 | | | | | | | | | | SR |
| MAP/MAHP | [1/2] | NA | | | | | | | | | | | | | MAP Prp |

**FIGURE 2.2.** Illustration of using underlying units and the Min/Max values on the Results printout. Reproduced from the Rorschach Performance Assessment System® (R-PAS®) Scoring Program (© 2010–2016) and excerpted from the *Rorschach Performance Assessment System: Administration, Coding, Interpretation, and Technical Manual* (© 2011) with copyrights by Rorschach Performance Assessment System, LLC. All rights reserved. Used by permission of Rorschach Performance Assessment System, LLC. Further reproduction is prohibited without written permission from R-PAS.

---

[4]For readers familiar with the CS, the new normative values and the implications for interpretation will require attention to adjusted benchmarks. For example, using Exner's CS (2003) norms, having no Texture (T) scores was considered a problem. However, numerous datasets from the United States and other countries have found that most people have Texture scores of 0 (Meyer, Erdberg, & Shaffer, 2007).

has an SR raw score of 1, and the coding of an additional SR is possible but uncertain, the underlying units can be viewed to determine the difference that coding an additional SR would make for this person. SR = 1 is in the Average range (SS = 102), and SR = 2 is High Average (SS = 113). Therefore, if another SR code is possible but uncertain, the interpreter should consider what it would mean if the examinee had a slightly elevated SR score. Because the underlying units are viewed as essential to accurate interpretation, they are the default setting for the results output. We do not recommend de-selecting them.

## Understanding and Using the Minimum/Maximum Values

The R-PAS interpreter should be aware of the minimum and maximum SSs for variables, which can be plotted on the printout by selecting the "Min/Max in Norms" option in the online scoring program. With that option selected, the output provides a hatched pattern on the upper or lower side of the SS distribution, as shown in Figure 2.2. On multiscale tests, there is a tendency for test interpreters to compare scale elevations in order to say what is the most important issue for the client. However, just like other tests (e.g., the MMPI-2 and WAIS-IV), there are limits as to how high and low the SSs can go for many R-PAS variables. Therefore, comparing R-PAS SSs to determine degrees of elevation or their potential level of importance for the client can be complicated. For instance, as shown in Figure 2.2, the maximum SS for MAP/MAHP is 123. If a client scored 132 on SR, one cannot conclude that SR is a more salient personality characteristic than MAP/MAHP because the MAP/MAHP score cannot be plotted any higher than 123.

## Understanding Complexity

As the first factor of the Rorschach, the complexity of a client's protocol is the main component that causes many individual scores to rise or fall and to potentially differentiate his or her protocol from that of others. R-PAS provides a measure of this task engagement using a composite score called Complexity. As described in the R-PAS manual, "Complexity is an aggregate measure involving information from several sections across all the responses. The three response components that contribute to its aggregate score are: (1) Location and Object Qualities contained in the Location, Space, Synthesis, and Vagueness sections, (2) Contents, and (3) Determinants" (Meyer et al., 2011, pp. 295–296). Additionally, the fact that these three response components are summed over all responses means that R is actually the fourth component of Complexity. When a case's Complexity score is more than one *SD* above or below the mean for his or her age group (i.e., < 85 SS or > 115 SS), one can click the box on the Results Output to apply Complexity Adjustment (CAdj) to the protocol. CAdj uses a regression equation to predict what a client's scores would look like if his or her protocol had an average level of Complexity.

A client's protocol can vary in Complexity for several reasons, affecting how Complexity will be interpreted and if and how CAdj scores will be interpreted. For example, a client's protocol could be low in Complexity because he or she is consciously withholding, as when a client constricts responses when attempting to dissimulate, or the low Complexity might be due to his or her low IQ and cognitive limitations that hinder engagement with the task. On the other hand, a client may have a high Complexity protocol due to a high IQ and typical sophisticated thinking; or, the client may be decompensating and the complexity may be due to confused, disinhibited thinking and reactivity. Therefore, the higher-order factor of Rorschach complexity has many different potential interpretations, yet it impacts many lower-order individual scores whose interpretation should be independent of it. For example, a client who is withholding responses in attempt to dissimulate or who produces a simplistic protocol due to cognitive deficits will be less likely to provide Vista responses (i.e., sophisticated responses that are less common in children and persons with low IQ). As such, the reason the client did not produce a Vista score is independent of the score's interpretation in the Stress and Distress section (i.e., critical self-evaluation). Therefore, R-PAS provides a way to predict what the person's protocol would look like if he or she had an average level of Complexity (or if everyone in the norms had that person's particular level of Complexity). However, it is important to keep in mind that CAdj scores are not more accurate or better than raw scores—they just provide different information. Furthermore, interpreting CAdj scores is an option, not a requirement.

Later in the chapter, we (1) describe how to interpret protocols with high or low Complexity and (2) refer to cases in chapters with high or low Complexity for various reasons. For further information, see the R-PAS manual, especially Chapter 10, "Recommendations for Interpretation," and Chapter 11, "Clinical Case Illustration" (Meyer et al., 2011), plus Chapter 3, this volume, "Using R-PAS Norms with an Emphasis on Children and Adolescents."

## Integrating with Other Assessment Data

Integrating R-PAS findings with other assessment data is briefly explicated in the manual (Meyer et al., 2001, pp. 329–330), but the clinician should be familiar with other key references (e.g., Finn, 1996; Ganellen, 1996; Meyer, 1996, 1997; Mihura, 2012; Mihura & Graceffo, 2014).[5] For example, clinicians should know how to understand results of scales ostensibly measuring similar characteristics that diverge from each other across methods. As Ganellen (1996) explains, when scores on similarly named MMPI-2 and Rorschach scales diverge from each other, the interpreter should ask the following two questions: Do the scales have similar names yet tap different aspects of the construct? Do the data indicate an emotional conflict, or does the client have limited self-awareness? For example, what does it mean when a male client has a high PAI Dominance score and a high R-PAS ODL% score? The client might be expressing his strong implicit dependency needs with "dominant" gender-congruent behaviors that put him at the center of attention and affection. Or the client's self-report may not reflect his actual behavior. Or perhaps the examiner coded ODL erroneously. When scores differ, there is a tendency to think that one score is right and the other is wrong. Although this may be the case, the divergences can also provide key insights into the client's personality dynamics (see also Meyer et al., 2017).

---

[5] One challenge when consulting sources published before R-PAS is the use of CS codes that must be translated to R-PAS codes. For assessors who were trained in the CS, Appendix D in the R-PAS manual provides a glossary of CS terms and their R-PAS counterparts.

## Steps of Interpretation with a Case Illustration

### Pre-Interpretation Tasks

Of course, assessors should be familiar with basic interpretive considerations, such as the nature and context of the evaluation (e.g., self-referred for psychotherapy vs. forensic) and demographic factors such as age, gender, and culture (see Brabender & Mihura, 2016; Hays, 2008), as well as how to formulate hypotheses. For other pre-interpretation tasks, see the R-PAS manual (Meyer et al., 2011, pp. 321–323, 385). As general guidelines:

1. Pre-R-PAS Administration Tasks
   a. Be aware of your personal biases and the natural human tendency to look for confirmation of your preexisting beliefs.
   b. Formulate expectations based on the client's characteristics observed in other performance situations (e.g., behavioral observations, intelligence tests, school or inpatient psychiatric records).
   c. Articulate what specific information you expect to gain from R-PAS compared to the client's self-reported characteristics.
   d. Formulate hypotheses that take into account the submethods of assessment embedded in R-PAS.
2. R-PAS-Specific Pre-Interpretation Tasks
   a. Make notes in the Comment sections of the scoring program to document any coding dilemmas (e.g., inadequate clarification, on-the-border coding decisions).
   b. Have all test data available (Responses with behavioral observations noted, Location Sheet, Code Sequence, and R-PAS results pages).

### Case Illustration

For illustrative purposes, we provide a focused overview of R-PAS interpretation using a fictive case example of an adult: "Mr. J," a 19-year-old, single, European American male. The referral question of psychosis was based on Mr. J's odd behaviors and social withdrawal after beginning his first semester of college. Mr. J entered college with an academic scholarship, and in high school had a history of mostly A's, good class attendance, and participation in sports and the debate team.

Mr. J was not attending his college classes, which his roommate reported to their resident assistant (RA). In addition, the roommate reported that Mr. J was acting "strange," and that he was starting to feel afraid of him—although not due to any overt aggression or threats. Mr. J's roommate said that Mr. J seems to actually be afraid of *him* and is quick to misinterpret what he says. The roommate explained that he doesn't get angry at Mr. J initially, but when Mr. J negatively misinterprets what he says, it *does* make him angry and he does not want to validate Mr. J's misperception. He stated that Mr. J's girlfriend had stopped by their dorm room a few times in the past few weeks, but Mr. J refused to see her. The girlfriend expressed concern for Mr. J, given that this behavior was unusual and he had said nothing to her about breaking up.

Mr. J's RA met with him and suggested that he talk to someone at the counseling center about his difficulty leaving his room and his lack of motivation to attend classes. The RA offered to help him make the first appointment and accompany him to it. After meeting with a student clinician, a referral was made for psychological testing at the university's Psychology Clinic. After the intake interview, the student clinician administered a multiscale self-report instrument. Mr. J was moderately elevated on scales that could suggest psychosis, but the items he endorsed on those scales targeted problems with attention, concentration, and organizing one's thoughts; he did not endorse psychosis markers such as thought insertion or control. Mr. J also reported elevated levels of distress. In the interview and on the self-report instrument, Mr. J denied ever using any substances. He explained that his family was Southern Baptist, and that drinking alcohol was forbidden. Using a collaborative assessment approach, the student clinician helped Mr. J formulate his own assessment questions. Mr. J said his main question was "Why is everyone turning against me?" With further encouragement, he added one other question: "Am I losing my mind?"

## Pre-R-PAS Administration Tasks

Because Mr. J formed a good working alliance with the RA at his dorm and voluntarily came for assessment and treatment, there was a higher likelihood that he would engage in the R-PAS task. Mr. J's cognitive sophistication, as assessed by his near straight-A record in high school, suggests that he has the cognitive capacity to engage in the R-PAS task, and we would expect an above-average level of Complexity. A lower than average level of Complexity could indicate one of the following: (1) He is shutting down as a general coping strategy, especially in unfamiliar situations like the Rorschach task; (2) he is shutting down due to psychopathology, such as severe depression or PTSD; (3) a good alliance was not formed with the examiner; or (4) situational reasons led to disengagement (e.g., he might experience qualities of the examiner as intrapsychically threatening to him, such as reminding him of a real or imagined threatening being).

Mr. J does not have a long history of maladjustment—to the contrary. Therefore, we might expect average or above-average scores on R-PAS variables assessing psychological resources, such as MC. Interpretation of two other R-PAS variables can hinge on knowing the client's history of functioning and the context of the assessment: Complexity and Critical Contents. Complexity can be high due to cognitive sophistication but also due to malingering or actual severe dysfunction. There is little evidence to suggest that Mr. J has motivation to malinger. Malingering is conceivable to "excuse" his poor class attendance and grades; however, during the informed consent period of the assessment, when Mr. J learned that some people might need to be hospitalized if their problems were severe enough, he was very averse to the idea of being hospitalized. Mr. J has not been functioning well lately, with the caveat that he made an alliance with his RA to come for psychological treatment. Therefore, it is possible that Mr. J's psychological condition is currently severe enough that he could elevate Complexity more than otherwise expected.

Critical Contents can be elevated under three major conditions: (1) a trauma history, (2) malingering, and (3) the presence of primitive cognitions as seen in borderline or psychotic levels of personality organization. Applying these three conditions to Mr. J: (1) he had denied a trauma history during the clinical interview; (2) he had no known incentives to malinger; and (3) persons with a borderline or psychotic level of personality organization typically exhibit a long history of poor or uneven functioning. On the contrary, Mr. J's functioning had only recently declined, although precipitously. Therefore, Mr. J did not obviously fit any of the three conditions that would lead us to expect a high Critical Contents score.

Regarding what we expect to gain from R-PAS compared to his self-report results, evidence suggests that the Rorschach is better at detecting psychosis than self-report instruments (e.g., Dao, Prevatt, & Horne, 2008; Mihura, Roy, Dumitrascu, & Meyer, 2016; Mihura et al., 2013, Table 3). We also know that Mr. J is having difficulty communicating, and perhaps understanding, what is happening with him or to him; therefore, a performance test whose responses are evaluated via a formal coding system, using empirically supported scores, should be helpful. The Rorschach is also unique in its ability to assess mental images; therefore, we might be able to see if disturbing or otherwise salient images occupy Mr. J's mind (e.g., Critical Contents).

### Orientation to Mr. J's Page 1 and 2 Results

Pages 1 and 2 of Mr. J's R-PAS results are shown in Figures 2.3a and 2.3b. The variables are listed in the far left column and abbreviated in the far right column. In the next three columns from the left are (1) his raw scores, (2) the percentiles and SSs corresponding to those raw scores, and (3) his Complexity Adjusted scores, which are grayed out by default and would remain that way because his case does not need Complexity Adjustment. The grid that follows contains Mr. J's results on the SS metric, with a mean of 100 and an *SD* of 15. His main results are interpreted in the subsequent sections.

### R-PAS-Specific Pre-Interpretation Tasks

Three main coding dilemmas to consider were noted and recorded in the Comment boxes of the scoring program. First, an instance of overclarification led to verbiage that could have been coded for FAB2; however, consistent with R-PAS coding guidelines for instances of overclarification (Meyer et al., 2011, p. 173), we did not assign the code. We can, however, consider it idiographically in regard to what happens when Mr. J is pushed too far to explain his experiences. In another instance, a key word was missed, and further appropriate clarification could have led to a coding of Vista, but his Vista score was already Very High. Finally, in a response that contained multiple objects, one of the objects that met criteria for FQ– was considered "important to the response," but this decision could be debated. Based on the R-PAS rules for how to assign FQ to multi-object responses, we coded down to FQ– (Meyer et al., p. 42) but noted the ambiguity about how central this object was to the response. With a 20 response protocol, 1 FQ– score equates to 5 percentage points, so it is possible his FQ–% is actually 5% lower than profiled.

Regarding whether to apply Complexity Adjustment (CAdj), Mr. J's Complexity score was not quite high enough to consider calculating his CAdj results. His Complexity SS was 110, and CAdj is not considered until it is higher than 115. Before we coded and reviewed Mr. J's results, we considered our potential personal and

## R-PAS Summary Scores and Profiles – Page 1

C-ID: Mr. J - Applications of R-PAS    P-ID: 50    Age: 19    Gender: Male    Education: 12

| Domain/Variables | Raw Scores | Raw %ile | Raw SS | Cplx. Adj. %ile | Cplx. Adj. SS | Standard Score Profile R-Optimized | Abbr. |
|---|---|---|---|---|---|---|---|
| **Admin. Behaviors and Obs.** | | | | | | 60 70 80 90 100 110 120 130 140 | |
| Pr | 1 | 62 | 104 | | | | Pr |
| Pu | 0 | 40 | 96 | | | | Pu |
| CT (Card Turning) | 1 | 38 | 95 | | | | CT |
| **Engagement and Cog. Processing** | | | | | | 60 70 80 90 100 110 120 130 140 | |
| Complexity | 89 | 76 | 110 | | | | Cmplx |
| R (Responses) | 20 | 21 | 88 | 4 | 73 | | R |
| F% [Lambda=0.18] (Simplicity) | 15% | 5 | 75 | 12 | 83 | | F% |
| Blend | 8 | 88 | 118 | 76 | 110 | | Bln |
| Sy | 11 | 87 | 117 | 72 | 109 | | Sy |
| MC | 9.5 | 75 | 110 | 54 | 102 | | MC |
| MC - PPD | -6.5 | 17 | 85 | 20 | 87 | | MC-PPD |
| M | 7 | 88 | 118 | 74 | 110 | | M |
| M/MC [7/9.5] | 74% | 84 | 115 | 83 | 114 | | M Prp |
| (CF+C)/SumC [2/2] | NA | | | | | | CFC Prp |
| **Perception and Thinking Problems** | | | | | | 60 70 80 90 100 110 120 130 140 | |
| EII-3 | 1.5 | 97 | 127 | 97 | 127 | | EII |
| TP-Comp (Thought & Percept. Com...) | 2.5 | 97 | 128 | 96 | 127 | | TP-C |
| WSumCog | 27 | 98 | 131 | 98 | 130 | | WCog |
| SevCog | 4 | 99 | 138 | 99 | 138 | | Sev |
| FQ-% | 20% | 93 | 122 | 92 | 121 | | FQ-% |
| WD-% | 24% | 98 | 132 | 96 | 126 | | WD-% |
| FQo% | 30% | 2 | 71 | 2 | 70 | | FQo% |
| P | 4 | 22 | 88 | 25 | 89 | | P |
| **Stress and Distress** | | | | | | 60 70 80 90 100 110 120 130 140 | |
| YTVC' | 10 | 92 | 122 | 88 | 117 | | YTVC' |
| m | 4 | 90 | 119 | 80 | 112 | | m |
| Y | 0 | 17 | 85 | 17 | 85 | | Y |
| MOR | 1 | 51 | 100 | 41 | 96 | | MOR |
| SC-Comp (Suicide Concern Comp.) | 5.0 | 65 | 106 | 53 | 101 | | SC-C |
| **Self and Other Representation** | | | | | | 60 70 80 90 100 110 120 130 140 | |
| ODL% | 40% | 98 | 133 | 98 | 131 | | ODL% |
| SR (Space Reversal) | 0 | 19 | 87 | 19 | 87 | | SR |
| MAP/MAHP [1/2] | NA | | | | | | MAP Prp |
| PHR/GPHR [7/11] | 64% | 91 | 120 | 91 | 120 | | PHR Prp |
| M- | 0 | 36 | 95 | 36 | 95 | | M- |
| AGC | 5 | 85 | 116 | 80 | 113 | | AGC |
| H | 6 | 94 | 123 | 89 | 119 | | H |
| COP | 1 | 54 | 102 | 45 | 98 | | COP |
| MAH | 1 | 64 | 105 | 34 | 93 | | MAH |

© 2010-2016 R-PAS

**FIGURE 2.3A.** Mr. J's Page 1 results. Reproduced from the Rorschach Performance Assessment System® (R-PAS®) Scoring Program (© 2010–2016) and excerpted from the *Rorschach Performance Assessment System: Administration, Coding, Interpretation, and Technical Manual* (© 2011) with copyrights by Rorschach Performance Assessment System, LLC. All rights reserved. Used by permission of Rorschach Performance Assessment System, LLC. Further reproduction is prohibited without written permission from R-PAS.

## R-PAS Summary Scores and Profiles – Page 2

C-ID: Mr. J - Applications of R-PAS  P-ID: 50  Age: 19  Gender: Male  Education: 12

| Domain/Variables | Raw Scores | Raw %ile | Raw SS | Cplx. Adj. %ile | Cplx. Adj. SS | Standard Score Profile R-Optimized | Abbr. |
|---|---|---|---|---|---|---|---|
| **Engagement and Cog. Processing** | | | | | | | |
| W% | 40% | 51 | 100 | 43 | 98 | | W% |
| Dd% | 15% | 56 | 102 | 61 | 104 | | Dd% |
| SI (Space Integration) | 2 | 38 | 96 | 39 | 96 | | SI |
| IntCont | 1 | 31 | 93 | 19 | 86 | | IntC |
| Vg% | 0% | 18 | 86 | 18 | 86 | | Vg% |
| V | 6 | >99 | 141 | >99 | 141 | | V |
| FD | 1 | 60 | 104 | 57 | 103 | | FD |
| R8910% | 30% | 37 | 95 | 39 | 96 | | R8910% |
| WSumC | 2.5 | 40 | 96 | 21 | 88 | | WSC |
| C | 1 | 82 | 114 | 82 | 114 | | C |
| Mp/(Ma+Mp) [6/7] | 86% | 95 | 125 | 95 | 125 | | Mp Prp |
| **Perception and Thinking Problems** | | | | | | | |
| FQu% | 50% | 95 | 125 | 95 | 125 | | FQu% |
| **Stress and Distress** | | | | | | | |
| PPD | 16 | 89 | 119 | 81 | 113 | | PPD |
| CBlend | 0 | 28 | 91 | 28 | 91 | | CBlnd |
| C' | 4 | 88 | 117 | 79 | 112 | | C' |
| V | 6 | >99 | 141 | >99 | 141 | | V |
| CritCont% (Critical Contents) | 25% | 68 | 107 | 64 | 105 | | CrCt |
| **Self and Other Representation** | | | | | | | |
| SumH | 9 | 81 | 113 | 72 | 108 | | SumH |
| NPH/SumH [3/9] | 33% | 13 | 83 | 14 | 84 | | NPH Prp |
| V-Comp (Vigilance Composite) | 4.6 | 85 | 115 | 75 | 110 | | V-C |
| r (Reflections) | 0 | 36 | 95 | 36 | 95 | | r |
| p/(a+p) [11/13] | 85% | 97 | 128 | 97 | 128 | | p Prp |
| AGM | 1 | 75 | 110 | 75 | 110 | | AGM |
| T | 0 | 28 | 91 | 28 | 91 | | T |
| PER | 0 | 30 | 92 | 30 | 92 | | PER |
| An | 2 | 71 | 108 | 71 | 108 | | An |

© 2010-2016 R-PAS

**FIGURE 2.3B.** Mr. J's Page 2 results. Reproduced from the Rorschach Performance Assessment System® (R-PAS®) Scoring Program (© 2010–2016) and excerpted from the *Rorschach Performance Assessment System: Administration, Coding, Interpretation, and Technical Manual* (© 2011) with copyrights by Rorschach Performance Assessment System, LLC. All rights reserved. Used by permission of Rorschach Performance Assessment System, LLC. Further reproduction is prohibited without written permission from R-PAS.

confirmation biases. We had a working hypothesis that Mr. J was experiencing psychotic symptoms, given his recent history and biological sex and age. As alternative hypotheses, we considered other medical disorders that could result in psychotic symptoms and whether Mr. J might be withholding evidence of drug use.

### Key Interpretations

Mr. J's slight Complexity elevation (SS = 110) was in line with his expected level of cognitive complexity, suggesting he was adequately engaged in the task and provided sufficient material for interpretation. Mr. J's results were indeed elevated on the scales associated with psychosis, including the aggregated measure (TP-Comp SS = 128) and its components of thought disturbance (SevCog SS = 138) and reality testing problems (FQ–% SS = 122), and a slightly elevated Vigilance Composite (V-Comp = 115). We noted that his CritCont% score was not elevated (SS = 107), which, in the context of this generally complex record, makes it less likely that he was malingering or experiencing misperceptions and disorganized thought processes that were trauma related. Other key findings were Very High elevations on Oral Dependent Language (ODL% SS = 133) and Vista (SS = 141), suggesting that Mr. J might be experiencing strong dependency needs in the face of feeling helpless about his emerging psychosis and that he is likely caught up in ruminating thoughts. It is important to know, however, that most of Mr. J's ODL images were religious figures that were coded poor Form Quality (FQ–), which in the context of the other data suggests that Mr. J might be experiencing religious delusions that he has not yet shared. These dependency needs and reliance on a higher power may have actually helped him form an alliance with his RA and the student clinician, whereas he had difficulty trusting his roommate and girlfriend. As an example of the Case-Based Interpretive Guide, Mr. J's general and case-based SevCog interpretations are provided in Table 2.1.

A more thorough interpretation of R-PAS results is the goal of the case chapters in this book. However, we briefly return to Mr. J's findings to illustrate the process of making treatment recommendations and communicating the results.

**TABLE 2.1. General and Case-Based Interpretations for Very High Severe Cognitive Score**

| R-PAS variable | Level | General interpretation |
|---|---|---|
| SevCog | General | SevCog captures significant or severe disruptions in thought processes. At least among adults and adolescents, these kinds of disruptions are typically most indicative of psychotic-level lapses in conceptualization, reasoning, communication, or thought organization.<br><br>If SevCog is elevated, as with WSumCog, one should ensure that this is not solely due to repeated speech patterns, mistaken scoring (overcoding DR2, PEC, or CON), or mild and concrete PEC codes. Finally, one should also consider whether playfulness with the examiner or the task, deliberate efforts to be shocking or provocative, or a penchant for narrative dramatization might be healthier processes contributing to an elevation in SevCog. |
| Scores | Level | Case-based interpretation |
| Raw Score = 3, SS ≥ = 131 | Very high | This person produced three or more responses incorporating suggestions of severe, psychotic-level disturbances in thinking, logic, and/or communication. This is a highly significant finding. Even one instance is atypical, and assuming coding accuracy is not an issue, the presence of three severe codes indicates that psychotic-like processes will be present in reasoning, conceptualization, communication, and thought organization. |

## Applying R-PAS Interpretation

### Making Treatment Recommendations

The interpreter should be aware of the major strengths that R-PAS can bring to treatment planning, as well as its limitations. Mihura and Graceffo (2014) discuss how different methods of assessment inform case conceptualization and treatment recommendations. In regard to R-PAS, Mihura and Graceffo make several key points: (1) A major strength of the Rorschach is its ability to detect psychosis, and clients with severe thinking disturbance (SevCog) might be particularly good candidates for antipsychotic medications; (2) research suggests the presence of some Complexity variables (e.g., higher Sy and Blends, lower F%) can serve as positive indicators of a client's ability to engage in and benefit from psychotherapy; (3) clients with reality testing problems (FQ–%) can understand situations very differently than others, including their experience with their therapist; and (4) the Rorschach is a unique assessment tool that can help therapists understand the images on a client's mind, such as traumatic imagery or flashbacks, nightmares, or obsessional images.

Further, the Self and Other variables and the interactive behaviors during the administration (including CT, Pr, Pu, and PER) can help predict what to expect in the therapy relationship in terms of transference, countertransference, enactments, and so forth. For example, one can predict the likelihood that a client will (1) experience ODL needs with his or her therapist; (2) "need my own space" (SR) from the therapist, which could be expressed in oppositional behaviors, independence strivings, or the need to creatively shape his or her own therapy process; (3) experience the therapy relationship as controlling or harmful (MAP/MAHP), and so on. Remember that the content on a client's mind does not necessarily reveal his or her attitude toward that content or his or her overt behaviors in response to it. For example, a client with strong ODL needs might cope by being counterdependent and therefore appear on the surface to be exceedingly independent. A client whose self and other representations are malevolent (MAP) might cope by using reaction formation and therefore behave in a way that appears to be exceedingly compliant and kind, yet use these behaviors in a passive–aggressive way. In general, Rorschach findings do not reveal how a client consciously *feels*. For conscious internal experience, one must ask the client either via a self-report instrument or interview.

### Communicating the Findings

There are several good sources on communicating assessment findings; we recommend an approach similar to that pioneered by Fischer (1985) and popularized by Finn (2007), referred to as collaborative/therapeutic assessment (C/TA; Finn, Fischer, & Handler, 2012). Because the C/TA model engages the client throughout the assessment process, there is not just one final feedback session in which R-PAS findings are communicated to the client; there is two-way communication and processing of the findings throughout the assessment. The C/TA approach views tests as "empathy magnifiers" for more fully understanding clients, and the assessment data as a way to "get in the client's shoes" (Finn et al., 2007, p. 14). Therefore, in addition to informing case conceptualization and treatment planning, the assessment data provide information to help the assessor communicate the assessment findings to the client in an empathic, therapeutic manner. For example, the assessor should use the assessment data to predict the best way to discuss the assessment findings with the client. Several chapter authors used the C/TA approach with their cases; for example, Lipkind and Fahy (Chapter 17) provide a good illustration of using this framework to communicate assessment findings in a way that considers the clients' readiness to hear the information.

For referral sources who are not familiar with the Rorschach, the assessor should (1) develop a standard way of describing the R-PAS task rather than just saying "administering the Rorschach" or calling it a "projective test," and, if applicable, (2) tell the referral source specifically why R-PAS is being used for the particular case. For example, one can refer to R-PAS as a "performance measure to assess disordered thinking," "a typical performance measure of cognitive strengths or resources," or "a broadband implicit measure of psychological functioning." When using R-PAS, the assessor should highlight its strong empirical base (e.g., Meyer, Viglione, & Mihura, 2017; Mihura et al., 2013), particularly for answering the referral questions.

Regarding the communication of specific findings, the assessor should stay as close as possible to the response process. Frequently consulting the Case-Based Interpretive Guide will help the assessor conceptualize and communicate interpretations that are tied closely to the response process, which should resonate with the client. For example, when interpreting MOR, instead of telling the client that the Rorschach suggests that he or she is "depressed," the interpretive guide stays closer to MOR's response process (in this case, morbid images) by saying "themes of damage, injury, or sadness are on their mind." The assessor can review the client's MOR responses to see what type of morbid images the client described. For example, if the client did not report the less common dysphoric or sad MOR images, then the assessor would not say that themes of "sadness" were on the client's mind.

## Mr. J: Treatment Recommendations and Communicating the Findings

Returning to our fictive case, Mr. J's R-PAS results showed some positive indications for an ability to profit from psychotherapy. His High Average Sy score and Low F% score may bode well for his ability to engage in therapy. The presence of a response with COP and MAH codes bodes well for an ability to envision and perhaps form a positive relationship with the therapist. However, his High Average V-Comp suggests that he is somewhat vigilant for threats and may at times question the clinician's motives. Therefore, the clinician should attempt to be as transparent as possible about what he or she is thinking and check in with Mr. J to see what he understands the clinician to mean. Also, Mr. J's High ODL% and p/(a+p) suggest that it may currently be difficult for him to actively pursue help on his own, without guidance. At the same time, the assessor should also be careful not to regress Mr. J by infantilizing him. Given that Mr. J's thinking is confused and disordered (SevCog), he will have more difficulty comprehending the assessment feedback. Therefore, during the feedback session, the assessor should intermittently stop and check in with Mr. J, asking him to summarize his understanding of the feedback so far. The assessor also should provide Mr. J with a focused written summary of the assessment feedback to refer to later.

Regarding treatment targets, Mr. J's high SevCog suggests he may be a good candidate for an antipsychotic medication. Research shows that early treatment of first-episode psychosis is vital for long-term adaptive functioning (Penttilä, Jääskeläinen, Hirvonen, Isohanni, & Miettunen, 2014). Answers to Mr. J's assessment questions "Why is everyone turning against me?" and "Am I losing my mind?" are closely tied to his psychotic symptoms. The clinician can empathize with the extreme fear and confusion he is experiencing (as expressed on the self-report testing and inherent in his assessment questions), and can formulate a way to tell him that people who experience psychosis for the first time are often terrified because it is very hard to make sense out of what is happening. Mr. J can be assured that antipsychotic medication is helpful for many people who experience similar symptoms, and that it is particularly good that he is addressing it early on, because it should result in a better outcome for him. Mr. J's desire to stay out of the hospital can be a good motivator for compliance with treatment. The treatment team at the counseling center offered to help Mr. J request a medical leave from his classes and to work with him to move in with his parents while he continued treatment, with the goal of getting back on his feet and eventually returning to college. The option was also explored to complete his first semester in college at a nearby junior college while living at home to see how things go.

## A Final Note on Interpreting Complexity-Adjusted Protocols

We used a fictive case that did not require Complexity Adjustment (CAdj) because most protocols will not require it. Our Case-Based Interpretive Guide provides direction regarding how to proceed if the client's Complexity score is outside the Average range. Here, we provide some basics and refer the reader to this book's chapters that contain cases with high or low Complexity.

Statistically speaking, interpreting CAdj protocols is similar to interpreting strengths and weaknesses on IQ subtests where the client's overall IQ score serves as the reference point. Conceptually, however, before considering CAdj scores, one must also understand the reasons for the statistically deviant score on Complexity itself. Analogously, one would never interpret strengths and weaknesses on the subtests of an IQ test without first thoroughly understanding the implications of the person's atypically high or low intelligence score. Considering Complexity in R-PAS interpretation also is similar to considering response styles when interpreting self-report instruments such as the MMPI-2 or PAI. Elevated scores on response style markers can be due to various reasons; for instance, underreporting can be due to faking good or to a characterological naiveté—both are very different processes. How to adjust the interpretation of the client's protocol thus depends on the reason the client is underreporting problems.

The PAI provides adjusted protocols that are roughly similar to CAdj protocols in R-PAS. Specifically, if a client has high scores on the PAI Positive or Negative Impression Management scales, one can use the scores on those scales to generate predicted profiles showing the degree of elevation or suppression that would be expected across all the other scales. One can then mentally compare the client's observed score to the predicted score. R-PAS takes this process a couple of steps further by computing the actual difference between the observed score and the score predicted by Complexity and then profiling that result as the CAdj score.

What follows is a concise guide on how to consider Complexity in the Scan, Sift, Synthesize, and Summarize interpretive steps:

1. *Scan*. There is nothing specific required for CAdj during the Scan.

2. *Sift*. After reviewing the Administration Behaviors and Observations, review the Complexity score to see whether the protocol is of low, average, or high complexity. Complex records are much more likely than simplistic records to elevate multiple scores; therefore, the absence of codes or low scores in complex records have stronger negative predictive power (i.e., you can be more confident the characteristic is absent). In contrast, simplistic records low in complexity suppress scores; therefore, the presence of codes or high scores has stronger positive predictive power (i.e., you can be more confident the characteristic is present). You should also consider whether Complexity is at the level you would expect for your client; for example, is it generally consistent with his or her IQ and level of education? If the Complexity score is particularly low (< 85) or high (> 115), you can use CAdj later in the interpretive process to evaluate Complexity's impact on other scores. The CAdj score icon is a square compared to the raw score icon, which is a circle. The CAdj score is only plotted on the Profile Pages when you have selected the CAdj option. We recommend that users not select this option in isolation, but rather use it in conjunction with the raw score profile. When doing so, the CAdj icons are shown if there are 8 SSs of difference between the CAdj and the raw score.

3. *Synthesize*. If you expect to plot and interpret CAdj scores, first review your client's protocol using the regular raw score (non-CAdj) interpretations. Afterward, when applying CAdj, interpret the profile keeping in mind that CAdj profiles estimate how the results would look if the person had a protocol with completely average Complexity. Also keep in mind that CAdj SSs are not more "valid" than raw scores; their meaning is just different. They simply show what scores are relatively high or low, given the person's level of Complexity. Therefore, each interpretive inference should be contextualized with the conditional statement, "given this person's level of Complexity." For instance, one might think, "This person has surprisingly few instances of Human Movement, given her level of Complexity." You should also be familiar with the scores that contribute to the Complexity formula (e.g., F%, Blend, Sy, MC) so you can better conceptualize their CAdj results.

Particular chapter cases can be reviewed to gain a better understanding of Complexity and how it is conceptualized. For examples of low Complexity, see Hughes, Piselli, and Berbary (Chapter 19); for high Complexity, see Kleiger and Khadivi (Chapter 5); Fantini and Smith (Chapter 8); Kaakinen, Muzio, and Säävälä (Chapter 11); and Lipkind and Fahy (Chapter 17). For an example of Complexity that is higher than expected, given the person's IQ, see Nørbech, Hartmann, and Kleiger (Chapter 12).

## Wrapping It All Up

The chapters of this casebook serve as an advanced interpretive guide to use in concert with the R-PAS manual (Meyer et al., 2011). We recommend that assessors consult the present chapter, Table 1.1 in Chapter 1, and Chapter 3 when interpreting their first several R-PAS cases, and then return to these resources a few months later to better consolidate learning. Chapter 3, by Meyer and Erdberg, discusses using the R-PAS norms, with a focus on children and adolescents, in particular. Chapters 4–19 contain a wide variety of R-PAS cases in various settings to give the reader a broad range of experience with different R-PAS applications.

## REFERENCES

Berant, E., Newborn, M., & Orgler, S. (2008). Convergence of self-report scales and Rorschach indexes of psychological distress: The moderating role of self-disclosure. *Journal of Personality Assessment, 90,* 36–43.

Bornstein, R. F. (1999). Criterion validity of objective and projective dependency tests: A meta-analytic assessment of behavioral prediction. *Psychological Assessment, 11,* 48–57.

Brabender, V. M., & Mihura, J. L. (Eds.). (2016). *Handbook of gender and sexuality in psychological assessment.* New York: Routledge.

Dao, T. K., Prevatt, F., & Horne, H. L. (2008). Differentiating psychotic patients from nonpsychotic patients with the MMPI-2 and Rorschach. *Journal of Personality Assessment, 90,* 93–101.

Diener, M. J., Hilsenroth, M. J., Shaffer, S. A., & Sexton, J. E. (2011). A meta-analysis of the relationship between the Rorschach Ego Impairment Index (EII) and psychiatric severity. *Clinical Psychology & Psychotherapy, 18,* 464–485.

Exner, J. E. (1989). Searching for projection in the Rorschach. *Journal of Personality Assessment, 53,* 520–536.

Exner, J. E. (2003). *The Rorschach: A comprehensive system: Vol. 1. Basic foundations* (4th ed.). New York: Wiley.

Finn, S. E. (1996). Assessment feedback integrating MMPI-2 and Rorschach findings. *Journal of Personality Assessment, 67,* 543–557.

Finn, S. E. (2007). *In our clients' shoes: Theory and techniques of therapeutic assessment.* Mahwah, NJ: Erlbaum.

Finn, S. E., Fischer, C. T., & Handler, L. (Eds.). (2012). *Collaborative/therapeutic assessment: A casebook and guide.* Hoboken, NJ: Wiley.

Fischer, C. T. (1985). *Individualizing psychological assessment.* Mahwah, NJ: Erlbaum.

Ganellen, R. J. (1996). *Integrating the Rorschach and the MMPI-2 in personality assessment.* Hillsdale, NJ: Erlbaum.

Graceffo, R. A., Mihura, J. L, & Meyer, G. J. (2014). A meta-analysis of an implicit measure of personality functioning: The Mutuality of Autonomy Scale. *Journal of Personality Assessment, 96,* 581–595.

Hays, P. A. (2008). *Addressing cultural complexities in practice: Assessment, diagnosis, and therapy* (2nd ed.). Washington, DC: American Psychological Association.

Hemphill, J. F. (2003). Interpreting the magnitudes of correlation coefficients. *American Psychologist, 58,* 78–79.

Hopwood, C. J., & Bornstein, R. F. (Eds.). (2014). *Multimethod clinical assessment.* New York: Guilford Press.

Leichtman, M. (1996). The nature of the Rorschach task. *Journal of Personality Assessment, 67,* 478–493.

McClelland, D. C., Koestner, R., & Weinberger, J. (1989). How do self-attributed and implicit motives differ? *Psychological Review, 96*, 690–702.

Meyer, G. J. (1996). The Rorschach and MMPI: Toward a more scientifically differentiated understanding of cross-method assessment. *Journal of Personality Assessment, 67*, 558–578.

Meyer, G. J. (1997). On the integration of personality assessment methods: The Rorschach and MMPI. *Journal of Personality Assessment, 68*, 297–330.

Meyer, G. J. (1999). The convergent validity of MMPI and Rorschach scales: An extension using profile scores to define response and character styles on both methods and a reexamination of simple Rorschach response frequency. *Journal of Personality Assessment, 72*, 1–35.

Meyer, G. J., Erdberg, P., & Shaffer, T. W. (2007). Toward international normative reference data for the Comprehensive System. *Journal of Personality Assessment, 89*(Suppl. 1), S201–S216.

Meyer, G. J., Finn, S. E., Eyde, L. D., Kay, G. G., Moreland, K. L., Dies, R. R., . . . Reed, G. M. (2001). Psychological testing and psychological assessment: A review of evidence and issues. *American Psychologist, 56*, 128–165.

Meyer, G. J., Hsiao, W., Viglione, D. J., Mihura, J. L., & Abraham, L. M. (2013). Rorschach scores in applied clinical practice: A survey of perceived validity by experienced clinicians. *Journal of Personality Assessment, 95*, 351–365.

Meyer, G. J., Huprich, S. K., Blais, M. A., Bornstein, R. F., Mihura, J. L., Smith, J. D., & Weiner, I. B. (2017). *From screening to integrative multimethod assessment: Implications for training and practice*. Manuscript submitted for publication.

Meyer, G. J., & Kurtz, J. E. (2006). Advancing personality assessment terminology: Time to retire "objective" and "projective" as personality test descriptors. *Journal of Personality Assessment, 87*, 223–225.

Meyer, G. J., Viglione, D. J., & Mihura, J. L. (2017). Psychometric foundations of the Rorschach Performance Assessment System (R-PAS). In R. Erard & B. Evans (Eds.), *The Rorschach in multimethod forensic practice* (pp. 23–91). New York: Routledge.

Meyer, G. J., Viglione, D. J., Mihura, J. L., Erard, R. E., & Erdberg, P. (2011). *Rorschach Performance Assessment System: Administration, coding, interpretation, and technical manual.* Toledo, OH: Rorschach Performance Assessment System.

Mihura, J. L. (2012). The necessity of multiple test methods in conducting assessments: The role of the Rorschach and self-report. *Psychological Injury and Law, 5*, 97–106.

Mihura, J. L., Dumitrascu, N., Roy, M., & Meyer, G. J. (2017). The centrality of the response process in construct validity: An illustration via the Rorschach space response. *Journal of Personality Assessment.* [Epub ahead of print]

Mihura, J. L., & Graceffo, R. A. (2014). Multimethod assessment and treatment planning. In C. J. Hopwood & R. F. Bornstein (Eds.), *Multimethod clinical assessment* (pp. 285–318). New York: Guilford Press.

Mihura, J. L., Meyer, G. J., Dumitrascu, N., & Bombel, G. (2013). The validity of individual Rorschach variables: Systematic reviews and meta-analyses of the comprehensive system. *Psychological Bulletin, 139*, 548–605.

Mihura, J. L., Roy, M., Dumitrascu, N., & Meyer, G. J. (2016, March 12). *A meta-analytic review of the MMPI (all versions) ability to detect psychosis*. Paper presented at the annual meeting of the Society for Personality Assessment, Chicago, IL.

Peebles-Kleiger, M. J. (2002). Elaboration of some sequence analysis strategies: Examples and guidelines for level of confidence. *Journal of Personality Assessment, 79*, 19–38.

Penttilä, M., Jääskeläinen, E., Hirvonen, N., Isohanni, M., & Miettunen, J. (2014). Duration of untreated psychosis as predictor of long-term outcome in schizophrenia: Systematic review and meta-analysis. *The British Journal of Psychiatry, 205*, 88–94.

Pianowski, G., Meyer, G. J., & Villemor-Amaral, A. E. (2016). Potential projective material on the Rorschach: Comparing Comprehensive System protocols to their modeled R-Optimized administration counterparts. *Journal of Personality Assessment, 98*, 398–407.

Schachtel, E. G. (1966). *Experiential foundations of Rorschach's test*. New York: Basic Books.

# CHAPTER 3

# Using R-PAS Norms with an Emphasis on Children and Adolescents

Gregory J. Meyer
Philip Erdberg

In many ways, the Rorschach is particularly well suited for assessing psychological characteristics in children and adolescents. The task provides a structured and standardized form of behavioral observation. Within the standardized context of providing responses to the fixed inkblot stimuli that answer the question "What might this be?," the child or adolescent provides a sample of behavioral problem solving in the form of visual attributions to the inkblot stimuli, verbal and nonverbal communications about these attributions, and interactive behaviors with the examiner, the inkblots, and other features in the assessment setting. The context of the problem-solving task is unique. It does not impose particular demands on the individual other than verbally responding to the visual stimuli. The inkblot stimuli have considerable structure built into them, but they also consist of contradictory critical bits that are suggestive and evocative of many things, none of which is perfectly or completely represented in the stimuli.

There is nothing in the process of responding to the task that requires the child or adolescent to engage in the higher-level cognitive processes that are necessary for effective use of the introspective self-report inventories that are used ubiquitously in adult assessment. Those measures require the respondent to reflect on personal characteristics and to judge how his or her characteristics compare to relevant other people in their magnitude, frequency, or generality. Once that judgment is made, the respondent also has to decide the degree to which he or she will share with the examiner what he or she thinks is true.

The Rorschach task, in contrast, puts the responsibility for comparative classification on the shoulders of the examiner. This is as true for adult assessments as it is for child and adolescent assessments. The examiner must evaluate the client's behavioral record of attributions, communications, and interactions to classify each response along dimensions of interest before aggregating those coded features across all responses and comparing the results to what relevant others see, say, and do when confronted with the same problem-solving task. Based on this aggregated and normatively referenced information, the examiner is able to make inferences about what the individual will likely do in everyday life when left to his or her own devices to understand, represent, and make meaning of complex environmental stimuli that validly can be seen from multiple and often very different perspectives. These parallel complex environmental stimuli include internal experiences and external experiences. *Internal experiences* encompass thoughts, feelings, impulses, and physiological reactions. *External experiences* encompass social relations with friends and peers and close relations with significant others, as well as management of developmental demands associated with achievement and mastery.

## The Importance of Norms

Embedded in the forgoing description of making assessment-based inferences is the role of normative data. Norms provide the yardstick against which everyone else is measured. As such, normative data are integral in the inference-making interpretive process. To understand any particular child, adolescent, or adult, we must understand how he or she is similar to and different from others at that age. Unfortunately, for the vast majority of Rorschach users, the Comprehensive System (CS; Exner, 2003) norms that were used over decades for children, adolescents, and adults have been wrong (Meyer, Erdberg, & Shaffer, 2007; Meyer, Shaffer, Erdberg, & Horn, 2015; Viglione & Hilsenroth, 2001; Wood, Nezworski, Garb, & Lilienfeld, 2001). Over time, evidence has accumulated that documents how the standard CS normative samples are notably different than other nonpatient samples for some important Rorschach variables; this is true when comparing the CS norms to other samples from the United States and to samples from other countries. Although it was initially thought that the problems were limited to Form Quality (FQ) scores (Meyer, 2001), in fact, the CS norms erroneously cause nonpatients to appear psychologically unhealthy across a much broader number of variables. And for some variables the standard CS norms are wrong by a wide margin. This extent of error in the norms is even more dramatically true for children and adolescents than for adults (Meyer et al., 2007; Viglione & Giromini, 2016).

The relevant literature for adult samples and for child and adolescent samples is briefly summarized here as context for understanding the Rorschach Performance Assessment System (R-PAS) norms that are available for anchoring interpretation. Subsequently, the practical use of those norms with children and adolescents is explained and illustrated with examples. Because the next section and its subsections are rather dense with methodological and statistical issues (i.e., it's the "pointy-headed researcher" section), readers with an interest in just the practical application of R-PAS to child and adolescent cases may wish to jump to the narrative in the section titled, "Practical Use of the R-PAS Norms for Children and Adolescents."

## Norms from the CS to R-PAS

### Problems with the Standard CS Norms for Children, Adolescents, and Adults

Beginning in the summer of 1997, Rorschach researchers from various countries started to compile their existing efforts to gather normative reference samples for the CS. That project was ultimately published in 2007 as a Special Supplement to the *Journal of Personality Assessment* (Shaffer, Erdberg, & Meyer, 2007). The internationally collected adult data encompassed 21 samples from 17 countries, and they were shown to be cohesive across countries, including the United States. However, as described above, they differed from the standard CS norms on a number of notable variables (Meyer et al., 2007; Meyer, Shaffer, et al., 2015). The internationally collected child and adolescent norms encompassing 31 samples from five countries were as cohesive as the adult norms on most variables, after excluding the standard CS reference data provided by Exner (2003). However, for 34 of 143 variables, cross-sample differences in the observed mean values were more notable.

The variability across samples in these 34 variables was due in part to (1) the relatively small number of samples available for analysis, (2) particular methodological decisions made by individual researchers, and (3) site-specific administration and coding conventions that were resolved in different ways by different groups as a result of ambiguities inherent in the CS reference books and training guides. For instance, there were only two countries (Italy and the United States) represented in the age range from 13 to 18 and just four or five countries at the other ages. In another case, a single examiner collected most of the U.S. reference data outside of that reported by Exner (2003) and imposed strict location use procedures that led to artificial elevations in Dd and FQ– codes, which in turn adversely affected the other variables dependent on location and form quality (e.g., P, PTI). Finally, the researchers from Japan did not extrapolate from the CS form quality tables but instead coded all objects that were not listed in the tables as FQ– (Meyer et al., 2007). Despite some of these limitations, the internationally collected normative data for children and adolescents still corrected for significant problems with the standard CS norms.

Nonetheless, the internationally collected normative data have been criticized because some of the data were collected by relatively inexperienced examiners (Ritzler & Sciara, 2009). Meyer, Shaffer, et al. (2015) investigated these concerns in three interrelated studies with adults. The first study documented that the international norms were virtually identical when organized into three groups differentiated by the quality of their data collection efforts, which included an optimal group of four samples that used multiple experienced examiners and provided ongoing quality control over administration and coding. Analyses showed that relative to the group of more optimal samples, the group of less optimal samples did not produce more variability in summary scores within or across samples or lower interrater reliability for coding.[1] The second study used the existing CS reference norms to generate T scores for the

---

[1]The absence of differences across the groups differentiated by quality does not indicate that training and experience are unimportant; it simply indicates that when samples were averaged at each level of quality, there were no discernible differences in those averaged values. All of the R-PAS authors believe very strongly in the importance and necessity of training and skill development for proper administration and accurate coding.

mean scores observed in the international norms. Doing so documented how the CS norms made other samples of healthy nonpatients look psychologically impaired in multiple domains. The third study used data from four different countries that each had two sets of normative data available as competing reference points to indicate what was typical or expected for people in that country. This study demonstrated how these contrasting within-country local norms produced notably different results on some variables—differences that compromise the ability of local norms to be used instead of the composite international norms. Taken together, these three studies provided strong support for using the international norms in clinical practice as norms that are generalizable across samples, settings, languages, and cultures and that account for the natural variability that is present when clinicians and researchers contend with the ambiguity contained in the standard CS administration and coding guidelines.

Giromini, Viglione, and McCullaugh (2015) demonstrated a similar point using a sample of 80 adult nonpatient protocols collected in San Diego, California, using CS administration and coding guidelines. The examiners were advanced doctoral students who had completed at least two courses with Rorschach training. The administration and coding were monitored closely by Viglione, and all protocols were independently coded twice. Giromini et al. determined whether the San Diego data were more likely to belong to a population defined by CS norms or a population defined by the international norms. They restricted their analyses to 28 variables that differed notably between the two sets of norms (Cohen's d $\geq$ |0.50|). The evidence clearly indicated that the San Diego sample most likely belonged to the international norms for 24 of the 28 variables. For the remaining four variables, neither normative sample provided a better fit. Even though one might assume that the San Diego sample would show a closer affinity to another U.S.-based sample than to an international standard, this was not the case. In addition, the CS norms made the San Diego nonpatients appear pathological on the same variables that the CS norms made the international sample of nonpatients appear pathological (Meyer, Shaffer, et al., 2015).

Expanding on their adult norm study, Viglione and Giromini (2016) conducted a second study comparing (1) the pattern of differences in Exner's (2003) CS norms for children and adolescents versus the international norms for children and adolescents (Meyer et al., 2007) to (2) the pattern of differences seen in the adult norms as summarized above. Using the same criteria as in the adult study, they identified 43 variables for the child and adolescent norms that differed notably across groups. This finding considerably exceeds the 28 notable differences found with adults, and it illustrates how the normative problems with the standard CS norms are worse for children and adolescents than for adults. As with adults, using the standard CS norms would result in pathological interpretations being applied to the nonpatient children and adolescents who comprise the international norms. Also, the pattern of differences between the CS standard and the internationally collected norms was very similar in the child and adolescent data and the adult data, producing a very large correlation ($r$ = .84). Thus, as with adults, there is a similar bias in Exner's existing CS norms for children and adolescents.

Overall, these data document how clinicians relying on the standard CS norms will incorrectly infer that nonpatients are prone to perceptual distortions, see the world in an atypical and idiosyncratic manner, tend to be simplistic, lack affective resources, lack coping resources in general, are prone to affective disturbances and dysregulation, and misunderstand others and misperceive relationships. These mistaken inferences will be present across all ages, but they are even more pronounced when working with children and adolescents than with adults (Meyer et al., 2007; Viglione & Giromini, 2016). For CS users, the only way to avoid making these mistaken inferences is to use the internationally collected normative values, rather than the standard CS values, as the foundation for interpretation. The international data do not make typical nonpatients look disturbed or pathological.

## The R-PAS Norms for Adults

For its adult norms, R-PAS uses a subset of the internationally collected protocols, consisting of up to 100 records from 15 different samples (Meyer, Viglione, Mihura, Erard, & Erdberg, 2011). Although these records were collected using CS administration guidelines, they were modeled so that the distribution of protocol-level responses (R) in these records matched the distribution of R found when using R-Optimized administration procedures. Although R-Optimized administration has been criticized as being a procedure that significantly alters the Rorschach task relative to CS administration (e.g., Mattlar, 2011; Ritzler, 2014), that argument is not consistent with the evidence. When using the modeling procedures, one observes what is expected by design, which is a small increase in the average number of responses and a notable reduction in its variability, accompanied by slight changes in several variables that are strongly correlated with R (Meyer et al., 2011). These findings were recently replicated in an independent sample of Brazilian nonpatients (Pianowski, Meyer, & Villemor-Amaral, 2016).

In addition, six studies encompassing children, adolescents, and adults, as well as patients and nonpatients, have randomly assigned people to receive either standard CS administration or a version of R-Optimized administration (Berant, 2009; Dean, Viglione, Perry, & Meyer, 2007; Meyer et al., 2011; Reese, Viglione, & Giromini, 2014; Resende, 2011; Viglione et al., 2015). Hosseininasab et al. (2017) recently completed a meta-analysis examining 51 variables across these studies. As expected, R has a slightly higher mean and a substantially reduced standard deviation (*SD*) when using the R-Optimized version of administration rather than CS administration. In addition, two variables derived from R, R8910% and Complexity, showed less variability. However, no other scores showed replicated differences across samples. Thus, R-Optimized administration and its modeling achieve the goal of reducing variability in R but otherwise have a trivial effect on other variables. This supports the use of the internationally collected records as norms for R-PAS.

When considering norms, a key question is to what extent various demographic variables are associated with variability in scores. Consistent with historical research, the most recent and systematic exploration on this topic showed that gender, adult age, and race or ethnicity were not associated with R-PAS scores across three large samples (*n*'s from 241 to 640) encompassing nonpatients, patients, children, adolescents, and adults (Meyer, Giromini, Viglione, Reese, & Mihura, 2015). However, consistent with previous research, Meyer, Giromini, et al. (2015) documented that there are two demographic factors that do have an important influence on Rorschach responding: level of education and youth age. Both of these variables are associated with the overall complexity and richness of a protocol in nonpatients, and youth age is also associated with perceptual accuracy and thought organization in clinical and nonclinical samples (Meyer, Giromini, et al., 2015; Stanfill, Viglione, & Resende, 2013).

To some extent, the use of Complexity Adjusted scores with adults can adjust for instances when a lower than normative level of education contributes to unsophisticated and simplistic responding. However, Complexity Adjusted scores would not be sufficient for children and adolescents because youth age is correlated with facets of Rorschach responding that go beyond typical markers of protocol complexity to include the conventionality of perceptions and thought organization. Thus, it is important to have age-stratified R-PAS norms available for children and adolescents.

## The R-PAS Transitional Child and Adolescent Norms

When the R-PAS manual was first published in August 2011, it provided only adult norms (Meyer et al., 2011). However, three months later, R-PAS began using child and adolescent norms derived from the previously described internationally collected data (Meyer et al., 2007), after omitting the problematic data from Japan (see also, *www.r-pas.org/InitialStatement.aspx*). However, the internationally collected data for children and adolescents were limited in several important ways. The data (1) used three rather broad age classifications (5–8, 9–12, and 13–18), (2) were based on standard CS administration rather than modeled R-Optimized administration, and (3) provided no normative data for R-PAS variables that were not included in the CS. Consequently, R-PAS needed new norms for children and adolescents. Although it took time, transitional R-PAS norms for children and adolescents were developed by January 2014 (Meyer, Viglione, & Giromini, 2014[2]). The norms make use of R-PAS protocols from 346 children and adolescents, ranging in age from 6 to 17, primarily from Brazil and the United States, with a smaller number also from Italy. The Brazilian data and most of the U.S. data were collected using standard R-Optimized administration; however, a small number of protocols were added from the United States ($n = 24$) and Italy ($n = 11$) using modeled R-Optimized administration. All 346 protocols were scored using R-PAS coding guidelines. Gender was approximately evenly balanced, though sample size varied by age and by country. To anchor the developmental continuum, the R-PAS adult normative sample of full-text records was used, which brought the full sample size to 463.

Because the individual, age-based subsamples were small, two statistical procedures were used to maximize the ability to detect genuine developmental changes. First, rather than estimating normative values by plotting mean scores in age-based bins or silos, as has traditionally been done (i.e., compute and compare Ms for those age 6, age 7, age 8, etc.), we used continuous inferential norming to fit polynomial regression curves to the developmental data (Oosterhuis, van der Ark, & Sijtsma, 2016; Zhu & Chen, 2011). Regression-based inferential norming is a dramatic

[2]Data and research contributions to these norms came from Ana Cristina Resende, Carla Hisatugo, Janell Crow, Daria Russo, and Jessica Swanson; scoring help came from Heidi Miller, Vanessa Laughter, and Andrew Williams.

improvement over traditional norming procedures, such that using samples of 50 per age group produces norms that are as accurate as norms produced the traditional way using samples of 200 per age group (Zhu & Chen, 2011).

Second, because our samples were relatively small and thus affected by fairly substantial sampling error (the natural variability that causes the observed data values to depart from their true population values), we used bootstrap resampling procedures (Efron & Tibshirani, 1993) to create 100 alternative possible versions of the existing age-based datasets for each R-PAS variable. These bootstrap samples provide 100 equally likely versions of what each age-based sample could have looked like, and they show how much the sample estimate for a variable (e.g., the mean for Sy) could vary by chance alone.

Regression equations were then fit to predict the means for all R-PAS variables from the linear, quadratic, and cubic functions of age (i.e., Age, $Age^2$, and $Age^3$). After predicting the means for each variable, we predicted the *SD*s. The goal of these analyses was to find the best-fitting linear or curvilinear model that made developmental sense. For inferential norming, a key step is to review the alternative results to see (1) how much prediction increases when moving from linear to curvilinear models, and (2) most importantly, to see which of the various regression models makes the most developmental sense. For the R-PAS norms, initial judgments about optimal fit were made by one researcher (Meyer) and then independently checked by two others (Viglione and Giromini), with disagreements resolved through discussion by all three people.

The resulting norms provide developmentally expected scores (i.e., *M*s and *SD*s) for each R-PAS variable at each age from 6 to 17. These norms are transitional and will ultimately be replaced by larger age-based samples from multiple countries. However, for the time being, they provide reasonable, developmentally sensitive expectations for what children and adolescents see, say, and do when completing the task at various ages.

## How the R-PAS Child and Adolescent Norms Correct Problems in the CS Norms

We have already established (Meyer et al., 2007; Viglione & Giromini, 2016) that for children and adolescents, the CS-based internationally collected norms correct for problems in the standard CS norms (Exner, 2003). However, the CS-based international norms possess irregularities. These irregularities are corrected when using the newer R-PAS child and adolescent norms. To determine this correction, we grouped the R-PAS normative data into three age categories (6–8, 9–12, and 13–17) that closely matched those used for the CS-based international norms (5–8, 9–12, and 13–18). We then compared the mean scores from the CS-based norms to the means of the R-PAS norms, using the R-PAS *SD*s to quantify how far apart the two means were.

Across the 40 variables that could be computed from the CS-based norms for the Page 1 and Page 2 Profiles, there were eight scores that differed by a half *SD* or more (i.e., Glass's *delta* ≥ 0.50) in at least one of the three age groups. Differences of this magnitude were considered meaningful. Across the three age groups, notable differences on these eight scores were observed 11 times. The teen group had a notable difference on all eight scores, but there was a notable difference for only one score in the 9- to 12-year-old group and two scores in the 6- to 8-year-old group. The reason the teen group had more notable differences is because the CS-based norms were derived from just two samples and thus provided less stable data than the other ages.

In 8 of the 11 instances when there was a notable difference between the R-PAS normative standard and the CS-based norms, the CS-based norms had previously been identified by Meyer et al. (2007) as unstable because the mean estimates were so different across samples. The most likely reason why the composite CS-based normative means were identified as being unstable is that problematic site-specific administration or coding conventions were being followed in one of the CS samples that did not generalize to other samples. In all 11 of the instances when there were notable differences between the R-PAS norms and the CS-based norms, the R-PAS norms corrected an irregularity in the CS-based norms. In almost all cases, the irregularity occurred in a determinant-related variable that showed developmental progressions with age (YTVC', PPD, Y, V, C', and r). However, the CS-based norms for the teen group notably overshot the adult reference norms, whereas the R-PAS norms showed a smooth dimensional progression across the age bands that intersected directly with the adult values.

For instance, in the adult norms that were used to anchor the developmental continuum for children and adolescents in the R-PAS norms, the mean for YTVC' was 4.2. When averaged across the three broad age categories, the new R-PAS norms for children and adolescents produced average values of 1.8, 2.4, and 2.9 for ages 6–8, 9–12, and 13–17, respectively. This steady increase reflects the cognitive maturation that is associated with the propensity to articulate these subtle nuances of the inkblot stimulus as a determinant of one's perception (Meyer, 2016; Stanfill et al., 2013). In the CS-based norms, there also is a developmental progression. However, the average values were 2.2, 3.1, and 5.7 for the three age groups. Note how the value of 5.7 for the teen group (and to a lesser extent, the second age group) is much higher than the R-PAS mean of 2.9, and also too high relative to adults (5.7 vs. 4.2). This discrepancy suggests that the CS-based normative data for teens is atypical for this variable.

One could make a counterargument stating that adolescence is a tumultuous period and thus maybe YTVC' should be more elevated in teens than in adults. However, if that is the case, it is an elevation that appears specific to just one of the two samples used to generate the CS-based normative estimate. The teen data that were collected in Italy (Lis, Salcuni, & Parolin, 2007) reported a mean for YTVC' of 7.1 for 12- to 18-year-olds, whereas the teen data collected in the United States (Van Patten, Shaffer, Erdberg, & Canfield, 2007) had a mean of just 2.9 for 15- to 17-year-olds. These are dramatically different benchmarks. More recently published CS data support the validity of the U.S. estimate by Van Patten et al. over the Italian estimate by Lis et al. (see Hosseininasab, Mohammadi, Weiner, & Delavar, 2015; Tibon Czopp, Rothschild-Yakar, & Appel, 2012).

The relevant information is summarized in Table 3.1, which provides mean scores for the two CS-based samples from Italy and the United States that contributed to the initial teen norms, the two more recently published CS studies from Israel and Iran, and the current R-PAS norms based on data from Brazil, the United States, and Italy. It can be seen rather easily that the R-PAS normative estimate of 2.9 for teens is quite consistent with the other three estimates from the United States, Israel,

**TABLE 3.1. Teenage Normative Reference Values from Five Available Samples for the YTVC' Variable**

| Sample | Teen $M$ for YTVC' |
|---|---|
| Initial CS-based norms (Italy and U.S.) | |
|     Lis et al. (Italy) | 7.1 |
|     Van Patten et al. (U.S.) | 2.9 |
| More recently published CS studies | |
|     Tibon Czopp et al. (Israel) | 2.6 |
|     Hosseininasab et al. (Iran) | 2.9 |
| R-PAS norms (Brazil, U.S., Italy) | 2.9 |

and Iran. However, the Italian mean is notably discrepant from all the others. This pattern supports the hypothesis that the initial Italian result was an outlier and that the current R-PAS norms provide better developmental standards than the older CS-based norms.

Another advantage that the current R-PAS norms have over the older CS-based norms is the use of age-specific normative data rather than normative data collapsed into three broad age groups. For the actual R-PAS norms, the means for YTVC' increase steadily at each year from age 6 to age 17, and they intersect seamlessly with the adult expected value.

## Practical Use of the R-PAS Norms for Children and Adolescents

For clinicians using R-PAS with children and adolescents, the first step when preparing to enter the coding in the R-PAS scoring program is to select the appropriate age from 6 to 17. The two coding interfaces (Tables format or Point-and-Click format) are the same for children and adolescents as they are for adults. Once the coding is completed, the user generates results output, just as for adults. The results output starts with the Code Sequence page followed by the Counts and Calculations page, neither of which differs from its adult counterpart. However, the Profile Pages for Page 1 and Page 2 variables, which are the main focus of interpretation, differ from the adult Profile Pages.

### Understanding the Profile Pages

The Profile Pages for children and adolescents show two things at once: how this person compares to others of the same age and how this person compares to adults. The details of this will be explained below. However, for readers interested in the rationale for this approach, we first address the question of "Why? Why not just show how this child or adolescent compares to others of the same age?" The answer to these questions is fairly technical; it is a function of how the transitional child and adolescent norms were generated relative to how they were generated for adults. If the answer to these questions is not your concern, just skip the next two paragraphs.

For these transitional norms, we generated expected normative means and *SD*s. We did not generate expected normative percentiles for each observed raw score value. In contrast, the adult norms were generated using percentiles associated with the exact distribution of raw score values for every variable; those percentiles were then transformed to their normal curve standard score (SS) equivalents. This was done to respect the non-normal distributions that are found with many Rorschach scores. Psychometrically, we believe it is more optimal to have the child and adolescent raw scores pattern themselves in the same general manner as the adult raw scores, such that, for example, variables with truncated distributions, like Pr, Pu, COP, MAH, T, and so on, provide the same patterning of scores for children and adolescents as for adults. Here, we are making the assumption that the relative frequency of each score for a variable is more important than the age of the person responding to the task. In other words, we took the position that the relative rarity of a variable such as MAH and its patterning from scores of 0 to 1, 1 to 2, 2 to 3, and so on, was generalizable from adults to children and adolescents.

If we did not take this approach, the alternative would have been to compute SS values for children and adolescents using their estimated means and *SD*s and treating those values as if they were continuous and normally distributed, like IQ scores or scores on the MMPI or PAI, of which most are reasonably normally distributed. A normal distribution justifies computing an SS based on how far it is from the mean in *SD* units. But this is not the case with many Rorschach scores, which are largely counts of behaviors observed in the microcosm of the task. As count variables, many of them are distributed according to non-normal distributions (e.g., Poisson or zero-inflated negative binomial distributions). Practically speaking, this means that often many scores have a large number of people with values of zero and an increasingly smaller subset with values of 1, 2, 3, or more. With these kinds of distributions, it is not optimal to simply use the mean and *SD* to estimate where a score falls on the normal curve. Rather, the patterning of scores from 0 to 1, 1 to 2, 2 to 3, and so on, is what is most important. It is because we wish to retain this patterning of scores that we superimpose the child and adolescent norms over the adult norms.

On the Profile Pages for children and adolescents, the most central information is the SS, which indicates how far their score is from the average score. SSs have a mean of 100 and an *SD* of 15. An SS of 85 is one *SD* below average, and an SS of 115 is one *SD* above average. As can be seen in the edited image in Figure 3.1, which shows parts of the Page 1 Profile for a 10-year-old, this information is presented in the "Raw" and "Cplx. Adj." (i.e., Complexity Adjusted) columns adjacent to the variable names for Complexity and R. (The Complexity variable is not itself adjusted for Complexity, so that area is blank in the image below.) There are two elements for the SSs: the grayed-out A-SS subcolumn, which provides the SS for this person relative to adults (Complexity = 81, R = 88), and the regular font C-SS subcolumn, which shows the SS for this person relative to children or adolescents of the same age (Complexity = 90, R = 88).

The right-side section of Figure 3.1 is where scores are profiled. There are two primary elements to the profile: the grid and the overlays. The *grid* refers to the vertical lines on the Profile Pages that range from 55 to 145 and are marked with SS values from 60 to 140 in 10-unit increments. This grid is structured for adults; the heavy dark line down the center of the profile page is at an A-SS value of 100; it indicates

| Domain/Variables | Raw Scores | Raw | | Cplx. Adj. | | Standard Score Profile R-Optimized | | | | | | | | | Abbr. |
|---|---|---|---|---|---|---|---|---|---|---|---|---|---|---|---|
| | | A-SS | C-SS | A-SS | C-SS | 60 | 70 | 80 | 90 | 100 | 110 | 120 | 130 | 140 | |
| Admin. Behaviors and Obs. | | | | | | | | | | | | | | | |
| Engagement and Cog. Processing | | | | | | 60 | 70 | 80 | 90 | 100 | 110 | 120 | 130 | 140 | |
| Complexity | 48 | 81 | 90 | | | 30 | | 40 | | 50 | 60 | 70 | 80 | 90 | 100 | | 120 | | 140 | 160 | Cmplx |
| R (Responses) | 20 | 88 | 88 | 97 | 96 | 16 | | | 18 | | 20 | 22 | 24 | 26 | 28 | 30 | 32 | 34 | 36 | 38 | R |

**FIGURE 3.1.** Edited portion of the Page 1 Profile illustrating the grid and overlays. Reproduced from the Rorschach Performance Assessment System® (R-PAS®) Scoring Program (© 2010–2016) and excerpted from the *Rorschach Performance Assessment System: Administration, Coding, Interpretation, and Technical Manual* (© 2011) with copyrights by Rorschach Performance Assessment System, LLC. All rights reserved. Used by permission of Rorschach Performance Assessment System, LLC. Further reproduction is prohibited without written permission from R-PAS.

the median score for an adult. Superimposed on the grid are the *overlays,* which show what is expected for a child or adolescent at a particular age. The overlay has two parts: an X and surrounding dashed lines or whiskers. The X designates the average value for respondents of that particular age, which corresponds to a C-SS value of 100. The whiskers extend one *SD* below the X to a C-SS value of 85, and one *SD* above the X to a C-SS value of 115.

The third important element of the profile area is the *icon,* which is placed at the raw score value that was obtained by this particular child or adolescent. That icon can be interpreted relative to both of the normative standards that are profiled: adults or others of the same age. When the icon is compared to the grid, it indicates how typical or atypical the score is compared to adults. This comparison is what produces the grayed-out numbers in the A-SS column. When the icon is compared to the overlays, it indicates how typical or atypical the score is compared to others of the same age. This comparison is what produces the regular font numbers in the C-SS column, which again are the SS values that quantify how far from average this child is, using the X to indicate what is average and the whiskers to indicate typical variability around that average for other children in the same age range. The colors and shapes of the icons on the child and adolescent profiles are keyed to the overlays, not to the grid. Thus, they are keyed to what is expected for someone of the same age and not keyed to what is expected for an adult. A green icon with no bars means that the result falls within the broad average range (C-SS: 85–115); a yellow icon with one bar means that the result falls between one and two *SD*s above or below the mean (C-SS: 70–84 or 116–130); a red icon with two bars means that the result falls between two and three *SD*s above or below the mean (C-SS: 55–69 or 131–145); and a black icon with complete fill means that the result is more than three *SD*s above or below the mean (C-SS: < 55 or > 145).

Some users like the overlays because they like being able to see both the adult reference standard and the age-specific reference standard. However, other users would prefer that R-PAS do away with the overlays and just present Profile Pages using the age-specific reference points, such that the grid itself would be keyed to the child or adolescent normative information. Although we have explained why the overlays are being used, at some point in the future, R-PAS may offer users the possibility of either option.

## The Key Summary Point

Because there are many components to the Profile Pages for children and adolescents, they can be challenging to use at the outset. However, based on the information just given, this is the key point to understand: The C-SS values are determined by the icon in relation to the data for the age-specific overlays, and the A-SS values are determined by the icon in relation to the data for the underlying adult grid. When focusing on the age-specific results, one should read the number in the C-SS column and note what type of icon it is and its relative distance from the X on the overlay.

## An Illustration

In the output shown in Figure 3.1, the C-SS value for Complexity is 90, which by definition falls in the broad average range. The icon is placed in the profile area at the examinee's raw score value of 48. Although it is a little difficult to see in Figure 3.1, the underlying units are shown in light gray font just below the overlay. Those underlying units are easier to read in Figure 3.2, where it can be more easily seen that the icon is placed at a raw score of 48.

From the profile it also can be seen that the icon is an open circle (and green when viewed in color) and that it falls on the lower whisker of the overlay. The green open circle icon and the fact that it falls on the whisker also indicate that it falls in the broad average range for a 10-year-old. But more specifically, we also can see that the icon is two-thirds of the whisker away from the X. Remember that the X equates to a C-SS value of 100 for 10-year-olds, and the whisker corresponds to 15 C-SS points. Because the icon is two-thirds of a whisker away and because two-thirds of a 15-point whisker is 10 points, the icon is placed 10 points below the C-SS value of 100 (i.e., the X) at a C-SS value of 90. This illustrates how to understand the results output and the placement of the icon relative to the overlay.

When understanding the child or adolescent relative to others the same age is the sole interest, one simply ignores the A-SS values that range from 60 to 140, marking the gridlines in the profile area. Those numbers correspond to the adult grid. Focus instead should be placed on the icon in relation to the overlay and its corresponding C-SS value (as given in the C-SS column). However, when there is an interest in understanding how the child or adolescent looks relative to an adult standard, one

**FIGURE 3.2.** Enlarged portion of the Page 1 Profile illustrating the underlying units and overlays. Reproduced from the Rorschach Performance Assessment System® (R-PAS®) Scoring Program (© 2010–2016) and excerpted from the *Rorschach Performance Assessment System: Administration, Coding, Interpretation, and Technical Manual* (© 2011) with copyrights by Rorschach Performance Assessment System, LLC. All rights reserved. Used by permission of Rorschach Performance Assessment System, LLC. Further reproduction is prohibited without written permission from R-PAS.

can attend to the A-SS values given in the score columns and the placement of the icon relative to the vertical lines of the profile grid.

## Three Advanced Points

Figure 3.3 provides an example of the top of the Page 1 Profile for a 10-year-old boy. Three more subtle or advanced points are worth noting. First, notice that each overlay appears in various places on the Profile grid. Wherever the X falls, that value is the mean for that child or adolescent's nonpatient reference group, even though the same score might be higher or lower than the median for the adult nonpatient reference group (i.e., above or below the A-SS value of 100 at the center of the profile). Second, notice that the whiskers surrounding the X's are sometimes longer or shorter than the 15 SS points on the grid for the adult norms. That is because the *SD*s of the raw scores for the child or adolescent reference group may be slightly larger or smaller than the *SD* equivalent for the adult reference group. Third, notice that the whiskers on the left side or right side are sometimes not the same length. This is due to floor or ceiling effects in the data, or to situations in which the size of the raw score intervals varies irregularly between the left and right sides. For instance, the whisker for Pu is shorter on the left side than the whisker on the right side. This is because 0 is the minimum value possible, and it imposes a floor effect on variability around the mean. Alternatively, consider the *M* variable. The raw score intervals are narrower on the right than the left, which causes the whisker to be narrower on the right than on the left.

| C-ID: X Y | | | P-ID: 135 | Age: 10 | | Gender: Male | Education: 5 | |
|---|---|---|---|---|---|---|---|---|
| **Domain/Variables** | **Raw Scores** | **Raw A-SS** | **Raw C-SS** | **Cplx. Adj. A-SS** | **Cplx. Adj. C-SS** | **Standard Score Profile R-Optimized** | **Abbr.** | |
| **Admin. Behaviors and Obs.** | | | | | | 60  70  80  90  100  110  120  130  140 | | |
| Pr | 1 | 104 | 105 | | | | Pr | |
| Pu | 0 | 96 | 95 | | | | Pu | |
| CT (Card Turning) | 5 | 104 | 104 | | | | CT | |
| **Engagement and Cog. Processing** | | | | | | 60  70  80  90  100  110  120  130  140 | | |
| Complexity | 48 | 81 | 90 | | | | Cmplx | |
| R (Responses) | 20 | 88 | 88 | 97 | 96 | | R | |
| F% [Lambda=1.50] (Simplicity) | 60% | 116 | 103 | 106 | 94 | | F% | |
| Blend | 0 | 73 | 86 | 92 | 99 | | Bln | |
| Sy | 2 | 81 | 89 | 98 | 105 | | Sy | |
| MC | 3.5 | 85 | 94 | 98 | 107 | | MC | |
| MC - PPD | -0.5 | 105 | 105 | 105 | 105 | | MC-PPD | |
| M | 3 | 97 | 103 | 105 | 112 | | M | |
| M/MC [3/3.5] | 86% | 123 | 120 | 126 | 122 | | M Prp | |
| (CF+C)/SumC [0/1] | NA | | | | | | CFC Prp | |

**FIGURE 3.3.** A portion of the Page 1 Profile for a 10-year-old to illustrate three advanced points. Reproduced from the Rorschach Performance Assessment System® (R-PAS®) Scoring Program (© 2010–2016) and excerpted from the *Rorschach Performance Assessment System: Administration, Coding, Interpretation, and Technical Manual* (© 2011) with copyrights by Rorschach Performance Assessment System, LLC. All rights reserved. Used by permission of Rorschach Performance Assessment System, LLC. Further reproduction is prohibited without written permission from R-PAS.

## Complexity Adjusted Scores

Complexity Adjusted scores (CAdj) follow the same conventions as raw scores; the only difference is that the CAdj scores are profiled using square icons. When this option is selected in the results output online, the placement of the square icons on the Profile Page indicates the raw score expected for this person after adjusting for his or her level of Complexity. That is, the icon shows the score this person would be expected to obtain if he or she had an average level of Complexity, or if everyone in the norms was as Complex as the examinee. The color and interior shape of the icons follow the same classification rules as for the raw score C-SS values (e.g., they are green and open squares when the CAdj C-SS fall in the range of 85–115). Paralleling the data in the "Raw" column, the "Cplx. Adj." column contains two sub-columns of SS values. The A-SS column shows what this person's CAdj score would be relative to adult norms (i.e., relative to the vertical lines of the underlying grid), and the C-SS column indicates what this person's CAdj score is relative to other children or adolescents of the same age (i.e., relative to the X's and whiskers of the overlays). When the option for CAdj scores is selected, the C-SS values in the "Cplx. Adj." column become easy-to-see regular black font, whereas the A-SS values remain in gray font.

## The R-PAS Profile Appendix

Finally, on the last page of the results output is the Profile Appendix showing summary scores for all variables. For children and adolescents, it contains a column for their raw score, followed by columns of SSs that correspond to that raw score and the CAdj version of that raw score. Within the SS columns are subcolumns that provide information about what the SS would be using adult norms (A-SS) and what it is relative to other children or adolescents of the same age (C-SS). This is the same information as is given on the Profile Pages; the only difference is that now the information is given for all variables. As with the Profile Pages, the A-SS column is always grayed out; it is present for assessors to consult if desired, but not prominent, as partially illustrated in Figure 3.4.

R-PAS Profile Appendix – Summary Scores for All Variables

C-ID: X Y    P-ID: 135    Age: 10    Gender: Male    Education: 5

| Section & Variable | Raw | Raw Scores A-SS | Raw Scores C-SS | Cplx. Adj. A-SS | Cplx. Adj. C-SS | Section & Variable | Raw | Raw Scores A-SS | Raw Scores C-SS | Cplx. Adj. A-SS | Cplx. Adj. C-SS | Section & Variable | Raw | Raw Scores A-SS | Raw Scores C-SS | Cplx. Adj. A-SS | Cplx. Adj. C-SS |
|---|---|---|---|---|---|---|---|---|---|---|---|---|---|---|---|---|---|
| R & Admin. | | | | | | FQ and Popular | | | | | | Cognitive Codes | | | | | |
| R | 20 | 88 | 88 | 97 | 96 | FQo | 11 | 91 | 102 | 95 | 106 | DV1 (1) | 0 | 93 | 91 | 93 | 91 |
| R8910 | 5 | 80 | 80 | 90 | 91 | FQu | 6 | 97 | 92 | 106 | 103 | DV2 (2) | 0 | 100 | 98 | 100 | 98 |
| Pr | 1 | 104 | 105 | | | FQ- | 3 | 108 | 90 | 114 | 94 | DR1 (3) | 0 | 94 | 94 | 94 | 94 |
| Pu | 0 | 96 | 95 | | | FQn | 0 | 97 | 94 | 97 | 94 | DR2 (6) | 0 | 99 | 99 | 99 | 99 |
| CT | 5 | 104 | 104 | | | WDo | 8 | 79 | 92 | 83 | 96 | PEC (5) | 0 | 97 | 95 | 97 | 95 |
| R8910% | 25% | 81 | 78 | 79 | 74 | WDu | 4 | 93 | 89 | 101 | 97 | INC1 (2) | 0 | 90 | 87 | 90 | 85 |
| | | | | | | WD- | 2 | 106 | 88 | 106 | 88 | INC2 (4) | 0 | 98 | 95 | 98 | 95 |

**FIGURE 3.4.** A portion of the Profile Appendix of Summary Scores for all variables for a 10-year-old. Reproduced from the Rorschach Performance Assessment System® (R-PAS®) Scoring Program (© 2010–2016) and excerpted from the *Rorschach Performance Assessment System: Administration, Coding, Interpretation, and Technical Manual* (© 2011) with copyrights by Rorschach Performance Assessment System, LLC. All rights reserved. Used by permission of Rorschach Performance Assessment System, LLC. Further reproduction is prohibited without written permission from R-PAS.

## Conclusion

This chapter has provided an overview of normative issues related to R-PAS interpretation in applied practice, with a focus on the R-PAS norms for children and adolescents. Also provided is a primer on how to interpret the results output for children and adolescents. Readers interested in child and adolescent assessment with R-PAS are encouraged to consult other chapters in this book with child and adolescent cases (Chapters 3, 4, 6, 12, 16, and 18), as well as the information available at *www.r-pas. org/ChildNorms.aspx.*

## REFERENCES

Berant, E. (2009). *CS and R-Optimized administrations* [Data files]. Herzliya, Israel: Baruch Ivcher School of Psychology, Interdisciplinary Center (IDC).

Dean, K. L., Viglione, D. J., Perry, W., & Meyer, G. J. (2007). A method to optimize the response range while maintaining Rorschach Comprehensive System validity. *Journal of Personality Assessment, 89,* 149–161.

Efron, B., & Tibshirani, R. T. (1993). *An introduction to the bootstrap.* New York: Chapman & Hall.

Exner, J. E. (2003). *The Rorschach: A comprehensive system: Vol. 1. Basic foundations* (4th ed.). Hoboken, NJ: Wiley.

Giromini, L., Viglione, D. J., & McCullaugh, J. (2015). Introducing a Bayesian approach to determining degree of fit with existing Rorschach norms. *Journal of Personality Assessment, 97,* 354–363.

Hosseininasab, A., Meyer, G. J., Viglione, D. J., Mihura, J. L., Berant, E., Resende, A. C., Reese, J., & Mohammadi, M. R. (2017). *The effect of CS administration or an R-Optimized alternative on R-PAS variables: A meta-analysis of findings from six studies.* Manuscript submitted for publication.

Hosseininasab, A., Mohammadi, M. R., Weiner, I. B., & Delavar, A. (2015). Rorschach Comprehensive System data for a sample of 478 Iranian children at four ages. *Journal of Personality Assessment, 97,* 123–135.

Lis, A., Salcuni, S., & Parolin, L. (2007). Rorschach Comprehensive System data for a sample of 116 preadolescent and 117 adolescent nonpatients from Italy. *Journal of Personality Assessment, 89,* S91–S96.

Mattlar, C.-E. (2011). The issue of an evolutionary development of the Rorschach Comprehensive System (RCS) versus a revolutionary change (R-PAS). Retrieved from *www.rorschachtraining.com/category/articles.*

Meyer, G. J. (2001). Evidence to correct misperceptions about Rorschach norms. *Clinical Psychology: Science and Practice, 8,* 389–396.

Meyer, G. J. (2016). Neuropsychological factors and Rorschach performance in children. *Rorschachiana, 37,* 7–27.

Meyer, G. J., Erdberg, P., & Shaffer, T. W. (2007). Towards international normative reference data for the Comprehensive System. *Journal of Personality Assessment, 89,* S201–S216.

Meyer, G. J., Giromini, L., Viglione, D. J., Reese, J. B., & Mihura, J. L. (2015). The association of gender, ethnicity, age, and education with Rorschach scores. *Assessment, 22,* 46–64.

Meyer, G. J., Shaffer, T. W., Erdberg, P., & Horn, S. L. (2015). Addressing issues in the development and use of the Composite International Reference Values as Rorschach norms for adults. *Journal of Personality Assessment, 97,* 330–347.

Meyer, G. J., Viglione, D. J., & Giromini, L. (2014). *Current R-PAS transitional child and adolescent norms.* Retrieved from *www.r-pas.org/CurrentChildNorms.aspx.*

Meyer, G. J., Viglione, D. J., Mihura, J. L., Erard, R. E., & Erdberg, P. (2011). *Rorschach Performance Assessment System: Administration, coding, interpretation, and technical manual.* Toledo, OH: Rorschach Performance Assessment System.

Oosterhuis, H. E. M., Andries van der Ark, L. A., & Sijtsma, K. (2016). Sample size requirements for traditional and regression-based norms. *Assessment, 23,* 191–202.

Pianowski, G., Meyer, G. J., & Villemor-Amaral, A. E. (2016). The impact of R-Optimized administration modeling procedures on Brazilian normative reference values for Rorschach scores. *Journal of Personality Assessment, 98,* 408–418.

Reese, J. B., Viglione, D. J., & Giromini, L. (2014). A comparison between Comprehensive System and an early version of the Rorschach Performance Assessment System administration with outpatient children and adolescents. *Journal of Personality Assessment, 96,* 515–522.

Resende, A. C. (2011). *R-PAS & CS Data* [Data file]. Goiânia, GO, Brasil: Pontifícia Universidade Católica de Goiás.

Ritzler, B. A. (2014). *Society for Personality Assessment (SPA).* March/April Newsletter, Vol. 6, # 2. Retrieved from *www.rorschachtraining.com/category/newsletters.*

Ritzler, B. A., & Sciara, A. (2009). Rorschach Comprehensive System international norms: Cautionary notes. Retrieved from *www.rorschachtraining.com/category/articles.*

Shaffer, T. W., Erdberg, P., & Meyer, G. J. (Eds.). (2007). International reference samples for the Rorschach Comprehensive System [Special issue]. *Journal of Personality Assessment, 89*(Suppl. 1).

Stanfill, M. L., Viglione D. J., & Resende, A. C. (2013). Measuring psychological development with the Rorschach. *Journal of Personality Assessment, 95,* 174–186.

Tibon Czopp, S., Rothschild-Yakar, L., & Appel, L. (2012). Rorschach Comprehensive System (CS) reference data for Israeli adolescents. *Journal of Personality Assessment, 94,* 276–286.

Van Patten, K., Shaffer, T. W., Erdberg, P., & Canfield, M. (2007). Rorschach Comprehensive System data for a sample of 37 nonpatient/nondelinquent adolescents from the United States. *Journal of Personality Assessment, 89,* S188–S192.

Viglione, D. J., & Giromini, L. (2016). The effects of using the international versus Comprehensive System norms for children, adolescents, and adults. *Journal of Personality Assessment, 98,* 391–397.

Viglione, D. J., & Hilsenroth, M. J. (2001). The Rorschach: Facts, fiction, and future. *Psychological Assessment, 13,* 452–471.

Viglione, D. J., Meyer, G., Jordan, R. J., Converse, G. L., Evans, J., MacDermott, D., & Moore, R. (2015). Developing an alternative Rorschach administration method to optimize the number of responses and enhance clinical inferences. *Clinical Psychology & Psychotherapy, 22,* 546–558.

Wood, J. M., Nezworski, M. T., Garb, H. N., & Lilienfeld, S. O. (2001). The misperception of psychopathology: Problems with norms of the Comprehensive System for the Rorschach. *Clinical Psychology: Science and Practice, 8,* 350–373.

Zhu, J., & Chen, H.-Y. (2011). Utility of inferential norming with smaller sample sizes. *Journal of Psychoeducational Assessment, 29,* 570–580.

# PART II

## Using R-PAS
## in Clinical Settings

# CHAPTER 4

# The Broken Zombie
## Using R-PAS in the Assessment of a Bullied Adolescent with Borderline Personality Features

Jan H. Kamphuis
Hilde De Saeger
Joni L. Mihura

One is likely to be made into a good, bad, valued, and hated figure, to be transported at magical speeds and unpredictably through a massive intrapsychic terrain. There is a constant search for alternative figures to serve as hosts for the alien self, which gives rise to the apparent "promiscuity" of these adolescents. Sadly, most people are not accepting of their projections, and experiences of profound rejection tend to dog these young people.
—FONAGY, GERGELY, JURIST, AND TARGET (2002, p. 339)

## Client Identifying Information and Referral Questions

Our client, "Jill," is a 15-year-old adolescent female who was referred by a center for child and adolescent psychiatry for a second opinion regarding diagnosis, treatment, and medication. In treatment for affective problems (severe depression and highly unstable mood), posttraumatic stress symptoms (PTSS), and possible personality pathology, Jill was not making sufficient progress. The center specifically requested therapeutic assessment (Finn, 2007) for Jill.

## Client Background

Jill had been living with both parents and her younger brother, age 3. Her parents were born in different foreign countries and had met through work. Her mother expatriated to join her father, and subsequently they lived in different countries together before coming to the Netherlands. Because of work, the family also relocated several times within the Netherlands, each time causing Jill to change schools and social networks. Jill's developmental history is nonetheless unremarkable, as she reached developmental milestones without major problems. She followed a multilingual education at an international school and generally received good grades. Her parents described her temperament as "rather quiet, perhaps a little anxious." By all accounts, Jill had a strong interest in horseback riding.

Jill's psychological problems started when she was severely bullied by a female peer at primary school. As a result, she became very fearful and mistrustful in social relations (especially with girls), and increasingly withdrew. She began experiencing nightmares and intrusive thoughts, typically related to the bullying, as well as intense mood changes and nighttime bingeing. Moreover, Jill began to hear voices telling her to harm herself, and she started engaging in deliberate self-harming behaviors (mostly cutting herself). Because of these problems, she could no longer attend school and continued her education through online classes. Always a strong student, her grades began to slip.

Jill was initially seen by a psychiatrist in private practice, who treated her for sleeping problems and bullying-related PTSS. After receiving an initial eye movement desensitization and reprocessing (EMDR) session for her PTSS, Jill reported that her rumination and restlessness intensified rather than lessened, particularly at night. She also experienced panic attacks when making an effort to return to school. For sleep, Jill was initially prescribed two 0.5 mg Risperdal twice a day, which the psychiatrist doubled after her restlessness increased. Concerned about a potential crisis, the psychiatrist referred her to a center for child and adolescent psychiatry for an observational inpatient admission.

At the center for child and adolescent psychiatry, a full clinical assessment was conducted for intellectual and neuropsychological functioning and personality development. The report concluded that Jill met criteria for major depressive disorder (MDD, single, severe) and PTSS (chronic) with rule-out diagnoses of dysthymia, panic disorder, and psychotic disorder. During this time, Jill told of a very shame-laden instance in which a much-trusted, same-age uncle had sexually assaulted her. This traumatic event occurred during the time she was being bullied. The clinic's treatment recommendations included continuing her current pharmacotherapy, EMDR, and cognitive-behavioral therapy (CBT), and for her parents to continue their parent counseling. However, several months later, Jill's mood and anxiety problems had not improved and her parents had grown increasingly worried. About 1 year later, Jill was in a severe emotional crisis. She was subsequently admitted to an inpatient unit for a period of 10 weeks, which she described to us as quite depersonalizing and traumatic.

## Previous Assessment

### Cognitive Performance Tests

Intellectual testing had been conducted with Jill at the child and adolescent psychiatry center at age 13, using the Dutch version of the Wechsler Intelligence Scale for Children—Third Edition (WISC-III). Her intellectual performance was in the high-average range (Full Scale IQ [FIQ] = 117), with harmonious Performance IQ (PIQ) and Verbal IQ (VIQ) profiles (118 and 115, respectively). She had a weakness in Processing Speed (PS = 108), which may have been due to her severe depressive symptoms at the time of testing.

## Structured Interview

On the Structured Clinical Interview for DSM Disorders–II (SCID-II; First, Gibbon, Spitzer, Williams, & Benjamin, 1997; Weertman, Arntz, & Kerkhofs, 2000), administered as part of the subsequent therapeutic assessment procedure, Jill met three criteria for borderline personality disorder (BPD) and received two threshold scores. She displayed *recurrent suicidal and self-mutilating behavior*. Three times during the past three years she had ingested overdoses of medication, and she had attempted to suffocate herself by pulling a plastic bag over her head. Her self-harm behaviors including cutting and (currently) scratching when feeling highly distressed. She reported *affective lability* consisting of recurrent intense rapid mood changes, sometimes without apparent reason. She also reported experiencing *transient, stress-related dissociative symptoms* at the time of her inpatient treatment. With mounting stress, Jill reported trouble with reality testing. Four years ago, these problems were most severe, when for about 6 months she heard voices and believed that she could communicate with plants.

Regarding subthreshold BPD criteria, Jane strongly resonated with the *feelings of emptiness*, but she was not sure if these were indeed chronic. She reported being consumed by thoughts about peers changing their opinion of her and abandoning her, and how she might stop this from happening, but this did not constitute "*frantic efforts*" to avoid abandonment.

Jill also had reported features of avoidant personality disorder. Most notably, she was preoccupied with being criticized or rejected in social situations and saw herself as socially inept, personally unappealing, and inferior to others.

## Personality Self-Report Tests

Jill's Minnesota Multiphasic Personality Inventory—Adolescent (MMPI-A; Butcher et al., 1992) scores yielded a valid profile; she had approached the test in a consistent (both VRIN and TRIN < T = 60) and open manner (L, T = 41; K, T = 42). Several indicators of general maladjustment as well as behavioral disinhibition were elevated, and her scores suggested significant social discomfort and immaturity (inspected Codetypes: 7–8/8–7; 7–9/9–7; 8–9/9–8; Archer, 2005). Her scores were indicative of a great deal of tension, anxiety, and rumination (Scale 7, T = 74; ANX T = 76). Poor stress tolerance and problems in emotion regulation are likely, as well as strong feelings of insecurity and inadequacy. Scores also suggested significant conflicts about dependency needs (greatly needing as well as resenting the neediness). Jill's results were consistent with acknowledgments of alcohol- or drug-related symptoms, attitudes, or beliefs (ACK T = 72) and a vulnerability to developing substance abuse problems (PRO T = 66). However, as there was no indication of current (or past) drug abuse, we inspected the content of the items she endorsed for these scales. A likely explanation was her preoccupation with food and eating, and feeling out of control in this domain. Further, it is of note that, given the outpatient clinic's diagnosis of severe depression (MDD), Jill's highest MMPI-A score was on Scale 9 (T = 78), followed by Scales 7 and 8 (both at T = 74), and her Scale 2 was not significantly elevated (T = 60). Therefore, it will be important to review results from the Rorschach Performance Assessment System (R-PAS; Meyer, Viglione, Mihura, Erard, & Erdberg, 2011) for scores related to reality testing and thought disorder (e.g., TP-Comp) to further evaluate for emerging bipolar or psychosis.

## Research Relevant to the Case

### Diagnosing Personality Disorders in Adolescence

Diagnosing adolescents with a personality disorder (PD) is a controversial issue. As noted in DSM-5 (American Psychiatric Association, 2013), PD categories may be applied to children or adolescents "in those relatively unusual instances in which the individuals' particular maladaptive personality traits appear to be pervasive, persistent, and unlikely to be limited to a particular developmental stage or another disorder" (p. 647). Critics caution that adolescence is period of great biological, psychological, and social transformation, and that a certain degree of adjustment difficulty is to be expected. Large numbers of "false positives" are therefore to be expected, and labeling costs are emphasized. Proponents argue that nothing magical happens at age 18, and that early diagnosis and intervention may prevent an array of personal suffering, and decrease suicide risk and mental health care cost (e.g., see Feenstra et al., 2012). Clearly, it is a major challenge to accurately distinguish enduring personality pathology from transient adjustment difficulties associated with this period of transformation.

Empirical research suggests there is major continuity between adolescent and adult PD. As reviewed in Emmelkamp and Kamphuis (2007), joint analyses of measures of normal personality variation and of dimensional representations of PD symptoms are quite similar for adult and adolescent groups (de Clercq & De Fruyt, 2003), and the structure of PDs in adolescents resembles the structure of PDs observed in adult samples (Durret & Westen, 2005). Importantly as well, Cluster B PD symptoms demonstrated high stability across an 8-year interval from adolescence to adulthood, beyond well-established psychiatric disorder symptom clusters (Crawford, Cohen, & Brook, 2001). Moreover, numerous studies now show that adolescent PDs are associated with impairment, distress, suicidality, disturbed family relationships, romantic partner conflict, and general poor outcomes during adulthood (Emmelkamp & Kamphuis, 2007).

### The Psychological Impact of Bullying

Many studies document that bullying is a prevalent problem in elementary and high school, with about 1 in 10 children being targets of repeated and severe bullying, and presumably many more experiencing less severe, more transient victimizations. Peer victimization can take on many shapes, including teasing, systematic exclusion, becoming the target of gossip campaigns, (threats of) physical violence, and bullying on social media. As now documented in a large body of research, bullying is associated with a vast array of psychosocial adjustment difficulties. In fact, two meta-analytic studies focusing on longitudinal research showed that prospective linkages exist between peer victimization and both internalizing and externalizing symptoms (Reijntjes, Kamphuis, Prinzie, & Telch, 2010; Reijntjes et al., 2011). Particularly pertinent to the present case are two meta-analytic reviews showing that childhood bullying is associated with increased odds of (1) subsequent development of psychotic symptoms (Cunningham, Hoy, & Shannon, 2015) and (2) suicidal ideation (Holt et al., 2014). Of course, it is difficult to discern the causal pathways between these associations, and the observed risks are likely moderated by a diversity of individual difference variables (e.g., emotional stability, social support) and stressor variables (e.g., intensity and duration of bullying), but the overall increased odds of developing significant psychopathology are quite alarming by themselves.

## The Current Assessment

A therapeutic assessment (TA) approach was used for Jill's assessment. TA is a semi-structured method of collaborative psychological assessment, which, in addition to regular information-gathering purposes, explicitly aims for therapeutic impact (Finn, 2007; Finn & Kamphuis, 2006). The TA assessor is a participating observer whose primary goal is to help the patient gain new information that may help him or her to improve the quality of his or her life. In the first session, patient and clinician collaboratively develop individualized assessment questions, which subsequently orient the testing phase and the interactive summary and discussion session. Recent research has documented that TA can lead to strong effects in treatment process variables (e.g., alliance, sense of progress and focus, positive therapy expectancies), but not to immediate symptom change in patients with PD (De Saeger et al., 2014). A qualitative follow-up study suggested that the most memorable TA experiences were (1) the relationship aspects of the model, (2) new insights into personal dynamics, (3) the sense of empowerment, and (4) the validation of self (De Saeger, Bartak, Eder, & Kamphuis, 2016).

Jill's assessment questions were:

- "Why do I have such problems sleeping?"
- "Why do I find it so hard to deal with intense emotions?"
- "Why do I find it so hard to go to school?"
- "What is my diagnosis?"
- "What kind of therapy might help me?"

Her parents were also invited to formulate questions for the assessment, which were:

- "What causes Jill to have such problems sleeping?"
- "To what extent does Jill think and feel differently as a result of the traumatic experiences, and should we be thinking in terms of personality problems?"
- "Which patterns do we have as a family in dealing with emotions that may affect Jill?"

## Behavioral Observations

Jill is a tall and slender girl with long dark-red hair, who looks slightly older than her age. To each session, she wore a T-shirt showing a different heavy metal rock group. She came across as serious and reflective, and was repeatedly rather slow to respond to questions. At times, this latency occurred because she could not find the exact word she wanted in the Dutch language, but at other times no such explanation was evident.

## Why Use R-PAS for Jill's Assessment?

On the first page, the R-PAS manual (Meyer et al., 2011) explains that Rorschach scores are performance-based, and thus form a "complement to the characteristics [persons] consciously recognize and willingly endorse on a self-report instrument" (p. 1). As suggested by Finn (1996), it can be helpful to think of different "levels of personality" that are being accessed by these two methods of assessment. This notion can be best understood when realizing the divergent processes that underlie the respective scores. Self-report tests are typically highly structured and administered in noninteractive fashion, and primarily elicit information consistent with self-presentation and conscious views of self. Rorschach scores, on the other hand, are derived from a testing process that is usually unfamiliar and relatively unstructured, interpersonal, and emotionally arousing to the individual being assessed. Particularly (but certainly not exclusively), this latter type of information can be of great value in the context of personality assessment with adolescent patients with PD, who may present with complex interpersonal and emotional issues, and have serious limitations in introspective capacity and/or have motivational conflicts to recognize and disclose.

Moreover, R-PAS taps a number of content domains that are hard to efficiently assess otherwise, were highly salient to the present case, and have strong support in the research literature (Mihura, Meyer, Dumitrascu, & Bombel, 2013). Specifically, self and other representations, emotional experience, and quality of reality testing were all central to the conceptualization of this case and to addressing the patient's assessment questions.

## The R-PAS Administration

R-PAS was introduced and administered at "de Viersprong," a specialized clinic for the assessment and treatment of PD in the Netherlands,[1] by a young male clinician who was extensively trained in TA. Consistent with TA, he stated that the test would likely be helpful in providing answers to Jill's personal questions about emotional issues. Jill was satisfied with this introduction and posed no further questions. During the R-PAS administration, Jill was cooperative and seemed to enjoy the process. She frequently turned the cards to inspect them from all angles. After the administration, she said that she liked having an opportunity to "express her creativity" in this test. The administration took about 50 minutes.

## Discussion of the R-PAS Results as Applied to the Case

Jill's R-PAS Responses, Location Sheet, Code Sequence, and Page 1 and 2 Profiles are presented in Appendix 4.1 at the end of the chapter. A quick *Scan* of her results revealed that Jill's most significant pathology was in the *Stress and Distress* and *Self and Other Representation* domains, which are discussed in the following material.

---

[1] The R-PAS administration was conducted in Dutch and translated for use in the present chapter.

## Administration Behaviors and Observations

Toward the end of the test, Jill had difficulty following the R-PAS instructions to "try to give two responses . . . or maybe three, to each card," requiring the examiner to intervene, due to both underproductive and overproductive behaviors (Prompts SS[2] = 118; Pulls SS = 123). This pattern rarely happens. These behaviors occurred in response to the last three colorful, emotionally activating cards. Her behaviors suggest poor regulation and behavioral control, especially in unstructured, emotionally stimulating environments, as is consistent with Jill's history. Jill also turned the cards to view them in different orientations more frequently than most people her age. This behavior can mean a number of different things depending on an array of contextual variables; in Jill's case, it is likely an expression of her engagement with the task as well as intellectual curiosity and ambition. Indeed, she spontaneously indicated that she enjoyed the test, as it gave her "an opportunity to express her creativity."

## Engagement and Cognitive Processing

Consistent with these observations, Jill's Complexity score was average,[3] and she provided an above-average number of responses (R = 29, SS = 120). Therefore, all indications point to her positive motivation and engagement with the task, which suggest that her results are valid for interpretation.

In general, Jill appears to possess an adequate level of enlivening thought and cognitive coping resources (average Complexity, Sy, and MC–PPD). However, her responses to stimulating environmental situations are likely to be spontaneous and absorbing, and may feel dangerous to her [(CF+C)/SumC SS = 128; Pure C SS = 134; R8910% SS = 120]. Illustrative responses are R6 "Looks like someone fired a shot and there was blood"; R19 "A rainbow"; followed by R20 "A gas mask"; R21 "A very large boat . . . coming your way"; and in the CP "That is one of my fears."

These responses indicate that Jill is likely to be more influenced by situational stressors than others, leading to emotional upset, fear, disruptions in concentration, and impulsive behavior, all of which would make her more unstable and unpredictable. Central to Jill's assessment questions, all of these findings clearly validate her sense of being unable to manage her internal experiences. Although these problems are not due to cognitive deficits, given Jill's intelligence (FIQ = 117) and her apparent introversive style, one would expect her to show more cognitive strengths in the ability to mentalize (M). For the Rorschach cards on which people are most likely to illustrate their mentalization abilities (i.e., Popular human responses Cards III and VII), Jill not only did not see humans in activity, but she saw no humans at all. The closest she came was "Aliens" on Card III, which is likely how Jill feels, given the ostracism she has faced.

## Perception and Thinking Problems

As one of the assessment questions was whether Jill had problems with thought disturbance or reality testing, the good news was that Jill's scores in these domains

---

[2] Standard scores (SS) have a mean of 100 and an *SD* of 15.

[3] This score also that there is no need to consider Complexity Adjusted scores.

were consistently average for her age (EII-3, TP-Comp, WSumCog, SevCog, FQ–%, WD–%). Therefore, at the time of testing, Jill had reasonably accurate thinking and reality testing.

## Stress and Distress

As noted earlier, Jill incorporated the dark and gloomy features of her environment ($C' = 7$) significantly more than the average adolescent. Further suggestive of emotional difficulties, Jill also reported significantly more morbid images (MOR SS = 130) than other adolescents, strongly suggesting a sense of being damaged and defective. Her response to Card IX, "a broken zombie . . . it looks like the skin is completely pulled down, the skin is torn," provides a rather dramatic illustration of the extent of the morbidity. We could also hypothesize that this broken zombie with its skin pulled down may represent the extent of inhumaneness—the damaged living dead—that Jill has at least implicitly experienced given the ostracizing bullying experience and the shameful loss of trust with her same-age uncle. Finally, Jill also scored above average on an implicit measure of suicide risk (SC-Comp = 6.6, SS = 124). In view of this score, certainly in the context of Jill's history of parasuicidality, the clinician is advised to explore current risk for self-harm with her.

Clearly, Jill's elevated scores on these implicit distress variables are key to understanding her current situation and assessment questions. Much akin to the concept of demoralization, Jill holds a very dark view of the world and a damaged and defective view of herself. Particularly noteworthy in this regard is her response to Card X, in which she imposes gray on the chromatically colored D7 area, akin to an inverse color projection that may be seen as highly illustrative of her demoralized state.

## Self and Other Representation

Jill's responses contained human and relational representations that help us understand more specifically where her strengths and pathologies lie. For example, the degree to which Jill had aggressive images on her mind was striking (AGC SS = 134). However, this is not surprising given the severe bullying she experienced that resulted in her leaving school, as well as the sexual assault by her trusted same-age uncle. But knowing the degree to which aggressive representations are on her mind is crucial to understanding her difficulties, how she is coping, and what needs to be addressed in her therapy and her life.

What is promising is that Jill reported a developmentally advanced relational response that shows good potential for her to be able to perceive mutual, healthy relationships (MAH = 1, SS = 111). However, the participants in her mutual relational response were insects (R28). In fact, Jill reported no mental representations of whole humans (H = 0, SS = 82), which suggests a developmental lag in understanding people as complex, complete, integrated individuals. Instead, she has a propensity to mentally represent self and others in incomplete, unrealistic, or fanciful ways (Non-Pure Human/SumH SS = 124). In Jill's case, images included several masks, witches, aliens, and the "broken zombie" with the "skin completely pulled down" described earlier, underscoring the predominance of mistrust, alienation, and vigilance in her object world.

Accordingly, relative to same-age peers, she exhibited a more general vigilant style of processing information; however, given the high elevation of the related scale (V-Comp SS = 129) and her generally good reality testing discussed in previous sections, her level and quality of vigilance did not qualify for a paranoid disorder. For Jill, her vigilance is likely associated with interpersonal distancing and wariness as well as anxious attentiveness to signs of interpersonal threats. Finally, Jill gave a few responses that could indicate oppositionality, independence-striving, and/or creativity (SR SS = 142). Importantly, these responses carried a distant, not a hostile, quality (R5, a UFO surrounded by the night air; R12, stars in the night sky; R16, a lamp).

## Case Conceptualization

One might ask, What caused the severe symptoms and dysfunction in this generally resourceful and high-functioning girl? Indeed, Jill's R-PAS scores were actually indicative of generally adequate psychological resources (MC SS = 110). From the R-PAS results it appears that she could not process the accumulation of deeply aversive interpersonal experiences (YTVC' SS = 127), and that she held a profound sense of being damaged, to the point of not even feeling human (MOR, Zombie response to Card IX). It also appears that these symptoms are *not* due to underlying psychotic vulnerabilities.

As we know from research, bullying occurs over time (i.e., not a single trauma) and can amount to a severe beating down of one's sense of connectedness, causing both internalizing and externalizing symptoms over time (e.g., see meta-analyses by Reijntjes et al., 2010, 2011). Especially in the crucial period of adolescence, dominated by the core business of identity, acceptance, and belonging, such experiences are extremely socially painful, to the point that people may no longer want to exist at all (risk of suicidality). Added to this intense ongoing assault on her interpersonal trust was the completely unexpected sexual assault by her uncle, who was a very trusted attachment figure. She may have reasoned, "If even he cannot be trusted, who can?" Perhaps of lesser importance, but worth mentioning, Jill had always been a strong performer in school, but presumably due to all of the factors above, she started having problems with concentration, which in turn caused problems with her scholastic achievement—posing another threat to her sense of self. Other stressors may be the repetitive relocations, complicating the formation of solid object relations, and a generally very busy and changing family environment.

We can see these experiences clearly reflected in her MMPI-A scores, as well as in her elevated V-Comp index; of course Jill is interpersonally hypervigilant, given her situation. It is also evident from her MAP/MAHP score; in three out of the four instances in which she characterized human interaction, she indicated expectations of exploitation, abuse of power, and malevolent intent (MAP = 3, SS = 145). As well, the high AGC score (SS = 134) and her reactivity to color/stimulating situations lend further support to this conceptualization.

Moreover, one might say that Jill was rather unlucky in terms of early treatment experiences. She did not build a positive alliance with her first treating psychotherapist. Next, her subsequent psychiatrist opted rather quickly for EMDR treatment. The selection of EMDR for her presenting ongoing interpersonal problems may not have been optimal, and she clearly did not respond well. One may surmise that she particularly needs connectedness (bolstering her lack of H), acceptance, guidance, and support that provide her with a sense of control, instead of more technique-driven change agents. Finally, Jill experienced the crisis inpatient admission as quite dehumanizing and traumatic. In fact, her brief stint with dissociative symptoms may have been her "solution" to the unbearable social pains she was experiencing in her life. Regardless, these experiences provided painfully little reason for any hope of the understanding, acceptance, and support that she needed. Feeling understood in TA may have somewhat restored her hope for getting her dependency needs met, which will need consolidation in subsequent treatment that should address her damaged sense of self. Clearly, she needs a reliable ally to help her navigate these deep waters, to come up with ways of coping with attending school, and to validate her as a person and her pain.

## BPD Characteristics and the Rorschach

It is perhaps impossible to be completely sure whether Jill meets or will meet DSM-5 criteria for BPD, because (1) we cannot tease apart the situational factors, (2) we did not hear of similar problems preexisting this extreme level of stress (i.e., bullying, sexual assault, and instability with peer relationships), (3) and research shows that teenagers may exhibit BPD-like symptoms in reaction to severe bullying. Ultimately, this question requires a longitudinal perspective, which is not the focus of the current chapter.

It may nonetheless be instructive to consider Jill's R-PAS scores vis-à-vis those theoretically most characteristic of patients with BPD. Mihura (2006) provided a scholarly discussion of the literature on Rorschach assessment of BPD. She distinguished four major sections that can easily be juxtaposed on Jill's R-PAS results, including (1) unstable identity/interpersonal relationships, (2) negative affective instability, (3) behavioral instability (self-destructive aggressive impulsivity), and (4) cognitive instability (psychotic-like thinking). In terms of BPD criterion for unstable identity/interpersonal relationships, Jill's responses were dominated by themes of malevolent control and influence (MAP), and she exhibited great difficulty seeing others as realistic, integrated individuals (H = 0). Consistent with BPD negative affective instability, her emotional experience was dominated by excessive dysphoria (C'), negative feelings about self (MOR), and themes of aggressiveness and dangerousness (AGC). Behavioral instability was also evident from her protocol, as well as signs of impulsivity [combination of Pu and Pr, (CF+C)/SumC, elevated SC-Comp]. Her elevated scores on MOR and AGC also suggest that her impulsivity may turn self-destructive. Fortunately, no significant indications were present for psychotic-like thinking, although these certainly were present at the time of her inpatient admission. Jill did show signs of hypervigilance (V-Comp), but it was not consistent with psychotic levels of paranoia. Taken together, Jill's R-PAS results are consistent with borderline features, but we need to remember, as Mihura (2006) put it, "the Rorschach is not designed to determine the BPD diagnosis (this is the job of the DSM interview), but Rorschach results can help to provide dynamic understanding of the particular BPD person's personality characteristics" (p. 190).

## R-PAS Contributions to Answering Jill's Assessment Questions

R-PAS contributed three key building blocks to conceptualizing Jill and her presenting problems. First, it provided reassuring information on her reality testing and cognitive processes. Her responses, certainly when combined with self-report and information from direct interactions, suggested that her difficulties were not due to a psychotic process. Second, both her formal R-PAS scores, but certainly also the vivid imagery (e.g., "the broken zombie . . . with the skin completely torn off") helped convey how damaged and defective she felt, and how negatively the bullying had affected her identity development. The third and final component to the case conceptualization was her apparent deficit in mentalization, or put differently, her very sketchy, poorly differentiated, but certainly negative sense of the intentions and motivations of others. We now review how these findings helped answer Jill's assessment questions.

- *"Why do I have such problems sleeping?"* In conjunction with the MMPI-A scores, SCID-II information, and self-reported history, the R-PAS scores suggest a great deal of rumination about themes of personal unattractiveness and the risk of being humiliated and rejected. Clearly, Jill was unable to process the intense emotions associated with her bullying victimization, and these are reexperienced at night. In sum, when alone and without distractions, these experiences haunt her the most.

- *"Why do I find it so hard to deal with intense emotions?"* From the R-PAS results, Jill comes across as a person who is certainly reactive to evocative, emotional situations and stimuli, and currently has difficulty regulating and controlling her behavior. She is consistently vigilant in interpersonal situations, and holds a profound sense of being damaged. She is unable to mentalize adequately, which leaves her vulnerable for emotional overload.

- *"Why do I find it so hard to go to school?"* Obviously, the R-PAS results cannot directly speak to this question. However, Jill's scores suggested intense mistrust and wariness of others, as well as a deep sense of being personally unattractive, defective, and damaged. She likely feels "like [a] broken zombie," and expects others to see her this way and to abuse her for it (see also all the malevolent, large eyes in her responses). In TA, feedback often includes such imagery, to let the client feel that the assessor has really "got it," and was indeed able to get into the client's shoes (Finn, 2007).

- *"What is my diagnosis?"* As mentioned previously, R-PAS is not in the business of assigning DSM diagnoses, but it can (and did) help rule out psychotic phenomena. Jill's R-PAS scores, particularly in the Stress and Distress domain but also in the Self and Other Representation domain, were consistent with the borderline features she exhibited behaviorally.

- *"What kind of therapy might help me?"* Above all, Jill's R-PAS scores are indicative of structural emotion regulation difficulties, as well as difficulties mentalizing in interpersonal situations. Certainly, these difficulties are expressed in her presenting problems, including her self-harm, rumination, sleeping problems, and general affective reactivity and malaise. Given the R-PAS evidence, getting back on track in terms of emotional development seemed like the primary target for treatment. Several evidence-based psychological treatments match this focus and, given local access and availability, we considered both mentalization-based treatment (MBT; Bateman & Fonagy, 2006) and dialectical behavior therapy (DBT; Linehan, 1993) to be good options. MBT conceptualizes BPD primarily as a failure to develop a robust self-structure, due to the absence of contingent and marked mirroring during development. The key functional deficit is called *mentalization,* and the focus of MBT is on stabilizing the patient's sense of self by strengthening his or her capacity for mentalization (see also Fonagy & Bateman, 2006, for an in-depth description of presumed mechanisms of change). DBT considers emotional dysregulation at the core of the borderline pathology. Emotional dysregulation leads to a cascade of dysregulation in other domains: cognitive dysregulation, a dysregulated sense of self, and interpersonal dysregulation. More specifically, patients with borderline pathology do not learn to adequately recognize, label, and modulate their intense emotional experiences and accordingly have not developed trust in their private experiences. As a consequence, a stable core sense of self does not fully evolve. Patients with these problems tend to experience the self as a vessel of conflicting, variable, and intense emotions and states, which in turn greatly complicates the formation of supportive long-term relationships. The DBT treatment protocol includes group-based specific skills modules to address these core deficits, as well as weekly individual sessions.

The above-mentioned findings and recommendations were shared in a TA so-called Summary and Discussion session. When all goes well, no major surprises emerge in this phase of TA, as the findings and recommendations are shared throughout the process. Indeed, the parents commented they finally felt that their daughter was accurately seen and understood, and readily accepted the answers to their TA questions. Jill particularly resonated with the image of "the broken zombie" as a reflection of her emotional state. Jill and her parents followed up on our recommendations, and opted for a DBT psychotherapy program near their place of residence. We learned from a follow-up phone conversation (part of the full TA model) that Jill continued to actively participate in the DBT program and was doing much better in terms of emotional distress.

## REFERENCES

American Psychiatric Association. (2013). *Diagnostic and statistical manual of mental disorders* (5th ed.). Arlington, VA: Author.

Archer, R. P. (2005). *MMPI-A: Assessing adolescent psychopathology* (3rd ed.). Mahwah, NJ: Erlbaum.

Bateman, A., & Fonagy, P. (2006). *Mentalization-based treatment for borderline personality disorder: A practical guide.* Oxford, UK: Oxford University Press.

Butcher, J. N., Williams, C. L., Graham, J. R., Archer, R. P., Tellegen, A., Ben-Porath, Y. S., & Kaemmer, B. (1992). *MMPI-A (Minnesota Multiphasic Personality Inventory—Adolescent): Manual for administration, scoring, and interpretation.* Minneapolis: University of Minnesota Press.

Crawford, T. N., Cohen, P., & Brook, J. S. (2001). Dramatic-erratic personality disorder symptoms: I. Continuity from early adolescence into adulthood. *Journal of Personality Disorders, 15,* 319–335.

Cunningham, T., Hoy, K., & Shannon, C. (2015). Does childhood bullying lead to the development of psychotic symptoms?: A meta-analysis and review of prospective studies. *Psychosis, 8,* 48–59.

De Clercq, B., & De Fruyt, F. (2003). Personality disorder symptoms in adolescence: A five-factor model perspective. *Journal of Personality Disorders, 17,* 269–292.

De Saeger, H., Bartak, A., Eder, E., & Kamphuis, J. H. (2016). Memorable experiences in Therapeutic Assessment: Inviting the patient's perspective following a pretreatment randomized controlled trial. *Journal of Personality Assessment, 98,* 472–479.

De Saeger, H., Kamphuis, J. H., Finn, S. E., Smith, J. D., Verheul, R., van Busschbach, J. J., . . . Horn, E. K. (2014). Therapeutic Assessment promotes treatment readiness but does not affect symptom change in patients with personality disorders: Findings from a randomized clinical trial. *Psychological Assessment, 26,* 474–483.

Durrett, C., & Westen, D. (2005). The structure of Axis II disorders in adolescents: A cluster-and factor-analytic investigation of DSM-IV categories and criteria. *Journal of Personality Disorders, 19,* 440–461.

Emmelkamp, P. M. G., & Kamphuis, J. H. (2007). *Personality disorders.* New York: Taylor & Francis.

Feenstra, D. J., Hutsebaut, J., Laurenssen, E. M. P., Verheul, R., Busschbach, J. J. V., & Soeteman, D. I. (2012). The burden of disease among adolescents with personality pathology: Quality of life and costs. *Journal of Personality Disorders, 26,* 593–604.

Finn, S. E. (1996). Assessment feedback integrating MMPI-2 and Rorschach findings. *Journal of Personality Assessment, 67,* 543–557.

Finn, S. E. (2007). *In our clients' shoes: Theory and techniques of Therapeutic Assessment.* Mahwah, NJ: Erlbaum.

Finn, S. E., & Kamphuis, J. H. (2006). Therapeutic Assessment with the MMPI-2. In J. N. Butcher (Ed.), *MMPI-2: A practitioner's guide* (pp. 165–191). Washington, DC: American Psychological Association.

First, M., Gibbon, M., Spitzer, R. L., Williams, J. B. W., & Benjamin, L. S. (1997). *User's guide for the Structured Clinical Interview for DSM-IV Axis II personality disorders (SCID-II).* Washington, DC: American Psychiatric Press.

Fonagy, P., & Bateman, A. W. (2006). Mechanisms of change in mentalization-based treatment of BPD. *Journal of Clinical Psychology, 62,* 411–430.

Fonagy, P., Gergely, G., Jurist, E. L., & Target, M. (2002). *Affect regulation, mentalization, and the development of the self.* New York: Other Press.

Holt, M. K., Vivolo-Kantor, A. M., Polanin, J. R., Holland, K. M., DeGue, S., Matjasko, J. L., . . . Reid, G. (2015). Bullying and suicidal ideation and behaviors: A meta-analysis. *Pediatrics, 135,* e496–e509.

Linehan, M. M. (1993). *Cognitive-behavioral treatment of borderline personality disorder.* New York: Guilford Press.

Meyer, G. J., Viglione, D. J., Mihura, J. L., Erard, R. E., & Erdberg, P. (2011). *Rorschach Performance Assessment System: Administration, coding, interpretation, and technical manual.* Toledo, OH: Rorschach Performance Assessment System.

Mihura, J. L. (2006). Rorschach assessment of borderline personality disorder. In S. K. Huprich (Ed.), *Rorschach assessment of the personality disorders* (pp. 171–203). Mahwah, NJ: Erlbaum.

Mihura, J. L., Meyer, G. J., Dumitrascu, N., & Bombel, G. (2013). The validity of individual Rorschach variables: Systematic reviews and meta-analyses of the comprehensive system. *Psychological Bulletin, 139,* 548–605.

Reijntjes, A., Kamphuis, J. H., Prinzie, P., Boelen, P. A., van der Schoot, M., & Telch, M. J. (2011). Prospective linkages between peer victimization and externalizing problems in children: A meta-analysis. *Aggressive Behavior, 37,* 215–222.

Reijntjes, A., Kamphuis, J. H., Prinzie, P., & Telch, M. J. (2010). Peer victimization and internalizing problems in children: A meta-analysis of longitudinal studies. *Child Abuse & Neglect, 34,* 244–252.

Weertman, A., Arntz, A., & Kerkhofs, M. (2000). *Handleiding Gestructureerd Klinisch Interview voor DSM-IV As-II Persoonlijkheidsstoornissen.* Lisse, The Netherlands: Swets Test.

**Jill's R-PAS Responses, Location Sheet, Code Sequence, and Page 1 and 2 Profiles**

**Rorschach Responses "Jill"**

| Respondent ID: Jill | Examiner: Roel |
|---|---|
| Location: De Viersprong | Date: **/**/**** |
| Start Time: 13:00 P.M. | End Time: 13:50 P.M. |

| Cd # | R # | Or | Response | Clarification | R-Opt |
|---|---|---|---|---|---|
| I | 1 | | A mask. (W) | E: (Examiner Repeats Response [ERR].)<br>R: The mouth here (points). A mask that is looking at me. The eyes (DdS30) look angry, like they are looking at me.<br>E: What makes it look like that?<br>R: Because of the shape. | |
| | 2 | | What is the name of that animal? Gray, an African rhinoceros. (W) | E: (ERR)<br>R: Because of the gray color, with a horn (D3) shape, because of shape. | |
| | 3 | | Or the head of a dinosaur. (W) | E: (ERR)<br>R: From the side, because of shape. There are two types of dinos that have on the side these big, can't think of the name . . . at the end there are these pointy things (D7), and you have the eyes here (DdS30) (points). | |
| II | 4 | | Looks like two dog heads. (D6) | E: (ERR)<br>R: The shape. You see the eyes, ears right here (points). | |
| | 5 | | Or a UFO. (D5, D6) | E: (ERR)<br>R: Because of the shape, and the white color. The dark color is the night, the air. | |
| | 6 | v | v Looks like someone fired a shot and there was blood. (D3) | E: (ERR)<br>R: Blood looks like it was smashed hard against the wall, red like blood. [E could have asked what made it look "smashed hard," targeting Diffuse Shading (Y) and form dominance of color.] | |
| III | 7 | | Aliens. (D9) | E: (ERR)<br>R: Here's the head (Dd32), the chin.<br>E: What makes it look like aliens?<br>R: Because of the unfamiliar shape of the head. | |
| | 8 | v | v Weird frog with a bug head with teeth (points to upper part of D8). (D1) | E: (ERR)<br>R: It has bug's eyes (Dd31); large, black circles. These are the legs here (D5, Dd32). | |
| | 9 | | A demon cat, pretty scary actually. . . . (D7) | E: (ERR)<br>R: Here's the mouth with teeth (lower D8). The eyes (Dd31) are large and black. Thought of demon because of large, empty eyes.<br>E: Scary?<br>R: Because of the pointy teeth, empty eyes. | |
| IV | 10 | v | v A bat. (W) | E: (ERR)<br>R: Because of the gray color, and the shape. | |
| | 11 | | A dragon. (W) | E: (ERR)<br>R: I rather like dragons, it looks like how I might draw a dragon; here are the wings (D6) and the head (D1), with eyes, the nose, horns. | |
| V | 12 | v | v Part of the sky, at night. (W) | E: (ERR)<br>R: Small little white dots here; in terms of color it looks like stars. | |
| | 13 | | A gull with a very large mouth. (W) | E: (ERR)<br>R: The shape. Here's the wings (D4), legs (Dd34), and beak (D9). Why do I keep seeing animals? | |

78

| Cd # | R # | Or | Response | Clarification | R-Opt |
|---|---|---|---|---|---|
| VI | 14 | | A guitar with fire. (D2, Dd22) | E: (ERR)<br>R: This part looks like the neck (D2); here's the fire (Dd22).<br>E: Fire?<br>R: It has the shape of flames. | |
| | 15 | | Skin of a bear; like when someone murders a bear and puts the skin on the ground. (D1) | E: (ERR)<br>R: There is a straight line in the middle. There is usually a black line on the back . . . here, darker than the rest. Here's the legs (Dd24). | |
| VII | 16 | v | v A lamp. (DS7) | E: (ERR)<br>R: Yes, a lamp with a shade (DS10); the shape. | |
| | 17 | | Looks like wet paint, and then it slides down because it is still wet or something. . . . (W) | E: (ERR)<br>R: Like the lamp; the gray is the wall, and down here you see little lines that go down; like paint on a wall goes down. | |
| | 18 | > | > Something with a very large mouth, and he is trying to swallow something. (W) | E: (ERR)<br>R: Here is the mouth (DS7). It is easier when there is color. [E could have clarified "Trying to swallow something?" to more firmly establish MAP coding.] | |
| VIII | 19 | | A rainbow. (W) (R starts to hand card back. E: Take your time and look some more. I'd like you to give two, maybe three responses.) | E: (ERR)<br>R: Lots of colors. | Pr |
| | 20 | v | v A gas mask. (W) | E: (ERR)<br>R: Here the eyes (DdS32), because of the shape. | |
| | 21 | v | v A boat that is coming your way. A very large boat; that you are in the water and a very large boat is coming your way. (D8) | E: (ERR)<br>R: That is one of my fears.<br>E: What makes it look like a boat?<br>R: It looks like a pointy object (D4) in the middle of the water (D5).<br>E: Water?<br>R: The blue. | |
| | 22 | | A dog with its tail. (D1)<br>E: Thank you, let's go the next one. Remember, I would like you to give me two, perhaps three responses. | E: (ERR)<br>R: Yes, here are the four legs, the way it is standing makes it looks like a dog. | Pu |
| IX | 23 | < | < Some kind of witch head with super large eyes. (D1) [R hands back the card] (E: We would like two, or maybe three responses to each card, so please try to give another.) | E: (ERR)<br>R: Because of the shape. You see the eye (DdS29), nose (Dd28), hair over here (points to Dd31). | Pr |
| | 24 | > | v > A zombie. (D3) | E: (ERR)<br>R: A broken zombie, here's the eye (white space within D3).<br>E: Broken?<br>R: It looks like the skin is completely pulled down; the skin is torn. | |
| | 25 | > | > An arrow. (Dd99 = D5 extended to either end of the image when viewed in the > orientation) | E: (ERR)<br>R: Because of the shape; the straight line. | |
| X | 26 | | A crab. (D7) | E: (ERR)<br>R: The shape of the body; legs here. | |
| | 27 | | A spider. (D7) | E: (ERR)<br>R: Here; because it is gray. | |
| | 28 | | Two little animals, like when you win something in a race, like a golden trophy, that they are holding on to. Two insects that are holding a trophy. (D11) | E: (ERR)<br>R: Eyes (white space), mouth, belly, legs, antennas. The long thing is the trophy (D14); they (D8) are holding it up. | |
| | 29 | | A wolf, two wolves. (Dd99 = D1 – most of extending lines) [R hands card back; E did not pull or give a reminder, as this was the last card.] | E: (ERR)<br>R: (Points and circles finger around Dd99.) They have their mouths wide open. | |

# Rorschach Performance Assessment System (R-PAS)®

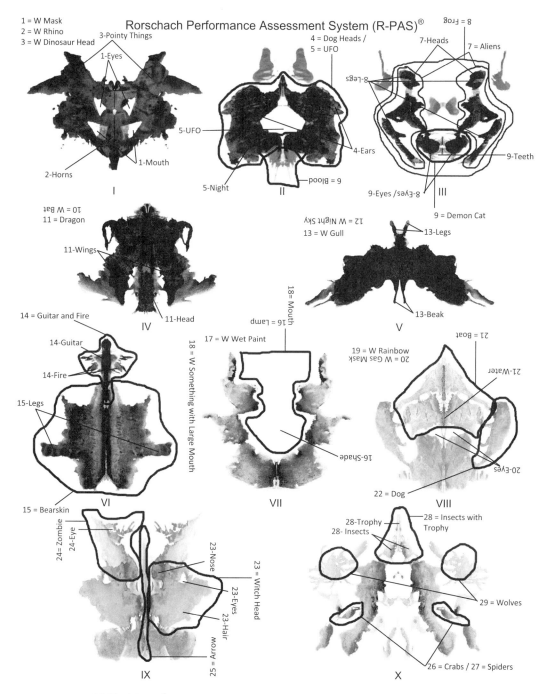

1 = W Mask
2 = W Rhino
3 = W Dinosaur Head

3-Pointy Things
1-Eyes
2-Horns
1-Mouth

I

4 = Dog Heads /
5 = UFO
5-UFO
4-Ears
6 = Blood
5-Night

II

8 = Frog
7-Heads
7 = Aliens
8-Legs
9-Teeth
9-Eyes / 8-Eyes
8-Eyes / 6-Eyes
9 = Demon Cat

III

10 = W Bat
11 = Dragon
11-Wings
11-Head

IV

12 = W Night Sky
13 = W Gull
13-Legs
13-Beak

V

14 = Guitar and Fire
14-Guitar
14-Fire
15-Legs
15 = Bearskin

VI

16 = Mouth
17 = W Wet Paint
18 = W Something with Large Mouth
16 = Lamp
16-Shade

VII

19 = W Rainbow
20 = W Gas Mask
21 = Boat
21-Water
20-Eyes
22 = Dog

VIII

24 = Zombie
24-Eye
23-Nose
23 = Witch Head
23-Eyes
23-Hair
25 = Arrow

IX

28-Trophy
28- Insects
28 = Insects with Trophy
29 = Wolves
26 = Crabs / 27 = Spiders

X

© 2012 R-PAS; Rorschach® trademarks and images are used with permission of the trademark owner, Hogrefe AG, Berne, Switzerland

80

# R-PAS Code Sequence: "Jill"

**C-ID**: Jill    **P-ID**: 103    **Age**: 15    **Gender**: Female    **Education**: NA

| Cd | # | Or | Loc | Loc # | SR | SI | Content | Sy | Vg | 2 | FQ | P | Determinants | Cognitive | Thematic | HR | ODL (RP) | R-Opt | Text |
|---|---|---|---|---|---|---|---|---|---|---|---|---|---|---|---|---|---|---|---|
| I | 1 | | W | | | SI | (Hd) | | | | o | | Mp | INC1 | AGM | PH | | | |
| | 2 | | W | | | | Ad | | | | u | | C' | | AGC | | | | |
| | 3 | | W | | | SI | Ad | | | | o | | F | | AGC | | | | |
| II | 4 | | D | 6 | | | Ad | | | 2 | o | P | F | | | | | | |
| | 5 | | D | 5,6 | SR | SI | NC | Sy | | | o | | C' | | | | | | |
| | 6 | v | D | 3 | | | Bl | | Vg | | o | | CF | | MOR,MAP | | | | * |
| Comment: E could have asked what made it look "smashed hard," targeting Diffuse Shading (Y) and form dominance of color. | | | | | | | | | | | | | | | | | | | |
| III | 7 | | D | 9 | | | (H) | | | 2 | o | | F | | | GH | | | |
| | 8 | v | D | 1 | | | A | | | | u | | C' | INC1 | | | ODL | | |
| | 9 | | D | 7 | | | (Ad) | | | | u | | C' | | AGC,MOR | | | | |
| IV | 10 | v | W | | | | A | | | | o | | C' | | | | | | |
| | 11 | | W | | | | (A) | | | | o | | F | | AGC | | | | |
| V | 12 | v | W | | SR | SI | NC | | Vg | | u | | C' | | | | | | |
| | 13 | | W | | | | A | | | | o | | F | | | | ODL | | |
| VI | 14 | | D | 2,22 | | | Fi,NC | Sy | | | u | | F | FAB1 | | | | | |
| | 15 | | D | 1 | | | Ad | | | | o | P | C' | DV1 | PER,MOR,MAP | | | | |
| VII | 16 | v | D | 7 | SR | | NC | | | | o | | F | | | | | | |
| | 17 | | W | | | | NC | | Vg | | u | | mp,Y | | | | | | |
| | 18 | > | W | | | | (Hd) | | | | - | | Ma | | MAP | PH | ODL | | * |
| Comment: E could have clarified "Trying to swallow something?" to more firmly establish MAP coding. | | | | | | | | | | | | | | | | | | | |
| VIII | 19 | | W | | | | NC | | Vg | | n | | C | | | | | Pr | |
| | 20 | v | W | | | SI | (Hd) | | | | u | | F | | | GH | | | |
| | 21 | v | D | 8 | | | NC | Sy | | | u | | ma,CF | | | | | | |
| | 22 | | D | 1 | | | A | | | | o | P | FMp | | | | | Pu | |
| IX | 23 | < | D | 1 | | SI | (Hd) | | | | - | | F | | AGC | PH | | Pr | |
| | 24 | > | D | 3 | | SI | (H) | | | | o | P | F | | AGC,MOR | PH | | | |
| | 25 | > | Dd | 99 | | | NC | | | | u | | F | | AGC | | | | |
| X | 26 | | D | 7 | | | A | | | 2 | o | | F | | | | | | |
| | 27 | | D | 7 | | | A | | | 2 | u | | C | | | | | | |
| | 28 | | D | 11 | | SI | A,NC | Sy | | 2 | o | | Ma | FAB1 | COP,MAH | GH | | | |
| | 29 | | D | 1 | | | A | | | 2 | - | | FMp | | AGC | | | | |

©2010-2016 R-PAS

## R-PAS Summary Scores and Profiles – Page 1

C-ID: Jill    P-ID: 103    Age: 15    Gender: Female    Education: NA

| Domain/Variables | Raw Scores | Raw A-SS | Raw C-SS | Cplx. Adj. A-SS | Cplx. Adj. C-SS | Abbr. |
|---|---|---|---|---|---|---|
| **Admin. Behaviors and Obs.** | | | | | | |
| Pr | 2 | 114 | 118 | | | Pr |
| Pu | 1 | 116 | 123 | | | Pu |
| CT (Card Turning) | 11 | 122 | 123 | | | CT |
| **Engagement and Cog. Processing** | | | | | | |
| Complexity | 68 | 98 | 102 | | | Cmplx |
| R (Responses) | 29 | 114 | 120 | 114 | 120 | R |
| F% [Lambda=0.71] (Simplicity) | 41% | 100 | 92 | 96 | 89 | F% |
| Blend | 2 | 91 | 94 | 92 | 95 | Bln |
| Sy | 4 | 91 | 94 | 95 | 98 | Sy |
| MC | 8.0 | 105 | 110 | 106 | 111 | MC |
| MC - PPD | -4.0 | 93 | 92 | 94 | 93 | MC-PPD |
| M | 3 | 97 | 100 | 96 | 98 | M |
| M/MC [3/8.0] | 38% | 91 | 93 | 92 | 94 | M Prp |
| (CF+C)/SumC [4/4] | 100% | 126 | 128 | 126 | 128 | CFC Prp |
| **Perception and Thinking Problems** | | | | | | |
| EII-3 | 0.8 | 118 | 112 | 120 | 115 | EII |
| TP-Comp (Thought & Percept. Com...) | 1.0 | 108 | 98 | 111 | 101 | TP-C |
| WSumCog | 13 | 113 | 111 | 114 | 112 | WCog |
| SevCog | 0 | 94 | 94 | 94 | 94 | Sev |
| FQ-% | 10% | 103 | 90 | 106 | 92 | FQ-% |
| WD-% | 11% | 108 | 94 | 106 | 93 | WD-% |
| FQo% | 52% | 93 | 103 | 87 | 98 | FQo% |
| P | 4 | 88 | 95 | 92 | 99 | P |
| **Stress and Distress** | | | | | | |
| YTVC' | 8 | 115 | 127 | 115 | 128 | YTVC' |
| m | 2 | 106 | 105 | 104 | 103 | m |
| Y | 1 | 99 | 101 | 99 | 101 | Y |
| MOR | 4 | 123 | 130 | 123 | 131 | MOR |
| SC-Comp (Suicide Concern Comp.) | 6.6 | 120 | 124 | 121 | 125 | SC-C |
| **Self and Other Representation** | | | | | | |
| ODL% | 10% | 101 | 107 | 102 | 109 | ODL% |
| SR (Space Reversal) | 3 | 122 | 142 | 122 | 142 | SR |
| MAP/MAHP [3/4] | 75% | 118 | 112 | 113 | 109 | MAP Prp |
| PHR/GPHR [4/7] | 57% | 116 | 107 | 116 | 107 | PHR Prp |
| M- | 1 | 113 | 110 | 113 | 110 | M- |
| AGC | 8 | 132 | 134 | 131 | 133 | AGC |
| H | 0 | 75 | 82 | 75 | 81 | H |
| COP | 1 | 102 | 101 | 105 | 105 | COP |
| MAH | 1 | 105 | 111 | 98 | 102 | MAH |

A-SS = Adult Standard Score; C-SS = Age-Based Child or Adolescent Standard Score

# R-PAS Summary Scores and Profiles – Page 2

C-ID: Jill  P-ID: 103  Age: 15  Gender: Female  Education: NA

| Domain/Variables | Raw Scores | Raw A-SS | Raw C-SS | Cpbk. Adj. A-SS | Cpbk. Adj. C-SS | Standard Score Profile R-Optimized | Abbr. |
|---|---|---|---|---|---|---|---|
| **Engagement and Cog. Processing** | | | | | | | |
| W% | 38% | 99 | 100 | 101 | 101 | | W% |
| Dd% | 3% | 80 | 84 | 80 | 84 | | Dd% |
| SI (Space Integration) | 8 | 130 | 146 | 131 | >150 | | SI |
| IntCont | 0 | 81 | 87 | 83 | 89 | | IntC |
| Vg% | 14% | 116 | 133 | 115 | 132 | | Vg% |
| V | 0 | 92 | 92 | 92 | 86 | | V |
| FD | 0 | 88 | 90 | 94 | 94 | | FD |
| R8910% | 38% | 117 | 120 | 116 | 119 | | R8910% |
| WSumC | 5.0 | 111 | 118 | 112 | 119 | | WSC |
| C | 2 | 124 | 134 | 124 | 134 | | C |
| Mp/(Ma+Mp) [1/3] | 33% | 94 | 93 | 94 | 93 | | Mp Prp |
| **Perception and Thinking Problems** | | | | | | | |
| FQu% | 34% | 106 | 103 | 109 | 106 | | FQu% |
| **Stress and Distress** | | | | | | | |
| PPD | 12 | 109 | 113 | 111 | 115 | | PPD |
| CBlend | 0 | 91 | 91 | 91 | 84 | | CBlnd |
| C' | 7 | 131 | >150 | 130 | >150 | | C' |
| V | 0 | 92 | 92 | 92 | 86 | | V |
| CritCont% (Critical Contents) | 24% | 106 | 111 | 108 | 113 | | CrCt |
| **Self and Other Representation** | | | | | | | |
| SumH | 6 | 101 | 100 | 104 | 103 | | SumH |
| NPH/SumH [6/6] | 100% | 127 | 124 | 126 | 123 | | NPH Prp |
| V-Comp (Vigilance Composite) | 5.6 | 122 | 129 | 125 | 132 | | V-C |
| r (Reflections) | 0 | 95 | 93 | 95 | 93 | | r |
| p/(a+p) [4/7] | 57% | 111 | 109 | 110 | 108 | | p Prp |
| AGM | 1 | 110 | 107 | 110 | 107 | | AGM |
| T | 0 | 91 | 91 | 91 | 91 | | T |
| PER | 1 | 109 | 104 | 109 | 104 | | PER |
| An | 0 | 85 | 87 | 85 | 87 | | An |

A-SS = Adult Standard Score; C-SS = Age-Based Child or Adolescent Standard Score

© 2010-2016 R-PAS

# CHAPTER 5

# When Wolves Fall from the Sky

## Using R-PAS in Early Detection of Psychosis in an Adolescent

James H. Kleiger
Ali Khadivi

Early detection of psychotically vulnerable patients has attracted a great deal of interest among diagnosticians and researchers (Addington & Heinssen, 2012; McGlashan, Walsh, & Woods, 2010; Yung & McGorry, 2007). Researchers argue that the neuropathological processes associated with the onset of psychosis appear long before the appearance of identifiable psychotic symptoms (Fenton & McGlashan, 1994). With an eye on early detection and intervention, clinical researchers have sought to identify vulnerable patients and prevent or minimize the traumatic effects of a first psychotic episode and the poor prognosis associated with late identification and delayed treatment. With secondary prevention at stake, researchers have developed operational criteria and assessment tools to identify clinical characteristics that precede an initial psychotic episode.

## The Rorschach and the Assessment of Psychosis: Why R-PAS?

Historically, psychologists have relied on the Rorschach as a reliable and valid instrument for assessing symptoms of psychosis (Holzman, Levy, & Johnston, 2005; Kleiger, 1999, 2017). Nearly 100 years ago, Hermann Rorschach's (1942/1921) identification of the characteristic disturbances in thought processes in people with schizophrenia, as revealed in their inkblot responses, is considered one of his greatest discoveries (Kleiger, 2015). Others, most notably Rapaport (Rapaport, Gill, & Schafer, 1946), developed Rorschach's seminal discoveries into a sophisticated set of scoring variables to identify forms of disordered thinking and perception, which formed the basis of all subsequent Rorschach scoring systems to assess thought disorder (Kleiger, 1999, 2017).

Recent meta-analyses by Mihura, Meyer, Dumitrascu, and Bombel (2013) found large effect sizes for the Rorschach's ability to detect psychosis in clinical settings, demonstrating convincingly that the Rorschach is a robust method for assessing the disordered thinking and impaired reality testing associated with psychotic conditions. The recent Rorschach Performance Assessment System (R-PAS; Meyer, Viglione, Mihura, Erard, & Erdberg, 2011) includes updated versions of the variables supported in Mihura et al.'s (2013) meta-analyses, as well as new empirically supported variables, and uses more accurate norms than the Comprehensive System (CS; Exner, 2003; see Meyer, Shaffer, Erdberg, & Horn, 2015). Importantly, R-PAS has identified problems with existing CS child and adolescent norms (Meyer, Erdberg, & Shaffer, 2007; Viglione & Giromini, 2016), which it has addressed with new R-PAS norms (Meyer & Erdberg, Chapter 3, this volume).

R-PAS variables that assess perception and thinking problems include (1) the Thought and Perception Composite (TP-Comp), which assesses reality testing and thought organization; (2) the Cognitive Codes (WSumCog and SevCog), which identify severe disruptions in communicating, thinking, conceptualizing, and reasoning; (3) the Form Quality scores (FQ–%, WD–%, and FQo%), which assess perceptual distortions that indicate problems in reality testing; and (4) the Ego Impairment Index–3 (EII-3), a composite index of psychopathology, which includes and extends beyond the previously mentioned scores.

## Early Detection Studies and the Rorschach

People interested in identifying psychosis risk have recently turned to the Rorschach as a method for early detection in vulnerable patients. Using early versions of R-PAS scores found in the CS, several studies provide a look at how clinical practitioners can use the Rorschach to detect emerging psychosis in young, at-risk patients (Ilonen, Heinimaa, Korkeila, Svirskis, & Salokangas, 2010; Inoue, Yorozuya, & Mizuno, 2014; Kimhy et al., 2007; Lacoua, Koren, & Rothschild-Yakar, 2015; Rothschild-Yakar, Lacoua, Brener, & Koren, 2015). In their seminal study, Kimhy and colleagues (2007) found that clinically high-risk patients displayed substantial deficits in visual form perception (Form Quality of responses) comparable to that found in patients with schizophrenia. In contrast, the high-risk patients did not show the level of disturbance in thinking and conceptualization (Cognitive Scores) as seen in the schizophrenic groups. Inoue and her colleagues (2014) recently replicated these findings. In contrast, Ilonen and colleagues' (2010) high-risk patients displayed substantial problems in both thinking and perception, similar to patients with schizophrenia and much higher than nonpsychotic patients.

In addition to examining Rorschach variables associated with psychosis risk, a team of Israeli researchers (Lacoua et al., 2015; Rothschild-Yakar et al., 2015) examined the role of theory of mind (ToM) and social cognition (Lysaker et al., 2011) in predicting psychosis risk. The researchers developed a new Rorschach measure of "self-reflectivity of perception and ideational accuracy," in which patients were asked to rate how much they thought others would either see what they saw or reason about the card in the same way they did. The researchers' preliminary investigations showed that deficits in social awareness of one's perceptual and thinking deviations added to the Rorschach's predictive ability of risk for psychosis prodrome.

While prospective longitudinal investigations are needed to determine the Rorschach variables that predict which patients actually develop psychosis, these studies of high-risk psychosis are promising. In addition to nomothetic approaches, idiographic investigations using the Rorschach can provide us with a window into the unique meaning of the emerging psychosis to the person experiencing it. The following clinical case provides an example of how R-PAS provided a unique contribution to the assessment of psychosis risk in ways that the routine clinical psychiatric and psychotherapeutic interview approaches did not.

## Chandra: A Case of Emerging Psychosis

"Chandra," a 17-year-old biracial high school junior with a lengthy and complicated history of behavioral, emotional, and social difficulties, presented with an 8-month history of functional deterioration, including a decline in her school performance, a neglect of her hygiene, and an increase in stealing from peers and family members. Her treating psychiatrist and psychotherapist referred Chandra for psychological assessment in order to clarify their diagnostic understanding and to make recommendations for treatment and educational planning. Previously diagnosed with attention-deficit/hyperactivity disorder (ADHD), major depressive disorder, anxiety disorder not otherwise specified, and a reactive attachment disorder, the referring clinicians wanted to understand more about Chandra's deterioration and whether their existing diagnostic formulations could account for her current level of functioning. Their principal referral question was "Is there anything else going on that would help explain the increase in Chandra's odd behavior and functional deterioration?" Neither referring clinician explicitly raised the question of whether Chandra might be exhibiting early signs of psychosis.

### Relevant Background Information

Life began in a harsh way for Chandra. Her birth mother, a homeless Haitian prostitute, reportedly suffered from a drug addiction and posttraumatic stress disorder (PTSD) as a result of traumatic abuse earlier in her life. Prior to Chandra's birth, her mother had reportedly been charged with neglect and sexual abuse of an older daughter, who had subsequently been removed from her care. In addition to abusing alcohol during her pregnancy with Chandra, her birth mother contracted syphilis. Following Chandra's birth, her mother lived with her on the streets until Chandra was 8 months old, at which point social services intervened. Chandra was immediately placed in foster care and eventually adopted at 18 months.

A developmental assessment at 9 months showed poor muscle tone and difficulty molding her body to her foster mother's arms. Chandra was unable to lift her head or sit up until she was 11 months old. She did not seek eye contact. Between the ages of 5 and 14, the list of psychosocial and behavioral problems multiplied. Adoptive parents indicated that she was distractible, impulsive, defiant, and deceitful. Additionally, they described her thinking as somewhat "odd" and regarded her behavior as "strange." For example, they once discovered that Chandra had put abrasive dental powder in their dog's food and, afterward, displayed little remorse or concern. Chandra was periodically encopretic, long after she had achieved control over her bowel functioning. She occasionally hid soiled underwear and spoiled food in her room. Her adoptive father described incidents when the encopresis and enuresis appeared willful, in response to parental limit setting.

During elementary school, Chandra had reportedly been involved in sex play with other girls in the bathroom. She frequently lied and stole. On one occasion, her teacher observed her rummaging through backpacks at school. During this time, Chandra remained on the edge of her peer group. She appeared to want friends but was not successful in making or keeping friendships. As a result, she was frequently rejected by peers and became socially isolated.

Several years after Chandra's parents had adopted her, they fostered and then adopted her younger biological sister Delsia. Chandra and her sister constantly fought, and Delsia later accused Chandra of sexually molesting her. Despite Chandra's significant behavioral difficulties, it was Delsia who commanded more psychiatric attention because of her violent temper, heightened anxiety, and subsequent auditory hallucinations. When Delsia was 12 (and Chandra was 15), she was hospitalized and given a diagnosis of schizophreniform disorder. Delsia improved after she was started on neuroleptic medication. Chandra seemed to gradually get worse.

Chandra began seeing mental health professionals as a child, first for her inattention and hyperactivity, and later for her lying and stealing. Since middle school, she had been treated by a psychotherapist and a psychiatrist, who initially prescribed Adderall and Prozac but broadened her regimen to include Concerta 72 mg A.M., Ritalin 10 mg, Prozac 60 mg, Abilify 7.5 mg, and Naltrexone 25 mg around the time she was referred for testing.

## Referral Questions

Chandra's parents and outpatient clinicians were interested in understanding the driving forces behind her worsening behavior and what more could be done to treat her. They had long viewed her psychosocial difficulties through the joint lenses of a mood and reactive attachment disorder. The referring clinicians wondered what they were missing. When asked what she had hoped to learn or accomplish through the testing, Chandra said that she had no questions for the evaluation. She politely stated that she felt she understood herself well enough.

## Summary of Non-Rorschach Test Results

During the structured interview of psychotic experiences (Child Unusual Belief Scale), when Chandra was directly questioned regarding the presence of key symptoms of psychosis (including hallucinatory experiences and bizarre ideas), she consistently denied these experiences. Furthermore, there was no indication of odd language or derailed thinking during the interview. On cognitive performance tests, Chandra obtained a High Average Full Scale IQ (Wechsler Adult Intelligence Scale—Fourth Edition [WAIS-IV]) and performed well on the tests of achievement (Woodcock–Johnson Achievement Test [WJ-ACH]), indicating that, despite her developmental delays and multitude of behavioral and social difficulties, her academic achievement had kept pace with grade-level expectations. On these and other cognitive measures, similar to the structured interview, Chandra evidenced no signs of disordered thinking or the intrusion of psychotic phenomena. Parent and teacher ratings reflected the known concerns about Chandra's behavioral dyscontrol, inattention, conduct problems, and social withdrawal, but they also reported odd thinking. For example, in a symptom checklist (the Developmental History Questionnaire), her parents endorsed the item "Odd Thinking." Additionally, the Behavior Assessment System for Children, Second Edition (BASC-2), Parent Rating Scales—Adolescent Atypicality score reached a T score of 94. Her parents later elaborated that occasionally Chandra said things that did not make sense to them. Although the Teacher BASC-2 Atypicality scale was not elevated, during an interview with the parents, they mentioned that Chandra's teacher had commented that, when she wrote essays or spoke up in class, her reasoning was sometimes difficult to follow.

In contrast to Chandra's self-reported experiences during the interview, when taking the Personality Assessment Inventory—Adolescent (PAI-A), she privately endorsed a number of positive psychotic symptoms (SCZ-P T = 78). Chandra's acknowledgment of these test items is consistent with the parent and teacher rating scales that identified "odd thinking" as a potential area of concern. But, interestingly, it is inconsistent with the fact she did not openly report or display these characteristics to her referring psychotherapist or psychiatrist.

On the PAI-A, Chandra's reported average levels of depression (DEP T = 53) and only slightly elevated levels of anxiety, which match the generally low level of emotional distress she communicated during the clinical interview. Her elevated PAI-A SOM-H (Health Concerns) subscale score indicates that she may focus a great deal on health-related concerns, specifically her frequent appointments with mental health professionals.

### Introducing R-PAS

Chandra was unfamiliar with the Rorschach. When it was introduced to her, she said that she had never heard of it or seen representations of it in the media or online. Her reaction to the introduction of R-PAS was unremarkable. She sat and listened, as she looked away from the examiner, while drawing designs on her legs with her pen.

Chandra followed the instructions and gave two to three responses to each card. Her reaction time to each card was unremarkable. However, she frequently turned the cards and looked briefly at each new orientation before giving her responses. The length of administration was just short of an hour.

### Behavioral Observations

During the R-PAS administration, Chandra glanced at the examiner briefly. She later commented that she felt uncomfortable looking at people because she was afraid of what they might be thinking about her. While delivering her responses, her affect was flat. She verbalized each response and responded appropriately to queries in the Clarification Phase (CP).

### Discussion of R-PAS Results as Applied to Chandra

Chandra's R-PAS results are summarized below, highlighting areas of potential strength, offset by significant vulnerabilities in thought organization, reality testing, affect management, and self–other relationships. The issue of prodromal features of psychosis is considered throughout the review of Chandra's R-PAS findings. See

Appendix 5.1 at the end of the chapter for Chandra's R-PAS Responses, Location Sheet, Code Sequence, and Page 1 and 2 Profiles.

## A Surprising and Revealing Level of Engagement

Given her flat affect, aloof demeanor, and laconic verbal expression, it was surprising to find that Chandra produced such a rich and revealing R-PAS record (Complexity $SS^1$ = 125), suggesting that she was deeply engaged in the task. On the one hand, her elevated Complexity score suggests the presence of developmentally mature cognitive processing and ideational productivity, which is consistent with her Full Scale IQ of 113. However, an elevated Complexity score should not be automatically taken as a de facto sign of psychological health. In the context of psychological disturbance, elevated Complexity might also signal ideational and affective dyscontrol, resulting in heightened anxiety, emotional flooding, and confusion. R-PAS interpretive guidelines prompt us to review the EII-3 as a global indicator of psychopathology, and Chandra's high EII-3 score (SS = 139) indicates the presence of significant psychopathology. Therefore, we will consider that her ideational complexity may go hand in hand with her pathology and not focus on her Complexity Adjusted scores.

## Thought Disorganization and Impaired Reality Testing

At the heart of the R-PAS results, we encounter extreme elevations on four of eight variables pertaining to thought organization and reality testing and slight elevations on two others. Compared to age-relevant norms, Chandra's scores in the Perception and Thinking Problems domain indicate severe disturbances in in her thinking and reasoning. Two key examples include her overall level of psychopathology (EII-3 SS = 139) and scores suggesting instances of psychotic-level thinking disturbance (SevCog SS = 147). At these extreme elevations, we would expect that when Chandra is left on her own to interpret and form inferences of ambiguous stimuli, she is prone to reason in markedly idiosyncratic and illogical ways. Based simply on these elevations, the presence of a thought disorder is a distinct possibility.

Illustrative examples of Chandra's responses that reflected severely disturbed thinking (Level 2 Cognitive Scores) are given in the following material. Each reflected severe boundary disruptions incompatible with reality.

Card III R11
*And this looks like there are wolves falling from the sky.* INC2

This evocative response combined an aggressive image with incompatible action. The response not only reflects a preoccupation with aggressive themes but also captures a sense of helplessness, as these aggressive figures are seized by illogical forces beyond their control.

Card VII R20
*Looks like two girls that are looking at each other intensely. Looks like there are surprised. Looks like they have worms coming out of their heads. Looks like they are pointing in different directions.*

---
[1] Standard scores (SS) have a mean of 100 and an *SD* of 15.

    CP: *They're looking at each other intensely like they're gonna start a fight or something.* (Worms coming out of their heads?) *These look like worms, like they were rotting.* FAB2

This is another highly evocative thought-disordered response, illogically combining separate images that flagrantly flout reality. The aberrant richness of this response not only brings in an intense, conflicted object relationship (Chandra's nemesis, Delsia?), but also poignantly reflects a graphic sense of mental decompensation.

Card X R31
    *And it looks like there is a rabbit in the middle of the figure. A rabbit where its eyes are, eyes that have green smoke coming out of them.*

    CP: *It's here and this is the smoke, like it's just been poisoned.* FAB2

Chandra completed her Rorschach with another graphic incompatible combination. The imagery combines a docile creature with smoke coming out of its eyes, "like it's just been poisoned." This is the impression that Chandra leaves us with: her final implicit communication of her confusion and struggle with what she may experience as a threatening world.

    In contrast to her severe thinking disturbance captured by the Cognitive Codes, R-PAS variables pertaining to reality testing were clinically within the Average range for her age (FQ−% SS = 114). This discrepancy suggests that whereas Chandra is capable of recognizing cues and forming more conventional impressions of events, her ability to reason and form inferences about what she perceives is disturbed.

    Finally, it is instructive to note that Chandra's style of scanning the environment is characterized by a propensity to focus on uncommon, idiosyncratic blot details (Dd% SS = 116; all Dd99s), and therefore perhaps becoming drawn to very arbitrary, idiographic, or personalized facts or clues. Thus, in addition to the illogical nature of her reasoning in an ambiguous problem-solving task, Chandra also seems to have an odd way of surveying her environment, focusing on idiosyncratic bits of information and often forming inaccurate impressions of what she notices (33% of her Dd responses were FQ−).

    The absence of disturbed language in Chandra's responses (i.e., she received no DRs or DVs) is consistent with why others who spoke with her had not readily identified an underlying disturbance in her thinking. Chandra's thought disorder was characterized by how she perceived the world and how she thought about what she saw. Her disturbance was not represented in disorganized speech or idiosyncratic language. Thus, the Rorschach was more uniquely suited than other measures to identify her difficulties.

### Lack of Awareness of Disturbance

Conducting a posttest inquiry into Chandra's awareness of her disturbed responses goes beyond standard R-PAS administration procedures, but R-PAS recognizes there may be occasions when follow-up questions after the administration is over may be valuable. For Chandra, a posttest inquiry was conducted using the previously described approach developed by Rothschild-Yakar and Lacoua (Lacoua et al., 2015; Rothschild-Yakar et al., 2015) using a 3-point scale (0–Others Would Not See It

This Way; 1–Others Might Agree to a Limited Extent; 2–Others Would See It the Same Way). Following the completion of formal R-PAS administration, the examiner selected Chandra's Level 2 response on Card VII (R20), and, paraphrasing Rothschild-Yakar et al.'s instructions, asked, "Regardless of the shape of the blot, *what might others think* about your response of 'two girls that are looking at each other intensely. . . . Looks like they have worms coming out of their heads'?" Without much pause, Chandra gave her response a rating of 2 and then explained, "It does make sense because logically it looks like worms are coming out of their heads and they're staring at each other. So I guess other people would see this too." Chandra's response suggested an inability to take distance from her thought-disordered response and achieve a realistic social perspective (Harrow & Quinlan, 1985) that would indicate an awareness of her disturbed thinking.

## Affect Management

Although Chandra had an average score on an R-PAS measure that could indicate that her psychological resources are sufficient to cope with distressing experiences (MC–PPD SS = 109), the interpretation of this score must take into account the quality of the related responses. Unfortunately, there were indications of internal turbulence and emotional volatility. For example, negative emotional themes were infused into many of her responses (MOR SS = 131; AGM SS = 125; CritCont% SS = 120). On Card IX, for example, she sees a "forest fire that's begun," followed by a volcano exploding; these together with her elevated [(CF+C)/SumC SS = 128] underscore the potential for poorly modulated primitive aggression. Although Chandra may experience negatively tinged affects in a matter-of-fact way (suggested by YTVC' SS = 84), these emotional themes seemed very much on her mind. A sense of damage, deterioration, conflict, and aggression thematically colored a number of her responses (e.g., R #s 11, 12, 17, 20, 21, 26, 31).

In addition, there are indications that, like Chandra's "wolves falling from the sky," she may be experiencing a vague sense of anxiety resulting from the impingement of external or internal forces, which she cannot control (m SS = 133). In particular, she may have the sense that something dangerous is being stirred within and is ready to emerge. This high degree of unwanted, distracting ideation can interfere with goal-directed thinking, though she may not recognize or be able to describe the stress-related cognitive disorganization.

The impact of early trauma cannot be denied, given what is known about the shocking circumstances of Chandra's early life. Her birth mother had been a victim of sexual abuse. With an older sibling, who was reportedly sexually abused by birth mother, one can only wonder whether Chandra's sexual abuse of her sister Delsia may have reflected the enactment of an earlier history of sexual trauma in Chandra's life as well.

## Experience of Self and Others

Chandra's underlying experience of self and others is seriously problematic in many ways. She seems to have a sense of herself as damaged and possibly deteriorating (MOR SS = 131), and her experiences of self and others are tinged with aggression (AGM SS = 125). As mentioned above, her "falling wolves" response condenses both an aggressive image of a predatory creature with a sense of powerless. Chandra had an elevated score that can indicate striving for autonomy and the ability to see things in a unique and creative manner (SR SS > 150); however, for Chandra, the degree of this score's elevation may reflect her oppositional stance vis-à-vis authority figures or anyone seeking to impose constraint or control on her. Given her own sense of being a victim of forces beyond her control, it is understandable that Chandra may seek ways to exert her control and resist the imposition of control from others.

There is evidence that Chandra exhibits instances of significant misperceptions and misunderstanding of others' experiences (M– SS = 128). Although she may be interested in others, as her high number of whole Human contents (SS = 127) would suggest, her ability to form accurate and realistic impressions of others' internal experiences is limited. Again, she demonstrated this gulf between how she thinks and perceives, on the one hand, and what she assumes other people would think, on the other, when she indicated that others would likely agree with the illogic behind her Card VII response of girls with "worms coming out of their heads."

Chandra surprised us in her attunement and responsivity to interpersonal cues, with above-average COP (SS = 126) and MAH (SS = 129). These are positive signs, which may prove helpful in her psychotherapy, suggesting an ability to perceive relationships as helpful and supportive. In some respects, this might reflect Chandra's ability to draw nurturing figures close to her. Unfortunately, her perception of relationships as benign and caring is offset by her relationally negative view of the world (MOR SS = 131), along with a possible sense of having been damaged at the hands of others. Chandra's ultimate R-PAS response, her final words to Card X, was her association that the "rabbit with green smoke coming out of its eyes" had just been poisoned. Clearly, "poisoning" has a prominent aggressive connotation (AGC, AGM). Thus, we have an encapsulated impression of a core feature of Chandra's paranoid preoccupation and its association to her idiosyncratic thinking.

## Discussion of Chandra's R-PAS Results

R-PAS identified severely disordered thinking and impaired reality testing, which supported a diagnostic impression that Chandra had an emerging psychotic disorder. What made this finding most significant is that disorganized speech, illogical thinking, hallucinations, and bizarre beliefs were not apparent in the clinical interview, nor were they reported by members of her treatment team. Although not notable in the clinical interview, these R-PAS findings were consistent with Chandra's response to a self-report measure of unusual perceptions and ideas that can include delusional beliefs (PAI-A: SCZ-P T = 78; MAN-G T = 75), though to a much more severe level.

Chandra's Rorschach findings were not consistent with Kimhy et al.'s (2007) results, which showed that visual form deficits, more than conceptual disorganization, were hallmark features of psychosis-risk patients. Although she had visual form deficits (FQ–%), her scores reflecting a disturbance in conceptual thinking and reasoning were even higher. However, Chandra's elevated scores in the Perception and Thinking Problems domain were consistent with Ilonen's finding that patients at clinically high risk scored similarly to patients diagnosed with psychotic disorders on the CS Perceptual Thinking Index (Ilonen et al., 2010). Interestingly, there was a significant gender difference among the subjects in the Kimhy and Ilonen studies, with Ilonen's subjects being primarily female. Thus, Chandra's elevated scores in the Perception and Thinking Problems domain, like those among female subjects in the Ilonen study, might also reflect a gender-based difference in thought disorder (Kleiger, 2016).

Finally, it was instructive to find that Chandra did not seem aware of her disturbed thinking or the extent to which others would find her reasoning illogical. According the findings of Israeli researchers (Lacoua et al., 2015; Rothschild-Yakar et al., 2015), Chandra's lack of awareness may be a predictive factor for psychosis risk.

## Impact of R-PAS on Chandra and Her Parents

At an interpretive session, the examiner first met with her parents and then with Chandra to review key assessment findings and recommendations. A detailed report was given to her parents and sent to members of her outpatient team. Additionally, the examiner prepared a brief summary for Chandra, which highlighted major findings in simple, experience-near language.

At a minimum, the recommendations included an individualized education program (IEP) to address Chandra's behavioral, processing, and social problems in school, all of which were having an adverse impact on her education. However, the more pressing issue had to do with finding an alternative educational and therapeutic placement because Chandra had demonstrated that she was unable to manage a large, conventional public high school setting. The principal problem was *not* her intellectual, cognitive, or academic capacities, but her ongoing disorganized thinking, behavioral dysregulation, inability to abide by structure and rules, and deterioration in all areas of psychosocial functioning.

Chandra's parents seemed relieved to have a diagnostic explanation for her deterioration, which went beyond known diagnoses of ADHD, attachment disorder, depression, and a pattern of oppositional behavior. The feedback about a possible emerging psychosis matched their own observations of "odd thinking," which they had acknowledged on rating scales. They further agreed that they were unable to provide a secure setting for Chandra in their home. They voiced an understanding of the recommendation for intensive treatment, beginning with a residential setting that could provide a range of treatment services, including individual, family, group, and milieu therapies, along with supervision and management of her medications. Meeting with a consultant to help them find a suitable residential program would be a first step toward reducing Chandra's risk for a full-blown psychotic episode and addressing her self-destructive behavior, damaged sense of self, and self-defeating pattern of relationships.

Chandra received her summary and feedback with little to no reaction. She asked no questions, even when encouraged to seek further explanation of the findings that indicated she was having difficulty controlling her thoughts and forming accurate impressions of others. When the examiner presented his recommendation for a residential treatment program, Chandra blinked but betrayed no visible affective reaction. She held her copy of a brief summary of the findings and recommendations, folded it when we had finished, and left the room with a brief "goodbye." Months after our last contact, her mother called to inform me that Chandra had been admitted to a residential program that had requested a copy of her testing report.

## Summary of R-PAS Contributions

The Rorschach, conducted according R-PAS procedures, detected impaired reality testing and a severe disturbance in Chandra's thinking that neither the parents nor clinicians had picked up. The fact that these adults in close contact with Chandra did not identify the severity of her thought disorder and disturbed reality testing was understandable, given her lack of peculiar language and the absence of florid psychotic symptoms. Essentially, R-PAS identified what was being masked by Chandra's and her sister's provocative behavior. After all, it was first Delsia's and then Chandra's dramatic behavior that drew all of the attention. Furthermore, Chandra was not complaining of significant depression or anxiety. Most importantly, despite her endorsement of positive symptoms of psychosis on the PAI-A (SCZ-P), she denied many of these experiences when questioned directly in a face-to-face interview format. Thus, one can see how her psychotherapist and psychiatrist might have overlooked more subtle signs of an emerging psychosis. This case also illustrates that in differential diagnosis, especially with adolescents and young adults, one must first rule out psychosis before considering other diagnosis (Kleiger & Khadivi, 2015).

In conclusion, the psychodiagnostic process with Chandra underscored the value of psychological assessment, and R-PAS in particular, in helping identify psychotic-level phenomena and their treatment implications. Recalling Appelbaum's (1977) findings from the Menninger Psychotherapy Research Program, psychological testing was found to be a more potent predictor of diagnosis and treatment outcome than either the clinical interview or the psychosocial history.

## REFERENCES

Addington, J., & Heinssen, R. (2012). Prediction and prevention of psychosis in youth at clinical high risk. *Annual Review of Clinical Psychology, 8,* 269–289.

Appelbaum, S. A. (1977). *The anatomy of change: A Menninger Foundation report on testing and the effects of psychotherapy.* New York: Plenum Press.

Exner, J. E. (2003). *The Rorschach: A Comprehensive System: Vol. 1. Basic foundations* (4th ed.). New York: Wiley.

Fenton, W. S., & McGlashan, T. H. (1994). Antecedents, symptom progression, and long-term outcome of the deficit syndrome in schizophrenia. *American Journal of Psychiatry, 151,* 351–356.

Giromini, L., Viglione, D. J., & McCullaugh, J. (2015). Introducing a Bayesian approach to determining degree of fit with existing Rorschach norms. *Journal of Personality Assessment, 97,* 354–363.

Harrow, M., & Quinlan, D. M. (1985). *Disordered thinking and schizophrenic psychopathology.* New York: Gardner Press.

Holzman, P. S., Levy, D. L., & Johnston, M. H. (2005). The use of the Rorschach technique for assessing formal thought disorder. In R. F. Bornstein & J. M. Masling (Eds.), *Scoring the Rorschach: Seven validated systems* (pp. 55–96). New York: Routledge.

Ilonen, T., Heinimaa, M., Korkeila, J., Svirskis, T., & Salokangas, R. K. R. (2010). Differentiating adolescents at clinical high risk for psychosis from psychotic and non-psychotic patients with the Rorschach. *Psychiatry Research, 179,* 151–156.

Inoue, N., Yorozuya, Y., & Mizuno, M. (2014, July). *Identifying comorbidities of patients at ultra-high risk for psychosis using the Rorschach Comprehensive System.* Paper presented at the XXI International Congress of Rorschach and Projective Methods, Istanbul, Turkey.

Kimhy, D., Corcoran, C., Harkavy-Friedman, J. M., Ritzler, B., Javitt, D. C., & Malaspina, D. (2007). Visual form perception: A comparison of individuals at high risk for psychosis, recent onset schizophrenia and chronic schizophrenia. *Schizophrenia Research, 97,* 25–34.

Kleiger, J. H. (1999). *Disordered thinking and the Rorschach.* Hillsdale, NJ: Analytic Press.

Kleiger, J. H. (2015). An open letter to Hermann Rorschach: What has become of your experiment? *Rorschachiana, 36,* 221–241.

Kleiger, J. H. (2016). Sex, gender identity, and the assessment of psychosis. In V. M. Brabender & J. L. Mihura (Eds.), *Handbook of gender and sexuality in psychological assessment* (pp. 233–255). New York: Routledge.

Kleiger, J. H. (2017). *Rorschach assessment of psychotic phenomena: Clinical, conceptual, and empirical developments.* New York: Routledge.

Kleiger, J. H., & Khadivi, A. (2015). *Assessing psychosis: A clinician's guide.* New York: Routledge.

Lacoua, L., Koren, D., & Rothchild-Yakar, L. (2015, March). *Poor awareness of problems in thought and perception and risk indicators of schizophrenia-spectrum disorders: A correlational study of nonpsychotic adolescents in the community.* Paper presented at the annual meeting of the Society for Personality Assessment, Brooklyn, NY.

Lysaker, P. H., Olesek, K. L., Warman, D. M., Martin, J. M., Salzman, A. K., Nicolo, G., . . . Dimaggio, G. (2011). Metacognition in schizophrenia: Correlates and stability of deficits in theory of mind and self-reflectivity. *Psychiatry Research, 190,* 18–22.

McGlashan, T. H., Walsh, B., & Woods, S. (2010). *The psychosis-risk syndrome: Handbook for diagnosis and follow-up.* New York: Oxford University Press.

Meyer, G. J., Erdberg, P., & Shaffer, T. (2007). Towards international normative reference data for the comprehensive system. *Journal of Personality Assessment, 89*(S1), S201–S216.

Meyer, G. J., Shaffer, T. W., Erdberg, P., & Horn, S. L. (2015). Addressing issues in the development and use of the Composite International Reference Values as Rorschach norms for adults. *Journal of Personality Assessment, 97,* 330–347.

Meyer, G. J., Viglione, D. J., Mihura, J. L., Erard, R. E., & Erdberg, P. (2011). *Rorschach Performance Assessment System: Administration, coding, interpretation, and technical manual.* Toledo, OH: Rorschach Performance Assessment System.

Mihura, J. L., Meyer, G. J., Dumitrascu, N., & Bombel, G. (2013). The validity of individual Rorschach variables: Systematic reviews and meta-analyses of the comprehensive system. *Psychological Bulletin, 139,* 548–605.

Rapaport, D., Gill, M. M., & Schafer, R. (1946). *Diagnostic psychological testing* (Vol. 2). Chicago: Year Book.

Rorschach, H. (1942). *Psychodiagnostik* (H. H. Verlag, Trans.). Bern, Switzerland: Bircher. (Original work published 1921)

Rothschild-Yakar, L., Lacoua, L., Brener, A., & Koren, D. (2015, March). *Impairments in interpersonal representations and deficits in social cognition as predictors of risk for schizophrenia in non-patient adolescents.* Paper presented at the annual meeting of the Society for Personality Assessment, Brooklyn, NY.

Viglione, D. J., & Giromini, L. (2016). The effects of using the International versus Comprehensive System norms for children, adolescents, and adults. *Journal of Personality Assessment, 98,* 391–397.

Yung, A. R., & McGorry, P. D. (2007). Prediction of psychosis: Setting the stage. *British Journal of Psychiatry, 191*(Suppl. 51), 1–8.

# APPENDIX 5.1. Chandra's Responses, Location Sheet, Code Sequence, and Page 1 and 2 Profiles

## Rorschach Responses "Chandra"

| Respondent ID: Chandra | Examiner: James H Kleiger |
|---|---|
| Location: Office, Private Practice | Date: **/**/**** |
| Start Time: 11:00 A.M. | End Time: 11:50 A.M. |

| Cd # | R # | Or | Response | Clarification | R-Opt |
|---|---|---|---|---|---|
| I | 1 | | It looks like two people holding onto to a pole. (D4) | E: (Examiner Repeats Response [ERR].)<br>R: In the middle there. One person on each side. There and there. | |
| | 2 | | Second is a man with wings who is going around in circles. Reminds me of one of those windmill things you can have on top of the house, and when the wind blows it goes around in circles. (D7) | E: (ERR)<br>R: Right there. The man and there is his wings. | |
| | 3 | < | < Am I allowed to put it at different angles?<br>E: Up to you.<br>R: Looks like the back part of a key. (W) | E: (ERR)<br>R: All of it. Just the way it was angled. | |
| | 4 | | >^ Now looking at it forward, it looks like Batman. A Batman design. (Dd99 = upper half of W)<br>E: (Remember, I asked for two, maybe three responses.) | E: (ERR)<br>R: Just here. Kind of looks like the design of Batman the way the wings are and the way the head (Dd22) had two humps on it. | Pu |
| II | 5 | | It looks like two ducks that are hi-fiving each other. (D2, D4) | E: (ERR)<br>R: All of this. [Circles upper part of the card.]<br>E: Ducks?<br>R: Just the shape of the head (D2) reminded me of a duck. | |
| | 6 | | In the center there is . . . looks like sort of a temple. (Dd99 = DS5 + more than D4) | E: (ERR)<br>R: You can see the shape of the temple (DS5) and there's the shape of a cross (D4) and there are stairs (protrusions into DdS29 and above) there where those bumps are leading up to the top. | |
| | 7 | | And also a mark in it that also looks like a butterfly. (D3) | E: (ERR)<br>R: Well, the way it is symmetrical on both sides and the way the top looks like the way a butterfly would look and the long tail at the end. A butterfly has that. | |
| III | 8 | | It looks like two women are holding onto a pot or making something. (D1) | E: (ERR)<br>R: Here they (D9) are, like they are stirring something (D7).<br>E: Pot?<br>R: Between them. The outline of it. | |
| | 9 | | But when you look in the middle, it looks like a bow. (D3) | E: (ERR)<br>R: It has that center piece and sort of a heart design that reminds me of a bow. | |
| | 10 | | And when I look below it, it looks like a river leading up to a castle. (D8) | E: (ERR)<br>R: (Respondent indicates D8).<br>E: River?<br>R: Kind of looks like a reflection in the white section from the top.<br>E: Castle?<br>R: In the white part, looks like a bridge leading up to something in the middle that's symmetrical on both sides.<br>E: Leading up?<br>R: It's next to it. | |
| | 11 | > | > And this looks like there are wolves falling from the sky. (D2)<br>E: (Remember, please give two, maybe three responses.) | E: (ERR)<br>R: Here are the wolves. It reminds me of them. I kind of saw ears and it looks like a long tail there. | Pu |

96

| Cd # | R # | Or | Response | Clarification | R-Opt |
|------|-----|----|----------|---------------|-------|
| IV | 12 | | A skeleton, no a praying mantis, and it looks like he is really angry. (D3, D4, D6) | E: (ERR)<br>R: The praying mantis. There are its pincers (D4) and head (D3). That's it, just the head.<br>E: You said angry?<br>R: The way he's standing with big feet (D6) kind of reminded me of anger.<br>E: You said just the head. Feet?<br>R: It's not part of the praying mantis.<br>E: I'm confused, can you help me with this?<br>R: Kind of looks like big feet that are sticking out of it that imply the praying mantis is angry.<br>[In a fragmented way, Chandra apparently used only D3, D4, and D6 to construct her response of the praying mantis.] | |
| | 13 | | When I look down here, there's a tree trunk. (D1) | E: (ERR)<br>R: The roots are at the bottom. There are the roots. | |
| | 14 | | And it looks like there are two horns sticking out of the side of it that belong to a bull. (D4) | E: (ERR)<br>R: The horns belong to the bull.<br>E: Bull?<br>R: Just the horns there. | |
| V | 15 | | Looks like a bat because the way the wings are formed. (W) | E: (ERR)<br>R: The whole thing. The wings (D4) are sorta webbed together. | |
| | 16 | > | > Sideways looks like a bird with its mouth open. (Dd99 = W – Dd34) | E: (ERR)<br>R: Just there (circles, omitting Dd34). The wings and mouth. | |
| VI | 17 | | It looks like a cat that is looking out the window and has a big bump on its head. (Dd99 = [W – lower ¼ of D1] + surrounding white space) | E: (ERR)<br>R: There's the cat (Dd99 = W– lower ¼ of D1), here.<br>E: Looking out the window?<br>R: The blank space kind of looked like a window (points to space between D3 and D1).<br>E: What about that?<br>R: It is blank there and you don't see the cat's eyes, which are looking forward, and it just looks like a cat looking out the window because that's what cats normally do.<br>E: Bump?<br>R: There.<br>[Bump = Dd23, Head = D3. Body = upper ¾ of D1] | |
| | 18 | V | V Upside down it looks like a tree that is beginning to grow out of the ground. (Dd99 = W – Dd22) | E: (ERR)<br>R: Trunk (D6) and the way the inkblot has a bushy top<br>E: Bushy?<br>R: It's wide and there are things sticking out of it like a tree would have. | |
| | 19 | | At top of the cat figure it looks like there is a bug, like a spider with wings. (D3) | E: (ERR)<br>R: Here I see eight legs and wings, and the only thing I know to have eight legs is a spider. | |
| VII | 20 | | Looks like two girls that are looking at each other intensely. Looks like they are surprised. Looks like they have worms coming out of their heads. Looks like they are pointing in different directions. (D2) | E: (ERR)<br>R: They're looking at each other intensely like they're gonna start a fight or something.<br>E: Worms coming out of their heads?<br>R: These look like worms (D5), like they were rotting.<br>E: Surprised?<br>R: It looks like their eyes were wide open like "Oh!" | |
| | 21 | | Looks like two ants that aren't sure where to go. They look confused. (W) | E: (ERR)<br>R: They're ants (Dd22s) because of the segments right here.<br>E: Confused?<br>R: The facial expressions, like "Wait, which way are we supposed to go?" | |
| | 22 | v | v Looks like there is a mushroom in the center of the two girls or ants. (DS7) | E: (ERR)<br>R: It has a cap (DS10) and stalk like mushrooms have. | |

| Cd # | R # | Or | Response | Clarification | R-Opt |
|---|---|---|---|---|---|
| VIII | 23 | | Looks like a beetle. The back of a beetle. (W) | E: (ERR)<br>R: All of it is kind of rounded at the edges, and it looks like the back of it is here and up here is the front. | |
| | 24 | | I see a skeleton of an antelope, and it looks like I see beavers crawling up the side of it and reaching. (W) | E: (ERR)<br>R: The skeleton is here (DS3).<br>E: Skeleton?<br>R: Its shape, and it just looks like beavers (D1) here. Looks like they're reaching up to something.<br>E: Crawling up the side?<br>R: A mountain (D6) or something. | |
| | 25 | v | v Upside down the white space in the middle looks like two people sitting down at the dinner table. (Dd99 = DdS28s+DdS32, D5) | E: (ERR)<br>R: (Respondent indicates DdS99). Here you see the people (both ½ of Dd32+28) and the table (D5).<br>E: Table?<br>R: It's rounded at top. | |
| IX | 26 | v | v It looks like a forest fire that's begun. (D11,6) | E: (ERR)<br>R: The greenery (D1) right here and there's the fire (D6) coming up.<br>E: Fire?<br>R: Because it's red and there is smoke.<br>E: Smoke?<br>R: The green. | |
| | 27 | v | v Also looks like a volcano is exploding. (Dd99 = W − D11) | E: (ERR)<br>R: The whole thing, no, it's just this part. It's tan down at the bottom (D3s) for rocky color and looks like it's erupting because of lava (D6) coming out of the center or epicenter. | |
| | 28 | v | v Looks like a girl that has bushy hair (D6) and a long dress (D3) and it looks like she has wings (D11). (W) | E: (ERR)<br>R: A girl because girls usually wear dresses.<br>E: Dress?<br>R: The way it's shaped at the edges. | |
| X | 29 | | Like two types of dust mites on the side of it. (D1) | E: (ERR)<br>R: I've seen dust mites before and they have many legs, and the way it was shaped reminded me of dust mites. | |
| | 30 | | And it looks like there are fleas on top of what look like two cliffs and they're holding onto what looks like a pole. (D11, 9) | E: (ERR)<br>R: Fleas (D8) are small and look like they have two legs for jumping.<br>E: Pole?<br>R: Up here (D14) and looks like they're holding on because their antennas are touching the pole. | |
| | 31 | < | < And it looks like there is a rabbit in the middle of the figure. A rabbit where its eyes are, eyes that have green smoke coming out of them. (D10) | E: (ERR)<br>R: It's here (D5) and this is the smoke (D4) like it's just been poisoned. | |

# Rorschach Performance Assessment System (R-PAS)®

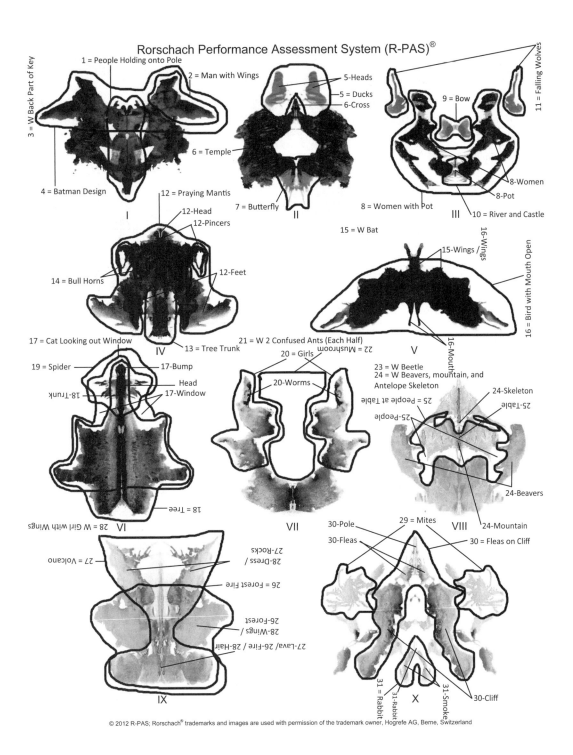

1 = People Holding onto Pole
2 = Man with Wings
3 = W Back Part of Key
4 = Batman Design
I

5-Heads
5 = Ducks
6-Cross
6 = Temple
7 = Butterfly
II

11 = Falling Wolves
9 = Bow
8-Women
8-Pot
8 = Women with Pot
10 = River and Castle
III

12 = Praying Mantis
12-Head
12-Pincers
12-Feet
14 = Bull Horns
13 = Tree Trunk
IV

15 = W Bat
16-Wings
15-Wings
16 = Bird with Mouth Open
16-Mouth
V

17 = Cat Looking out Window
19 = Spider
17-Bump
Head
17-Window
18-Trunk
18 = Tree
28 = W Girl with Wings
VI

21 = W 2 Confused Ants (Each Half)
20 = Girls
20-Worms
22 = Mushroom
VII

23 = W Beetle
24 = W Beavers, mountain, and Antelope Skeleton
25 = People at Table
24-Skeleton
25-Table
25-People
24-Beavers
24-Mountain
VIII

27 = Volcano
28-Dress / 27-Rocks
26 = Forest Fire
26-Forest
28-Wings / 26-Forest
27-Lava/ 26-Fire / 28-Hair
IX

30-Pole
30-Fleas
29 = Mites
30 = Fleas on Cliff
31 = Rabbit
31-Rabbit
31-Smoke
30-Cliff
X

# R-PAS Code Sequence: "Chandra"

**C-ID**: Chandra      **P-ID**: 159      **Age**: 17      **Gender**: Female      **Education**: 11

| Cd | # | Or | Loc | Loc # | SR | SI | Content | Sy | Vg | 2 | FQ | P | Determinants | Cognitive | Thematic | HR | ODL (RP) | R-Opt |
|---|---|---|---|---|---|---|---|---|---|---|---|---|---|---|---|---|---|---|
| I | 1 | | D | 4 | | | H,NC | Sy | | 2 | o | | Mp | | | GH | | |
| | 2 | | D | 7 | | | H,Art | | | | u | | Mp | | | GH | | |
| | 3 | < | W | | | | NC | | | | - | | F | | | | | |
| | 4 | | Dd | 99 | | | (A),Art | | | | u | | F | | | | | Pu |
| II | 5 | | Dd | 99 | | | A | Sy | | 2 | u | | Ma | FAB1 | COP,MAH | GH | | |
| | 6 | | Dd | 99 | SR | SI | NC | Sy | | | u | | F | | | | | |
| | 7 | | D | 3 | | | A | | | | o | | F | | | | | |
| III | 8 | | D | 1 | | | H,NC | Sy | | 2 | o | P | Ma | | COP,MAH | GH | | |
| | 9 | | D | 3 | | | Cg | | | | o | | F | | | | | |
| | 10 | | D | 8 | SR | SI | NC | Sy | | | - | | F | | | | | |
| | 11 | > | D | 2 | | | A | | | 2 | - | | FMp | INC2 | AGC | | | Pu |
| IV | 12 | | D | 3,4,6 | | | A | | | | u | | Ma | INC1 | AGM,AGC | PH | ODL | |
| | 13 | | D | 1 | | | NC | | | | o | | F | | | | | |
| | 14 | | D | 4 | | | Ad | | | 2 | u | | F | | AGC | | | |
| V | 15 | | W | | | | A | | | | o | P | F | | | | | |
| | 16 | > | Dd | 99 | | | A | | | | u | | FMp | | | | ODL | |
| VI | 17 | | Dd | 99 | | SI | A,NC | Sy | | | - | | FMp | | MOR | | | |
| | 18 | v | Dd | 99 | | | NC | | | | u | | ma | | | | | |
| | 19 | | D | 3 | | | A | | | | o | | F | INC1 | | | | |
| VII | 20 | | D | 2 | | | H,A | Sy | | 2 | u | P | Ma,mp | FAB2 | AGM,MOR,MAP | PH | | |
| | 21 | v | W | | | | A | | | 2 | - | | Mp | INC1 | | PH | | |
| | 22 | v | D | 7 | SR | | NC | | | | o | | F | | | | | |
| VIII | 23 | | W | | | | A | | | | - | | F | | | | | |
| | 24 | | W | | SR | | A,An,NC | Sy | | | u | P | FMa | | MOR | | | |
| | 25 | v | Dd | 99 | SR | SI | H,NC | Sy | | 2 | - | | Mp | | COP | PH | ODL | |
| IX | 26 | v | D | 6, 11 | | | Fi,NC | Sy | | | u | | ma,CF | | AGC,MAP | | | |
| | 27 | v | Dd | 99 | | | Ex,NC | Sy | | | u | | ma,CF | | AGC | | | |
| | 28 | v | W | | | | H,Cg | Sy | | | u | | F | INC1 | | PH | | |
| X | 29 | | D | 1 | | | A | | | 2 | o | | F | | PER | | | |
| | 30 | | D | 9, 11 | | | A,NC | Sy | | | o | | FMp | FAB1 | | | | |
| | 31 | < | D | 10 | | | A,Fi | | | | u | | mp,CF | FAB2 | MOR,MAP | | | |

©2010-2016 R-PAS

## R-PAS Summary Scores and Profiles – Page 1

C-ID: Chandra   P-ID: 159   Age: 17   Gender: Female   Education: 11

| Domain/Variables | Raw Scores | Raw A-SS | Raw C-SS | Cplx. Adj. A-SS | Cplx. Adj. C-SS | Standard Score Profile R-Optimized | Abbr. |
|---|---|---|---|---|---|---|---|
| **Admin. Behaviors and Obs.** | | | | | | 60 70 80 90 100 110 120 130 140 | |
| Pr | 0 | 89 | 91 | | | | Pr |
| Pu | 2 | 125 | 150 | | | | Pu |
| CT (Card Turning) | 11 | 122 | 122 | | | | CT |
| **Engagement and Cog. Processing** | | | | | | 60 70 80 90 100 110 120 130 140 | |
| Complexity | 105 | 118 | 125 | | | | Cmplx |
| R (Responses) | 31 | 120 | 127 | 109 | 111 | | R |
| F% [Lambda=0.82] (Simplicity) | 45% | 104 | 96 | 114 | 106 | | F% |
| Blend | 4 | 102 | 103 | 78 | 86 | | Bln |
| Sy | 13 | 123 | 126 | 108 | 110 | | Sy |
| MC | 11.0 | 115 | 122 | 100 | 102 | | MC |
| MC - PPD | 1.0 | 111 | 109 | 114 | 112 | | MC-PPD |
| M | 8 | 122 | 129 | 109 | 111 | | M |
| M/MC [8/11.0] | 73% | 114 | 114 | 112 | 113 | | M Prp |
| (CF+C)/SumC [3/3] | 100% | 126 | 128 | 126 | 128 | | CFC Prp |
| **Perception and Thinking Problems** | | | | | | 60 70 80 90 100 110 120 130 140 | |
| EII-3 | 2.3 | 135 | 139 | 132 | 136 | | EII |
| TP-Comp (Thought & Percept. Com…) | 3.2 | 142 | 132 | 142 | 128 | | TP-C |
| WSumCog | 34 | 136 | >150 | 135 | 147 | | WCog |
| SevCog | 3 | 131 | 147 | 131 | 147 | | Sev |
| FQ-% | 23% | 126 | 114 | 124 | 111 | | FQ-% |
| WD-% | 22% | 127 | 114 | 119 | 109 | | WD-% |
| FQo% | 32% | 72 | 79 | 73 | 80 | | FQo% |
| P | 4 | 88 | 94 | 87 | 93 | | P |
| **Stress and Distress** | | | | | | 60 70 80 90 100 110 120 130 140 | |
| YTVC' | 0 | 73 | 84 | 73 | 71 | | YTVC' |
| m | 5 | 125 | 133 | 115 | 117 | | m |
| Y | 0 | 85 | 89 | 85 | 79 | | Y |
| MOR | 4 | 123 | 131 | 120 | 125 | | MOR |
| SC-Comp (Suicide Concern Comp.) | 4.7 | 103 | 101 | 91 | 91 | | SC-C |
| **Self and Other Representation** | | | | | | 60 70 80 90 100 110 120 130 140 | |
| ODL% | 10% | 101 | 106 | 95 | 99 | | ODL% |
| SR (Space Reversal) | 5 | 132 | >150 | 132 | >150 | | SR |
| MAP/MAHP [3/5] | 60% | 102 | 101 | 106 | 105 | | MAP Prp |
| PHR/GPHR [5/9] | 56% | 115 | 108 | 115 | 108 | | PHR Prp |
| M- | 2 | 123 | 128 | 123 | 128 | | M- |
| AGC | 5 | 116 | 113 | 111 | 109 | | AGC |
| H | 6 | 123 | 127 | 115 | 115 | | H |
| COP | 3 | 120 | 126 | 114 | 117 | | COP |
| MAH | 2 | 116 | 129 | 104 | 108 | | MAH |

A-SS = Adult Standard Score; C-SS = Age-Based Child or Adolescent Standard Score

C-ID: Chandra   P-ID: 159   Age: 17   Gender: Female   Education: 11

| Domain/Variables | Raw Scores | Raw A-SS | Raw C-SS | Cplx. Adj. A-SS | Cplx. Adj. C-SS | Standard Score Profile R-Optimized | Abbr. |
|---|---|---|---|---|---|---|---|
| **Engagement and Cog. Processing** | | | | | | | |
| W% | 19% | 85 | 85 | 74 | 79 | | W% |
| Dd% | 26% | 114 | 116 | 115 | 119 | | Dd% |
| SI (Space Integration) | 4 | 111 | 113 | 108 | 109 | | SI |
| IntCont | 2 | 100 | 104 | 91 | 93 | | IntC |
| Vg% | 0% | 86 | 88 | 87 | 89 | | Vg% |
| V | 0 | 92 | 91 | 92 | 77 | | V |
| FD | 0 | 88 | 90 | 88 | 85 | | FD |
| R8910% | 29% | 92 | 94 | 94 | 96 | | R8910% |
| WSumC | 3.0 | 99 | 101 | 84 | 87 | | WSC |
| C | 0 | 95 | 92 | 95 | 92 | | C |
| Mp/(Ma+Mp) [4/8] | 50% | 104 | 103 | 104 | 103 | | Mp Prp |
| **Perception and Thinking Problems** | | | | | | | |
| FQu% | 45% | 120 | 118 | 117 | 114 | | FQu% |
| **Stress and Distress** | | | | | | | |
| PPD | 10 | 103 | 107 | 87 | 93 | | PPD |
| CBlend | 0 | 91 | 90 | 91 | 72 | | CBlnd |
| C' | 0 | 84 | 86 | 84 | 74 | | C' |
| V | 0 | 92 | 91 | 92 | 77 | | V |
| CritCont% (Critical Contents) | 32% | 113 | 120 | 109 | 114 | | CrCt |
| **Self and Other Representation** | | | | | | | |
| SumH | 6 | 101 | 100 | 87 | 87 | | SumH |
| NPH/SumH [0/6] | 0% | 65 | 59 | 66 | 62 | | NPH Prp |
| V-Comp (Vigilance Composite) | 4.0 | 110 | 109 | 95 | 95 | | V-C |
| r (Reflections) | 0 | 95 | 92 | 95 | 92 | | r |
| p/(a+p) [10/18] | 56% | 110 | 109 | 111 | 109 | | p Prp |
| AGM | 2 | 121 | 125 | 121 | 125 | | AGM |
| T | 0 | 91 | 90 | 91 | 90 | | T |
| PER | 1 | 109 | 104 | 109 | 104 | | PER |
| An | 1 | 99 | 102 | 99 | 102 | | An |

A-SS = Adult Standard Score; C-SS = Age-Based Child or Adolescent Standard Score

© 2010-2016 R-PAS

# CHAPTER 6

# An Inpatient R-PAS Case
# with a Recent Suicide Attempt

## Ali Khadivi

### Introduction and Reason for the Referral

"I took rat poison to die." This was the first thing "Mary," a 32-year-old Caucasian married woman, verbalized, with sadness, as she woke up in a medical emergency room of a major urban hospital. She was admitted after medical clearance to the inpatient psychiatric service following a near-lethal suicide attempt. One week into Mary's hospitalization, the inpatient treatment team requested a psychological assessment to assist in developing a suicide risk formulation. Suicide has a low base rate, and, as a result, the goal of a suicide risk assessment is not prediction; rather, the aim is to identify individualized risk and protective factors, and to develop case-specific treatment strategies to mitigate the risk (American Psychiatric Association, 2003; Jacobs & Brewer, 2006). Therefore, the treatment team was interested in identifying case-specific suicide risk and protective factors, as well as determining how best to manage her suicide risk postdischarge. Although Mary denied current symptoms of depression and suicidal ideation, she did appear to the treatment team as "internally preoccupied with severe flat affect." As a result, the treatment team wanted to know if there was an underlying psychotic process and, if so, to what extent psychosis played a part in her suicide risk.

### Mary's Suicide Attempt

Based on the psychiatric evaluation, consisting of a record review, collateral information from her family, a direct psychiatric evaluation, and observation of her behavior on the ward, the inpatient psychiatric treatment team's initial diagnostic impression was that Mary was clinically depressed and had multiple suicide risk factors. They identified two major precipitants for her suicide attempt. Approximately 3 months prior to Mary's hospitalization, her 7-year-old son had developed a severe seizure condition. According to the family, Mary was "devastated" to see her son develop a neurological condition at such an early age. Her husband responded to the stress of his son's medical condition by drinking and engaging in online gambling, a long-standing habit that he had kept secret from Mary. One day prior to her suicide attempt, she found out that her husband had lost the modest savings that she had accumulated, to gambling. They proceeded to argue and she reportedly "felt stressed out" and was "not thinking straight." She started having intense suicidal ideation throughout that evening, which continued on to the next day.

On the day of her suicide attempt, after her husband went to work, she went to the kitchen and consumed a whole container of rat poison that her family had purchased long ago for a rodent problem. She then texted her husband and told him that she was not feeling well, and that he should pick their son up from school. Her husband reportedly became concerned when she did not reply to his text in the afternoon and decided to come home. He called 911 when he saw her on the kitchen floor.

From the time of the admission to her arrival on the inpatient unit, Mary denied any current depression or suicidal thoughts, plan, or intention. She indicated to the staff that she was stressed out and her suicide attempt was "a mistake" and she "never again would do such a thing." The treatment team also noted that Mary had difficulty identifying and expressing her emotions. Nursing staff described her as a pleasant, cooperative woman who appeared depressed and socially withdrawn, and preoccupied with seeing her son and being discharged from the hospital. Although her family, including her husband, visited her regularly, she felt unsupported by them. She perceived her mother to be "depressed and self-absorbed" and felt "betrayed" by her husband's actions.

## Client Background

Mary described her childhood as a "living hell," indicating that her alcoholic father was emotionally abusive, and, more importantly, that he would verbally "lash out" at the family without any apparent reason. She and her younger sister, who corroborated the history, indicated that the family was always in a "terrified state of mind." Mary reported that despite frequent displays of unpredictable rage, her father never physically abused the family. She reported no other traumatic history.

Mary described her mother as "overwhelmed and depressed," and reported that she was on antidepressive medication. Her parents divorced when she was 16 years old because her mother could not take the verbal abuse anymore; her father, she reported, died in a car accident shortly thereafter. According to the family, the father hit a parked trailer truck when he was exiting the highway. Mary is not sure if her father's death was an accident or a suicide. Mary's mother reported that the father was distraught over the divorce. According to the family, the father's autopsy results revealed high levels of PCP (angel dust). In addition, the family reported that the police found empty beer bottles in his car.

Mary indicated that she was an average student. She had attended regular classes and obtained her high school diploma at age 18. She had worked in a supermarket as a cashier for 3 years before accepting a job as a home attendant.

Mary described herself as a cautious person who has few friends but cares deeply for her friends and family. Although not religious, she described herself as having a strong sense of "right and wrong." She reported no history of substance abuse, impulsivity, or high-risk behavior. With regard to her intimate relationships, she stated that she had dated one man when she was 20 years old and married her high school boyfriend at age 24.

Mary reported that she has periodically struggled with sad mood but had not sought help until age 25, when she developed postpartum depression after giving birth to her son. Her mother told the treatment team that Mary was very depressed, with intense feelings of self-deprecation, loss of interest in daily life, severe insomnia, and loss of appetite. Mary indicated that she was treated with Prozac 20 mg and once-per-week supportive therapy for 6 months. She reported that her postpartum depression responded well to treatment, and that by end of the 6 months, she was symptom-free. Both Mary and her family reported that she had made no past suicide attempts. However, Mary reported that she has had suicidal ideation throughout her life.

## Psychological Assessment of the Case

A multimethod psychological evaluation is essential to answering the referral questions for Mary's assessment, which, in this case, was to develop a suicide risk formulation and to clarify the possibility of underlying psychosis. In addition to the unstructured clinical interview and records review (which included access to collateral information and hospital records), a multiscale self-report inventory—the Personality Assessment Inventory (PAI)—was used to assess her general level of psychopathology, extent of suicide ideation, and response style. A structured interview-based suicide risk assessment tool—the Columbia-Suicide Severity Rating Scale (C-SSRS; Posner et al., 2011)—was used to systematically gather lifetime and current evidence-based suicide risk factors. Finally, a performance-based broad personality measure—the Rorschach Performance Assessment System (R-PAS; Meyer, Viglione, Mihura, Erard, & Erdberg, 2011)—was used.

## Testing and Clinical Interview Findings

Mary was cooperative and well engaged with the psychological assessment. She reportedly was feeling better and her affect was no longer flat. At the time of the assessment, Mary was in full adherence with her psychiatric treatment, which in addition to milieu therapy, consisted of antidepressants (Prozac 20 mg), supportive therapy by her resident psychiatrist, and family meetings with her social worker.

The psychological assessment was conducted 1 week into her inpatient hospitalization. During the clinical interview, Mary did not display any overt depressive or psychotic symptoms; she also gave no history consistent with manic or psychotic symptoms.

The association between suicide and negative emotions such as humiliation, shame, anger, loss, and severe anxiety is well documented (American Psychiatric Association, 2003; Simon, 2004). Understanding and identifying the emotional triggers for suicidal behavior can potentially guide the clinician to help patients recognize the negative emotional state and to develop strategies to reduce its impact.

Using the unstructured clinical interview, Mary was invited to explore and explain how she was feeling prior to her suicide attempt and what about the fight with her husband had triggered her to ingest rat poison. Mary had difficulty articulating her feeling state, but she did indicate that during the course of the argument with her husband, he told her that she had brought a "damaged child" into this world. Mary recalls that she was "very upset" by that comment but could not elaborate what it meant to her. Her husband reportedly apologized immediately after making the comment, but it was too late.

The C-SSRS, a structured interview, systematically assesses lifetime suicidal behavior, including aborted and interrupted attempts, degree of past and current suicidal ideation or planning, and other related suicide risk factors. Mary reported that when she had suffered from postpartum depression 7 years ago, she seriously considered killing herself and admitted that she had aborted a suicide attempt, in which she opened a bottle of Tylenol but decided not to go through with it. On the C-SSRS, she revealed that the severity of her suicidal ideation prior to her current attempt was the worst ever.

On the PAI, Mary produced a valid profile with no evidence of inconsistencies (INC T = 52 & INF T = 55). She also did not engage in any symptom overreporting (NIM T = 59) or underreporting (PIM T = 50).

Mary's PAI profile indicates that she is currently experiencing significant stress (STR T = 89) and very limited perceived support (NON T = 88). Surprisingly, she showed only one significant elevation on the clinical scales and subscales. The PAI scales that measure anxiety (ANX T = 47), depression (DEP T = 48), anxiety-related disorders and trauma (ARD T = 56, ARD-T T = 58), manic symptoms (MAN T = 53, MAN-A T = 57, MAN-G T = 40), and schizophrenia and psychotic experiences (SCZ T = 42, SCZ-P T = 43, SCZ-T T = 43) were all well below a T score of 70. The most elevated clinical scale was PAR-P, a Persecution scale (T = 72), suggesting that Mary is prone to interpersonal sensitivity and to feel that others are trying to undermine her efforts or interests. However, given her history and her recent experiences with her husband, her elevated score is understandable.

With regard to suicide risk, Mary showed moderate elevations on a PAI scale that measures varying degrees of suicidal ideation ranging from passive to active (SUI T = 66). Consistent with her clinical presentation on the unit, she did not endorse any items measuring active suicidal ideation. Her Suicide Potential Index (SPI), which is not comprised of suicidal ideation items but is instead made up of the PAI scales and subscales that are associated with increased suicide risk, was not elevated (T = 59).

On a positive side, Mary demonstrated good treatment prognostic signs. She reported being motivated to make changes (RXR T = 35) and her Treatment Progress Index (TPI), which measures negative treatment indicators, was well below the recommended cutoff of 7 (i.e., 2, T = 55). Consistent with her history, she had no clinical elevations on scales assessing substance abuse (DRG T = 48, ALC T = 41) or severe personality disorders (ANT T = 38, BOR T = 53).

## Summary of Suicide Risk Factors in Non-R-PAS Assessment Findings

The PAI findings indicated that Mary is experiencing significant environmental and situational stress, and feels alone and unsupported. She perceives others as uncaring and does not believe that they are there for her. She is quick to feel that others might be rejecting of her and may undermine her efforts and interests. The PAI revealed a moderate elevation of suicidal ideation.

The clinical interview and C-SSRS indicated that Mary has multiple suicide risk factors, including a recent near-lethal suicide attempt, a past aborted attempt, intense recent suicidal ideation, a past proclivity toward major depression, financial stress and family problems, and a family history of depression and possible suicide. More importantly, the stressors that triggered her suicide attempt are still unresolved.

Mary lacks social support and has limited protective factors. For instance, she has no cultural or religious belief against suicide. Furthermore, although she has a child living with her at home (which is usually considered to be a protective factor), in her case, having her son at home did not prevent her from attempting suicide, and his presence should not be considered a protective factor. However, on the positive side, she has no evidence of substance abuse or of borderline or antisocial personality features.

## Mary's Assessment Question

Mary had only one assessment question. She wondered, "What is wrong with me, how could I try to kill myself? I love my son."

## Why R-PAS for Mary's Suicide Risk Assessment?

As indicated before, the aim of a suicide risk assessment is to identify case-specific risk factors and develop management and treatment plans to mitigate the risk. The suicide risk factors are divided into two groups: (1) static risk factors such as gender, past suicide attempt, family history of suicide; and (2) dynamic risk factors such as level of depression, anxiety, reality testing, and emotional dysregulation. Assessing dynamic risk factors is essential because they are the ones that potentially can be modified to reduce suicide risk (American Psychiatric Association, 2003). The Rorschach can contribute to the assessment of suicide risk by identifying relevant dynamic psychological risk factors that go beyond introspective self-report. Recent meta-analyses by Mihura and colleagues (Mihura, Meyer, Dumitrascu, & Bombel, 2013) demonstrated that the Rorschach is an empirically robust method for assessing a number of personality and psychological functioning variables that have behavioral correlates—psychosis, in particular.

R-PAS (Meyer et al., 2011), with a more solid empirical base than any other Rorschach method, can significantly contribute to the development of a suicide risk formulation in three important ways. First, R-PAS has a general measure for suicide risk (the Suicide Concern Composite, SC-Comp). This empirically validated measure is related to completed suicide or serious suicidal behavior with intent to die. A notable elevation on this index indicates that the individual has characteristics similar to people who are at an increased risk for suicide or serious self-harm behavior. The fact that this index correlates with suicidal behavior rather than suicidal ideation or self-mutilation makes it particularly useful in suicide risk assessment.

There is a growing body of literature on suicide risk assessment that has determined that many individuals either (1) commit suicide impulsively without fully expressing suicidal ideation (Simon, 2004) or (2) have suicidal ideation that they choose not to reveal to an examining clinician (Shea, 2009). For example, in a review of inpatient suicides (patients who killed themselves while on the unit), 77% did not express any suicidal ideation in their last contact with inpatient staff before killing themselves. However, most were severely agitated. Another study found that 25% of patients in a psychiatric emergency room denied suicidal ideation to their examining psychiatrists, but nearly all had reported suicidal thoughts to their family members (Simon, 2004). Therefore, elevated SC-Comp informs the examiner that a further risk assessment, which goes beyond self-report of suicidal ideation, is required.

Second, R-PAS has an empirically validated measure (YTVC') that, when used with less psychologically healthy individuals, can identify implicit distress, characterized by negative emotions including anxiousness, irritation, dysphoria, loneliness, or helplessness. In addition, Morbid (MOR) responses on R-PAS can identify underlying dysphoric ideations and perceptions of the self as being damaged or flawed—all of which are important dynamic suicide risk factors.

Third, R-PAS has a robust number of empirically supported measures that assess the capacity for psychological adaptation, including (1) the degree of internal resources (MC) and stress tolerance (MC–PPD), (2) the capacity for reality testing (FQ–%), (3) the extent to which thinking is organized and logical (WSumCog and SevCog), and (4) the degree of sophistication in interpersonal templates, including healthy versus pathological internal representations of others (MAP/MAHP) and the capacity to understand people and relationships (PHR/GPHR). These psychological functions are essential in understanding and developing suicide risk management strategies.

In this case, one of the key referral questions concerned the presence of psychosis, which is a significant suicide risk factor (American Psychiatric Association, 2003). The use of R-PAS is especially indicated to answer the referral question because it has strong empirical support for assessing reality testing impairment and thinking disturbance, which are core features of psychosis (Mihura et al., 2013).

## Introducing R-PAS to Mary

R-PAS was introduced to Mary using the recommended R-PAS instructions. Mary did not have any visible reactions and offered no comments. She appeared attentive to the instruction and seemed interested. She said she had never heard of the Rorschach nor seen it online or in the media.

## The R-PAS Administration

Mary was evaluated on the inpatient unit. R-PAS was the last test administered. At the time of the evaluation, there was a good assessment alliance as evidenced by Mary's engagement with previous tests and her openness during the clinical interview. Mary followed the R-PAS instructions and gave two to three responses to each card. Her reaction time to each card was unremarkable. However, she appeared overly cautious and after she accepted the card, made no attempt to turn it (CT SS[1] = 86). The length of administration was approximately 1 hour.

## The R-PAS Case Findings[2]

Mary produced R-PAS results that were valid for interpretation; she gave an average number of responses (R = 26) and they were sufficiently elaborated (F% SS = 91). The overall complexity of her responses was slightly above average (Complexity SS = 111), suggesting that she was well engaged with the task and had provided a sufficiently rich Rorschach protocol to interpret.

With regard to suicide risk, Mary scored above average on the SC-Comp (raw = 6.2, SS = 117), indicating that she is at an increased risk for suicide or serious self-harm, which is consistent with the fact that she had a recent near-lethal suicide attempt. However, it is still a lower score than that obtained by most people who commit suicide or engage in serious self-harm (i.e., raw ≥ 7; Fowler, Piers, Hilsenroth, Holdwick, & Padawer, 2001). Mary's psychological characteristics that contribute to her increased suicide risk are described in the subsequent sections.

With regard to stress management, although Mary has the potential for having good psychological resources (MC SS = 120), most of her cognitive and emotional capacities are fraught with disturbing feelings, thoughts, and images (most M and Color codes are accompanied by either MOR, MAP, AGC, AGM; Critical Contents SS = 131) or unmet dependency needs (ODL). In general, Mary is experiencing considerable implicit distress in the form of anxiousness, dysphoria, loneliness, and helplessness (YTVC' SS = 122; Y SS = 120). Simply reading through Mary's R-PAS responses is impactful as to their troubling nature. For example, her first response (Card I), "A woman in a solitary confinement in chains," metaphorically captures her experience of isolation, helplessness, and ineffectiveness. Her sense of feeling stuck in a bad situation with no clear direction is also reflected symbolically in her responses "two women stuck in the mud" (R6) and "a road to nowhere" (R13). Consistent with the interview and the PAI (STR T = 89), the R-PAS results indicate that at the present time, Mary is experiencing the effects of an above-average level of situational stressors that are likely leading to the aforementioned implicit distress of which Mary is either unaware or does not want to or cannot communicate.

In addition to the significant impact of implicit distress, Mary's R-PAS results show that she is flooded with severe dysphoric ideation and a sense of being damaged or injured (MOR SS = 146). A review of the thematic content of her responses further supports the interpretation that Mary is someone who feels she has been harmed by life. As a result, she feels flawed, like "a leaf in the fall losing its color" (R20) or "a shield, looks like it has holes in it" (R21); and damaged, like a fragile "leaf about to break" (R2), "two people fighting . . . bleeding from their knees" (R4), or "pigs'

---

[1] Standard scores (SS) have a mean of 100 and an *SD* of 15.

[2] See Appendix 6.1 at the end of the chapter for Mary's R-PAS Responses, Location Sheet, Code Sequence, and Page 1 and 2 Profiles.

heads after being slaughtered" (R16). The R-PAS findings also show that Mary is vulnerable to experiencing mixed positive and negative affective states, and her positive emotions can be tarnished easily by negative ones (CBlend SS = 117). A common reaction to cope with this experience is to restrict any spontaneous expression of emotions in order to avoid uncomfortable affect. However, Mary's results suggested that she had only a modest degree of cognitive control over becoming absorbed in emotionally tinged situations [(CF+C)/SumC SS = 119]. Mary's fear of losing control in the face of emotional situations may explain, at least in part, her observed difficulty in expressing her emotions and her severely flat affect after her suicide attempt (i.e., the need to shut down all emotion until she felt safe again).

Mary's R-PAS results indicate that she is capable of good reality testing, and there is no evidence of disturbance in her thinking. She is likely to exhibit logical, organized, and accurate thinking. These findings were consistent with both the clinical interview and PAI results, suggesting no evidence of impairment in reality testing or thought disorder. However, the R-PAS results indicate that Mary engages in a highly conventional interpretation of her environment (P SS = 132). Although this can be adaptive, especially for someone who is in an inpatient psychiatric setting, it can also suggest an overly cautious, stereotyped view of the world. Her behavior of not turning any of the cards during the Rorschach administration further supports this cautious, overly conformist approach, which may be a coping strategy to prevent evoking anger in others, especially her father's unpredictable rage. Furthermore, her implicit dependency (ODL% SS = 118) and sensitivity to rejection is likely to increase her anxiety about others' aggression. Her anxiety about aggression is perhaps captured by her responses to Card IV, "A furry monster coming at you," and to Card VIII, "looks like a giant grabbing the animals," and her fear of aggressive forces (AGC SS = 116) is further supported by her PAI profile, indicating suppressed aggression and lack of assertiveness (AGG-A T = 38; AGG-V T = 35).

Mary's R-PAS results revealed that although she has an average ability to understand people as complex and complete individuals (Pure H SS = 98), she has difficulty envisioning her interactions with others in a mutually rewarding and autonomous manner (MAH = 0; MAP/MAHP SS = 123). As previously noted, there are indications that Mary's sense of being damaged and her dysphoric view of herself potentially color her interactions with others, in which she feels vulnerable and anticipates aggression. This fear of aggression, coupled with her sense of being damaged, further diminishes her interpersonal effectiveness.

## Discussion of R-PAS Results as Applied to the Case

In contrast to the PAI and clinical interview results, the R-PAS findings suggest that Mary is experiencing clinically significant implicit distress characterized by negative emotions that include anxiousness, dysphoria, loneliness, and helplessness. R-PAS findings also capture Mary's underlying depression and feelings of isolation that appear to stem from a sense of being damaged and flawed. Although both the PAI and the interview had captured Mary's interpersonal difficulties and a marked perceived lack of support, the R-PAS findings more specifically identified a pattern of problematic interpersonal relationships in which Mary's feelings of vulnerability, fear of aggression, and her implicit dependency needs compromised her ability to effectively deal with and negotiate her relationships.

The PAI, interview, and R-PAS findings also converge. All three assessment methods found no evidence of any underlying psychotic processes. Given how empirically robust and sensitive the Rorschach is in detecting psychosis (Mihura et al., 2013), the absence of any thought disorder or impairment in reality testing further clarified the referral questions for the treatment team. Since suicidal behavior is often a response to a recent crisis, the findings from R-PAS, the PAI, and the clinical interview all identified Mary's marked situational stress. However, as indicated previously, R-PAS was the only measure to capture the extent of distress, underlying dysphoria, and negative emotion associated with it.

## Impact of the R-PAS Experience on Mary

Mary appeared as engaged in assessment feedback as she was in the whole assessment processes. The feedback from the PAI and interview resonated with her, but she indicated that she was most interested to know what the R-PAS findings were. She had some awareness that some of her responses to the Rorschach were "disturbing and dark." Given her difficulty in identifying and expressing her feelings verbally, some of her Rorschach responses with morbid themes were read to her. It was through this process that she was able to show sadness, and on one occasion became tearful and indicated that she felt "sad" while at the same time felt "relieved and understood."

Mary's R-PAS findings had a significant impact in developing a suicide risk formulation for her. The R-PAS results were integrated with other risk factors from the C-SSRS, PAI, and interview. Both Mary and the treatment team were told that her suicide attempts were in the context of depression, and that she was experiencing and continues to experience significant implicit distress in the form of dysphoria, anxiety, and helplessness. More importantly, Mary's underlying feeling of being damaged was most likely a trigger for her suicide. In particular, it is very likely that her husband's comment that she had brought a damaged child into this world activated her own underlying concern about being flawed. As a result, Mary's risk of suicide is likely to increase if she has life experiences or interactions that exacerbate her self-perception as a damaged person. Therefore, working through her feelings of being a damaged person should be the major focus of her treatment.

As a result of the R-PAS findings, the treatment team decided to extend Mary's hospitalization with a focus on treating her depression and her distorted sense of self. The rationale to initiate therapy on an inpatient unit was to alleviate some of Mary's distress, provide her with some positive experiences of therapy, help her to feel more hopeful, and make it easier for her to transition to individual outpatient psychotherapy. In addition, given the nature of Mary's interpersonal dynamics, it was recommended to the treatment team that the focus of family sessions should change from providing psychoeducation and support to couple therapy with the aim of continuing treatment postdischarge.

Mary was discharged after approximately 4 weeks of hospitalization. In addition to psychopharmacological treatment, she agreed to enter individual and couples therapy. Her husband also accepted the recommendation to enter treatment for his gambling problems. It was further recommended that the hospital mobile crisis team monitor Mary's postdischarge adjustment by visiting her at home for the first 2 weeks. One-month follow-up by the treatment team indicated that Mary was doing well and was engaged in her outpatient treatment. Her husband was also attending their joint sessions regularly.

## REFERENCES

American Psychiatric Association. (2003). Practice guideline for assessment and treatment of patients with suicidal behavior. *American Journal of Psychiatry, 160*(Suppl.), 1–44.

Fowler, J. C., Piers, C., Hilsenroth, M. J., Holdwick, D. J., & Padawer, J. R. (2001). The Rorschach Suicide Constellation: Assessing various degrees of lethality. *Journal of Personality Assessment, 76,* 333–351.

Jacobs, D. G., & Brewer. M. L. (2006). Application of APA practice guidelines on suicide to clinical practice. *CNS Spectrum, 11,* 447–454.

Meyer, G. J., Viglione, D. J., Mihura, J. L., Erard, R. E., & Erdberg, P. (2011). *Rorschach Performance Assessment System: Administration, coding, interpretation, and technical manual.* Toledo, OH: Rorschach Performance Assessment System.

Mihura, J. L., Meyer, G. J., Dumitrascu, N., & Bombel, G. (2013). The validity of individual Rorschach variables: Systematic reviews and meta-analyses of the comprehensive system. *Psychological Bulletin, 139,* 548–605.

Posner, K., Brown, G. K., Stanley, B., Brent, D. A., Yershova, K. V., Oquendo, M. A., . . . Mann, J. J. (2011). The Columbia–Suicide Severity Rating Scale: Initial validity and internal consistency findings from three multisite studies with adolescent and adults. *American Journal of Psychiatry, 168,* 1266–1277.

Shea, S. C. (2009). Suicide assessment part 1: Uncovering suicidal intent—a sophisticated art. *Psychiatric Times, 26,* 2–4.

Simon, R. I. (2004). *Assessing and managing suicide risk: Guidelines for clinically based risk management.* Washington, DC: American Psychiatric Publishing.

### Rorschach Responses "Mary"

| Respondent ID: Mary | Examiner: Ali Khadivi |
|---|---|
| Location: Inpatient Unit | Date: **/**/**** |
| Start Time: 4:00 P.M. | End Time: 4:55 P.M. |

| Cd # | R # | Or | Response | Clarification | R-Opt |
|---|---|---|---|---|---|
| I | 1 | | A woman in a solitary confinement in chains. (D4) | E: (Examiner Repeats Response [ERR].)<br>R: Here is her body; she is wearing a black dress, her head (Dd22) and she has her hands (D1) up as if she is tied up with chains.<br>E: Solitary confinement?<br>R: She is standing alone, and the way she is holding her arms. | |
| | 2 | | A leaf about to break. (W) | E: (ERR)<br>R: The whole thing. The lines here and different dark colors makes it look fragile. | |
| | 3 | | A black bat. (W) | E: (ERR)<br>R: The whole thing, the wings (D2). | |
| II | 4 | | Looks like two people fighting; they are bleeding from their knees. (W) | E: (ERR)<br>R: Here are the people (D1). This part, I see it as blood (D3) because it is red . . . looks like it is dripping out. | |
| | 5 | | A red butterfly flying. (D3) | E: (ERR)<br>R: I see it down here, the wings and the color. | |
| III | 6 | | Two women stuck in the mud looking at each other. (D1) | E: (ERR)<br>R: Here are the two women (D9) with shoes (Dd33).<br>E: Mud?<br>R: The darkish color and it has no shape to it (D7). | |
| | 7 | | Two pieces of meat hanging from the ceiling. (D2) | E: (ERR)<br>R: The way it is shaped and different colors. | |
| IV | 8 | | A furry monster coming at you. (W) | E: (ERR)<br>R: The size of it; it has big feet (D6).<br>E: Furry?<br>R: The dark and light colors. | |
| | 9 | | Could also be a creature; it's missing its arms. (W) | E: (ERR)<br>R: The whole thing, here (points to D4). It looks like it has no arms. | |
| V | 10 | | A bat. It is all black. (W) | E: (ERR)<br>R: Here are the wings (D4). | |
| | 11 | | Crocodiles on both sides with their mouth open. (D4) | E: (ERR)<br>R: It looks like heads of crocodiles, shaped like a mouth and here is the neck area. | |
| VI | 12 | | An old rug. (D1) | E: (ERR)<br>R: The edges and the wide shape.<br>E: Old?<br>R: Looks a bit torn. I don't know, the light and dark colors make it look torn and faded. | |
| | 13 | | A road to nowhere. (D5) | E: (ERR)<br>R: The long shape. It looks like it just ends. | |
| | 14 | | A ditch. (D12) | E: (ERR)<br>R: The white line here and light and dark make it look like a ditch; it looks caved in. | |

| Cd # | R # | Or | Response | Clarification | R-Opt |
|---|---|---|---|---|---|
| VII | 15 | | Two girls with weird hair staring at each other. (D1) | E: (ERR)<br>R: The shape.<br>E: Weird hair?<br>R: The way the hair (D5) is drawn. | |
| | 16 | | Pigs' heads after being slaughtered. I have seen that—it is gross; I lived near a slaughter house. (D3) | E: (ERR)<br>R: Looks like pigs' cheeks; I see the ears. I just see the heads not the body. | |
| | 17 | | A stone, down here. (D4) | E: (ERR)<br>R: Shaped like it. | |
| VIII | 18 | | Two animals climbing a mountain. (W) | E: (ERR)<br>R: Here are the animals (D1). I see their legs and here is the head. This part looks like a mountain (D6)—all the different colors and the shape. | |
| | 19 | | Looks like a giant grabbing the animals. (D4, D1) | E: (ERR)<br>R: Here are giant arms (Dd22), here is the body of it (rest of D4), and it looks like it is grabbing the two animals (D1) on the side. | |
| | 20 | | Reminds me of a leaf in the fall losing its color. (W) | E: (ERR)<br>R: The whole thing, all the colors spreading, it gives the impression that is fading. | |
| | 21 | | I guess it be could be a shield; looks like it has holes in it. (W) | E: (ERR)<br>R: The whole thing and these white areas (DdS28, 32) look like they have holes in them. | |
| IX | 22 | | Explosion. (W) | E: (ERR)<br>R: All the colors, the way they are shaped, the whole thing. | |
| | 23 | | Two monsters wearing a hood. (D3) | E: (ERR)<br>R: Here on the side the orange things. The way they are shaped. | |
| | 24 | | Looks like a needle that junkies use. I know about it; I went out with a guy who used heroin. (D5) | E: (ERR)<br>R: It looks thin and long. | |
| X | 25 | | Two crabs. (D1) | E: (ERR)<br>R: The two blue things are the crabs. The shape and the legs. | |
| | 26 | | Two pieces of red meat. (D9) | E: (ERR)<br>R: The color and long shape. | |

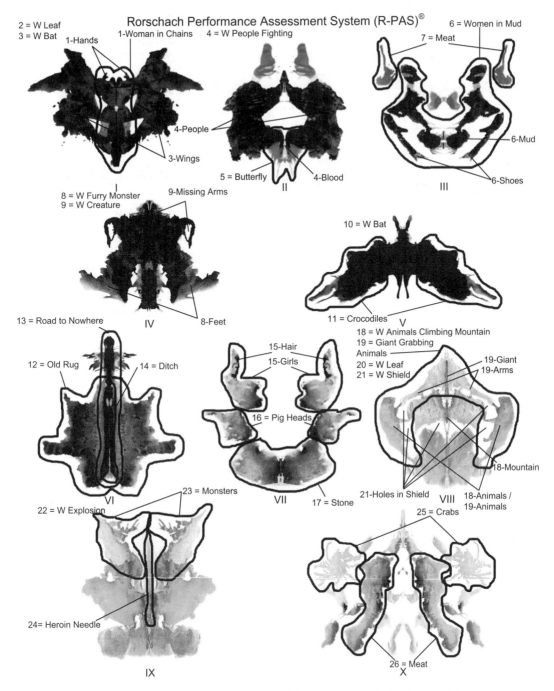

# Rorschach Performance Assessment System (R-PAS)®

2 = W Leaf
3 = W Bat
1-Hands
1-Woman in Chains
4 = W People Fighting
6 = Women in Mud
7 = Meat

4-People
3-Wings
5 = Butterfly
4-Blood
6-Mud
6-Shoes

I
II
III

8 = W Furry Monster
9 = W Creature
9-Missing Arms
10 = W Bat

13 = Road to Nowhere
8-Feet
11 = Crocodiles
IV
V

18 = W Animals Climbing Mountain
19 = Giant Grabbing Animals
20 = W Leaf
21 = W Shield
19-Giant
19-Arms

12 = Old Rug
14 = Ditch
15-Hair
15-Girls
16 = Pig Heads
18-Mountain

21-Holes in Shield
18-Animals /
19-Animals
VI
VII
17 = Stone
VIII

23 = Monsters
25 = Crabs
22 = W Explosion

24= Heroin Needle
26 = Meat
IX
X

© 2012 R-PAS; Rorschach® trademarks and images are used with permission of the trademark owner, Hogrefe AG, Berne, Switzerland

# R-PAS Code Sequence: "Mary"

**C-ID**: Mary    **P-ID**: 6    **Age**: 32    **Gender**: Female    **Education**: 12

| Cd | # | Or | Loc | Loc # | SR | SI | Content | Sy | Vg | 2 | FQ | P | Determinants | Cognitive | Thematic | HR | ODL (RP) | R-Opt |
|---|---|---|---|---|---|---|---|---|---|---|---|---|---|---|---|---|---|---|
| I | 1 | D | | 4 | | | H,Cg | Sy | | | o | | Mp,C' | | MOR,MAP | PH | ODL | |
| | 2 | W | | | | | NC | | | | o | | Y | | MOR | | | |
| | 3 | W | | | | | A | | | | o | P | C' | | | | | |
| II | 4 | W | | | | | H,Bl | Sy | | 2 | o | | Ma,mp,CF | | AGM,MOR,MAP | PH | | |
| | 5 | D | | 3 | | | A | | | | o | | FMa,FC | | | | | |
| III | 6 | D | | 1 | | | A,Cg,NC | Sy | | 2 | o | P | Mp,C' | | MAP | GH | ODL | |
| | 7 | D | | 2 | | | NC | Sy | | 2 | u | | mp,CF,Y | | | | ODL | |
| IV | 8 | W | | | | | (H) | | | | o | P | Ma,T | | AGM,AGC,MAP | GH | | |
| | 9 | W | | | | | (H) | | | | o | P | F | | MOR | PH | | |
| V | 10 | W | | | | | A | | | | o | P | C' | | | | | |
| | 11 | D | | 4 | | | Ad | | | 2 | u | | FMp | | AGC | | ODL | |
| VI | 12 | D | | 1 | | | NC | | | | o | | Y | | MOR | | | |
| | 13 | D | | 5 | | | NC | | | | o | | F | | | | | |
| | 14 | D | | 12 | | | NC | | | | u | | V | | MOR | | | |
| VII | 15 | D | | 1 | | | Hd | Sy | | 2 | o | P | Ma | | | GH | | |
| | 16 | D | | 3 | | | Ad | | | 2 | o | | F | | PER,MOR,MAP | | | |
| | 17 | D | | 4 | | | NC | | | | o | | F | | | | | |
| VIII | 18 | W | | | | | A,NC | Sy | | 2 | o | P | FMa,CF | | | | | |
| | 19 | D | | 1,4 | | | (H),A | Sy | | 2 | u | P | Ma | | AGM,MAP | PH | | |
| | 20 | W | | | | | NC | | | | u | | CF,Y | | MOR | | | |
| | 21 | W | | | | SI | NC | | | | o | | F | | AGC,MOR | | | |
| IX | 22 | W | | | | | Ex | | Vg | | o | | CF | | AGC | | | |
| | 23 | D | | 3 | | | (H),Cg | Sy | | 2 | o | P | F | | AGC | GH | | |
| | 24 | D | | 5 | | | NC | | | | o | | F | | PER | | ODL | |
| X | 25 | D | | 1 | | | A | | | 2 | o | P | F | | | | | |
| | 26 | D | | 9 | | | NC | | | 2 | u | | CF | | | | ODL | |

©2010-2016 R-PAS

# R-PAS Summary Scores and Profiles – Page 1

C-ID: Mary    P-ID: 6    Age: 32    Gender: Female    Education: 12

| Domain/Variables | Raw Scores | Raw %ile | Raw SS | Cplx. Adj. %ile | Cplx. Adj. SS | Standard Score Profile R-Optimized | Abbr. |
|---|---|---|---|---|---|---|---|
| **Admin. Behaviors and Obs.** | | | | | | | |
| Pr | 0 | 24 | 89 | | | | Pr |
| Pu | 0 | 40 | 96 | | | | Pu |
| CT (Card Turning) | 0 | 18 | 86 | | | | CT |
| **Engagement and Cog. Processing** | | | | | | | |
| Complexity | 90 | 77 | 111 | | | | Cmplx |
| R (Responses) | 26 | 69 | 107 | 49 | 100 | | R |
| F% [Lambda=0.44] (Simplicity) | 31% | 28 | 91 | 40 | 96 | | F% |
| Blend | 8 | 88 | 118 | 75 | 110 | | Bln |
| Sy | 8 | 64 | 106 | 44 | 97 | | Sy |
| MC | 12.5 | 91 | 120 | 78 | 112 | | MC |
| MC - PPD | -2.5 | 46 | 99 | 52 | 101 | | MC-PPD |
| M | 6 | 82 | 113 | 61 | 104 | | M |
| M/MC [6/12.5] | 48% | 43 | 97 | 43 | 97 | | M Prp |
| (CF+C)/SumC [6/7] | 86% | 90 | 119 | 90 | 119 | | CFC Prp |
| **Perception and Thinking Problems** | | | | | | | |
| EII-3 | -0.9 | 17 | 86 | 16 | 85 | | EII |
| TP-Comp (Thought & Percept. Com...) | -0.9 | 1 | 64 | 1 | 64 | | TP-C |
| WSumCog | 0 | 8 | 79 | 8 | 79 | | WCog |
| SevCog | 0 | 35 | 94 | 35 | 94 | | Sev |
| FQ-% | 0% | 7 | 78 | 7 | 78 | | FQ-% |
| WD-% | 0% | 11 | 82 | 11 | 82 | | WD-% |
| FQo% | 77% | 89 | 118 | 88 | 117 | | FQo% |
| P | 10 | 98 | 132 | 99 | 133 | | P |
| **Stress and Distress** | | | | | | | |
| YTVC' | 10 | 92 | 122 | 87 | 117 | | YTVC' |
| m | 2 | 66 | 106 | 39 | 96 | | m |
| Y | 4 | 91 | 120 | 87 | 117 | | Y |
| MOR | 9 | >99 | 146 | >99 | 146 | | MOR |
| SC-Comp (Suicide Concern Comp.) | 6.4 | 87 | 117 | 81 | 113 | | SC-C |
| **Self and Other Representation** | | | | | | | |
| ODL% | 23% | 88 | 118 | 87 | 116 | | ODL% |
| SR (Space Reversal) | 0 | 19 | 87 | 19 | 87 | | SR |
| MAP/MAHP [6/6] | 100% | 94 | 123 | 97 | 136 | | MAP Prp |
| PHR/GPHR [4/8] | 50% | 76 | 111 | 76 | 111 | | PHR Prp |
| M- | 0 | 36 | 95 | 36 | 95 | | M- |
| AGC | 5 | 85 | 116 | 80 | 113 | | AGC |
| H | 2 | 45 | 98 | 21 | 88 | | H |
| COP | 0 | 21 | 88 | 21 | 88 | | COP |
| MAH | 0 | 26 | 90 | 26 | 90 | | MAH |

© 2010-2016 R-PAS

C-ID: Mary    P-ID: 6    Age: 32    Gender: Female    Education: 12

| Domain/Variables | Raw Scores | Raw %ile | Raw SS | Cplx. Adj. %ile | Cplx. Adj. SS | Standard Score Profile R-Optimized | Abbr. |
|---|---|---|---|---|---|---|---|
| **Engagement and Cog. Processing** | | | | | | | |
| W% | 38% | 47 | 99 | 40 | 96 | | W% |
| Dd% | 0% | 5 | 75 | 7 | 77 | | Dd% |
| SI (Space Integration) | 1 | 18 | 86 | 18 | 86 | | SI |
| IntCont | 0 | 11 | 81 | 11 | 81 | | IntC |
| Vg% | 4% | 46 | 99 | 46 | 99 | | Vg% |
| V | 1 | 72 | 109 | 54 | 102 | | V |
| FD | 0 | 21 | 88 | 21 | 88 | | FD |
| R8910% | 35% | 72 | 109 | 75 | 110 | | R8910% |
| WSumC | 6.5 | 90 | 119 | 82 | 114 | | WSC |
| C | 0 | 36 | 95 | 36 | 95 | | C |
| Mp/(Ma+Mp) [2/6] | 33% | 36 | 94 | 36 | 94 | | Mp Prp |
| **Perception and Thinking Problems** | | | | | | | |
| FQu% | 23% | 27 | 91 | 27 | 90 | | FQu% |
| **Stress and Distress** | | | | | | | |
| PPD | 15 | 86 | 116 | 76 | 110 | | PPD |
| CBlend | 2 | 88 | 117 | 74 | 110 | | CBlnd |
| C' | 4 | 88 | 117 | 79 | 112 | | C' |
| V | 1 | 72 | 109 | 54 | 102 | | V |
| CritCont% (Critical Contents) | 54% | 98 | 131 | 97 | 129 | | CrCt |
| **Self and Other Representation** | | | | | | | |
| SumH | 7 | 65 | 106 | 49 | 99 | | SumH |
| NPH/SumH [5/7] | 71% | 71 | 108 | 72 | 109 | | NPH Prp |
| V-Comp (Vigilance Composite) | 3.0 | 45 | 98 | 27 | 91 | | V-C |
| r (Reflections) | 0 | 36 | 95 | 36 | 95 | | r |
| p/(a+p) [5/11] | 45% | 57 | 103 | 56 | 103 | | p Prp |
| AGM | 3 | 98 | 131 | 98 | 131 | | AGM |
| T | 1 | 68 | 107 | 68 | 107 | | T |
| PER | 2 | 89 | 118 | 89 | 118 | | PER |
| An | 0 | 16 | 85 | 16 | 85 | | An |

© 2010-2016 R-PAS

# CHAPTER 7

# Understanding a Therapetutic Impasse

## *Using R-PAS in a Multimethod Assessment*
## *of Alliance Dynamics and Underlying Developmental Disruption*

### Anthony Bram

In their landmark evidentiary review of the psychological and medical test literature, Meyer et al. (2001) identified several conditions under which psychological evaluations should provide the greatest clinical yield. Such conditions include when "(a) the treating clinician or patient has salient questions, (b) there are a variety of treatment approaches from which to choose and a body of knowledge linking treatment methods to patient characteristics, (c) the patient has had little success in prior treatment, or (d) the patient has complex problems and treatment goals must be prioritized" (p. 129). Meyer et al. also highlighted the factors associated with psychological assessment that have the optimal therapeutic impact, including when "initial treatment efforts have failed" (p. 129). This point applies to assessments conducted as a consultation to a patient and therapist who are embroiled in a therapeutic impasse, that is, in a "stalemate or plateau in the process of achieving a therapeutic objective" (Whitaker, Warkentin, & Johnson, 1950, p. 641).

In this chapter, I illustrate the value of such a psychological assessment in the outpatient treatment of a 15-year-old adolescent female with an array of difficulties that included impediments to forming lasting and beneficial alliances with her treaters. My primary goal is to demonstrate the utility of the Rorschach Performance Assessment System (R-PAS; Meyer, Viglione, Mihura, Erard, & Erdberg, 2011) in a multimethod assessment to untangle a therapeutic impasse.

## Therapeutic Impasse: The Importance of the Case Study

Although the idea that a psychological assessment is beneficial in cases of therapeutic impasse is embedded in clinical wisdom, there has been a paucity of empirical research on this proposition. Until recently, there have also been few published case illustrations of the benefit of psychological assessment as consultation to understand and address impasses.

Fortunately, in part spurred by the surging interest in collaborative/therapeutic assessment (C/TA; Finn, Fischer, & Handler, 2012) and its emphasis on pragmatic links between evaluation and treatment, there have been more case reports published in recent years, contributing to the beginnings of an evidence base for practice (American Psychological Association Presidential Task Force on Evidence-Based Practice, 2006). Such case studies have emanated from both a more explicit C/TA perspective (Finn, 2003; Fowler, 2012) and a more traditional approach (albeit with a collaborative emphasis) to psychological assessment (Bram, 2015; Bram & Yalof, 2015).

## Introduction to the Case

### Context of the Assessment Referral

"Heidi" was a 15-year-old female in the 10th grade who had been in outpatient psychotherapy and pharmacotherapy for many years to address an array of long-standing symptoms, including depression with self-harm and suicidality, binge eating, potentially dangerous sexualized online activity, volatile mood, anxiety, pervasive relational conflicts, attentional problems, and academic struggles. Central to the focus of this chapter, Heidi had a history of difficulties in forming alliances and sustaining progress with treaters and educators.

### Brief History of Development, Education, and Treatment

Heidi lived with her parents and older brother. There was a history of depression and substance abuse on both sides of the family. Heidi did not report a history of trauma, and there were no data from her parents, therapist, and previous evaluators indicating otherwise. Her parents reported delays in her speech/language, fine motor, and basic self-regulatory (e.g., feeding, sleeping) and self-help skills (dressing, toileting), for which she had received early intervention. In elementary school, Heidi struggled academically and socially, despite the provision of special education services. Neuropsychological testing revealed borderline-to-low-average intellectual functioning, a nonverbal learning disorder, attention-deficit/hyperactivity disorder (ADHD) and executive functioning weaknesses, and learning disabilities in expressive language, reading, writing, and math. Since third grade, she'd had an out-of-district placement at a school specializing in learning disabilities. Recently, the school team reported that they could no longer meet her emotional needs, and the family and school district were at odds in the process of determining an appropriate placement.

Increasingly, Heidi had difficulty remaining in class and was prone to tearfulness, angry outbursts, and intense conflict with classmates, teachers, and her soccer coach and teammates. She rejected the academic and emotional supports offered. The school district remained unconvinced of the seriousness of her emotional difficulties and needs and maintained a stance that the solution was to implement more limits and behavioral consequences. Meanwhile, her parents and their attorney were advocating for a placement at a therapeutic school.

Heidi went through a series of outpatient therapists, all of whom she ultimately dismissed as unhelpful, incompetent, or uninteresting. In the year before this assessment, Heidi had begun with a new therapist, Dr. Y, who wisely recognized this history as a cautionary tale likely to be recapitulated, especially if not better understood. Indeed, after about a 3-month honeymoon phase in which Heidi idealized the new therapist, she complained to her parents and therapist that the therapy and therapist were "annoying" and "useless," and she battled with her parents around coming to sessions.

## Questions for the Assessment

Dr. Y noted that previous evaluations did not illuminate what made it so difficult for Heidi to access the help offered to her. In early sessions, Dr. Y was struck by Heidi's (1) difficulty internalizing the experience of others as helpful, (2) presentation as emotionally and cognitively much younger than her age, (3) vulnerability to severe emotional dysregulation, and (4) occasional confusing and illogical verbal communications. Dr. Y posited that understanding these psychological factors would illuminate how to work through the current, recapitulated impasse. Dr. Y wondered about the extent to which these difficulties might be indicative of an undiagnosed autism spectrum disorder (ASD), emerging characterological problems, incipient bipolar illness, or some other variant of thought disorder.

I understood there to be two fundamental questions essential to understanding the impasse and how to overcome it: (1) Given Heidi's pattern of failed engagement with previous treaters (and educators), what are the factors and conditions that might impede and facilitate her capacity for therapeutic (and educational) alliances? And, (2) how can Heidi's *underlying developmental disruption(s)* (structural weakness, maladaptive character, trauma, conflict, or splits; Bram & Peebles, 2014; Peebles, 2012) be conceptualized so that treatment could be appropriately focused? Autism spectrum, bipolar, and thought disorders are specific types of structural weakness that could be evaluated in the test data. Note that this referral met all of Meyer et al.'s (2001) indications for psychological assessment.

## Pragmatics of Assessment Administration

I worked with Heidi for four sessions of 1 or 2 hours each, over a 2-week span. All sessions were held in my private practice office. Heidi's medications included the antidepressant Zoloft and the antipsychotic and mood stabilizer Abilify.[1]

## Heidi's Non-R-PAS Assessment Findings

The findings from the non-R-PAS data are organized according to the two primary referral questions involving (1) alliance dynamics and (2) underlying developmental disruption.

---

[1]Because antipsychotics have been shown to attenuate the most severe Rorschach signs of thought disorder (Gold & Hurt, 1990), I had hoped to test Heidi off the Abilify. Efforts to taper, however, were associated with exacerbation of her suicidality, so it made clinical sense for her to resume taking Abilify throughout the evaluation.

## Alliance Dynamics

Heidi's self-reported attitudes and experiences on the Millon Adolescent Clinical Inventory (MACI) pointed to mistrust that could elicit the rejection she anticipates and fears (Oppositional BR = 77, Self-Demeaning BR = 73). Further, her story narratives on the Thematic Apperception Test (TAT) revealed implicit relational expectations that potential helpers would be punitive, rejecting, and unsympathetic. However, Heidi's TAT responses included one glimmer of helpful alliance potential: On Card 3BM, a suicidal girl has "had enough," feels alone, and rants that "no one listens." But as the story unfolds, the character's mother is not behaviorally or emotionally reactive and remains available to talk. The girl shares what is troubling her, and the mother is able to "get [her daughter] the help she needs," suggesting Heidi's implicit premise that help can be accessed if the helper remains available, steady, and containing, and does not respond in kind to her dismissiveness and provocation.

Patient–examiner hypothesis testing revealed that fostering collaboration included (1) showing interest in less conflictual aspects of her life, notably sports; (2) carefully pacing and breaking down tasks to mitigate against feeling overwhelmed (e.g., a few TAT cards at a time); (3) helping her save face around areas of known cognitive weakness (e.g., volunteering to read MACI items aloud to her); (4) allowing "movement breaks" to provide sensory soothing and discharge tension; and (5) playful, self-effacing humor, aimed at leveling her experience of feeling one-down. In contrast, explicit encouragement to be curious and reflective resulted in her agitation and shutting down.

## Underlying Developmental Disruption

Non-R-PAS findings bearing on the question of underlying developmental disruption are organized according to the three of the four models[2]: (1) structural weakness, (2) maladaptive character patterns, and (3) conflict or splits.

### Evidence for Structural Weaknesses

Heidi's results suggested structural weaknesses in emotional regulation and interpersonal relatedness but not in reasoning or reality testing. In terms of *emotional regulation*, her self-reported subjective experience included intense and overwhelming depression, suicidal thoughts, and anxiety (e.g., MACI Depressive Affect BR = 83, Anxious Feelings BR = 78). Heidi's performance on the TAT, both in content and her feeling overwhelmed by the task, underscored the extent to which she was lacking in basic capacities to manage feelings. Her non-R-PAS findings were mixed as to whether her structural weakness in emotional regulation was consistent with a bipolar spectrum condition. Heidi did not report elevated mood, impulsivity, or grandiosity on the MACI. However, her parents' ratings on the Child Mania Rating Scale yielded a score that exceeded the research-based diagnostic threshold for mania.

---

[2]There was no compelling evidence for the trauma model, so that is not addressed here. Heidi did not endorse trauma items on the MACI, and her parents did not report trauma in the developmental questionnaires. Other clinicians had evaluated Heidi previously, with no findings of trauma.

Multiple methods of assessment illuminated Heidi's structural weaknesses in *relatedness*, both in (1) social skills (parent ratings of Social Awareness, Social Cognition, and Social Communication on the Social Responsiveness Scale—2nd Edition) and (2) in capacity for basic trust (MACI, Oppositionality and Self-Demeaning elevations; TAT themes of implicit expectations of disappointment, misunderstanding, mistreatment, and loss). Although her weaknesses in social skills resembled adolescents on the autism spectrum, the performance-based Autism Diagnostic Observation Scale (ADOS) suggested that Heidi possessed strengths inconsistent with autism (Module 4, Overall Total = 2 [Cutoff = 7]), notably her capacity for conversational reciprocity, eye contact, and emotional expressiveness.

### Evidence for Maladaptive Character Patterns

Clinicians had consistently remarked that Heidi exhibited behaviors characteristic of a much younger child. She exuded these characteristics through her sing-song speech, intense focus on immediate gratification, challenges with perspective taking, and the degree to which she required external scaffolding to mitigate meltdowns and outbursts. On a task eliciting a series of wishes, she expressed longings to be 5 years old again with freedom from demands, responsibility, and complex relationships. As a behavioral example, when queried about an MACI item in which she acknowledged frequently losing her temper, she smiled and explained that outbursts or the threat of them helped her get her way. Although Heidi's extreme immaturity was certainly rooted in her pervasive neurodevelopmental delays, the present findings suggested a characterological component as well.

### Evidence for Intrapsychic Conflicts or Splits

Heidi showed indications of a split related to struggles with accepting and integrating her sexual feelings. There was a striking disconnect between her potentially dangerous online sexualized behavior and her conscious self-concept. Her MACI self-report minimized sexual concerns, and her strong disavowal was even clearer from her response to the TAT. To a card of a Picasso painting with two unclothed figures,[3] she immediately covered the card, exclaiming: "Inappropriate! . . . I can't describe it—it's too disgusting. Now you're going to scar me for life!" Given her cognitive and emotional limitations, one can imagine how difficult it was for her to sort out healthy, expectable sexual thoughts and feelings, leaving her at risk for acting on feelings that she cannot consciously own.

## Why R-PAS for Heidi's Evaluation?

The Rorschach was deemed central to the evaluation because it illuminates a range of psychological capacities and associated dynamics bearing on the referral questions. R-PAS was selected not only for its sound psychometric properties and normative data but also because its R-Optimized approach to administration seemed a better

---

[3] *La Vie*; Card 8 from Series B and the Menninger set.

match for Heidi than that of the Comprehensive System (CS; Exner, 2003). Given Heidi's lower intellectual functioning and history of difficulty sustaining engagement, I viewed her as at risk of a constricted, uninterpretable protocol. I was concerned that in such an event (fewer than 14 responses), the CS readministration procedure (i.e., readministering all 10 cards) would be experienced by her as critical (Yalof & Rosenstein, 2014), leading to shutting down not only on the Rorschach but also on the collaboration needed to complete the evaluation.

## The R-PAS Administration

In our fourth and final session, I introduced the Rorschach, as delineated in the R-PAS manual (Meyer et al., 2011), and emphasized the need for two or three responses to each card. The R-PAS administration took 55 minutes. As discussed in the next section, Heidi had initial difficulty grasping the requirement for two or three responses to each card.

## Discussion of Heidi's R-PAS Scores and Findings[4]

### Heidi's Profile of Administration Behaviors and Engagement: Implications for Alliance

How Heidi engaged with the complex cognitive, emotional, and interpersonal task of the Rorschach had implications for how she would engage around similar challenges in therapy. Both her Card Prompts (SS[5] = 114) and Pulls (SS = 116) were in the above-average range for her age, suggesting that optimal engagement requires some regulating activity on the part of the other (e.g., therapist).

Occurring on the first and last cards, her two Prompts were understood in the context of her cognitive limitations, problems with collaboration, and challenges with emotional regulation. Heidi's providing only a single unprompted response to Card I was likely due to her difficulty attending to and understanding the instructions (given her documented attentional and learning problems and lower intellectual functioning) and to her difficulties with interpersonal engagement (see above and below for discussion of impediments to alliance).

But there were emotional factors as well. On Card I, in fewer than 5 seconds, she responded with the Popular butterfly and then trailed off, pausing for over 20 seconds before the Prompt. She followed, however, with dysphoric (MOR; "broken wing") and illogical (INC1, "hand") *elaborations of her first response* rather than offering a second response. Given that the second "new" response was "It looks like depression," it is likely that her pause after the first response reflected self-protective efforts to inhibit the dysphoria that soon followed.[6] On Card X, it was hypothesized

---

[4]See Appendix 7.1 at the end of the chapter for Heidi's R-PAS Responses, Location Sheet, Code Sequence, and Page 1 and 2 Profiles.

[5]Standard scores (SS) have a mean of 100 and an SD of 15.

[6]There could have been an additional Prompt on Card IX (raising her score to High). During the response phase it appeared she offered three separate responses, but later she indicated that all were part of a single response.

that her need for a Prompt and subsequent inability or unwillingness to provide an additional response reflected a similar need to shut down after a sequence of negative emotional intensity (two pure C's, two AGM's, and an MOR) and cognitive destabilization (an INC1, INC2, and FQ none) on the fully chromatic cards (VIII-X). These dynamics highlighted that to establish and maintain an alliance, treaters and educators should recognize that Heidi's manifest constriction (also evident in R8910% SS = 59), which could be mistaken as primarily oppositional, serves a self-protective, self-regulatory function.

Heidi had one Pull on Card VII. By this point, Heidi was engaged but was using a strategy of focusing on unusual details (Dd's), perhaps in an effort to steer away from more emotionally evocative aspects of the blot. It may have been that she lost the set as she involved herself in this approach, which did prove successful insofar as it provided a respite from the dysphoric and aggressive themes that had predominated prior to and resuming after Card VII. Again, to ally with Heidi, treaters would need to recognize the self-protective functions that can be associated with her apparent loss of focus or off-task behavior.

Even with her need for the examiner's Prompts and Pulls, it was to Heidi's credit that she was able to engage in the Rorschach, offering some hope that with adequate support, she could do the same in therapy. Heidi's Complexity score was in the average range for her age, reflecting a solid number of Responses (SS = 105), use of multiple Determinants (F% SS = 103), Blends (SS = 97), and efforts to integrate different aspects of the blots (Sy SS = 86). Thus, there was no need to adjust interpretation of other variables for high or low Complexity.

## Additional R-PAS Findings Related to Alliance Dynamics

Notice in the R-PAS data the *absence* of evidence of an ability to experience others in realistic, complex, multidimensional ways (H = 0, SS = 75; NPH/Sum H = 5/5, SS = 127) or to expect that relationships will be cooperative and mutually enriching (COP = 0, SS = 88; MAH = 0, SS = 90). Further inspection of her profile revealed not only an absence of realistic and benign relational representations (which in the cases of COP and MAH were still normative for her age), but, more importantly, the presence of human representations that were confused, inaccurately perceived, and/or tainted by concerns about aggression, malevolence, or injury (PHR/GPHR SS = 132; MAP/MAHP SS = 123; AGM SS = 131). Consider these responses garnering MAP scores (again, in the absence of any MAH): "a broken heart" (R3), "death . . . the world wants to get them and kill it" (R8), and "dead rat . . . the cat ate it" (R16). Such responses offered a window into how prospective relationships are laden with expectations of painful disappointment and rejection or, even worse, malevolence and predation. This is not a template that lends itself to openness to and acceptance of a clinician's or teacher's offer to help. Thus, the R-PAS results converged with those from the MACI and TAT, indicating that Heidi does not readily access benign introjects—a crucial component for anticipating that new relationships, including therapeutic ones, will be safe and sustaining. Fortunately, recall that the TAT did offer a hint of conditions under which Heidi might experience help as accessible.

## R-PAS Findings Related to Underlying Developmental Disruption

*Evidence for Structural Weaknesses*

The R-PAS results made a significant contribution to clarifying the nature and extent of Heidi's structural weaknesses. In terms of *emotional regulation,* Heidi's R-PAS profile highlighted the degree to which affect floods her capacity to use cognition to contextualize and deintensify her emotional experience [(CF+C)/SumC SS = 126]. Heidi exhibited a notable absence of frontal lobe or ego involvement to organize and contain her raw, intense experience of emotion (C SS = 138, *and* all C's were marked by FQn). Converging with these structural findings, R-PAS content revealed how unable she was to screen out of awareness emotionally intense primary-process concerns (Critical Contents SS = 136; MOR SS = 146; AGM SS = 131). Heidi's response content was laden with dysphoria and aggression, such as a butterfly with a "broken wing," "depression," "broken heart," "elephants fighting," "death," "fallen angel," "grim reaper," among others. Although Heidi's Suicide Concern Composite was not elevated (SC-Comp SS = 106), the presence of such dark preoccupations, plus her aforementioned vulnerability to emotional flooding and slips in reasoning (the latter described below)—not to mention the TAT and MACI data cited earlier—underscored concerns about her suicide risk.

The R-PAS data suggested that Heidi's structural weakness in *relatedness* was not so much a lack of interest in people (SumH SS = 96; M SS = 103), a finding that converges with ADOS findings that her relational difficulties were not on the autism spectrum. Her relational challenges had more to do with (1) how she experienced people in incomplete and unrealistic ways (NPH/SumH SS = 127) and (2) her vulnerability to interpersonal confusion and misperception (PHR/GPHR SS = 132; 5 of her 9 PHR's were driven by cognitive scores and/or poor or absent Form).

Consistent with the other measures, Heidi's R-PAS profile did not point to a major structural weakness in her *reality testing,* even under relatively unstructured conditions (FQ–% SS = 112; WD–% SS = 106; FQo% SS = 83; P SS = 111). However, R-PAS did underscore just how confused and illogical her *reasoning* could become under conditions when she was more on her own, that is, without much in the way of externally provided rules, expectations, monitoring, and feedback (WSumCog SS = 134; SevCog SS = 138). There was some evidence that this vulnerability in her reasoning was exacerbated to the extent that she also experienced greater emotional stirring (e.g., R24, her most confused response, garnering a Level 2 cognitive score, occurred on the fully chromatic, highly unstructured Card IX). Additionally, it was notable that even when perceiving situations accurately and conventionally (showing good reality testing), Heidi was still apt to subject such perceptions to faulty logic (see I-R1, II-R5, VIII-R22 for cognitive scores associated with P's). In other words, although she might perceive a situation accurately, she was vulnerable to drawing unsound conclusions about it.

Heidi's lapses in reasoning were specifically marked by her (1) putting ideas together in ways that do not make sense (FABs and INCs), (2) strained logic and jumping to unfounded conclusions (PECs), and (3) thinking that slips off track (DR1 on III-R8). In addition, although not quite captured by R-PAS scoring, Heidi also exhibited a vulnerability to confabulatory reasoning, that is, the tendency to read undue meaning into situations or to overly embellish meaning with internal fantasies (e.g., III-R8: "death . . . the world wants to get them and kill it"; IX-R24: "the rainbow is sad and depressing because it has no friends"; Bram & Peebles, 2014; Kleiger, 2017).

These R-PAS findings suggested that Heidi could be considered to have a "thought disorder" that manifests under particular conditions. Note that she exhibited significant vulnerabilities in her reasoning, despite taking antipsychotic medication, which is believed to mute more severe signs of thought disorder on the Rorschach (Gold & Hurt, 1990). This finding answers one component of an original referral question, but recall that there was a more specific question about the possibility that Heidi's challenges with affect regulation might be understood as an emerging bipolar spectrum illness. The nature of her R-PAS scores and Rorschach verbalizations did *not* point in that direction: Her combinative and confabulatory reasoning did not contain the overly playful, jocular qualities often associated with bipolar conditions (Kleiger, 2017). Instead, for Heidi, such illogical reasoning tended to be associated with malevolent, hostile, or rejecting interpersonal content (e.g., see II-R5, III-R8, VI-R15), which is more characteristic of borderline conditions (Kleiger, 2017).[7]

### Evidence for Maladaptive Character Patterns

Whereas the non-R-PAS findings pointed to the infantile elements of Heidi's character style, the R-PAS profile highlighted two other implicit aspects of Heidi's personality that were automatic, unquestioned, and rigidly held. The first involved her sense of herself as damaged, upended, and defeated (MOR = 10, SS = 146), conveyed in responses such as a "butterfly with broken wing," "broken heart," "fallen angel," and "fallen star." Second was how inflexibly negative her implicit relational expectations were. Consider again Heidi's absence of Rorschach representations of positive, cooperative, or mutually beneficial relationships juxtaposed with a preponderance of aggressive, hostile, or rejecting representations (MAP/MAHP SS = 123; COP = 0, SS = 88; AGM SS = 131). Moreover, in a testing-the-limits patient–examiner intervention (Bram & Peebles, 2014), she was encouraged to reflect on the relational contents of her Rorschach responses and what they might say about her: Heidi did not show signs of curiosity, question the responses, or indicate that she was troubled by them. It was this rigidity in her implicit relational expectations and how invested she was in these negative representations that suggested a characterological component contributing to the difficulty of engaging her therapeutically and educationally.

### Evidence for Conflict and Splits

On the Rorschach, evidence of conflicts or splits is discerned when there are contradictory data reflecting competing internal states (sometimes within the same response or within a sequence; contradictions can be among contents and/or determinants), or when there is recurrent straining or destabilization of ego functioning associated with

---

[7]Adding support for a borderline condition was her defensive style and object relations marked by splitting. Consider, for example, her poor integration of positively and negatively toned elements in II-R5 ("elephants fighting . . . they're happy"), IV-11 ("black pixie"), and IX-R24 ("rainbow . . . it looks sad . . . [and] lonely"; see Cooper & Arnow, 1986).

particular thematic content (Bram & Peebles, 2014). Careful inspection of Heidi's R-PAS Code Sequence revealed some evidence of such patterns. First, there was a hint of convergence with the non-R-PAS finding indicating a split involving difficulties with accepting and integrating her sexuality: Note the cognitive (Vg, FQn) and emotional destabilization (pure C, Bl, laughing) in her Card II-R4 response of "a period . . . because of the red." Second, her poorly integrated Card II-R5 response of "elephants . . . fighting over meat . . . they're happy," plus the R22 to R23 sequence from "too happy" to "fighting" suggested similar splits around aggression (see also Footnote 7).

## Integration of R-PAS and Non-R-PAS Findings to Answer Referral Questions

Heidi's contribution to her impasse with Dr. Y involved (1) a structural weakness in her capacity for basic relatedness, exacerbated by (2) maladaptive character patterns marked by her hostile and rejecting implicit relational expectations (which she is prone to enact) and reluctance to relinquish immature, maladaptive behaviors. Though there was no evidence of an autism spectrum condition, these factors made it extraordinarily challenging for Heidi to establish the collaborative alliances necessary for meaningful engagement and change. The data did, however, point to conditions facilitative of an alliance, particularly the importance of the helper's general stance of steadiness and containment in the face of Heidi's dismissal and provocation (Gabbard & Wilkinson, 1994). Other facilitative factors in sessions included space for discussion of her interests; use of self-effacing humor so she is less apt to feel one-down; careful pacing and breaking down of tasks to decrease her feeling cognitively or emotionally overwhelmed; supporting her face-saving efforts; and giving her access to sensory soothing and tension discharge (e.g., through clay, fidget toys).

Other domains indicating Heidi's structural weakness included her severe emotional dysregulation as well as her vulnerability to slips in logical reasoning. Her weakness in emotional regulation manifested in her feeling overwhelmed, depressed, and preoccupied with death and suicide. Lapses in her reasoning—constituting a thought disorder in a broad sense—were evident under conditions of less external structure and greater emotional press. Data were equivocal about whether Heidi's emotional dysregulation and thought disorder were consistent with a bipolar spectrum illness. A bipolar diagnosis could not be ruled out, but there was some evidence that her thought disorder was more consistent with a borderline condition. Heidi was also having difficulty accepting and integrating her aggression and burgeoning sexuality into her sense of self, and instead, splitting them off, which increases the likelihood of acting on such feelings or impulses when she does not consciously consider them.

It was clear why personnel in a school specializing in learning disabilities concluded that they could no longer safely and effectively meet Heidi's emotional needs, for she was a youngster with a highly complex amalgam of severe learning *and* emotional vulnerabilities. She was in need of a school with central psychiatric and therapeutic, as well as learning disability, components. Heidi required therapeutic interventions above and beyond the more routine outpatient psychotherapy-plus-medication management regimen. Based on the severity and complexity of her needs and the precariousness of her functioning, intensive in-home services and the possibility of a residential placement were worthy of strong consideration. Whether residential or day, her therapeutic school placement needed to include provision of individual and group interventions (informed by cognitive-behavioral therapy [CBT] and dialectical behavior therapy [DBT]) aimed at building social and coping skills.

Traditional individual therapy would also have a prominent role in her treatment plan. Given her interest in people but immense difficulty managing emotions in relationships, she would derive benefit from a relationally based psychotherapy with the alliance carefully tended. In addition to the facilitative alliance factors described above, addressing inevitable ruptures (e.g., frustrations, misunderstandings, disagreements) in the therapeutic dyad could model for her how unsatisfying and strained relationships can be worked through, repaired, and strengthened (Safran, Muran, & Eubanks-Carter, 2011). Individual therapy would also be necessary to offer her a safe space to verbalize, make better sense of, and consider more adaptive strategies to cope with such experiences as her (1) interpersonal challenges with peers, teachers, and family; (2) fears and ambivalences about growing up; and (3) confusing thoughts and feelings about sexuality and intimacy. With the strengthening of the alliance over time, there would be opportunities to gradually help her see the costs *to her* of maladaptive behaviors she is invested in maintaining. For example, the threat of tantrums—sometimes attaining what she wanted in the short-term—also undermined her exposure to more desired age-appropriate responsibilities and privileges.

## Impact of the Assessment

The assessment findings and report were shared and discussed in detail with Dr. Y and Heidi's parents. Unfortunately, there was no formal feedback session with Heidi because in the weeks following the evaluation, her symptoms exacerbated and she was in and out of the hospital and subsequently expressed a lack of interest in meeting with me.

More than a year after the evaluation, Dr. Y reported its positive impact both on resolving their impasse in psychotherapy and the overall course of the treatment and educational plans. Dr. Y cited that the findings assisted her to keep her central focus on the state of the alliance, including the importance of containment (resisting the urge to react in kind or defensively to dismissiveness and devaluation) and rupture–repair work. Dr. Y recounted that the specific finding that Heidi's thought disorder had more of a borderline than bipolar quality was crucial in helping her tune into borderline relational dynamics that required careful management of countertransference (Gabbard & Wilkinson, 1994). Dr. Y believed that this understanding contributed to Heidi's staying with this therapy far longer than previous ones, and consequently, Heidi's slow but meaningful gains in the ability to sit with and verbalize painful emotions that she would have previously been overwhelmed by and acted out impulsively.

The evaluation also played a key role in clarifying Heidi's needs for a therapeutically oriented educational placement. Dr. Y recounted that the rule-out of autism was vital in identifying which types of schools were more and less appropriate. Moreover, the clarification of the nature of Heidi's relational difficulties and needs was instrumental in countering the school district's push for a "tough-love" placement involving behavior modification. Ultimately, the assessment report assisted Heidi's parents to advocate successfully for a therapeutic day school placement as well as for state-supported in-home services, all of which have bolstered Heidi's movement toward greater emotional stabilization.

## REFERENCES

American Psychological Association Presidential Task Force on Evidence-Based Practice. (2006). Evidence-based practice in psychology. *American Psychologist, 61,* 271–285.

Bram, A. D. (2015). To resume a stalled psychotherapy?: Psychological testing to understand an impasse and reevaluate treatment options. *Journal of Personality Assessment, 97,* 241–249.

Bram, A. D., & Peebles, M. J. (2014). *Psychological testing that matters: Creating a road map for effective treatment.* Washington, DC: American Psychological Association.

Bram, A. D., & Yalof, J. (2015). Quantifying complexity: Personality assessment and its relationship with psychoanalysis. *Psychoanalytic Inquiry, 35*(Suppl.), 74–97.

Cooper, S. H., & Arnow, D. (1986). *The Rorschach Defense Scales.* Unpublished scoring manual, Department of Psychology, Cambridge Hospital, Cambridge, MA.

Exner, J. E. (2003). *The Rorschach: A comprehensive system: Vol. 1. Basic foundations* (4th ed.). New York: Wiley.

Finn, S. E. (2003). Therapeutic assessment of a man with "ADD." *Journal of Personality Assessment, 80,* 115–129.

Finn, S. E., Fischer, C. T., & Handler, L. (Eds.). (2012). *Collaborative/therapeutic assessment: A casebook and guide.* Hoboken, NJ: Wiley.

Fowler, J. C. (2012). Therapeutic assessment for a treatment in crisis following multiple suicide attempts. In S. E. Finn, C. T. Fisher, & L. Handler (Eds.), *Collaborative/therapeutic assessment: A casebook and guide* (pp. 113–132). Hoboken, NJ: Wiley.

Gabbard, G. O., & Wilkinson, S. M. (1994). *Management of countertransference with borderline patients.* Washington, DC: American Psychiatric Press.

Gold, J. M., & Hurt, S. W. (1990). The effects of haloperidol on thought disorder and IQ in schizophrenia. *Journal of Personality Assessment, 54,* 390–400.

Kleiger, J. H. (2017). *Rorschach assessment of psychotic phenomena: Clinical, conceptual, and empirical developments.* New York: Routledge.

Meyer, G. J., Finn, S. E., Eyde, L. D., Kay, G. G., Moreland, K. L., Dies, R. R., . . . Reed, G. M. (2001). Psychological testing and psychological assessment: A review of evidence and issues. *American Psychologist, 56,* 128–165.

Meyer, G. J., Viglione, D. J., Mihura, J. L., Erard, R. E., & Erdberg, P. (2011). *Rorschach Performance Assessment System: Administration, coding, interpretation, and technical manual.* Toledo, OH: Rorschach Performance Assessment System.

Peebles, M. J. (2012). *Beginnings: The art and science of planning psychotherapy* (2nd ed.). New York: Routledge.

Safran, J. D., Muran, J. C., & Eubanks-Carter, C. (2011). Repairing alliance ruptures. *Psychotherapy, 48,* 80–87.

Whitaker, C. A., Warkentin, J., & Johnson, N. (1950). The psychotherapeutic impasse. *American Journal of Orthopsychiatry, 20,* 641–647.

Yalof, J., & Rosenstein, D. (2014). Psychoanalytic interpretation of superego functioning following CS readministration procedures: Case illustration. *Journal of Personality Assessment, 96,* 192–203.

## Rorschach Responses "Heidi"

| Respondent ID: Heidi | Examiner: Anthony Bram, PhD |
|---|---|
| Location: Private Practice Office | Date: |
| Start Time: 10:15 A.M. | End Time: 11:10 A.M. |

| Cd # | R # | Or | Response | Clarification | R-Opt |
|---|---|---|---|---|---|
| I | 1 | | A butterfly (5″ pause); it looks like it's flying. (15″ pause) E: Remember, try to give two to three responses. R: And it has a broken wing. (5″ pause) E: Try to give two to three *different* responses. R: And it has a tail (5″ pause), and it has hands. That's it. (W) E: Again, try to see two or three things; can you see something other than a butterfly? | E: (Examiner Repeats Response [ERR].) R: Hands (D1), butterfly, broken wing (D2), tail (D3). | Pr |
| | 2 | | It looks like depression. (W) | E: (ERR) R: I don't know, just looks like it. E: What about the inkblot looks like that? R: The whole thing. E: Why depression? R: Because it's all black. | |
| II | 3 | | A broken heart (laughs). (D3) | E: (ERR) R: Because it looks like a heart form. E: What about it looks broken? R: It's . . . I don't know. [E could have queried "heart" for color.] | |
| | 4 | | A period (laughs). (D3) | E: (ERR) R: (She laughs.) Same area. E: Period? R: I don't know, it just looks like it. E: What about the inkblot looks like that? R: I don't know, it just looks like it. E: Help me see it—why a period? R: Because of the red. | |
| | 5 | | Elephants. That's it. (D6) | E: (ERR) R: Right there. They're fighting over meat. E: Meat? R: But the meat ain't there. E: Why does it look like elephants? R: 'Cause they look like it; they're happy. | |
| III | 6 | | Aliens. (Dd34) | E: (ERR) R: (She points.) E: Why aliens? R: 'Cause they're weird. E: Weird? R: Just the inkblot looks weird. | |
| | 7 | | Ravens. (D9) | E: (ERR) R: (She points.) E: What about it looks like ravens? R: The beak (protrusion on Dd32). E: Show me? R: Here. | |
| | 8 | | And death. (D3) | E: (ERR) R: Just does. The world wants to get them and kill it. E: What there makes it look like death? R: Because it just does, because it looks like blood. E: Blood? R: 'Cause it's red. | |

| Cd # | R # | Or | Response | Clarification | R-Opt |
|---|---|---|---|---|---|
| IV | 9 | | The grim reaper. (W) | E: (ERR)<br>R: The whole thing.<br>E: Grim reaper?<br>R: Because it looks spooky and deathly.<br>E: What about the blot makes it look like that?<br>R: It just does. | |
| | 10 | | The fallen angel. (D7) | E: (ERR)<br>R: (She traces blot.)<br>E: Fallen angel?<br>R: Because she's falling in midair.<br>E: Angel?<br>R: I already showed you the wings (D4). (She looks at clock.) 10:40. I can't believe we've been working so long. | |
| | 11 | | A black pixie. (D1) | E: (ERR)<br>R: This area (points) because it's small.<br>E: Where?<br>R: Right here.<br>E: What about it looks like a black pixie?<br>R: It just does; it looks like a black pixie. | |
| V | 12 | | A bat. (W) | E: (ERR)<br>R: (She traces whole blot.)<br>E: What about it makes it look like that?<br>R: The wings (D4) and body (D7) size. | |
| | 13 | | A moth. (W) | E: (ERR)<br>R: Same.<br>E: Why a moth?<br>R: It has wings (D4) and it looks like it, just does. | |
| | 14 | | A flying thing-a-ma-jig. (W) | E: (ERR)<br>R: Yeah. It looks like a flyin' thing-a-ma-jig. The whole thing looks so weird.<br>E: Thing-a-ma-jig?<br>R: Yeah.<br>E: Weird?<br>R: Just the whole thing. [Although the content is not specified, animal rather than inanimate movement seemed likely.] | |
| VI | 15 | | A dead cat. (W) | E: (ERR)<br>R: 'Cause the whiskers (Dd26) and the ears (Dd22), and the four legs (Dd25, Dd24) and the tail (Dd23).<br>E: Dead?<br>R: It has no heartbeat and it's . . . (she spreads own arms out to gesture that the percept is sprawled out). | |
| | 16 | | A dead rat. (W) | E: (ERR)<br>R: The same thing.<br>E: Rat?<br>R: I don't know. It just does.<br>E: Help me see it.<br>R: The whole thing looks like a dead rat.<br>E: Not sure what about it looks like a dead rat.<br>R: Just dead.<br>E: Dead?<br>R: It's not alive. The cat ate it. | |
| | 17 | | A fallen star. (D1) | E: (ERR)<br>R: Right here looks like a fallen star.<br>E: Why a fallen star?<br>R: It just does.<br>E: Fallen?<br>R: Because it is falling. | |

| Cd # | R # | Or | Response | Clarification | R-Opt |
|---|---|---|---|---|---|
| VII | 18 | | Faces. (D1) | E: (ERR)<br>R: Right here (pointing).<br>E: What makes it look like faces?<br>R: Just the whole structure (points to D1). | |
| | 19 | | Wings. (D3) | E: (ERR)<br>R: Just here. It just looks they're flying (flaps her arms). | |
| | 20 | | Tail. (Dd99 = outermost 1/8th of Dd23) | E: (ERR)<br>R: (She points to the blot.)<br>E: Tail?<br>R: It just does.<br>E: Help me see what makes it look like that.<br>R: It looks like a tail, just plain old tail. | |
| | 21 | | Moon. (Dd99 = crescent shape in lower half of DS10, curve mirroring curve of lower DS10)<br>E: (extends hand for card) Remember, try to give two or three responses. | E: (ERR)<br>R: Right in here, crescent moon.<br>E: What about the blot makes it look like that?<br>R: Just does when you tilt your head. | Pu |
| VIII | 22 | | Too happy! Too colorful! (W) | E: (ERR)<br>R: The whole thing.<br>E: Too happy?<br>R: All the colors are so bright. Like *too* happy. Every animal is smiling in happy land, *not my happy land*.<br>E: Animals?<br>R: Two happy animals (D1).<br>E: Did you see the animals the first time?<br>R: Yes. | |
| | 23 | | Rats fighting. (D1) | E: (ERR)<br>R: Right there (points to D1).<br>E: What makes them look like rats fighting?<br>R: They just do. | |
| IX | 24 | | Looks like a rainbow. (5″ pause)<br><br>It looks sad and depressing. (7″ pause)<br><br>It looks lonely.<br><br>[It initially appeared that these verbalizations reflected three separate responses, so E did not Prompt]. (W) | E: (ERR)<br>R: The whole thing, because of bright colors! The rainbow is sad and depressing because it has no friends.<br>E: Sad and depressing?<br>R: The rainbow is sad and depressing.<br>E: What about the blot makes it look sad and depressing?<br>R: All the colors do. Yeah! It has no friends (she begins speaking in a babyish, sing-song voice); nobody wants to be its friend.<br>E: Help me understand: You said a rainbow, sad and depressing, and looks lonely. Are these separate or part of the same thing?<br>R: Yeah, rainbow is sad and depressed and lonely, all one thing. | |
| X | 25 | | Looks like crabs fighting.<br>E: Remember, try to give two or three responses<br>R: (25″ pause) That's it.<br>E: Keep looking.<br>R: (20″ pause) Nothin'. (Dd99 = D1+12) (She hands card back.) | E: (ERR)<br>R: Right here (pointing).<br>E: Show me where.<br>R: (She traces D1 + D12.) | Pr |

# Rorschach Performance Assessment System (R-PAS)®

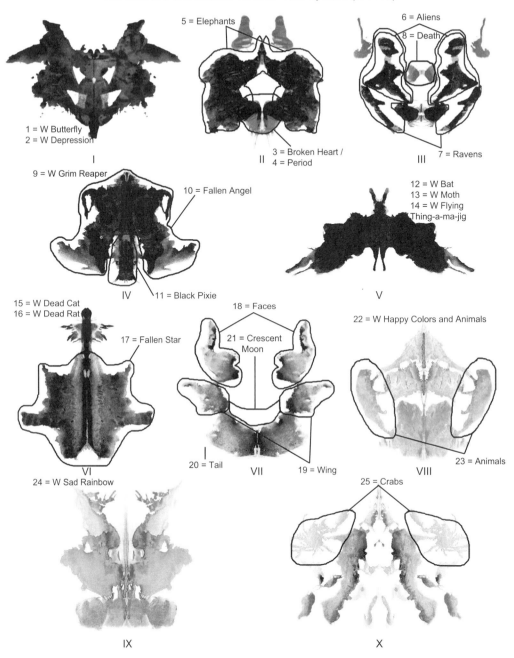

5 = Elephants

6 = Aliens

8 = Death

1 = W Butterfly
2 = W Depression

I

3 = Broken Heart /
4 = Period

II

7 = Ravens

III

9 = W Grim Reaper

10 = Fallen Angel

IV

11 = Black Pixie

12 = W Bat
13 = W Moth
14 = W Flying
Thing-a-ma-jig

V

15 = W Dead Cat
16 = W Dead Rat

17 = Fallen Star

VI

18 = Faces

21 = Crescent
Moon

20 = Tail

VII

19 = Wing

22 = W Happy Colors and Animals

23 = Animals

VIII

24 = W Sad Rainbow

IX

25 = Crabs

X

© 2012 R-PAS; Rorschach® trademarks and images are used with permission of the trademark owner, Hogrefe AG, Berne, Switzerland

134

# R-PAS Code Sequence: "Heidi"

**C-ID**: Heidi    **P-ID**: 7    **Age**: 15    **Gender**: Female    **Education**: 10

| Cd | # | Or | Loc | Loc # | SR | SI | Content | Sy | Vg | 2 | FQ | P | Determinants | Cognitive | Thematic | HR | ODL (RP) | R-Opt | Text |
|---|---|---|---|---|---|---|---|---|---|---|---|---|---|---|---|---|---|---|---|
| I | 1 | | W | | | | A | | | | o | P | FMa | INC1 | MOR | | | | Pr |
| | 2 | | W | | | | NC | | Vg | | n | | Mp,C' | | MOR | PH | | | |
| II | 3 | | D | 3 | | | An | | | | o | | F | | MOR,MAP | | | | * |
| Comment: E could have queried "heart" for color. | | | | | | | | | | | | | | | | | | | |
| | 4 | | D | 3 | | | Bl | | Vg | | n | | C | | | | | | |
| | 5 | | D | 6 | | | A | Sy | | 2 | o | P | FMa | FAB1 | AGM | PH | | | |
| III | 6 | | Dd | 34 | | | (H) | | | 2 | u | | F | | | GH | | | |
| | 7 | | D | 9 | | | A | | | 2 | u | | F | | | | | | |
| | 8 | | D | 3 | | | Bl,NC | | Vg | | n | | C | DR1 | MOR,MAP | | | | |
| IV | 9 | | W | | | | (H) | | | | o | P | F | | AGC,MOR | PH | | | |
| | 10 | | D | 7 | | | (H) | | | | o | | Mp | PEC | MOR | PH | | | |
| | 11 | | D | 1 | | | (H) | | | | - | | C' | | | PH | | | |
| V | 12 | | W | | | | A | | | | o | P | F | | | | | | |
| | 13 | | W | | | | A | | | | o | | F | | | | | | |
| | 14 | | W | | | | NC | | | | u | | FMa | | | | | | * |
| Comment: Although the content is not specified, animal rather than inanimate movement seemed likely. | | | | | | | | | | | | | | | | | | | |
| VI | 15 | | W | | | | A | | | | u | | F | PEC | MOR | | | | |
| | 16 | | W | | | | A | | | | u | | F | | MOR,MAP | | | | |
| | 17 | | D | 1 | | | NC | | | | - | | mp | PEC | MOR | | | | |
| VII | 18 | | D | 1 | | | Hd | | | 2 | o | P | F | | | GH | | | |
| | 19 | | D | 3 | | | Ad | | | 2 | u | | FMa | | | | | | |
| | 20 | | Dd | 99 | | | Ad | | | | - | | F | | | | | | |
| | 21 | | Dd | 99 | SR | | NC | | | | - | | F | | | | | Pu | |
| VIII | 22 | | W | | | | A,NC | | | 2 | o | P | Mp,C | INC1 | | PH | | | |
| | 23 | | D | 1 | | | A | Sy | | 2 | o | P | FMa | | AGM | PH | | | |
| IX | 24 | | W | | | | NC | | Vg | | n | | Mp,C | INC2 | MOR | PH | | | |
| X | 25 | | Dd | 99 | | | A | Sy | | 2 | o | | FMa | | AGM | PH | | Pr | |

©2010-2016 R-PAS

C-ID:    P-ID: 7    Age: 15    Gender: Female    Education: 9

| Domain/Variables | Raw Scores | Raw %ile | Raw SS | Cplx. Adj. %ile | Cplx. Adj. SS | Abbr. |
|---|---|---|---|---|---|---|
| **Admin. Behaviors and Obs.** | | | | | | |
| Pr | 2 | 82 | 114 | | | Pr |
| Pu | 1 | 86 | 116 | | | Pu |
| CT (Card Turning) | 0 | 18 | 86 | | | CT |
| **Engagement and Cog. Processing** | | | | | | |
| Complexity | 57 | 23 | 89 | | | Cmplx |
| R (Responses) | 25 | 62 | 105 | 70 | 108 | R |
| F% [Lambda=0.79] (Simplicity) | 44% | 59 | 103 | 37 | 95 | F% |
| Blend | 3 | 43 | 97 | 59 | 103 | Bln |
| Sy | 3 | 17 | 86 | 43 | 97 | Sy |
| MC | 10.0 | 78 | 112 | 88 | 118 | MC |
| MC - PPD | 1.0 | 76 | 111 | 76 | 111 | MC-PPD |
| M | 4 | 58 | 103 | 67 | 107 | M |
| M/MC [4/10.0] | 40% | 30 | 92 | 34 | 94 | M Prp |
| (CF+C)/SumC [4/4] | 100% | 96 | 126 | 96 | 126 | CFC Prp |
| **Perception and Thinking Problems** | | | | | | |
| EII-3 | 2.1 | 98 | 132 | 99 | 136 | EII |
| TP-Comp (Thought & Percept. Com...) | 1.5 | 88 | 117 | 92 | 122 | TP-C |
| WSumCog | 30 | 99 | 134 | 99 | 135 | WCog |
| SevCog | 4 | 99 | 138 | 99 | 138 | Sev |
| FQ-% | 16% | 79 | 112 | 87 | 117 | FQ-% |
| WD-% | 10% | 65 | 106 | 65 | 106 | WD-% |
| FQo% | 44% | 13 | 83 | 5 | 76 | FQo% |
| P | 7 | 77 | 111 | 85 | 117 | P |
| **Stress and Distress** | | | | | | |
| YTVC' | 2 | 23 | 89 | 35 | 95 | YTVC' |
| m | 1 | 42 | 97 | 46 | 98 | m |
| Y | 0 | 17 | 85 | 25 | 89 | Y |
| MOR | 10 | >99 | 146 | >99 | 146 | MOR |
| SC-Comp (Suicide Concern Comp.) | 5.0 | 65 | 106 | 72 | 109 | SC-C |
| **Self and Other Representation** | | | | | | |
| ODL% | 0% | 4 | 74 | 7 | 78 | ODL% |
| SR (Space Reversal) | 1 | 56 | 102 | 56 | 102 | SR |
| MAP/MAHP [3/3] | 100% | 94 | 123 | 92 | 122 | MAP Prp |
| PHR/GPHR [9/11] | 82% | 98 | 132 | 98 | 132 | PHR Prp |
| M- | 0 | 36 | 95 | 36 | 95 | M- |
| AGC | 1 | 17 | 86 | 19 | 87 | AGC |
| H | 0 | 5 | 75 | 11 | 80 | H |
| COP | 0 | 21 | 88 | 40 | 96 | COP |
| MAH | 0 | 26 | 90 | 26 | 90 | MAH |

© 2010-2015 R-PAS

C-ID:      P-ID: 7      Age: 15      Gender: Female      Education: 9

| Domain/Variables | Raw Scores | Raw %ile | Raw SS | Cplx. Adj. %ile | Cplx. Adj. SS | Standard Score Profile R-Optimized | Abbr. |
|---|---|---|---|---|---|---|---|
| **Engagement and Cog. Processing** | | | | | | | |
| W% | 40% | 51 | 100 | 63 | 105 | | W% |
| Dd% | 16% | 60 | 104 | 58 | 103 | | Dd% |
| SI (Space Integration) | 0 | 4 | 74 | 18 | 86 | | SI |
| IntCont | 0 | 11 | 81 | 23 | 88 | | IntC |
| Vg% | 16% | 89 | 118 | 88 | 117 | | Vg% |
| V | 0 | 29 | 92 | 29 | 92 | | V |
| FD | 0 | 21 | 88 | 43 | 97 | | FD |
| R8910% | 16% | <1 | 59 | <1 | 58 | | R8910% |
| WSumC | 6.0 | 86 | 116 | 91 | 121 | | WSC |
| C | 4 | 99 | 138 | 99 | 138 | | C |
| Mp/(Ma+Mp) [4/4] | 100% | 98 | 130 | 98 | 130 | | Mp Prp |
| **Perception and Thinking Problems** | | | | | | | |
| FQu% | 24% | 29 | 92 | 42 | 97 | | FQu% |
| **Stress and Distress** | | | | | | | |
| PPD | 9 | 51 | 101 | 69 | 107 | | PPD |
| CBlend | 0 | 28 | 91 | 28 | 91 | | CBlnd |
| C' | 2 | 62 | 105 | 62 | 105 | | C' |
| V | 0 | 29 | 92 | 29 | 92 | | V |
| CritCont% (Critical Contents) | 64% | 99 | 136 | 99 | 138 | | CrCt |
| **Self and Other Representation** | | | | | | | |
| SumH | 5 | 40 | 96 | 59 | 103 | | SumH |
| NPH/SumH [5/5] | 100% | 96 | 127 | 95 | 125 | | NPH Prp |
| V-Comp (Vigilance Composite) | 2.4 | 28 | 91 | 47 | 99 | | V-C |
| r (Reflections) | 0 | 36 | 95 | 36 | 95 | | r |
| p/(a+p) [5/11] | 45% | 57 | 103 | 53 | 101 | | p Prp |
| AGM | 3 | 98 | 131 | 98 | 131 | | AGM |
| T | 0 | 28 | 91 | 28 | 91 | | T |
| PER | 0 | 30 | 92 | 30 | 92 | | PER |
| An | 1 | 47 | 99 | 47 | 99 | | An |

© 2010-2015 R-PAS

# Using R-PAS in the Therapeutic Assessment of a University Student with Emotional Disconnection

Francesca Fantini
Justin D. Smith

## Introduction to the Case

"Cristina" was a 22-year-old student who was self-referred to the Student Counseling Service at the Catholic University of Milan, Italy, where she was completing an undergraduate degree in foreign languages. She sought a psychological consultation due to distress about her parents' divorce, which had occurred 1 year prior when her father discovered that her mother was having an affair with another man. Cristina participated in a therapeutic assessment (TA; Finn, 2007), which is the standard method of conducting brief consultations at the counseling service. She completed a five-session TA (see Figure 8.1), with a follow-up session conducted 3 weeks later, which included:

1. Initial session (Session 1): Assessment questions were collected along with background information related to the questions.
2. Test administration and extended inquiry (EI) sessions (Sessions 2–4): The Minnesota Multiphasic Personality Inventory–2 Restructured Form (MMPI-2-RF; Ben-Porath & Tellegen, 2008), the Early Memories Procedure, and the Rorschach Performance Assessment System (R-PAS; Meyer, Viglione, Mihura, Erard, & Erdberg, 2011) were administered. EIs were conducted to deepen the personal meaning of selected responses.
3. Summary and discussion session (Session 5): Cristina and the clinician discussed the results of her testing and the answers to her assessment questions.

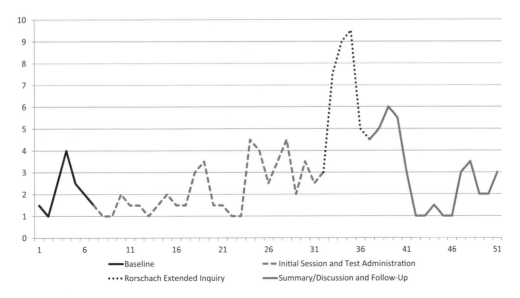

**FIGURE 8.1.** Cristina's composite daily rating and phases of the assessment and research design. Values on the X-axis indicate the day of symptom reporting. Values on the Y-axis indicate symptom severity (scale of 1–10).

## The Initial Interview

Cristina was a talkative and energetic young woman who appeared to be quickly at ease in disclosing that she was seeking help to deal with the impact her parents' separation had on her. She told the story of how, 1 year earlier, she learned that her mother was dating another man when she was eavesdropping on a conversation between her parents. Cristina recalled feeling angry at her mother at the time, but in the month that followed, she was able to pretend that she did not know of the affair. During this time, Cristina was able to remain focused on her studies and successfully pass eight exams. Eventually, her parents decided to tell her that they were separating. Cristina remembered that, at first, her parents only told her that they were having marital difficulties, but omitted mention of her mother's affair. So, she confronted her mother directly about her infidelity. She remembered talking with her tearful mother, but said she did not recall feeling anything in that moment. She had a calm and reasonable attitude, while trying to put herself in her "mother's shoes" to understand her reasons. After that conversation, her mother left the family home and Cristina continued to live there with her father.

In the following days and weeks, Cristina's anger toward her mother progressively intensified—particularly, she said, after realizing how much her father was suffering. After the separation, Cristina's father became very moody. He would stop talking to anyone for days at a time, including Cristina, if they mentioned his estranged wife. It was hard for Cristina to live in the house with her father this way, and she felt angry at her mother for being responsible for the situation. At the same time, Cristina was disturbed by her own anger, as she felt it was an unproductive feeling that put her at risk of hurting her mother. Cristina's mother, on the contrary, was acting as if nothing had happened; she was as calm and cheerful as she had always been. According to Cristina, her mother had always been a kind woman who never became angry or argued with anyone. Cristina felt that her mother's attitude was fueling the anger she felt toward her because she wanted her mother to regret what she had done, and instead she appeared utterly unremorseful. In this context, after the parents' separation, neither Cristina nor her parents talked again about the family situation or its impact on each of them. Cristina said she did not think that talking to her parents would be useful, as it would not change what had happened.

## Cristina's Assessment Questions

At the time of the assessment, Cristina's difficulty concerned being around her mother. Despite Cristina's best efforts to hide the anger she felt toward her mother, she realized it was coming out, albeit indirectly. For example, Cristina often had strong angry reactions to minor misunderstandings that frequently occurred between her and her mother, and she ended up feeling bad for being aggressive and difficult. She hoped that as time went by, her anger would just fade away, but she came to realize that this was not happening and her anger continued to be intense and disturbing to her. Her first assessment question then was, "How can I get rid of the anger I feel toward my mother?" While describing her family situation and her difficult feelings toward her mother, Cristina became progressively more energetic in her nonverbal behavior and obviously started to feel some of the anger she was describing. Otherwise, no distressing feelings, such as sadness or sense of loss, appeared to surface.

Cristina also sought help for the frequent times that she felt "disconnected from her emotions." She described how, since the crisis in her family, it became fairly common that she would listen with a rational attitude to her best friend talking about her problems, without feeling any emotion. Other times, while she was interacting with her boyfriend, she realized that she felt distant and emotionally disconnected from him, and she was worried that over time this could result in the end of their 4-year-long relationship. In recalling the year since her parents' separation, Cristina had a general impression of herself as falling into apathy and feeling distant from others, even though she had trouble remembering clearly what she was thinking or feeling, as her memories were fuzzy. Her second question was, "Why do I often feel disconnected from my emotions?"

## Cristina's Non-R-PAS Assessment Findings

Cristina's MMPI-2-RF main profile was valid and showed no elevations above the cutoff (T score > 65) in any of the test scales. The highest elevation was a T score of 68 on the Anger Proneness (ANP) scale, indicating a tendency to internalize anger, which was bottled up and not expressed. However, in understanding Cristina's self-perception through her responses to this self-report measure, there were various interesting low scores that were worth consideration. Cristina reported not experiencing much emotional distress (Emotional/Internalizing Dysfunction, EID = 49; Demoralization, RCd

= 51), except for the anger that disturbed her a great deal. She instead depicted herself as being very able to manage life difficulties without feeling overwhelmed (Helplessness/Hopelessness, HLP = 38), and as being a self-confident person (Self-Doubt, SFD = 42; raw score = 0) with very strong feelings of engagement in and ability to find pleasure in life (Low Positive Emotions, RC2 = 40). Such low scores suggested that dysphoric, depressive, or sad feelings did not seem to be present in her emotional world, as might normally be expected given the situation. She also described herself as very behaviorally controlled (Behavioral/Externalizing Dysfunction, BXD = 39), particularly constricted in behavioral expressions of anger (Aggression, AGG = 36) and prone to renounce her assertive strivings to reach her goals if it might hurt others (Aggressiveness-Revised, AGGR-r = 43). Such scores, together with the aforementioned elevation on the ANP scale, were consistent with her self-report in the interview, suggesting that Cristina was experiencing strong conflicts around the expression of anger, and she therefore tended to avoid conflict in interpersonal relationships. These scores also seemed to indicate that Cristina's conflict around the expression of anger could be a more general issue, going beyond her mother and the current family situation. Her recent family circumstances seemed to be pushing her to feel distressing emotions, such as anger, and probably also sadness, which she felt unable to manage. The emotional disconnection she felt most likely represented avoidant mechanisms put in place to protect her against having distressing feelings surface related to the loss of her intact family. She was not able at that time to avoid feeling angry, but this left her feeling very uncomfortable and wishing to find a way to "get rid" of these feelings as soon as possible, as was reflected in her first assessment question.

On the Early Memories Procedure, Cristina described various childhood experiences representing variations on the theme of facing emotionally distressing situations (i.e., being ill in the nurse's office at a camp [age 6], breaking a finger and feeling a lot of pain [age 7]) without the support that she was longing for (her parents were far away or at work). In such situations, she felt overwhelmed by painful and distressing emotions that she was dealing with alone. As a result, as is often the case with children (Weiss, 1993), she was not able to be critical toward her unavailable parents, and she began to feel that there was something wrong with her for not being able to just stop feeling the emotions that led her to need support. According to Bruhn's (1992) theory, such memories and the way they are recalled represent prototypical examples of a core unresolved issue facing the client. Cristina's memories revealed what she learned to believe or expect from herself and the world as a result of experiencing distressing emotions such as loneliness, sadness, or fear; she expected that her need for support would go unfulfilled. Her solution seemed to be to simply stop feeling these emotions altogether.

It was clear from Cristina's MMPI-2-RF results that she had no insight into the hypothesized emotional regulation difficulties. She saw herself as a cheerful and resourceful woman, caring for others, and able to face life's difficulties without losing her optimism and hope—which could represent an identification with her mother. The ongoing anger she was experiencing toward her mother, and the emotional disconnection and apathy she was experiencing in her significant relationships, were very concerning for her because they jeopardized her self-narrative. During the EI of the Early Memories Procedure, Cristina began to accept the notion that her psychological strengths helped her deal with very stressful situations even without the support she needed and for which she was longing. She described frequent experiences of making herself available to others (and even soliciting others) to listen to and support them, but these others tended not to see Cristina's own difficulties in dealing with her family situation. It appeared that everyone saw her as positive and strong. She seemed to begin accepting the idea that what happened in her family had been more than she could deal with alone. At the same time, she minimized the influence of her earlier experiences of learning to rely on herself in the face of distressing situations. While discussing her early memories, Cristina strongly refused to explore the idea that her parents could have been more available when she needed them. In fact, Cristina idealized her parents, whom she described as always supportive and caring throughout her childhood, even though she said that her mother was often away for weeks on work trips and she described her father, who was her main attachment figure, as emotionally closed up and prone to anger and criticism. This idealization contributed to Cristina's feeling shocked about the affair and dissolution of their marriage. It also made it difficult for her to develop a more compassionate narrative concerning her difficulties dealing with the emotions triggered by her family crisis.

## Why R-PAS for Cristina's Therapeutic Assessment?

At this point in the TA, answering Cristina's assessment questions would have required delivering a lot of information to her that fundamentally conflicted with her narrative about herself and others. In doing so, the clinician probably would have triggered even more overwhelming and traumatizing emotions or a defensive and avoidant reaction (i.e., dropping out) in Cristina. In either case, the TA likely would have failed. Thus, there were two goals for using R-PAS:

1. *To better understand Cristina's emotional processing and sense of self.* The results of the MMPI-2-RF provided information about aspects of Cristina's psychological functioning that she was aware of and that were more likely to be evident in familiar situations in which she was less emotionally activated (Finn, 1996; Meyer, 1997). It was important to further assess Cristina's ways of dealing with distressing emotions in the context of a performance-based test such as the Rorschach, which assesses clients' implicit processes that automatically influence their behavior in a situation with more emotional stimulation than the self-report task (Bornstein, 2002; Finn, 1996, 2012; Meyer et al., 2011). In this case, the Rorschach could give the clinician more insight into (a) the origins of Cristina's inability to report distressing emotions other than anger and (b) the pervasiveness of the psychological mechanisms that prevented such emotions to surface. In using R-PAS, the clinician expected that the Stress and Distress domain would give more detailed information about Cristina's way of dealing with the distressing emotions possibly stirred up by her parents' separation and the traumatic impact that this seemed to have on her. Also, the data related to the Self and Other Representation domain could elucidate Cristina's ambivalence about asking for support.

2. *As a way to help Cristina express her implicit needs and motives* through the test in the here-and-now experience of the session. This would provide the clinician with what was needed to collaboratively work with her (i.e., through an EI) to

become more aware of and eventually reintegrate what she had previously disavowed (Finn, 2007).

## Cristina's R-PAS Administration

Cristina arrived at the session when the clinician intended to administer the Rorschach eager to discuss a "stupid" fight she'd had with her mother concerning the possible breakup of a couple with whom she was friends. It was important to give Cristina the time to express her anger and disdain for her mother's attitude toward her friends' problems. Her mother was calm and understanding of the reasons why the couple was separating, and Cristina felt angry with her for not taking into account the pain that a separation could produce for each of the partners. The clinician supported Cristina in expressing her angry feelings, and she eventually became visibly calmer. Then, it was possible to introduce the Rorschach. The test was presented as an instrument to better understand her assessment question, "Why do I often feel disconnected from my emotions?" Cristina did not have prior knowledge of the test and she readily accepted taking it without showing any resistance or asking specific questions. The administration took place in the office where Cristina and the clinician had met in previous sessions. Cristina did not show any sign of distress or any noteworthy emotional reaction at any point during the administration. She was observably at ease and willing to collaborate in giving the requested number of two or three responses per card. The test administration took 1½ hours.

## Cristina's R-PAS Results[1]

### Administration Behaviors and Observations with Engagement and Cognitive Processing

Cristina produced a very complex and elaborated protocol (Complexity SS = 123; F% SS = 90), showing that she was very engaged with the task. She was attentive and responsive to the test and the clinician's instructions, providing a high number of responses (R = 31, SS = 120) and requiring neither solicitation (Pr = 0, SS = 89) nor interruptions from the clinician (Pu = 0, SS = 96). The high number of responses contributed to the complexity of the protocol. Cristina's Complexity score was also related to her elevated scores in the Location, Space, and Object Quality Complexity score (LSO SS = 125) and Content Complexity score (Cont SS = 125). These scores suggested an unusually high ability to organize information from and make sense of her environment through conceptualizing the relations between different aspects of her experience, and a highly developed capacity of holding in mind and expressing multiple ideas in a context where multiple interpretations were possible.

Cristina showed many psychological resources to manage life challenges that were not easily challenged by situational stressors (MC SS = 138; MC–PPD = 148). Such resources seemed related to an above-average level of reflectiveness, ability to

---

[1] See Appendix 8.1 at the end of the chapter for Cristina's R-PAS Responses, Location Sheet, Code Sequence, and Page 1 and 2 Profiles.

think before acting, and a strong capacity to mentalize (M SS = 129). However, her scores indicated that she could also, on occasion, fall into significant misunderstanding or misperception of people (M– = 1, SS = 113), discussed below. Cristina also displayed an acute awareness of stimulating environmental features (WSumC SS = 131) that contributed to her high psychological resources. Her highly developed coping and thinking capacities suggested by her Complexity index could, however, become a weakness given her tendency to take an unconventional and individualistic approach to interpreting the environment and the people around her—making her ideas, motivations, and behaviors difficult to understand (FQo% SS = 79; FQu% SS = 123; M– SS = 113).

Given Cristina's high Complexity score, it was helpful to plot her R-PAS Complexity Adjusted scores. Her Complexity Adjusted scores showed that her ability to respond to and synthesize different aspects of her environment was commensurate with her general level of complexity (R CAdj SS = 106; Sy CAdj SS = 99). However, her responses were more simplistic than expected, indicating that she attended to multiple channels of information less often than expected given her level of Complexity (Blend CAdj SS = 73). On the other hand, compared to others with a similar level of Complexity, she displayed a highly developed ability to reflect and mentalize (M CAdj SS = 115) and to be receptive to evocative stimuli coming from events in the environment, including that from other people (WSumC CAdj SS = 120). She seemed to be able to balance her choices by using both her thinking abilities and her emotional reactions (M/MC SS = 100). However, she showed a proclivity to respond to emotionally arousing situations in a direct way, without much mental filtering [(CF+C)/SumC SS = 116]. Therefore, her preference for not talking to her parents could have been an adaptive effort to minimize the risk of losing control over her reactions if the situation became too emotionally stimulating.

## Perception and Thinking Problems

Cristina's R-PAS had no signs of severe perception and thinking problems (EII-3 SS = 105; TP-Comp SS = 106; SevCog SS = 94; FQ–% SS = 103). However, her thinking and reasoning could be more immature and ineffective than expected (WSumCog SS = 117), especially in situations that activated her affective reactions (four of the five Cognitive Codes appear in responses involving chromatic color; see R4, R6, R27, and R30). Cristina also seemed to oscillate between a strong tendency to perceive events in an unconventional or personalized way (FQu% SS = 123) and a highly stereotyped, conformist view of the world (P SS = 126). The latter tendency was especially visible in sessions when she was talking about her view of family and couple relationships, which seemed to be rigidly anchored to stereotyped ideas (i.e., betrayals are not acceptable or understandable under any circumstances, partners with large age differences are not compatible). Her rigidity related to these issues most likely had a role in her experiencing a stronger shock when an affair happened in her own family.

## Stress and Distress

Cristina's coping resources were extremely high even when adjusted for her general level of complexity of responding (MC–PPD CAdj SS = 148). This result seemed related to both her high psychological resources (MC CAdj = 122) and her significantly low sensitivity to the nuances and subtleties of her inner life (YTVC' CAdj SS = 81) given her level of Complexity. Cristina did not appear to be experiencing the expected level of normal sadness, helplessness, and distress that are common in individuals who are in contact with their emotional world (Y SS = 85; m SS = 84; MOR SS = 86; PPD CAdj SS = 59). These results seemed to strengthen what had been already found with the MMPI-2-RF. That is, Cristina was more stable, reliable, and resilient than most people in handling stressful or upsetting situations. A clear example was her ability to successfully focus on her studies for a month after uncovering her mother's affair. However, her very high coping capacities were, in part, a consequence of a numbed sensitivity to distressing emotions (low related scores on both the MMPI-2-RF and R-PAS), which had the downside of making her feel emotionally disconnected from herself and others.

## Self and Other Representation

Cristina seemed to have the capacity for interpersonal competence and skills in managing and understanding self, others, and relationships (PHR/GHR SS = 95). She appeared to be very interested in and attentive to people, which she tended to see in integrated, intact ways, without notable signs of vigilance or guardedness, particularly given her level of Complexity (H CAdj SS = 113; SumH CAdj SS = 116; V-Comp CAdj SS = 98). She seemed to have developed the ability to view relationships as cooperative and positive, and showed an average or above-average ability to envision mature and healthy interpersonal relationships, even after adjusting for her level of Complexity (COP CAdj SS = 112; MAH CAdj SS = 102). She also did not show notable signs of implicit dependency needs in general and given her level of Complexity (ODL% CAdj SS = 98). However, her way of thinking about others and relationships could be immature at times, especially when she was emotionally activated (in R6 FAB1 and potential INC1 connected to chromatic color, COP and MAH).

Her scores also supported the idea that Cristina could fall into misperceptions of others on occasion (M– = 1, SS = 113). In fact, on Card V she gave an M– response, when she saw "a person trying to wrap me . . . arms; they are spreading out like something that would wrap around me" (R14). In this response, she had a distorted perception of a human figure (FQ–) in relationship to the implied aggressive ideation that was present (the way she described the action did not meet full criteria for coding AGM). It is also noteworthy that Cristina lost distance from the card and began to describe the percept from an egocentric frame of reference that seemed to indicate a lowered capacity to think clearly and effectively. A similar process had already appeared in Card IV (R10), when Cristina saw a monster (AGC) in a similar position to the human in Card V, and lost distance from the card in a very similar way. In the sequence of scores, these responses came shortly after repeated, positive connotations attributed to human relationships (COP and MAH scores), which were concentrated in the first three cards. In the rest of the protocol, Cristina gave responses with three other thematic codes related to aggression (AGC in R25 and R30, AGM in R27), and in two of them she again showed clearer signs of ineffective and immature thinking (FAB1 in R27 and R30). Therefore, Cristina's scores seemed to indicate that the emergence of aggressive ideation or preoccupations around aggression had a negative impact on her ability to think clearly and effectively and might lead to distortions in the accuracy of her perception of others.

Although her total scores related to aggression were not elevated compared to the norms (AGC SS = 100; AGM SS = 110), on two occasions she gave quasi-aggressive descriptions of movements that were not elaborated enough to meet the coding criteria for AGM (in addition to the already discussed R14, this also happened on R16). It could be hypothesized that Cristina's aggressive pulls might be stronger overall than what was clearly elaborated in the Rorschach and that the discomfort she felt in relating to aggression, already detected by the MMPI-2-RF, was preventing her from elaborating some responses into clearly aggressive actions.

Overall, Cristina seemed to have the interest and the skills to build positive and mutual relationships. However, when she was emotionally aroused and in contact with her aggression, there was a higher likelihood that her thinking capacities would become less effective and more immature, and she could even misperceive others in significant ways. In terms of giving and asking for support, it could be hypothesized that when Cristina was undergoing personal difficulties, in which there was a high likelihood of being angry or emotionally aroused, she was less able to reach out to others. When she was less personally involved, she was able to use her elevated potential for empathy (M CAdj SS = 115) and her social skills to be a good support for others.

The clinician conducted an EI on response 27 by asking Cristina to describe any personal meaning related to the "inkblots trying to get somewhere, but they are pulled back by other inkblots underneath"[2] (scored CF, FAB1, AGM, PHR). Reflecting upon this response, Cristina easily identified with the victim of the aggressive movement, and disclosed that she often felt trapped by her parents' expectations that had left her feeling inadequate as a consequence of not being able to reach their desired standards. A clear example she gave was the repeated experience of feeling criticized for her weight and her body appearance, as her parents desired that she be thinner and more feminine. Their attitude made her angry but also left her feeling inadequate and insecure regarding her personal worth. She also felt trapped by her father's need of her support. In more than one instance, her father expressed the fear of also being abandoned by Cristina, saying things to her like, "Please, don't run away from me." Cristina felt that the pull to take care of her father's pain clearly conflicted with her desire for independence to the point that she felt guilty thinking about planning her summer vacations with her friends and boyfriend. While discussing the personal meaning to response 27, Cristina expressed a mix of anger and distress regarding her parents, which the clinician again validated. When she expressed a sense of helplessness for not being able to fix the situation, tears came into her eyes.

Personal meanings also provided the background for interpreting Cristina's very high Anatomy content (An SS = 128), which seemed to indicate the presence of strong worries about her body that were perhaps connected to feeling inadequate and criticized about her appearance.[3] The EI also opened the door for a deidealization of Cris-

---

[2] This response is thematically similar to R16, where an ambiguous object with "very little" wings is "trying to get out" and is "running away from darkness, fog" that apparently threatens to envelop it.

[3] Four of her five An responses were of lungs. Although unusual, it was not clear what significance this pattern may hold for her.

tina's parents that was tied to her critique about her relationship with them (their way of diminishing her, her sense of falling lower than their standards) and about their actual incapacity to deal with their marital issues in a way that did not negatively impact Cristina emotionally.

## Summary and Conceptualization

In summary, R-PAS highlighted important aspects of Cristina's functioning that were related to her questions. It helped the clinician further understand that Cristina had a general difficulty in managing emotionally arousing situations, including situations involving anger and aggressive pulls, as she could react in unfiltered ways and lose her ability to think clearly and effectively. This self-perceived troubling response led her to use avoidant strategies to protect herself from the risk of losing control and from the fear of acting in destructive ways toward important people and relationships. Therefore, Cristina faced a dilemma in finding effective ways to discharge anger because she was unsure of her ability to manage such emotionally arousing situations. The systemic piece was also relevant. Cristina was also holding and expressing her father's anger, which he too was not able to effectively manage, and she felt stymied by her mother's naïveté, which Cristina sensed as indicating that she would have difficulty witnessing or accepting Cristina's anger or pain about the affair and divorce.

An alternative way of interpreting Cristina's stuck emotional place is to consider her difficulties in the framework of the necessity to grieve her past idealized intact family by using Elisabeth Kübler-Ross' model of the stages of grief: denial, anger, bargaining, depression, and acceptance (Kübler-Ross, 1969; Mercer & Wennechuk, 2010). After discovering her mother's affair, Cristina was successfully able to deny the reality of the situation. However, when her parents decided to separate, she began resenting her mother for causing pain to her father and to her and for leaving the family. Cristina had been in the bargaining stage of grief, when she repeatedly thought about the various ways her parents could have handled the situation differently, so that everyone would have felt respected and the separation would have been less painful. And her efforts to be present at home for her father were also a way she tried to keep control of the suffering. By being supportive, she hoped to reduce the family's pain. What Cristina had not been able to do, in order to progress to the acceptance stage, was to enter the stage of depression. The R-PAS results helped the clinician understand that she tended to split off such emotional states. In this way, she was able to cope with the situation much better, but it left her with a sense of disconnection from herself and the world around her. It could be hypothesized that the sadness associated with grieving the loss of her intact family and of the idealization of her parents would have been too much for Cristina to tolerate, given her tendency to manage the distress alone. The assessment revealed that Cristina was prone to split off distressing emotions well before the family crisis. However, in the aftermath of the crisis, the disconnection from such emotions became stronger and distressing in and of itself. In particular, her YTVC' score suggested that in a subsequent psychotherapy, Cristina could be helped to better recognize and articulate her emotions in a way that she was not able to do at the time of the assessment.

## Feedback Session and Follow-Up

In this session, Cristina and the clinician discussed the answers to her assessment questions. The clinician's description of her dilemma of change resonated with Cristina. In order to feel less emotionally disconnected, she had to feel the bad emotions associated with her parents' separation, and doing so could be overwhelming and even retraumatizing. However, to protect herself from dealing with such emotions and to continue to function at her usual high level, she needed to numb herself to those emotions. Cristina disclosed that she recently began to think about what had definitely changed in her life when she suddenly said to herself, "You can't think about this now," and found a way to distract herself. The option of expressing her anger to her mother was also discussed. She expected it would be difficult, as the anger tended to affect her ability to think clearly and she had a desire to avoid hurting others in any way.

Three weeks after the summary/discussion session, Cristina participated in a follow-up session. She told the clinician that a few days before she had been able to confront her mother about the family situation and to disclose her angry feelings toward her. Afterward she felt less bottled up with anger and less fake in relating to her mother. Cristina said she was also feeling less disconnected, although she still tended to try to distract herself when she began feeling sadness. For this reason, she was considering initiating psychotherapy.

## An Empirical Test of the Impact of the Rorschach Extended Inquiry

Cristina consented to participate in a research study where repeated measures were collected to assess the effectiveness of the intervention. She met a research assistant 1 week before beginning the TA to develop individualized rating scales that captured salient aspects of her psychological functioning that she felt were problematic. Cristina then completed the rating scales throughout the TA and for 2 weeks afterward (see Figure 8.1). Single-subject experiments with daily measures have been used previously to evaluate the effectiveness of the TA model with adult clients (e.g., Aschieri & Smith, 2012; Smith & George, 2012; Tarocchi, Aschieri, Fantini, & Smith, 2013). In this case, Cristina's daily measures were used to probe the potential effectiveness of the Rorschach EI session in particular. This type of study has been done to evaluate the effects of the family intervention session in a child TA case (Smith, Nicholas, Handler, & Nash, 2011).

We tested the hypothesis that the Rorschach EI would serve as a catalyst in getting Cristina to experience the negative affective states that she had split off in the year since her parents' divorce. This strategy is consistent with evidence-based treatments for posttraumatic stress grounded in affect exposure and coping skill development (Foa, Keane, Friedman, & Cohen, 2008). The hypothesized model consisted of a relatively flat symptom trajectory from the baseline period through the initial meeting and test administration sessions, followed by a spike in symptom severity beginning at the Rorschach EI session and a rapid return to baseline levels from the summary/discussion session through the follow-up.

We tested this model using the CUSTOM VECTOR function of the simulation modeling analysis (SMA) program for time-series data (Borckardt et al., 2008), which allows the researcher to specify an a priori model and to test the fit of the data to that model. Although Cristina reported on two indices, the high and statistically significant concordant cross-correlation ($r = .44$, $p < .001$) between them supported evaluating a daily mean score. The model provided good fit to the data: $r = .73$, $p = .008$. We then conducted two supplemental analyses to determine whether the rapid spike and decline around the EI were statistically significant. Using a level-change analysis in SMA, which determines the exact probability of observing a given mean difference between two streams of data, the results indicated a significant increase in symptom severity after the EI compared to before (Phase means: 2.22, 7.10; $r = .80$, $p = .0001$) and a significant decrease following the summary/discussion session (Phase means: 7.10, 2.75; $r = -.73$, $p = .024$). These findings support the effectiveness of the intervention strategy with the Rorschach EI.

## Summary of R-PAS Contributions with Christina

In summary, the use of R-PAS allowed the clinician to articulate a more accurate hypothesis about Cristina's emotional disconnection and difficulty in dealing with her anger. It confirmed and expanded the knowledge about Cristina's psychological strengths, while putting them in the context of her difficulties in dealing with emotions and of dissociating important aspects of her emotional functioning. Also, the EI conducted on her Rorschach responses helped Cristina get in contact with and express attitudes and feelings toward her parents and her family that she had previously disowned. This shift opened up the possibility of her getting closer to some of the sadness and sense of loss from which she was distancing herself and helped her become more aware of her avoidant strategies in dealing with such feelings.

## REFERENCES

Aschieri, F., & Smith, J. D. (2012). The effectiveness of therapeutic assessment with an adult client: A single-case study using a time-series design. *Journal of Personality Assessment, 94*, 1–11.

Ben-Porath, Y. S., & Tellegen, A. (2008). *MMPI-2-RF (Minnesota Multiphasic Personality Inventory–2 Restructured Form): Manual for administration, scoring, and interpretation.* Minneapolis: University of Minnesota Press.

Borckardt, J. J., Nash, M. R., Murphy, M. D., Moore, M., Shaw, D., & O'Neil, P. (2008). Clinical practice as natural laboratory for psychotherapy research. *American Psychologist, 63*, 77–95.

Bornstein, R. F. (2002). A process dissociation approach to objective–projective test score interrelationships. *Journal of Personality Assessment, 78*, 47–68.

Bruhn, A. R. (1992). The Early Memories Procedure: A projective test of autobiographical memory: Part 1. *Journal of Personality Assessment, 58*, 1–15.

Finn, S. E. (1996). Assessment feedback integrating MMPI-2 and Rorschach findings. *Journal of Personality Assessment, 67*, 543–557.

Finn, S. E. (2007). *In our clients' shoes: Theory and techniques of therapeutic assessment.* Mahwah, NJ: Erlbaum.

Finn, S. E. (2012). Implications of recent research in neurobiology for psychological assessment. *Journal of Personality Assessment, 94*, 440–449.

Foa, E. B., Keane, T. M., Friedman, M. J., & Cohen, J. A. (2008). *Effective treatments for PTSD: Practice guidelines from the International Society for Traumatic Stress Studies* (2nd ed.). New York: Guilford Press.

Kübler-Ross, E. (1969). *On death and dying.* New York: Routledge.

Mercer, D., & Wennechuk, K. J. (2010). *Making divorce work: 8 essential keys to resolving conflict and rebuilding your life.* New York: Penguin.

Meyer, G. J. (1997). On the integration of personality assessment methods: The Rorschach and MMPI. *Journal of Personality Assessment, 68*, 297–330.

Meyer, G. J., Viglione, D. J., Mihura, J., Erard, R. E., & Erdberg, P. (2011). *Rorschach Performance Assessment System: Administration, coding, interpretation, and technical manual.* Toledo, OH: Rorschach Performance Assessment System.

Smith, J. D., & George, C. (2012). Therapeutic Assessment case study: Treatment of a woman diagnosed with metastatic cancer and attachment trauma. *Journal of Personality Assessment, 94*, 331–344.

Smith, J. D., Nicholas, C. R. N., Handler, L., & Nash, M. R. (2011). Examining the potential impact of a family session in therapeutic assessment: A single-case experiment. *Journal of Personality Assessment, 93*, 204–212.

Tarocchi, A., Aschieri, F., Fantini, F., & Smith, J. D. (2013). Therapeutic Assessment of complex trauma: A single-case time-series study. *Clinical Case Studies, 12*, 228–245.

Weiss, J. (1993). *How psychotherapy works: Process and technique.* New York: Guilford Press.

**Cristina's R-PAS Responses, Location Sheet, Code Sequence, and Page 1 and 2 Profiles**

**Rorschach Responses "Cristina"**

| Respondent ID: Cristina | Examiner: Francesca Fantini |
|---|---|
| Location: Counseling Service for University Students, Ente per il diritto allo studio dell'Università Cattolica (EDUCatt), Milan, Italy | Date: **/**/**** |
| Start Time: 2:30 P.M. | End Time: 4:00 P.M. |

| Cd # | R # | Or | Response | Clarification | R-Opt |
|---|---|---|---|---|---|
| I | 1 | | A butterfly. (W) | E: (Examiner Repeats Response [ERR].)<br>R: Body (D4), wings (D2), and antennae (D1). | |
| | 2 | | A bat. (Dd99 = upper half of W) | E: (ERR)<br>R: For the wings (D7), the shape of the wings right here, this part of the blot (respondent indicates). | |
| | 3 | | A person going toward something with the hands in this way (respondent mimics); this seems like a woman's dress. (D4) | E: (ERR)<br>R: Hands (D1), the dress (Dd24) is tighter here at the belt line, and the boots (Dd31). | |
| II | 4 | | A face. (W) | E: (ERR)<br>R: Strange eyes (D2), nose with the round shape of the nostrils (DdS30), mouth (DS5), cheeks (D6), chin under here (D3).<br>E: What made them look like strange eyes?<br>R: Maybe the color; here's the mouth and the nose in the white, and the eyes, colored; in a normal face the eyes are colored. | |
| | 5 | | Two people joining their hands, in front of each other. (D6) | E: (ERR)<br>R: Body, feet, knees (Dd28), joining their hands here (D4; she mimics the action), and the other person is the same. | |
| | 6 | | Two people who are meeting each other and they are looking at each other; in the previous one they were looking down. (W) | E: (ERR)<br>R: They seem to have roosters' heads (D2), but the body is of a person, body (D1), joined hands (D4), and here the roosters are looking at each other and talking to each other.<br>E: What made them look like roosters' heads?<br>R: They have a red crest and their beak is open. | |
| III | 7 | | Two women, they seem to be dancing; they're holding on to a table and are moving backward. (D1) | E: (ERR)<br>R: Two women's bodies (D9). I imagined a table or something they could hold on to (D7), to move their bottom backward.<br>E: What made it look like a table?<br>R: No, I didn't really see a table; I just imagined it could be a table or something. | |
| | 8 | | Two lungs. (D3) | E: (ERR)<br>R: The blot here, the color and the shape. | |
| | 9 | | It could be a uterus. (Dd35) | E: (ERR)<br>R: This is the ending part where the baby would come out (D7). I imagined in the upper part it would be tighter, and this could be the ovaries (Dd32) that are connected.<br>E: What made them look like ovaries?<br>R: The round shape. | |

| Cd # | R # | Or | Response | Clarification | R-Opt |
|------|-----|----|----------|---------------|-------|
| IV | 10 | | A monster looking at me, so it's like in front of me. (D7) | E: (ERR)<br>R: Two feet (D6), legs, body, head (D3), in front of me because he seems to be in this position (respondent mimics a still position with open legs and arms). | |
| | 11 | | A clown. (D7) | E: (ERR)<br>R: It's similar to the previous one but has shoes and trousers.<br>E: Similar to the previous one?<br>R: I imagined the head (D3) here and then it's not clear, but the lower part and the feet (D6) are those of a clown. | |
| | 12 | | A tree in the darkness. (W) | E: (ERR)<br>R: The trunk (D1) and the round-like shape (central portion of D7, not including D6, 3, 4) in the darkness because of the color—it reminds me when the trees don't have clear outlines and shade into the darkness (outer parts of D7). | |
| V | 13 | | A bat. (W) | E: (ERR)<br>R: Feet (D9), lower part of the body, wings (D4), and upper part with ears (D6). | |
| | 14 | | A person trying to wrap me, in front of me. (W). | E: (ERR)<br>R: Head (D6), body, feet (D9), arms (D4); they are spreading out like something that would wrap around me. | |
| | 15 | | A butterfly. (W) | E: (ERR)<br>R: Body (D7), lower part, antennae (Dd34), wings (D4). | |
| VI | 16 | | Somebody, an animal trying to get out, run away. (W) | E: (ERR)<br>R: I don't know which kind of animal this is; body (D3), some sort of wings (Dd22), it's running away from darkness, fog; it's going out from a cloud (D1).<br>E: What made it look like darkness, fog, cloud?<br>R: For the color, the shape of the blot and the color.<br>E: What made them look like some sort of wings?<br>R: They are very little, like bees' wings. | |
| | 17 | | Lungs. (Dd99 = central portion of D1) | E: (ERR)<br>R: In the middle, the shape of the middle part. | |
| | 18 | | A god that is above everything else. (W)<br>[She hands the card back and then she asks "Can I tell you one more thing?" and she gives R19. Because she had already returned the card and asked permission, she seemed aware of the guidelines, so E did not provide a reminder.] | E: (ERR)<br>R: The body (D3), in front of me, in this position (respondent mimics open arms), above everything because this seems to be a cloud on which he is standing (D1).<br>E: What made it look like a god?<br>R: Double arms (Dd22), face not clear; seems like Anubis.<br>E: What made it look like a cloud?<br>R: The blot, in this case not the color, just the shape. | |
| | 19 | | A female genital organ. (D12) | E: (ERR)<br>R: The labia and the slit, the way the vagina is made.<br>E: What made it look like a slit?<br>R: The color and the space here, darker color in the inside and two separate parts. | |
| VII | 20 | | Two people looking at each other; two faces with something on their heads. (D1) | E: (ERR)<br>R: Faces, eyes, nose, mouth, looking at each other and this thing on their head could be a feather (D5), I don't know.<br>E: What made it look like a feather?<br>R: The shape. | |
| | 21 | | Two people with a point where they are in contact with each other, but they seem to be searching for something else behind them with their hands. (W) | E: (ERR)<br>R: Face (D1), the body is uniting with the other person with the feet; their hand (Dd21) is searching for something behind them.<br>E: Uniting with the other person?<br>R: They are touching each other. | |
| | 22 | | The nutshell—the part that is in the middle and separates the two parts. (W) | E: (ERR)<br>R: Final part (D2), middle part (Dd26), and lateral part (rest of Dd23); this is the softer part that separates the nut, the whole thing.<br>E: What made it look like the softer part?<br>R: This is the softer part (Dd23 – Dd26), and this is the harder part (Dd26).<br>E: What made it look softer and harder?<br>R: It's darker and is the part that you touch where the two parts are joining. | |

| Cd # | R # | Or | Response | Clarification | R-Opt |
|------|-----|----|----------|---------------|-------|
| VIII | 23 | | The sternum and the lungs; here I see also the sternum. (Dd21,1) | E: (ERR)<br>R: The sternum (Dd21) for the shape and these are the lungs (D1) because of the color, the same color as before. | |
| | 24 | | A mask. (W) | E: (ERR)<br>R: First of all the colors. This part (D5) covers the eyes and this is the mouth (D2). I say a *mask* because it doesn't seem to be a face but something that might cover a face. | |
| | 25 | | Various animals. (D1, D7, Dd33) | E: (ERR)<br>R: Raccoons . . . no, marmots (D1), elephants (D7), and lions (Dd33), the shape, all profiles. | |
| IX | 26 | | A stemmed glass. (Dd99 = D6 + DS8) | E: (ERR)<br>R: The base (D6) has one color and the glass stem has a lighter color; both the shape and the color. | |
| | 27 | | These are creatures, neither animals nor humans; they are inkblots trying to get somewhere, but they are pulled back by other inkblots underneath. (W) | E: (ERR)<br>R: I don't see animals or humans, so they are really inkblots. These (D3) are inkblots trying to get here, and these in the middle (D11) and beneath (D6) are trying to catch them.<br>E: I'm not sure I see it as you see it.<br>R: This (Dd25) is an extension to touch something, and this part of the color is trying to pull down the upper color. | |
| | 28 | | The trachea or the sternum—no, the trachea (D5) at the opening of the lungs. (D9) | E: (ERR)<br>R: This seems like the upper part (D5), because it's longer, and this seems like the color of the lungs (D6), until here. | |
| X | 29 | | A butterfly. (W) | E: (ERR)<br>R: The colors, a little bit the shape, like stylized, but mainly the colors make me think of a butterfly. | |
| | 30 | | A group of animals united. (W) | E: (ERR)<br>R: Abstract, seahorses (D9), two of them; seems like a Chinese dragon (D8), fake, some sort of lions (D2), an ant (D7), crab (D1) like abstract; they touch each other because they are near each other; they are united in a sort of way.<br>E: What made them look like seahorses?<br>R: The color and the shape.<br>E: And the Chinese dragon?<br>R: The upper part has decorations coming out of the head and the eyes and the mouth that seem like those of a Chinese dragon.<br>E: Lions?<br>R: Yellow color and it seems to be stretching.<br>E: Crabs?<br>R: Claws and legs. | |
| | 31 | | The Eiffel Tower. (DdS99 = space between D9 and D10 + D11) | E: (ERR)<br>R: The two parts joining (DdS31 between D9 and D10) and going up (DdS29); the last part (D11) is the edge. | |

# Rorschach Performance Assessment System (R-PAS)®

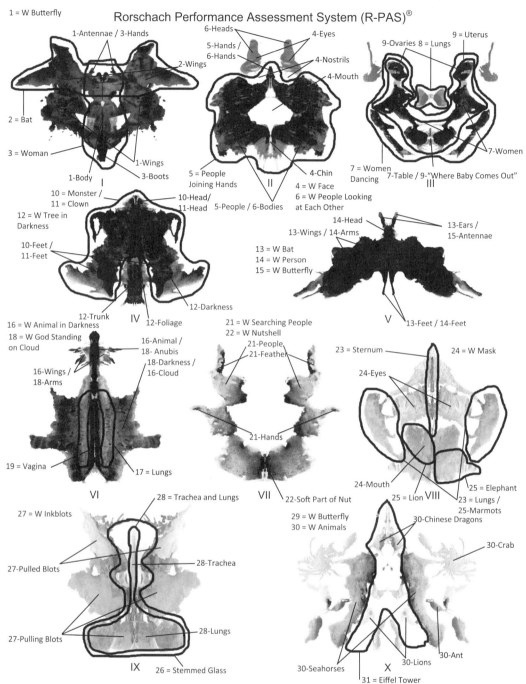

1 = W Butterfly

1-Antennae / 3-Hands
2-Wings
2 = Bat
3 = Woman
1-Wings
1-Body
3-Boots
I

6-Heads
4-Eyes
5-Hands / 6-Hands
4-Nostrils
4-Mouth
5 = People Joining Hands
4-Chin
4 = W Face
6 = W People Looking at Each Other
5-People / 6-Bodies
II

9-Ovaries  8 = Lungs
9 = Uterus
7-Women
7 = Women Dancing
7-Table / 9-"Where Baby Comes Out"
III

10 = Monster / 11 = Clown
12 = W Tree in Darkness
10-Feet / 11-Feet
10-Head/ 11-Head
12-Trunk
12-Foliage
12-Darkness
IV

14-Head
13-Wings / 14-Arms
13-Ears / 15-Antennae
13 = W Bat
14 = W Person
15 = W Butterfly
13-Feet / 14-Feet
V

16 = W Animal in Darkness
18 = W God Standing on Cloud
16-Wings / 18-Arms
16-Animal / 18- Anubis
18-Darkness / 16-Cloud
19 = Vagina
17 = Lungs
VI

21 = W Searching People
22 = W Nutshell
21-People
21-Feather
21-Hands
22-Soft Part of Nut
VII

23 = Sternum
24 = W Mask
24-Eyes
24-Mouth
25 = Lion
25 = Elephant
23 = Lungs / 25-Marmots
VIII

27 = W Inkblots
28 = Trachea and Lungs
28-Trachea
27-Pulled Blots
27-Pulling Blots
28-Lungs
IX
26 = Stemmed Glass

29 = W Butterfly
30 = W Animals
30-Chinese Dragons
30-Crab
30-Ant
30-Seahorses
30-Lions
X
31 = Eiffel Tower

154

# R-PAS Code Sequence: "Cristina"

**C-ID**: Cristina    **P-ID**: 5    **Age**: 22    **Gender**: Female    **Education**: NA

| Cd | # | Or | Loc | Loc # | SR | SI | Content | Sy | Vg | 2 | FQ | P | Determinants | Cognitive | Thematic | HR | ODL (RP) | R-Opt | Text |
|----|---|----|-----|-------|----|----|---------|----|----|---|----|---|--------------|-----------|----------|----|----------|-------|------|
| I | 1 | | W | | | | A | | | | o | P | F | | | | | | |
| | 2 | | Dd | 99 | | | A | | | | u | | F | | | | | | |
| | 3 | | D | 4 | | | H,Cg | Sy | | | o | | Ma | | | GH | | | |
| II | 4 | | W | | | SI | Hd | | | | o | | FC | INC1 | | PH | | | |
| | 5 | | D | 6 | | | H | Sy | | 2 | o | | Ma | | COP,MAH | GH | | | |
| | 6 | | W | | | | H | Sy | | 2 | o | | Mp,FC | FAB1 | COP,MAH | GH | | | * |

*Comment:* INC1 for people with rooster heads. But only FAB1 is applied since they are interrelated.

| Cd | # | Or | Loc | Loc # | SR | SI | Content | Sy | Vg | 2 | FQ | P | Determinants | Cognitive | Thematic | HR | ODL (RP) | R-Opt | Text |
|----|---|----|-----|-------|----|----|---------|----|----|---|----|---|--------------|-----------|----------|----|----------|-------|------|
| III | 7 | | D | 1 | | | H,NC | Sy | | 2 | o | P | Ma | | COP | GH | | | |
| | 8 | | D | 3 | | | An | | | | o | | CF | | | | | | |
| | 9 | | Dd | 35 | | | An,Sx | | | | u | | F | | | | ODL | | |
| IV | 10 | | D | 7 | | | (H) | | | | o | P | Mp | | AGC | GH | | | * |

*Comment:* Described from an egocentric frame of view and almost treats the card as real, but not quite DR1.

| Cd | # | Or | Loc | Loc # | SR | SI | Content | Sy | Vg | 2 | FQ | P | Determinants | Cognitive | Thematic | HR | ODL (RP) | R-Opt | Text |
|----|---|----|-----|-------|----|----|---------|----|----|---|----|---|--------------|-----------|----------|----|----------|-------|------|
| | 11 | | D | 7 | | | (H),Cg | Sy | | | o | P | F | | | GH | | | |
| | 12 | | W | | | | NC | Sy | | | u | | C' | | | | | | |
| V | 13 | | W | | | | A | | | | o | P | F | | | | | | |
| | 14 | | W | | | | H | | | | - | | Ma | INC1 | | PH | | | * |

*Comment:* Described from an egocentric view and almost treats the card as real, but not quite DR1. Near AGM.

| Cd | # | Or | Loc | Loc # | SR | SI | Content | Sy | Vg | 2 | FQ | P | Determinants | Cognitive | Thematic | HR | ODL (RP) | R-Opt | Text |
|----|---|----|-----|-------|----|----|---------|----|----|---|----|---|--------------|-----------|----------|----|----------|-------|------|
| | 15 | | W | | | | A | | | | o | P | F | | | | | | |
| VI | 16 | | W | | | | A,NC | Sy | | | u | | FMa,C' | | | | | | * |

*Comment:* There is an AGM and even MAP quality to the darkness and fog, though both below threshold.

| Cd | # | Or | Loc | Loc # | SR | SI | Content | Sy | Vg | 2 | FQ | P | Determinants | Cognitive | Thematic | HR | ODL (RP) | R-Opt | Text |
|----|---|----|-----|-------|----|----|---------|----|----|---|----|---|--------------|-----------|----------|----|----------|-------|------|
| | 17 | | Dd | 99 | | | An | | | | - | | F | | | | | | |
| | 18 | | W | | | | (H),Ay,NC | Sy | | | u | | Mp | | | GH | ODL | | |
| | 19 | | D | 12 | | | Hd,Sx | | | | u | | V | | | PH | | | |
| VII | 20 | | D | 1 | | | Hd,Cg | Sy | | 2 | o | P | Mp | | | GH | | | |
| | 21 | | W | | | | H | Sy | | 2 | u | P | Ma | | | GH | | | |
| | 22 | | W | | | | NC | | | | u | | T | | | | ODL | | |
| VIII | 23 | | Dd | 21,1 | | | An | | | | - | | CF | | | | | | |
| | 24 | | W | | | | (Hd) | | | | o | | CF | | | GH | | | |
| | 25 | | Dd | 1,7,33 | | | A,Ad | | | 2 | u | | F | | AGC | | | | |
| IX | 26 | | Dd | 99 | | | NC | | | | u | | CF | | | | ODL | | |
| | 27 | | W | | | | NC | Sy | | 2 | u | | Ma,CF | FAB1 | AGM | PH | | | |
| | 28 | | D | 9 | | | An | | | | u | | CF | | | | | | |
| X | 29 | | W | | | | A | | | | u | | CF | | | | | | |
| | 30 | | W | | | | A,(A),Ay | Sy | | 2 | u | P | FMa,CF | FAB1 | AGC | | | | |
| | 31 | | Dd | 99 | SR | SI | Ay | | | | u | | F | | | | | | |

C-ID: Cristina     P-ID: 5     Age: 22     Gender: Female     Education:

| Domain/Variables | Raw Scores | Raw %ile | Raw SS | Cplx. Adj. %ile | Cplx. Adj. SS | Standard Score Profile R-Optimized | Abbr. |
|---|---|---|---|---|---|---|---|
| **Admin. Behaviors and Obs.** | | | | | | | |
| Pr | 0 | 24 | 89 | | | | Pr |
| Pu | 0 | 40 | 96 | | | | Pu |
| CT (Card Turning) | 0 | 18 | 86 | | | | CT |
| **Engagement and Cog. Processing** | | | | | | | |
| Complexity | 114 | 94 | 123 | | | | Cmplx |
| R (Responses) | 31 | 90 | 120 | 65 | 106 | | R |
| F% [Lambda=0.41] (Simplicity) | 29% | 24 | 90 | 62 | 104 | | F% |
| Blend | 4 | 56 | 102 | 4 | 73 | | Bln |
| Sy | 12 | 91 | 120 | 48 | 99 | | Sy |
| MC | 19.0 | 99 | 138 | 93 | 122 | | MC |
| MC - PPD | 13.0 | >99 | 148 | >99 | 148 | | MC-PPD |
| M | 10 | 97 | 129 | 84 | 115 | | M |
| M/MC [10/19.0] | 53% | 51 | 100 | 46 | 99 | | M Prp |
| (CF+C)/SumC [8/10] | 80% | 85 | 116 | 85 | 116 | | CFC Prp |
| **Perception and Thinking Problems** | | | | | | | |
| EII-3 | 0.1 | 64 | 105 | 50 | 100 | | EII |
| TP-Comp (Thought & Percept. Com...) | 0.9 | 66 | 106 | 49 | 100 | | TP-C |
| WSumCog | 16 | 88 | 117 | 77 | 111 | | WCog |
| SevCog | 0 | 35 | 94 | 35 | 94 | | Sev |
| FQ-% | 10% | 57 | 103 | 45 | 98 | | FQ-% |
| WD-% | 4% | 24 | 89 | 11 | 82 | | WD-% |
| FQo% | 42% | 8 | 79 | 15 | 85 | | FQo% |
| P | 9 | 96 | 126 | 94 | 124 | | P |
| **Stress and Distress** | | | | | | | |
| YTVC' | 4 | 49 | 100 | 11 | 81 | | YTVC' |
| m | 0 | 14 | 84 | 14 | 84 | | m |
| Y | 0 | 17 | 85 | 17 | 85 | | Y |
| MOR | 0 | 18 | 86 | 18 | 86 | | MOR |
| SC-Comp (Suicide Concern Comp.) | 3.9 | 29 | 92 | 3 | 72 | | SC-C |
| **Self and Other Representation** | | | | | | | |
| ODL% | 13% | 66 | 106 | 46 | 98 | | ODL% |
| SR (Space Reversal) | 1 | 56 | 102 | 56 | 102 | | SR |
| MAP/MAHP [0/2] | NA | | | | | | MAP Prp |
| PHR/GPHR [4/14] | 29% | 36 | 95 | 36 | 95 | | PHR Prp |
| M- | 1 | 81 | 113 | 81 | 113 | | M- |
| AGC | 3 | 49 | 100 | 38 | 96 | | AGC |
| H | 6 | 94 | 123 | 80 | 113 | | H |
| COP | 3 | 91 | 120 | 79 | 112 | | COP |
| MAH | 2 | 86 | 116 | 56 | 102 | | MAH |

# R-PAS Summary Scores and Profiles – Page 2

C-ID: Cristina  P-ID: 5  Age: 22  Gender: Female  Education:

| Domain/Variables | Raw Scores | Raw %ile | Raw SS | Cplx. Adj. %ile | Cplx. Adj. SS | Standard Score Profile R-Optimized | Abbr. |
|---|---|---|---|---|---|---|---|
| **Engagement and Cog. Processing** | | | | | | | |
| W% | 48% | 65 | 106 | 43 | 97 | | W% |
| Dd% | 23% | 77 | 111 | 82 | 114 | | Dd% |
| SI (Space Integration) | 2 | 38 | 96 | 24 | 89 | | SI |
| IntCont | 3 | 67 | 107 | 41 | 96 | | IntC |
| Vg% | 0% | 18 | 86 | 21 | 87 | | Vg% |
| V | 1 | 72 | 109 | 43 | 98 | | V |
| FD | 0 | 21 | 88 | 21 | 88 | | FD |
| R8910% | 29% | 29 | 92 | 37 | 95 | | R8910% |
| WSumC | 9.0 | 98 | 131 | 91 | 120 | | WSC |
| C | 0 | 36 | 95 | 36 | 95 | | C |
| Mp/(Ma+Mp) [4/10] | 40% | 47 | 99 | 47 | 99 | | Mp Prp |
| **Perception and Thinking Problems** | | | | | | | |
| FQu% | 48% | 94 | 123 | 90 | 119 | | FQu% |
| **Stress and Distress** | | | | | | | |
| PPD | 6 | 26 | 90 | <1 | 59 | | PPD |
| CBlend | 0 | 28 | 91 | 28 | 91 | | CBlnd |
| C' | 2 | 62 | 105 | 30 | 91 | | C' |
| V | 1 | 72 | 109 | 43 | 98 | | V |
| CritCont% (Critical Contents) | 26% | 71 | 108 | 54 | 102 | | CrCt |
| **Self and Other Representation** | | | | | | | |
| SumH | 13 | 97 | 129 | 85 | 116 | | SumH |
| NPH/SumH [7/13] | 54% | 37 | 94 | 46 | 99 | | NPH Prp |
| V-Comp (Vigilance Composite) | 4.5 | 83 | 114 | 43 | 98 | | V-C |
| r (Reflections) | 0 | 36 | 95 | 36 | 95 | | r |
| p/(a+p) [4/12] | 33% | 36 | 95 | 38 | 96 | | p Prp |
| AGM | 1 | 75 | 110 | 75 | 110 | | AGM |
| T | 1 | 68 | 107 | 68 | 107 | | T |
| PER | 0 | 30 | 92 | 30 | 92 | | PER |
| An | 5 | 97 | 128 | 97 | 128 | | An |

# CHAPTER 9

# How Individual R-PAS Protocols Illuminate Couples' Relationships

## The Role of a Performance-Based Test in Therapeutic Assessment with Couples

Filippo Aschieri
Alessandra Chinaglia
Andrea B. Kiss

The health of a romantic relationship can be analyzed on various levels. Self-report tests allow assessors to investigate the conscious representations that partners have of themselves and each other. Performance tests, on the other hand, allow for the investigation of the implicit processes responsible for individual behaviors and interactions within the couple. The aim of this chapter is to illustrate the value of the Rorschach Performance Assessment System (R-PAS; Meyer, Viglione, Mihura, Erard, & Erdberg, 2011) in understanding how the functioning of the individual impacts the health of the couple.

## Introduction to Fred and Nora

"Nora" and "Fred," ages 65 and 64, respectively, were referred for Therapeutic Assessment with couples (TA-C) by their son's therapist, who suspected that some of the couple's difficulties were negatively influencing his client. During the first session, Nora and Fred disclosed a serious relational trauma: the recent discovery of Fred's betrayal of Nora. At the time of the assessment, Fred and Nora vacillated between short-lived quiet periods marked by the denial of the betrayal and days of continuous arguing. Ferocious fights between the two would climax with Nora's threats to break off the marriage; subsequent apologies from Fred seemed only to increase Nora's anger with him.

Fred and Nora had been married for more than 30 years. Some positive aspects they described about their marriage included a satisfying sex life; however, this ended when Fred became impotent due to a metabolic dysfunction 7 years prior to the present assessment. They reported enjoying traveling and visiting places together. On the other hand, they stated that communication was never their forte. Nora complained that Fred was emotionally distant and withdrawn and chose to keep most personal matters to himself. His lack of self-disclosure made Fred's betrayal even harder for Nora to contend with as she learned that the online relationships he was engaging in with at least two women were platonic in nature. Nora said she would have at least understood and preferred a sexual relationship, rather than a relationship based on communication and sharing of personal information, which she could not fathom.

## Research and Clinical Data Relevant to Marital Infidelity

Reviewing relevant literature, Snyder, Baucom, and Gordon (2007) stress that marital infidelity is common for couples. Physical or emotional infidelity is reported in up to 44% of males and 21% of females. Infidelity is the most common reason for couple separation and divorce, with 42% of divorcing couples reporting at least one extramarital sexual affair in the course of their marriage. Marital infidelity is considered a disruptive traumatic experience for the couple because of the undermining impact on a partner's sense of predictability of the other's behavior, as well as on the stability of the relationship. It also impacts both partners' psychological functioning; the betraying partner is at risk of experiencing increased levels of guilt, anxiety, and depression, whereas the betrayed partner often shows symptoms similar to those found in clients with posttraumatic stress. The treatment of couples presenting with this issue of infidelity focuses on reducing the disruptive cycles of negative emotionality, while exploring the relational problems that set the context for the betrayal. The construction of a coherent and convincing narrative that accounts for the betrayal is crucial if partners are to develop a new and more balanced view of each other and of their relationship (Snyder et al., 2007).

In recent years, a growing number of publications have focused on TA-C (Finn, 2015; Provenzi, Menichetti, Coin, & Aschieri, 2017). Finn (2015) provides a description of the goals and basic steps for this model of assessment. First, the couple and therapist collaboratively formulate questions to be answered through the assessment process. TA-C alternates individual sessions with couples' sessions. Individual sessions consist of assessment and processing experiences in the assessment. In couples' sessions, partners share insights gained during individual sessions, and assessors support them in developing a new understanding of their relational problems.

The insights and shared understanding that the couple reaches with the help of the therapist are reviewed in an oral summary and discussion session that generally addresses individual assessment questions first, followed by questions that regard both partners. Finally, the therapist provides the couple with written feedback that addresses the partner's assessment questions and all the assessment results, as they were discussed in the summary and discussion session.

TA-C can be a promising approach to cases involving betrayal. Some of the advantages of this method include: (1) a flexible format of the sessions that allows for therapeutic intervention as necessary to interrupt cycles of negative emotionality and to improve interpersonal communication skills; (2) an assessment of the current conflict and psychological consequences as well as long-standing, unresolved issues; and (3) active participation of both partners in the development of an interpretation of the assessment results and a convincing and coherent narrative, which allows for individual accounts of the reasons for and consequences of the betrayal.

## Other Assessment Data

### Nora's and Fred's Assessment Questions and Backgrounds

During the first session of the TA-C, the assessors helped Nora and Fred formulate assessment questions. Nora took the lead and expressed how perplexed she was when she learned about Fred's betrayal. Despite Nora's attempts to engage him, Fred remained aloof and silent about his motivations for emotional betrayal, leaving Nora to become even more enraged. They reported that their discussion began as a constructive effort to "talk about what happened," yet as soon as Nora challenged Fred about details of his betrayal (How had he met the women? How long had they lasted? What did he like in his parallel relationships?), he "closed up." Nora's feelings of betrayal increased with Fred's silence, and she became more intense in her demands for explanation. This resulted in his breaking down and crying without being able to give her any answers. The assessors inquired more about Fred's lack of responsiveness to Nora's requests, as well as about her interpretation of his silence. Fred disclosed how hard it was for him to sit during this session and feel forced or expected to talk about himself. He revealed that he could not make sense of his behavior, indicating that "95%" of him did not want to betray Nora. However, for reasons he could not understand, "5%" of him took the lead and made him do things he couldn't make sense of. When asked if the partners were curious about any aspects of this pattern, Fred inquired whether the assessment could help him find a reason for his actions. Thus he defined his first assessment questions: "Where is the 5% of myself that made me betray Nora coming from? What relation does it have with the remaining 95% of me?"

Nora seemed surprised that Fred was genuinely unable to account for his behavior, and said this might be another example of a recurrent feature of their marriage. They concurred that they were not used to talking about feelings and agreed to posing two couples' questions for the assessment. The first was, "How did we end up being so distant from each other?" The second was, "How has the betrayal affected our current relationship?"

By the end of the first session, both individuals were able to step back and reflect on their marriage and their individual selves, and to develop good assessment questions. Nora came to understand that Fred's silences were not intentional but because he was unable to account for his actions in that period of time. She said she felt good seeing Fred taking the risk to explore this part of himself via assessment. However, right before scheduling the following session, Nora started crying and violently attacking her husband again for the same reasons the assessors had been exploring. After validating her anger, the assessors asked if this was a process that they went through at home as well. Fred answered, "It seems her crying is never enough for her." She agreed, and said that even if it was painful, crying had a positive function for her. Even though her behavior was counterproductive in her commnication with Fred, and left her feeling dysregulated, she said it felt good to delve into her pain. Reflecting on this pattern, she asked a further individual assessment question: "Why does it feel so good to bask in my pain?"

## Initial Testing Results Prior to the Rorschach

In keeping with the TA-C model, the assessors decided to start administering testing instruments that were clearly connected to Nora's and Fred's assessment questions. The first question the assessors addressed concerned the current functioning of the couple ("How has the betrayal affected our current relationship?"). The first assessment tool administered was the Experiences in Close Relationships—Revised (ECR-R; adapted in Italian by Busonera, San Martini, Zavattini, & Santona, 2014). Fred scored 3.01 ($M = 2.28$, $SD = 0.80$) and 3.96 ($M = 3.09$; $SD = 0.96$) on fear of intimacy and separation anxiety, respectively, suggesting a fearful dyadic attachment. Fred agreed with the testing results. He said that prior to this crisis, he had felt much less separation anxiety, but that at the time of the assessment, he felt he was constantly on the verge of being overwhelmed by emotions. The assessors mirrored how uncomfortable this must be for him to be in touch with such strong emotions. They praised his courage to attend two sessions in which he had to "dive and swim in a new pool," a "pool" that included feelings of abandonment yet discomfort with opening up.

Nora's testing results revealed low fear of intimacy (1.84; $M = 2.30$; $SD = 1.04$) and moderate levels of separation anxiety (3.85; $M = 3.08$; $SD = 0.98$). The results suggested that she was approaching her relationship with preoccupied defenses. Nora disclosed that had she filled out this questionnaire prior to the betrayal, her answers might have been similar. Discussing the behavioral significance of her results, Nora disclosed that her resentment about being "let down" had turned into a "shield on her skin." Her "shield" made her feel strong, self-reliant, and aggressive in response to Fred's lack of attention. The assessors speculated that regardless of the reasons for Fred's silence, Nora might have experienced significant loneliness during their marriage. Nora agreed and added that her current loneliness was even harder to bear because she had stopped attending her women's peer support group due to the shame she felt around Fred's impotence and subsequent betrayal.

## The Choice of Using R-PAS

The assessors chose to administer R-PAS (Meyer et al., 2011) because of the utility of performance-based tests and the specifics of the couple's assessment questions. Prior to the R-PAS administration, Fred and Nora had actively collaborated with the assessment, reporting their conscious "narratives" about themselves and their relationship. As Finn states, "With those clients whose problems in living are due to insecure attachment or developmental trauma, [the Rorschach] often provide[s] a window—that is not readily available otherwise—into their right-hemisphere disorganization and subcortical dysregulation" (2012, p. 442). In this way, assessing other aspects of Fred's and Nora's individual functioning that might be less accessible to their awareness could enrich the systemic conceptualization of their relationship and provide them with a more accurate understanding of their difficulties.

In the case of Nora and Fred, emotional regulation seemed to play an important role in their marital functioning. The Rorschach might provide information around the psychological mechanisms underlying Nora's outbursts toward Fred. Was it anger against Fred that was igniting their fights? Which other emotions were so pressing to her that she felt she "needed to delve" into her pain and suffering? Were there signs of other traumatic experiences in her background that might have been stirred up by the betrayal? In addition, the Rorschach might be able to shed light on the difficulties Fred had in connecting with and expressing his emotions and the processes that were responsible for his need for "shelters." Would the Rorschach be able to shed light on the "5%" that was, according to Fred, responsible for the betrayal and that seemed to act outside of his other "95%" awareness? Was he genuinely unable to connect to himself, as observed in sessions, or was he deliberately withholding details of the betrayal, as Nora had previously suspected?

In addition to the demonstrated empirical support for R-PAS, its administration was uniquely suited in this context because of its ability to contain the variance in the number of responses (R), especially with the likelihood of receiving a short defensive protocol from Fred. To address the aforementioned issues and questions for the assessment, the following R-PAS variables were expected to provide valuable information: Engagement and Cognitive Processing (e.g., M, MC, M/MC), Perception and Thinking Problems (e.g., EII-3, TP-Comp), Stress and Distress (e.g., YTVC', MOR, CritCont%), and Self and Other Representation (e.g., ODL%, MAP/MAHP, PHR/GHR, AGC, and AGM).

## Fred's and Nora's Rorschach Protocols

The R-PAS task was introduced to each partner in individual sessions. After welcoming the clients and hearing their thoughts and reactions to the assessment process, the assessors proposed to use the Rorschach to address their assessment questions. Neither Nora nor Fred had prior knowledge of or experience with the test; however, both welcomed the possibility to further understand the way they manage their emotions. Whereas Nora expressed interest and curiosity about the task, Fred's approach was reserved, considering his participation as one of the "hard things" he had to do to save his marriage. (See Appendices 9.1 and 9.2 at the end of the chapter for Fred's and Nora's R-PAS Responses, Location Sheets, Code Sequences, and Page 1 and 2 Profiles.)

### Fred's Rorschach

#### Validity

Despite a cautious approach to the test (CT SS[1] = 86; completing the task in less than half an hour and using short verbalizations), Fred provided a valid (Responses [R] = 21, SS = 92) and sufficiently elaborated protocol (Complexity SS = 107; F% SS = 93).

---

[1]Standard scores (SS) have a mean of 100 and an *SD* of 15.

## Engagement and Cognitive Processing

Fred appeared to have adequate coping skills to adaptively contend with external demands (Complexity SS = 107; MC SS = 101; MC–PPD SS = 114), particularly by synthesizing and integrating his ideas and perceptions (Sy SS = 117). Further, he demonstrated an above-average ability to mentalize human experience and reflect upon his actions (M SS = 118). These results were consistent with his successful work as a manager for a software company and with his proclaimed talent for playing poker, as he said, " . . . remembering all the cards other players have previously used, so I am basing my choices on that data."

His coping style showed potential limitations in two areas of functioning: enjoying spontaneity in his life and relating to others' distress. The absence of color-based determinants (M/MC SS = 135; WSumC SS = 70), along with Fred's propensity for creative problem-solving strategies, suggested that he was at risk of "living in his head," with reduced ability to react appropriately in the moment and to consider and respond to emotions. Also, Fred seemed to be somewhat insensitive to the discomfort and disruptions others may experience due to his limited access to his own underlying distressing emotions (PPD SS = 86).

## Thinking and Cognition

Fred's reality testing and thinking processes appeared to be functioning within the average range (TP-Comp SS = 110), with evidence of conventional judgments about the environment (FQo% SS = 108; P SS = 96) and a relative absence of distorted perceptions (FQ–% SS = 110; WD–% SS = 97). His reality testing and clarity of thought seemed to diminish in two contexts. The first context was signaled by the slight elevation of the EII-3 (SS = 113), mainly due to the presence of an M– response. His M– response provides an example of instances in which his understanding of self and other may become unclear, possibly in connection with implicit experiences of dependency, helplessness, and powerlessness (R16, "two mice, rodents, stretching their paws to cling on to a man . . . the man is bent down and tries to hold them"; also coded FAB1, COP, ODL). The second context was signaled by the Form Quality difference between the black and white cards and the colored cards. Fred's perception of reality was appropriate in black and white cards, yet his three FQ– responses and his two cognitive codes all occurred on colored cards, suggesting that the quality of his reality testing and ability to think clearly were influenced by situations that pull for emotional processing.

## Stress and Distress

Fred's responses suggested that he was less sensitive than the average person to subtleties and nuances (YTVC' SS = 89) in terms of features of his own internal psychological world and aspects of his environment. This facet of his functioning, similar to alexithymia, could make him appear overly concrete and insensitive or unable to emotionally relate to others' requests for help. He also tended to avoid contact with depressive or dysphoric feelings connected to personal inadequacy (MOR SS = 86). Nonetheless, Fred's imagery suggested negative feelings of guilt and shame linked to sexuality. All of his dimensionality responses involved human content and included sexual contents or people hiding or being hidden (V+FD SS = 131). Although these percepts are not the traditional perspective-taking imagery, they may suggest that perspective taking for Fred is intertwined with a tendency to hide himself from others and maybe even from himself. If so, this tendency would be consistent with Fred's difficulty in sharing and knowing himself in the way he described himself in the interview, which was witnessed by his wife and the assessors. Both of his Vista determinants were accompanied by Sex content (V SS = 119; Sx SS = 128; see R12 and R15), and Response 17 ("one of those anatomic representations where you see all the anatomy . . . the penis is not fully depicted") conveys a sense of incompleteness with regard to his sexuality, likely connected to his impotence.

### Self and Other Representation

Fred's results indicated that he has interest in others (H SS = 113; SumH SS = 126), prone to expect collaborative interactions with people (COP SS = 120), and able to view relationships as mutually enhancing (MAH SS = 105, R2: "two people hugging . . . close . . . holding their arms behind each other's back"). On the other hand, Fred's R-PAS results revealed ambivalence regarding interpersonal relationships. He tended to be overly preoccupied and guarded (V-Comp SS = 118) and, as previously noted, he had a strong interpersonal theme of hiding or observing without being seen (e.g., R4, "the face of a woman . . . the black part made me think that the woman's mouth is behind it"; R7, "big tree, with two characters—maybe two witches— peeking from behind its trunk"; R19, "a person hidden in the mud . . . he opens his eyes"). Therefore, his R-PAS data suggested that Fred tended to oscillate between openness and guardedness in his relationships.

## Nora's Rorschach

### Validity

Nora started the administration of her Rorschach with curiosity for the test, yet from the first card, needed more support than typical to engage with the task and comply with the instruction of providing "two responses . . . or maybe three, to each card" (Pr SS = 119). In the first card, the Prompt was followed by an Anatomy response (R2, "a pelvis"). At Cards II and VII, the Prompt followed responses that each contained sexual content as well as dependency needs (R4, "a womb with a vagina and . . . the hips containing the uterus and vagina") and a cognitive special score (FAB2, R14, "African women; they are attached through their vaginas"). The analysis of responses following the Prompt for Card I suggested that Nora was reluctant to articulate what she was seeing. In contrast, the Prompts on later cards suggested that Nora needed external support from the examiner to step out from an unusual degree of absorption with the responses she had just given. In both cases, she might have associated anatomy and sexual representations with conflicts around sexuality and physical integrity. The additional support from the clinician to complete the Rorschach task allowed her to provide an open and interpretable protocol (Complexity SS = 107), with an average capacity to flexibly perceive the environment from different vantage points (Responses [R] = 23, SS = 99).

## Engagement and Cognitive Processing

The Complexity of Nora's responses (SS = 107) suggested a normal involvement in the task and elaboration of the stimuli. Nora displayed a higher than average effort to synthesize and integrate features of the stimulus field (Sy SS = 113; SI SS = 111) and to process the whole stimulus (W% SS = 114). The results suggested an average capacity for imagination and reflection (M SS = 97), but with control over her emotional reactions [(CF+C)/SumC SS = 75] and an occasional tendency to significantly misunderstand people (M– = 1 and 1 M with a FAB2). Although, on the surface, Nora's coping skills could appear adequate (MC–PPD SS = 102), she dealt effectively with internal and external demands only as long as her distressing emotions were limited in quantity (PPD SS = 90) and variety (only signs of loneliness and dysphoria were present, respectively, for the variables T SS = 118 and C' SS = 105). At the time of the assessment, her tendency to search for meaningful links between information (Sy SS = 113) might subsequently turn into an anxiously driven and taxing behavior.

## Perception and Thinking Problems

Nora's protocol suggested that she experienced a significant level of disturbances in her thinking (EII-3 SS = 136) when faced with the unstructured, emotionally arousing features of the Rorschach. The type of thinking disturbances that were particularly problematic for Nora were the logic and coherence of her thought processes (WSumCog SS = 135), an excess of disturbing thought content (CritCont% SS = 140), and problematic understandings of interpersonal exchanges (PHR Prop SS = 127)— all of which can compromise effective day-to-day functioning.

Closer scrutiny of the EII-3 components suggested, however, that Nora's impairment might not be as pervasive as a first screening would suggest. Among the components that increased the EII-3 score, the CritCont index was markedly elevated (SS = 140) due largely to an elevated number of Sex (Sx = 8, SS = 148) and Anatomy contents (An = 5, SS = 128). Nora provided some context to this elevation stating, "I keep on seeing sexual parts because I'm studying the pelvic floor and I know very well how these things are done." Nevertheless, Nora's clarification does not explain the profound cognitive disorganization co-occurring with the sexual and anatomy contents, including three Level 2 Fabulized Combinations (FAB2). These could be interpreted as cognitive slips triggered by crude and vivid sexual imagery that accompanied the theme of femininity and female identity (R5, "the moment of the delivery, the vagina, the hips, the legs, and the child in the white with her bow"; R14, "two women's faces, standing one in front of the other, and they are attached by their vaginas"; R23, "A woman . . . bra, legs, breast, head and fur coat. It's very colored, very beautiful, but I'm disturbed by these four insects that are attacking the woman from every side. She is surrounded by the insects, but the coat protects her because it is thick. She is protected except from the insect that is attacking her at the head. Wow! What am I saying?"). The disorganizing role of female anatomic and sexual contents was additionally exhibited in Nora's inability to further verbalize responses for Card II after having seen "the skeleton of the belly [sic], a womb with a vagina" (with a DV code). In this context, the struggles Nora was facing with the Rorschach resembled posttraumatic quasi-flashbacks. The Rorschach test data suggested that these experiences could be connected with her identity as a woman and/or with sexual or bodily preoccupations.

The TP-Comp (SS = 130) suggested severe problems in thinking clearly and logically as well as in forming accurate perceptions, making Nora vulnerable to psychotic, quasi-psychotic, or borderline states. However, the TP-Comp elevation actually may indicate a less pervasive problem. As with the EII-3 elevation, the three observed FAB2 scores seem to signal traumatic experiences. In terms of the quality of reality testing, Nora had an above-average proportion of responses that were inaccurate because they did not match the shape of the inkblots. Specifically, Nora had an above-average number of instances in which unique, idiosyncratic, or individualized ways of perceiving events interfered with her perceptual accuracy (FQ–% SS = 114), which indicates a misperception of her external environment. This was the case even when attending to common, obvious, and conventional features of the environment (WD–% SS = 114). However, one of her four FQ– responses indicated an increased level of disturbance and disorganization (R4), and two of the others were accompanied by AGM scores, suggesting that preoccupations with anger and aggression might interfere with her reality testing. Despite the psychological disturbance noted in emotionally arousing contexts, an average number of Popular responses (SS = 96) suggested that Nora has the capacity to see the most conventional and obvious features of her environment.

### Stress and Distress

Nora's results contain an average number of markers of implicit emotional distress (YTVC' SS = 100). In the framework of her fragile psychological stability, her low reactivity to subtleties in the environment that could trigger anxiety (Y SS = 85), distracting ideation (m SS = 84), and self-doubt (V SS = 92) might serve to protect her from additional psychological burden. However, Nora's fragile coping skills were not sufficient to contend with the abundance of crude and primary images (CritCont% SS = 140) against which she had no adequate resources to cope.

### Self and Other Representation

Despite seeing an average number of images suggestive of a negative and flawed self-image (MOR = 2, SS = 110), these percepts contained poignant representations of a damaged, ugly self (R8, "a bird, worn out, really in bad shape . . . broken wings . . . decayed. It's ugly"; R10, "an ugly baby bird . . . broken wings"), which reinforced the hypothesis that Nora had experienced incidents in which she felt "broken," leading her to develop a "decayed" and unattractive sense of self. Thus her difficulty in processing the recent betrayal was likely due to the possibility that rejected and painful aspects of herself might come to the surface.

These themes of ugliness and an unattractive sense of self were also visible in other variables related to her self-image and self-worth. Her Rorschach protocol contained two reflection responses (r SS = 122), both of which occurred with "ugly" contents (R9, "dragonfly . . . wings are particularly ugly"; R10, "ugly baby bird"). This finding suggested that Nora needed mirroring support from others to protect her from feeling ugly and unattractive. Interpersonal ruptures are experienced as painful, and given her tendency to externalize blame, she might defend against those experiences by shaming or attacking the needed other. Nora's frequent verbalization of "ugly" elements throughout the protocol referred both to contents she saw (R7, R8, R9, R10) and to the way contents were displayed in the responses (R11, R16), which demonstrates both her internalization and projection of blame.

Nora's Rorschach protocol had themes of nurturance (R6, R23, "breast"), primitive dependency, and birth (R4, R5, R15, R20, "uterus"), leading to elevated levels of oral dependency (ODL% SS = 124). Test evidence suggested that Nora has above-average implicit dependency needs, which have important implications for her interpersonal functioning. Her responses further indicated a strong sense of loneliness and a preoccupation with seeking closeness (T SS = 118). Nora additionally evidenced signs of oppositionality (SR SS = 113), in response to her own insecurities with aggrandizing and self-justifying defensive reactions (PER SS = 118), which can be experienced by others as defensive, self-centered, and irritating. She envisions attacks and aggression as possible outcomes in relationships (AGM SS = 121), and such preoccupation could lead to faulty judgments toward others (M– SS = 113; R23, coded M– with AGM content code).

The conflicting needs and stances with which Nora relates to others are coupled with her view of relationships as negative, unsatisfying, and problematic (PHR/GPHR SS = 127) due to concerns with aggression, sexuality, and her female identity (all her PHR responses include a Sx content or an AGM code). Therefore, Nora's interpersonal style and behavior can be characterized by high dependency needs for nurturance, guidance, support, and closeness. These needs are complicated by a sense of personal unattractiveness, oppositionality, defensiveness, and preoccupation with anger or aggression.

## Integrating Background Information with R-PAS Findings into a Case Formulation

R-PAS results played an important role in illuminating Fred and Nora's problems with communicating and processing the betrayal without external support. Fred's psychological functioning featured avoidance of emotional processing. Fred's imaginative problem-solving style and good interpersonal skills enabled him to successfully manage relations without processing distressing emotions and pain. However, due to his avoidance of strong feelings, Fred lacked the emotional intelligence necessary to explain the motives of his behavior to himself and to his wife. Conversely, Nora's protocol suggested prominent features of emotional dysregulation due to psychological trauma. Fred became emotionally activated and overwhelmed in response to Nora's emotional meltdowns, controlled by the strong feelings he was working to avoid. Addressing Nora directly would require Fred to regulate her negative feelings while tolerating the painful affect that her display triggered within him, namely, feelings of inadequacy and the inability to provide support and virility. Fred was unable to regulate or empathize for several reasons: his abilities to think clearly and provide coherent responses during provoking situations was suspended in the presence of strong emotions. Further, during their discussions, Fred's explanations were ineffective in calming Nora, as her emotional flooding prevented her from making sense of his actions and resulted in her highly disorganized states.

To preserve his good will and positive attitude toward Nora and to defend against the painful feelings that her emotional displays triggered, Fred was only able to experience Nora as vindictive. Fred's need to protect himself manifested as both avoidance and deliberate defensive behaviors. Fred's "hiding" behaviors, resulting from his anticipation of negative interactions with Nora (warranted or unwarranted), would then become the target of Nora's attacks, thus affirming Fred's fears and reinforcing a vicious cycle.

At the end of such a cycle, Nora is left struggling with the painful internal conflict of both needing and fearing Fred, while Fred is left isolated and overwhelmed by feelings of inadequacy and hopelessness.

## Impact of R-PAS on Nora and Fred, Individually and as a Couple

The subsequent sessions were devoted to discussing Fred's and Nora's R-PAS protocols and administering the Early Memories Procedure. The assessors first met with Fred and Nora individually, and then conducted a summary and discussion session with the couple.

### Discussion of Assessment Results with Nora

In accordance with the R-PAS results observed in Nora's case, the assessors decided to explore with her some of the response imagery expressed in her Critical Content percepts. Nora related that she had found the test interesting and was puzzled by the number of anatomy and sexual responses she had provided. The assessors explained that such contents can be indicative of severe traumatic experiences, still vividly impressed in subjects' memories to the point of blurring their contact with reality. Assessors offered the latter interpretation as a hypothesis and indicated that other explanations could be possible. Nora smiled and said, "Well, the test is right; that's exactly a picture of my life," and continued recalling in a very detailed manner the traumas she had experienced in her life. The eldest sister in her family, Nora had grown up without a father from the age of 1, as her father abandoned the family shortly after his second child was born. Her mother, unable to take care of the two sisters, decided to place them in a religious residential center for children, where they could keep in contact while receiving room and board and have their educational and basic care needs met with the help of the nuns.

At age 6, one of Nora's aunts proposed to adopt either Nora or her sister. Nora decided to remain in the center while her sister was adopted, hoping that once alone, her mother would take her back home. Unfortunately, Nora's mother couldn't afford to take care of a child; therefore, Nora stayed in the center until the age of 15, when she went to live with her godmother's family. Here, she was sexually and physically abused by her godmother's husband. At the same time, she found a job and, after saving enough money, secured a place to live on her own. In the following years, she had various sexual partners, was sexually and physically abused on several occasions, and used heroin (intravenous). At the age of 17, Nora was arrested but escaped from the police station prior to being transferred to jail.

In her early 20s, she became involved with a left-wing organization where she met a partner 13 years her senior who had a daughter from a previous relationship. They married and, shortly after, had a daughter. After a few years, they separated, and she ended up taking care of her stepdaughter while her husband maintained custody of their biological child. In the late 1970s, Nora reached some form of life stability, thanks to her joining the feminist movement. She described the female awareness groups she attended in the community as an invaluable source of support through which she could feel understood and share some of her adverse life experiences.

Assessors mirrored the extraordinary traumas she has suffered, acknowledged how incredibly well functioning she has been despite these unfortunate experiences, and noted the lack of emotion in her voice when she recounted these experiences. Nora agreed and explained that from an early age, she had learned to distance herself from feelings so that they would not overwhelm her. Assessors disclosed to her that the defense style she was describing was apparent in her Rorschach results and inquired whether her negative experience seeing Fred cry was a result of her difficulties withholding her emotions. Nora agreed and was curious to learn what other relevant information had emerged from her test results. Given that there was no need for a formal administration of the Early Memories Procedure at that point, the assessors turned to providing her with informal feedback about her R-PAS results.

Nora and the assessors discussed how the R-PAS results could help answer her assessment questions. The assessors reviewed the R-PAS findings with Nora, receiving confirmation from her regarding the accuracy of some of the observations made. The betrayal was hard to cope with because it unexpectedly "stirred up" other feelings and emotions connected with her previous life, which she had erroneously believed were somehow under control through her attendance at the women's support group discussions. Unfortunately, ashamed of Fred's impotence and of being betrayed, Nora stopped attending her support group meetings and found herself alone in dealing with her current and past problems.

## Discussion of Assessment Results with Fred

Fred's individual session was dedicated to a discussion of the Early Memories Procedure and a memory of himself at age 5 when he was hiding under the table, not knowing what to do to comfort his crying mother after her husband's passing. This memory was offered as an example of an image able to capture both a crucial element of his past and a reflection of the way he was feeling toward Nora at the time of this assessment. The assessors discussed with Fred the possibility that he adapted to emotionally overwhelming experiences by "numbing" his emotional reactivity to his environment. Fred agreed and commented that during his life course, he often felt powerless, desiring to help others (as his M, COP, and MAH indicated) and not knowing how to do it. The assessors discussed the role of emotional availability, of attuning and supporting others emotionally, and how this is a quality "learned" in interactions with adults who mirror emotional responses to children's needs. Fred disclosed that for the most part, his mother "was emotionally dead" after his father's passing, until the point she remarried, when Fred was in his mid-20s.

The assessors addressed with Fred the 5% and 95% divide that he thought was responsible for the betrayal, suggesting that his relationship with Nora, despite having been fulfilling in various aspects, did not contain much affective attunement and exchange. The assessors wondered if the betrayal and the way it happened might have communicated that his emotional life, rather than being absent, was segregated outside of his awareness, and for some reasons, took the lead on his behavior when he started to feel the need to talk with the two women via online chat. Fred said this was a new way of seeing things and that he had never thought about that possibility. Despite not being sure this observation was true for him, he agreed to give it more thought before the next session, when Nora would be present as well. The plan for that session included discussing all individual assessment questions the partners had while also addressing their couple's questions.

## Summary and Discussion Session with Fred and Nora

In the following couple session, Fred and Nora revealed that things were already starting to get better. During the week, they had talked about their individual Rorschach protocols and started to make positive changes in their interactions around the betrayal. Nora said that she tried to "take [her] foot off the pedal" when she noticed signs of distress in Fred. She was able to do this because she kept reminding herself that she was upset both about Fred's betrayal but also because of her mother's betrayal when she was only a child. Fred stated that he felt much more comfortable interacting with Nora and even proposed that they spend a weekend away, which they enjoyed.

The assessors praised these changes and discussed with Fred and Nora how the assessment results illuminated their couple's questions: how they ended up being so distant from each other, and what impact the betrayal had had on their marriage. Nora and Fred agreed that they had met, fallen in love, and decided to marry on the basis of deep emotional needs identified in their Rorschach protocols. Nora, having experienced a traumatic childhood deprived of mirroring needs, felt it was important to marry the gentle, collaborative, stable, rational, and calm man who was also known for being the "best poker player in their group." Fred, unable to process joy and emotions and feeling frustrated that he had not provided help to his depressed mother, felt that Nora's disinhibited behaviors would enliven his life and help him feel useful by sustaining her fight against her problematic past.

Later, two children arrived, and for more than 25 years they focused on their rearing and education, sharing mutual admiration for their parenting skills and keeping their marriage alive through a pleasurable intimate sexual life. During that period, however, the intimacy derived from sharing personal feelings by talking about their experiences decreased. While Nora found someone to listen and mirror her experiences in her woman's support group, Fred distanced himself from his emotions by focusing on his work.

Suddenly, two events shook the foundation of their marital life: Both children went to live on their own, and Fred's medical conditions brought sexual problems to the surface. Instead of coping with these events appropriately by processing the changes and talking about their feelings, they "forgot along the way" what was necessary to keep their marriage alive. Fred felt incapable of helping Nora and worthless due to his impotence. Nora felt "cursed": After surviving the first part of her life, how was it possible that things would have turned problematic again?

The betrayal revealed three relevant points for Fred and Nora, and they now had the chance to decide whether or not to go forward with their marriage. First, Fred had an absolute need to integrate his emotions in his life. His betrayal of Nora served as a clear indication that Fred's suppression of emotion had overtaken his judgment. Nora's past attempts to make him talk about himself had probably failed because she was too dysregulated for him to feel safe disclosing sensitive or vulnerable matters. Second, Nora's past still needed to be worked through. Despite the fact that she had processed some of her experiences in informal meetings and by attending a women's group support, what happened to her was simply too significant and overwhelming to cope with without professional support. Third, by betraying Nora, Fred provided an occasion for Nora to bring to the forefront her unbearable pain. The TA-C became an opportunity to repair some of the damage and relieve the pain she was experiencing, thus making him feel helpful again. They decided they would give their relationship another chance and would follow recommendations from the assessment (i.e., individual therapy for both partners prior to attending couple therapy). When commenting on their experience with the assessment, they both acknowledged the value of the Rorschach in helping them make these decisions with awareness and hope.

## Utility of R-PAS with Nora and Fred

The case of Nora and Fred illustrates the advantages of integrating a performance-based test with the other psychological assessment tools used with couples. The R-PAS coding and interpretation disentangled the elements of the partners' individual histories and indicated how such elements were interacting in their current functioning as a couple.

In particular, the R-PAS results helped Fred gain a better understanding of the origins of his resistance to discussing and processing his betrayal with Nora. His struggles were beyond just "unwillingness" to make their relationship work. The R-PAS results provided insights as to what would have allowed him to surpass such difficulty and openly discuss his emotions. Also, the R-PAS results validated Fred's cognitive strengths and interpersonal abilities, providing a more nuanced and dynamic appraisal of both the adaptive and maladaptive implications of his cognitive coping style.

The R-PAS results provided valuable information that helped Nora configure her difficulties in regulating emotions within the framework of a long-standing traumatic background. The assessors felt compelled to explore this background due to the results that surfaced on R-PAS. The individualized interpretation of R-PAS data helped to make sense of reality distortions and issues with clarity in thinking that otherwise would have pointed to a much more severe situation.

For the couple, the R-PAS results confirmed partners' observations regarding their individual functioning and also what they were experiencing in their interactions. The presentation during the TA-C of the relevant findings in simple terms, connected to their everyday life experiences, prompted spontaneous discussion for the couple and allowed the partners to identify, without the direct support of the assessors, new and more adaptive ways of relating to each other.

## ACKNOWLEDGMENT

The first author acknowledges Patrizia Bevilacqua who assessed the couple with him and helped the process to be therapeutic.

## REFERENCES

Busonera, A., San Martini, P., Zavattini, G. C., & Santona, A. (2014). Psychometric properties of an Italian version of the Experiences in Close Relationships—Revised (ECR-R) Scale. *Psychological Reports, 114,* 785–801.

Finn, S. E. (2012). Implications of recent research in neurobiology for psychological assessment. *Journal of Personality Assessment, 94,* 440–449.

Finn, S. E. (2015). Therapeutic Assessment with couples. *Pratiques Psychologiques, 21*(4), 345–373.

Janus, S. S., & Janus, C. L. (1993). *The Janus Report on Sexual Behavior.* New York: Wiley.

Meyer, G. J., Viglione, D. J., Mihura, J. L., Erard, R. E., & Erdberg, P. (2011). *Rorschach Performance Assessment System: Administration, coding, interpretation, and technical manual.* Toledo, OH: Rorschach Performance Assessment System.

Provenzi, L., Menichetti, J., Coin, R., & Aschieri, F. (2017). Psychological assessment as an intervention with couples: Single case application of collaborative techniques in clinical practice. *Professional Psychology: Research and Practice, 48,* 90–97.

Snyder, D. K., Baucom, D. H., & Gordon, K. C. (2007). Treating infidelity: An integrative approach to resolving trauma and promoting forgiveness. In P. Peluso (Ed.), *Infidelity: A practitioner's guide to working with couples in crisis* (pp. 99–125). Philadelphia: Routledge.

**Rorschach Responses "Fred"**

| Respondent ID: Fred | Examiner: Filippo Aschieri |
|---|---|
| Location: Private Practice, Milano, Italy | Date: **/**/**** |
| Start Time: 5:00 P.M. | End Time: 5:30 P.M. |

| Cd # | R # | Or | Response | Clarification | R-Opt |
|---|---|---|---|---|---|
| I | 1 | | It could be an angelic figure, because of the shape of its wings. (W) | E: (Examiner Repeats Response [ERR].)<br>R: The wings (D2) are spread out and they also look like wings, just like the way you see them in some paintings. | |
| | 2 | | In this central part there could also be two people hugging, they are close; it looks like they are holding their arms behind each other's back. (D4) | E: (ERR)<br>R: It's a strong hug; they are together and you see their hands (D1) coming out from behind. | |
| II | 3 | | The heads of two animals, touching each other's nose; maybe they are bears. (D6) | E: (ERR)<br>R: These are the animals (D1s), their noses (D4); they are rubbing their noses. | |
| | 4 | | In this part I see the face of a woman. (Dd99) | E: (ERR)<br>R: The small red dots are her eyes; you don't see the face very clearly.<br>E: Could you help me see the face the way you see it?<br>R: The face is in the white part; the black part (D4) made me think that the woman's mouth is behind it. | |
| III | 5 | | I see two people (D9) that are putting two trays (top of D7) on a table (rest of D7). (Dd99) | E: (ERR)<br>R: There is nothing to interpret here; you see their faces (Dd32), the body leaning forward; there is something in their hands. | |
| | 6 | | I can't interpret this part of the card (D2). That one in the middle looks like a bow tie. (D3) | E: (ERR)<br>R: I see the shape of a bow tie. | |
| IV | 7 | | A big tree, with two characters—maybe two witches—peeking from behind its trunk. (W) | E: (ERR)<br>R: This part is the trunk (central D1), a weeping willow.<br>E: You said two witches?<br>R: Yes, you see the chin; they look like witches (lighter outer part of D1). | |
| | 8 | | The whole card looks like some sort of ogre—a giant with big feet. (W) | E: (ERR)<br>R: This is the body—big feet (D6), the arms (D4), and its head (D3) are very small. [E missed a query on "giant" for FD.] | |
| V | 9 | | A type of animal that can fly. (W)<br>E: Like I said, I would like two, maybe three responses for each card. Could you please try to give me one more? | E: (ERR)<br>R: It sort of looks like a prehistoric butterfly the way it is drawn; it is something that can move with two big protuberances or antennae (Dd34), making it look mythological. | Pr |
| | 10 | | R: A man hiding behind a bush. (W) | E: (ERR)<br>R: The darker part looks like a protuberance coming out of the bush (Dd34); you see the head of the person (Dd30) . . . coming out of the bush. The vegetation doesn't permit a view of the shape of the person. | |

| Cd # | R # | Or | Response | Clarification | R-Opt |
|---|---|---|---|---|---|
| VI | 11 | | It reminds me of a totem from Native Americans. (D3) | E: (ERR)<br>R: Just this upper part. It has many arms, and it's decorated and indented.<br>E: Decorated?<br>R: All these outgrowths look like things that were put on the totem to make it look better. | |
| | 12 | | The lower part looks like the female genitalia. (D12) | E: (ERR)<br>R: In this part you sort of see a slit.<br>E: A slit?<br>R: The central part is darker and it looks like some sort of opening. | |
| VII | 13 | | The mirror image of an old lady. (D9) | E: (ERR)<br>R: You see the shape of the face of the old lady . . . her chin is prominent. | |
| | 14 | | Just below two masks that remind me of a pig. (Dd99 = D3 – Dd21) | E: (ERR)<br>R: These two parts—I don't consider the horn—remind me of the face of the pig.<br>E: Could you please help me see them the way you do?<br>R: This is the shape of the mask, the eyes, and the nose with the typical pig nose. | |
| | 15 | | The bottom part, again, female genitalia. (D6) | E: (ERR)<br>R: Like I said before . . . the shape of the central part reminds me of an opening.<br>E: You said opening?<br>R: This lighter part in the center reminds me of the pinkish part in contrast with the darker external part covered with hair. | |
| VIII | 16 | | Two mice, rodents, stretching their paws to cling on to a man; in this upper part, the man is bent down and tries to hold them. (D1,4) | E: (ERR)<br>R: These are the mice (D1); they're stretching one of their paws toward the hands (Dd22) of the man (D4). The man is leaning toward the mice and tries to catch them. | |
| | 17 | | The central part looks a little bit like the male genital organ. (Dd99 = D3, D5, Dd99) | E: (ERR)<br>R: It looks like one of those anatomic representations where you see all the anatomy of the chest (D3), the lungs (D5), and the penis is not fully depicted (ink outside DdS29). | |
| IX | 18 | | It looks like a fountain with gargoyles, mythological animals; they squirt water from their fingers. (W) | E: (ERR)<br>R: The bottom and the central parts (D6 with D11) look like the base of the fountain; these are the gargoyles (D3) and these are their fingers (Dd34) spraying the water. | |
| | 19 | | The central part looks like a person hidden in the mud. (DdS22) | E: (ERR)<br>R: It looks like the face of a person (Dd22), covered with mud; he opens his eyes (DdS23).<br>E: Help me see it the way you do.<br>R: You don't see the shape, just the eyes, and all the face is covered by this brownish mud (outer Dd22). | |
| X | 20 | | The blue part looks like two spiders. . . . They have some sort of weapon in their hands. (D1, 12) | E: (ERR)<br>R: They are spiders (D1) or crabs . . . these things; it looks like they are holding two spears (D12). | |
| | 21 | | This looks like architecture, like the Eiffel Tower. (D11) | E: (ERR)<br>R: The shape of the Eiffel Tower. | |

# Rorschach Performance Assessment System (R-PAS)®

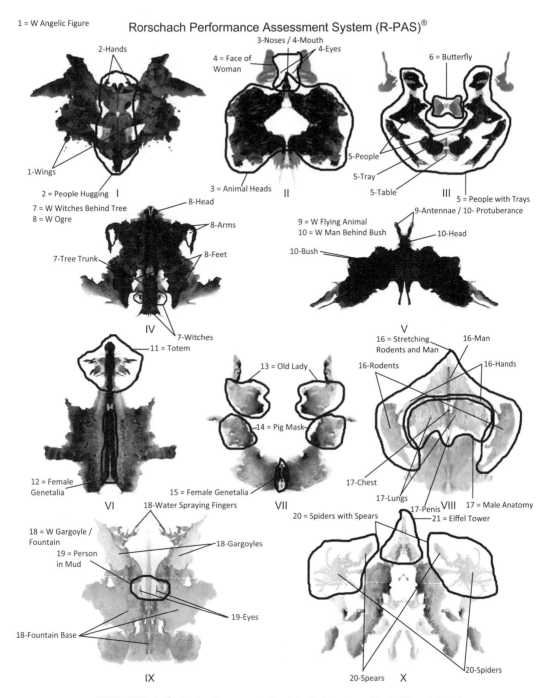

1 = W Angelic Figure

2-Hands

1-Wings

2 = People Hugging    I

7 = W Witches Behind Tree
8 = W Ogre

8-Head

8-Arms

7-Tree Trunk

8-Feet

7-Witches

IV

3-Noses / 4-Mouth

4 = Face of Woman

4-Eyes

3 = Animal Heads    II

9 = W Flying Animal
10 = W Man Behind Bush

9-Antennae / 10- Protuberance

10-Head

10-Bush

V

6 = Butterfly

5-People

5-Tray

5-Table

III

5 = People with Trays

11 = Totem

13 = Old Lady

14 = Pig Mask

12 = Female Genetalia

VI

15 = Female Genetalia

18-Water Spraying Fingers

VII

16 = Stretching Rodents and Man

16-Rodents

16-Man

16-Hands

17-Chest

17-Lungs

17-Penis

17 = Male Anatomy

VIII

18 = W Gargoyle / Fountain

19 = Person in Mud

18-Gargoyles

19-Eyes

18-Fountain Base

IX

20 = Spiders with Spears

21 = Eiffel Tower

20-Spears

20-Spiders

X

© 2012 R-PAS; Rorschach® trademarks and images are used with permission of the trademark owner, Hogrefe AG, Berne, Switzerland

175

# R-PAS Code Sequence: "Fred"

C-ID: Fred    P-ID: 3    Age: 64    Gender: Male    Education: NA

| Cd | # | Or | Loc | Loc # | SR | SI | Content | Sy | Vg | 2 | FQ | P | Determinants | Cognitive | Thematic | HR | ODL (RP) | R-Opt | Text |
|----|---|----|----|------|----|----|---------|----|----|---|----|---|--------------|-----------|----------|----|----|------|------|
| I | 1 | W | | | | | (H) | | | | o | | Mp | | | GH | | | |
| | 2 | D | 4 | | | | H | Sy | | 2 | o | | Ma | | COP,MAH | GH | | | |
| II | 3 | D | 6 | | | | Ad | Sy | | 2 | o | P | FMp | | COP | GH | | | |
| | 4 | Dd | 99 | | SR | SI | Hd | Sy | | | - | | FD | | | PH | | | |
| III | 5 | Dd | 99 | | | | H,NC | Sy | | 2 | o | P | Ma | | | GH | | | * |

*Comment*: An ODL code was debated for "trays." However a tray is for carrying things and does not necessarily imply it is for serving food or drink.

| Cd | # | Or | Loc | Loc # | SR | SI | Content | Sy | Vg | 2 | FQ | P | Determinants | Cognitive | Thematic | HR | ODL (RP) | R-Opt | Text |
|----|---|----|----|------|----|----|---------|----|----|---|----|---|--------------|-----------|----------|----|----|------|------|
| | 6 | D | 3 | | | | Cg | | | | o | | F | | | GH | | | |
| IV | 7 | W | | | | | (H),NC | Sy | | 2 | u | | Mp,FD | | AGC | GH | | | |
| | 8 | W | | | | | (H) | | | | o | P | F | | | GH | | | |
| V | 9 | W | | | | | (A) | | | | o | | F | | | | | Pr | |
| | 10 | W | | | | | H,NC | Sy | | | u | | FD | | | GH | | | |
| VI | 11 | D | 3 | | | | Art,Ay | | | | o | | F | | | | ODL | | |
| | 12 | D | 12 | | | | Hd,Sx | | | | u | | V | | | PH | | | |
| VII | 13 | D | 9 | | | | Hd | Sy | | | o | P | r | | | GH | | | |
| | 14 | Dd | 99 | | | | (Ad) | | | 2 | o | | F | | | | | | |
| | 15 | D | 6 | | | | Hd,Sx | | | | o | | V | | | PH | | | |
| VIII | 16 | D | 1, 4 | | | | H,A | Sy | | 2 | - | | Ma,FMa | FAB1 | COP | PH | ODL | | |
| | 17 | Dd | 5,99 | | | | An,Sx | | | | - | | F | | | | | | |
| IX | 18 | W | | | | | (A),NC | Sy | | 2 | u | | ma | | | | | | |
| | 19 | Dd | 22 | | | SI | Hd,NC | Sy | | | o | | Mp,FD | | | PH | | | |
| X | 20 | D | 1, 12 | | | | A,NC | Sy | | 2 | o | P | Mp | FAB1 | AGC | PH | | | |
| | 21 | D | 11 | | | | Ay | | | | o | | F | | | | | | |

©2010-2016 R-PAS

C-ID: Fred  P-ID: 3  Age: 64  Gender: Male  Education:

| Domain/Variables | Raw Scores | Raw %ile | Raw SS | Cplx. Adj. %ile | Cplx. Adj. SS | Standard Score Profile R-Optimized | Abbr. |
|---|---|---|---|---|---|---|---|
| **Admin. Behaviors and Obs.** | | | | | | | |
| Pr | 1 | 62 | 104 | | | | Pr |
| Pu | 0 | 40 | 96 | | | | Pu |
| CT (Card Turning) | 0 | 18 | 86 | | | | CT |
| **Engagement and Cog. Processing** | | | | | | | |
| Complexity | 83 | 68 | 107 | | | | Cmplx |
| R (Responses) | 21 | 30 | 92 | 14 | 84 | | R |
| F% [Lambda=0.50] (Simplicity) | 33% | 32 | 93 | 38 | 95 | | F% |
| Blend | 3 | 43 | 97 | 23 | 89 | | Bln |
| Sy | 11 | 87 | 117 | 79 | 112 | | Sy |
| MC | 7.0 | 53 | 101 | 35 | 94 | | MC |
| MC - PPD | 2.0 | 83 | 114 | 86 | 116 | | MC-PPD |
| M | 7 | 88 | 118 | 78 | 112 | | M |
| M/MC [7/7.0] | 100% | 99 | 135 | 99 | 142 | | M Prp |
| (CF+C)/SumC [0/0] | NA | | | | | | CFC Prp |
| **Perception and Thinking Problems** | | | | | | | |
| EII-3 | 0.4 | 80 | 113 | 81 | 113 | | EII |
| TP-Comp (Thought & Percept. Com...) | 1.1 | 75 | 110 | 75 | 110 | | TP-C |
| WSumCog | 8 | 62 | 104 | 57 | 102 | | WCog |
| SevCog | 0 | 35 | 94 | 35 | 94 | | Sev |
| FQ-% | 14% | 75 | 110 | 75 | 110 | | FQ-% |
| WD-% | 6% | 43 | 97 | 25 | 90 | | WD-% |
| FQo% | 67% | 71 | 108 | 68 | 107 | | FQo% |
| P | 5 | 39 | 96 | 45 | 98 | | P |
| **Stress and Distress** | | | | | | | |
| YTVC' | 2 | 23 | 89 | 13 | 83 | | YTVC' |
| m | 1 | 42 | 97 | 19 | 86 | | m |
| Y | 0 | 17 | 85 | 17 | 85 | | Y |
| MOR | 0 | 18 | 86 | 18 | 86 | | MOR |
| SC-Comp (Suicide Concern Comp.) | 3.7 | 26 | 90 | 20 | 87 | | SC-C |
| **Self and Other Representation** | | | | | | | |
| ODL% | 10% | 52 | 101 | 47 | 99 | | ODL% |
| SR (Space Reversal) | 1 | 56 | 102 | 56 | 102 | | SR |
| MAP/MAHP [0/1] | NA | | | | | | MAP Prp |
| PHR/GPHR [6/14] | 43% | 65 | 106 | 65 | 106 | | PHR Prp |
| M- | 1 | 81 | 113 | 81 | 113 | | M- |
| AGC | 2 | 34 | 94 | 29 | 92 | | AGC |
| H | 4 | 81 | 113 | 71 | 108 | | H |
| COP | 3 | 91 | 120 | 90 | 119 | | COP |
| MAH | 1 | 64 | 105 | 38 | 94 | | MAH |

© 2010-2016 R-PAS

# R-PAS Summary Scores and Profiles – Page 2

C-ID: Fred  P-ID: 3  Age: 64  Gender: Male  Education:

| Domain/Variables | Raw Scores | Raw %ile | Raw SS | Cplx. Adj. %ile | Cplx. Adj. SS | Standard Score Profile R-Optimized | Abbr. |
|---|---|---|---|---|---|---|---|
| **Engagement and Cog. Processing** | | | | | | | |
| W% | 29% | 30 | 92 | 27 | 91 | | W% |
| Dd% | 24% | 79 | 112 | 80 | 113 | | Dd% |
| SI (Space Integration) | 2 | 38 | 96 | 43 | 98 | | SI |
| IntCont | 3 | 67 | 107 | 61 | 104 | | IntC |
| Vg% | 0% | 18 | 86 | 18 | 86 | | Vg% |
| V | 2 | 89 | 119 | 83 | 115 | | V |
| FD | 4 | 97 | 129 | 97 | 129 | | FD |
| R8910% | 29% | 29 | 92 | 30 | 92 | | R8910% |
| WSumC | 0.0 | 2 | 70 | 2 | 70 | | WSC |
| C | 0 | 36 | 95 | 36 | 95 | | C |
| Mp/(Ma+Mp) [4/7] | 57% | 69 | 107 | 69 | 107 | | Mp Prp |
| **Perception and Thinking Problems** | | | | | | | |
| FQu% | 19% | 21 | 88 | 22 | 89 | | FQu% |
| **Stress and Distress** | | | | | | | |
| PPD | 5 | 17 | 86 | 9 | 79 | | PPD |
| CBlend | 0 | 28 | 91 | 28 | 91 | | CBlnd |
| C' | 0 | 14 | 84 | 14 | 84 | | C' |
| V | 2 | 89 | 119 | 83 | 115 | | V |
| CritCont% (Critical Contents) | 19% | 52 | 101 | 49 | 99 | | CrCt |
| **Self and Other Representation** | | | | | | | |
| SumH | 12 | 96 | 126 | 94 | 123 | | SumH |
| NPH/SumH [8/12] | 67% | 61 | 104 | 61 | 104 | | NPH Prp |
| V-Comp (Vigilance Composite) | 5.0 | 89 | 118 | 85 | 116 | | V-C |
| r (Reflections) | 1 | 81 | 113 | 81 | 113 | | r |
| p/(a+p) [5/10] | 50% | 66 | 106 | 65 | 106 | | p Prp |
| AGM | 0 | 31 | 93 | 31 | 93 | | AGM |
| T | 0 | 28 | 91 | 28 | 91 | | T |
| PER | 0 | 30 | 92 | 30 | 92 | | PER |
| An | 1 | 47 | 99 | 47 | 99 | | An |

© 2010-2016 R-PAS

## Rorschach Responses "Nora"

| Respondent ID: Nora | Examiner: Filippo Aschieri |
|---|---|
| Location: Private Practice, Milano, Italy | Date: **/**/**** |
| Start Time: 2:25 P.M. | End Time: 3:25 P.M. |

| Cd # | R # | Or | Response | Clarification | R-Opt |
|---|---|---|---|---|---|
| I | 1 | | A butterfly. (W)<br>E: Like I said I would like two, maybe three responses for each card. Could you please try to give me another? | E: (Examiner Repeats Response [ERR].)<br>R: The body (D4) and the wings (D2). | Pr |
| | 2 | | A pelvis. (W) | E: (ERR)<br>R: Just the shape. The shape of the pelvis. | |
| | 3 | | Two insects; they are symmetrical. (W) | E: (ERR)<br>R: These are the two bodies (each a half of D4), in the middle, and these are their wings (D2). | |
| II | 4 | | The skeleton of the belly [sic], a womb with a vagina and . . . the hips containing the uterus and vagina. (long pause) It's something symmetrical, like in the previous card. (D6) (She starts to hand the card back.)<br>E: Like I said, I would like two maybe three responses for each card. Could you please try to give me one more?<br>R: No, I can't see anything else. | E: (ERR)<br>R: Hips (D6), containing the vagina (D3) and the uterus (DS5).<br>E: Can you help me see it the way you do?<br>R: Yes, the hips are symmetrical, vagina, uterus (points to the parts). | Pr |
| III | 5 | | Theoretically, I would see the moment of the delivery, the vagina, the hips, the legs (D9), and the child in the white with her bow. (lower Dd24) | E: (ERR)<br>R: Uterus (D7), opened vagina (upper D8).<br>E: Not sure I see it the way you do.<br>R: The kid is already grown up, but is still part of the delivery. You see the bow (D3) of the child and below her there is the butt and the vagina; both are opened up. | |
| | 6 | | Two women with breasts and high heel shoes. (D9) | E: (ERR)<br>R: They might have also been two men, because I see two penises (Dd26), but they are mainly women. | |
| IV | 7 | | A monster (long pause), an insect, cheap high heel shoes—very ugly. (W) | E: (ERR)<br>R: Insect with high heel shoes (D2) . . . it looks furry. One of those insects in fantasy movies with a lot of fur (rubs the card); ugly species of insect. | |
| | 8 | v | (v) A bird, worn out, really in bad shape. The big legs (D4) look like those from a duck; the broken wings (D6) belong to another kind of bird. (W) | E: (ERR)<br>R: The bill is here (D1); the bird is worn out, decayed. It's ugly. It's all black. | |
| V | 9 | | A dragonfly and its mirror image; this is its body [with] butterfly-like wings. On the head it has a very ugly horn (Dd31); it has no color. (W) | E: (ERR)<br>R: It's ugly, all black, the body (half D7), the head (half D6), and the tail (Dd32). The wings (D4) are particularly ugly. | |
| | 10 | < | (<) An ugly baby bird; the beak is not well drawn—just half of the bird. One bird on each side of the card, like he was reflected in the mirror. One is the true bird [and] the other is the mirror image. (W) | E: (ERR)<br>R: Half of the card, you see the bird, ugly, the mirror (i.e., the other side), the wing (D4), and the body (half D7).<br>E: Ugly?<br>R: Yes, it's worn out.<br>E: Worn out?<br>R: Broken wings, not well drawn. | |

| Cd # | R # | Or | Response | Clarification | R-Opt |
|---|---|---|---|---|---|
| VI | 11 | v | (v) A bearskin, like a carpet, symmetrical. (W) | E: (ERR)<br>R: I have one similar at home. The legs behind (Dd25) are poorly cut, in an irregular way, while the front legs (Dd24) are cut well. | |
| | 12 | v | (v) The back of a person; two persons, back to back; they are keeping their arms open. The fur of the animal; they are wearing fur coats.(W) | E: (ERR)<br>R: Nose (Dd99), mouth (middle Dd29), arms (Dd24) are open, arms sticking out from the fur coat (rest of D4).<br>E: Fur?<br>R: The coat has shades that make it look soft. | |
| | 13 | | This part looks like an otter. (D3) | E: (ERR)<br>R: The whiskers (Dd26), small head (Dd23), and legs (Dd22). | |
| VII | 14 | | Two African women looking at each other, but it could also be a porch swing for children. But I really see two women's faces, standing one in front of the other and they are attached by their vaginas. (W)<br>E: Like I said, I would like two, maybe three responses for each card. Could you please try to give me one more? | E: (ERR)<br>R: I see a part of their hair (D5) and the profile of the face (D9), the typical long neck of African women; they are attached through their vaginas (D6). | Pr |
| | 15 | | Nothing else. I still think of the human body: I see the uterus, the vagina in the middle, and the neck of the uterus. (W) | E: (ERR)<br>R: The neck of the uterus (D7), vagina (D6). I keep on seeing sexual parts because I'm studying the pelvic floor and I know very well how these things are done. | |
| VIII | 16 | v | (v) A beautiful color! An ugly flower drawn in a very inaccurate way. (W) | E: (ERR)<br>R: Just half of this—not finished . . . the corolla. Carnations have this shape, but they are missing many parts. The petals and the colors, but there are many parts missing. | |
| | 17 | | A vagina in the middle. (Dd30) | E: (ERR)<br>R: Just the shape. | |
| | 18 | | Two animals. (D1) | E: (ERR)<br>R: Just the shape. | |
| | 19 | | Two squirrels climbing on a mirror . . . no, just two squirrels. (D1) [R casually gave this response while handing E the card; E was surprised and did not provide a Pull.] | E: (ERR)<br>R: Their shape and they have beautiful colors. | |
| IX | 20 | | Ovaries, uterus, other parts of the body, and the spine. (W) | E: (ERR)<br>R: The vagina, the uterus, ovaries, and the back of the body. | |
| | 21 | @ | (>v <∧) Two insects fighting. (D3) | E: (ERR)<br>R: These two, one in front of the other . . . looks like they are fighting. | |
| X | 22 | | The Eiffel Tower. (D11) | E: (ERR)<br>R: For the shape. | |
| | 23 | | A woman wearing a coat (D9), bra (D6), legs (D10), breast (D6), head (DdS99), and fur coat. It's very colored, very beautiful, but I'm disturbed by these four insects that are attacking the woman from every side (D11, D1+12, D7+15, D13). She is surrounded by the insects, but the coat protects her because it is thick. She is protected except from the insect that is attacking her at the head. Wow! What am I saying? (W) | E: (ERR)<br>R: The insects are attacking the coat (D9); these are the parts of the woman (head, upper part of DdS29; legs, D10); she has a red fur coat that protects her.<br>E: Insects?<br>R: The legs and the bodies (points to D1).<br>[E missed a query of fur for T.] | |

180

# Rorschach Performance Assessment System (R-PAS)®

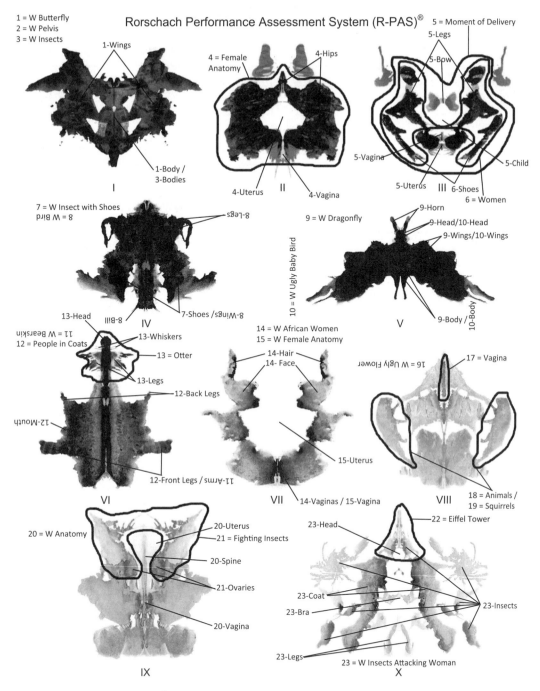

1 = W Butterfly
2 = W Pelvis
3 = W Insects

1-Wings

1-Body / 3-Bodies

I

4 = Female Anatomy

4-Hips

4-Uterus

4-Vagina

II

5 = Moment of Delivery

5-Legs

5-Bow

5-Vagina

5-Uterus

5-Child

6-Shoes

6 = Women

III

7 = W Insect with Shoes
8 = W Bird

8-Legs

8-Bill

7-Shoes / 8-Wings

IV

9 = W Dragonfly

9-Horn

9-Head/10-Head

9-Wings/10-Wings

9-Body / 10-Body

10 = W Ugly Baby Bird

V

13-Head

13-Whiskers

13 = Otter

13-Legs

12-Back Legs

12-Mouth

12-Front Legs / 11-Arms

11 = W Bearskin
12 = People in Coats

VI

14 = W African Women
15 = W Female Anatomy

14-Hair

14- Face

15-Uterus

14-Vaginas / 15-Vagina

VII

16 = W Ugly Flower

17 = Vagina

18 = Animals / 19 = Squirrels

VIII

20 = W Anatomy

20-Uterus

21 = Fighting Insects

20-Spine

21-Ovaries

20-Vagina

IX

22 = Eiffel Tower

23-Head

23-Coat

23-Bra

23-Insects

23-Legs

23 = W Insects Attacking Woman

X

**C-ID**: Nora    **P-ID**: 4    **Age**: 65    **Gender**: Female    **Education**: NA

| Cd | # | Or | Loc | Loc # | SR | SI | Content | Sy | Vg | 2 | FQ | P | Determinants | Cognitive | Thematic | HR | ODL (RP) | R-Opt | Text |
|---|---|---|---|---|---|---|---|---|---|---|---|---|---|---|---|---|---|---|---|
| I | 1 | | W | | | | A | | | | o | P | F | | | | | Pr | |
| | 2 | | W | | | | An | | | | o | | F | | | | | | |
| | 3 | | W | | | | A | | | 2 | u | | F | | | | | | |
| II | 4 | | D | 5,6 | | SI | An,Sx | | | | u | | F | DV1 | | | ODL | Pr | |
| III | 5 | | Dd | 1,3,24 | SR | SI | H,Hd,An,Cg,Sx | Sy | | | - | | Ma | FAB2 | | PH | ODL | | |
| | 6 | | D | 9 | | | H,Cg,Sx | Sy | | 2 | o | | F | | | GH | ODL | | |
| IV | 7 | | W | | | | (A),Cg | Sy | | | o | | T | FAB1 | AGC | | | | |
| | 8 | v | W | | | | A | | | | u | | C' | INC1 | MOR | | | | |
| V | 9 | | W | | | | A | Sy | | | u | | C',r | INC1 | | | | | |
| | 10 | < | W | | | | A | Sy | | | u | | r | | MOR | | ODL | | |
| VI | 11 | v | W | | | | Ad | | | | o | P | F | | PER | | | | |
| | 12 | v | W | | | | H,Cg | Sy | | 2 | u | | Mp,T | | | GH | | | |
| | 13 | | D | 3 | | | A | | | | - | | F | | | | | | |
| VII | 14 | | W | | | | H,Sx | Sy | | 2 | u | P | Mp | FAB2 | | PH | | Pr | |
| | 15 | | W | | SI | | An,Sx | | | | u | | F | | PER | | ODL | | |
| VIII | 16 | v | W | | | | NC | | | | o | | FC | | | | | | |
| | 17 | | Dd | 30 | | | Hd,Sx | | | | u | | F | | | PH | | | |
| | 18 | | D | 1 | | | A | | | 2 | o | P | F | | | | | | |
| | 19 | | D | 1 | | | A | Sy | | 2 | o | P | FC | INC1 | | | | | |
| IX | 20 | | W | | | | An,Sx | | | | o | | F | | | | ODL | | |
| | 21 | @ | D | 3 | | | A | Sy | | 2 | - | | FMa | | AGM | PH | | | |
| X | 22 | | D | 11 | | | Ay | | | | o | | F | | | | | | |
| | 23 | | W | | SR | SI | H,A,Cg,Sx | Sy | | 2 | - | | FMa,FC | FAB2 | AGM | PH | ODL | | * |

*Comment*: This response verges on CF based on the statement "It's very colored, very beautiful." However, the response itself, including the colored coat are articulated in very form determined ways. For this reason it was coded FC. However, this protocol may have one more CF and one less FC than was actually coded.

©2010-2016 R-PAS

# R-PAS Summary Scores and Profiles – Page 1

C-ID: Nora          P-ID: 4     Age: 65     Gender: Female     Education: NA

| Domain/Variables | Raw Scores | Raw %ile | Raw SS | Cplx. Adj. %ile | Cplx. Adj. SS | Standard Score Profile R-Optimized (60–140) | Abbr. |
|---|---|---|---|---|---|---|---|
| **Admin. Behaviors and Obs.** | | | | | | | |
| Pr | 3 | 90 | 119 | | | | Pr |
| Pu | 0 | 40 | 96 | | | | Pu |
| CT (Card Turning) | 6 | 68 | 107 | | | | CT |
| **Engagement and Cog. Processing** | | | | | | | |
| Complexity | 83 | 68 | 107 | | | | Cmplx |
| R (Responses) | 23 | 46 | 99 | 31 | 93 | | R |
| F% [Lambda=1.09] (Simplicity) | 52% | 74 | 110 | 78 | 111 | | F% |
| Blend | 3 | 43 | 97 | 23 | 89 | | Bln |
| Sy | 10 | 81 | 113 | 71 | 109 | | Sy |
| MC | 4.5 | 25 | 90 | 10 | 81 | | MC |
| MC - PPD | -1.5 | 56 | 102 | 59 | 104 | | MC-PPD |
| M | 3 | 43 | 97 | 23 | 89 | | M |
| M/MC [3/4.5] | 67% | 74 | 110 | 74 | 110 | | M Prp |
| (CF+C)/SumC [0/3] | 0% | 5 | 75 | 5 | 75 | | CFC Prp |
| **Perception and Thinking Problems** | | | | | | | |
| EII-3 | 2.4 | 99 | 136 | >99 | 143 | | EII |
| TP-Comp (Thought & Percept. Com...) | 2.6 | 98 | 130 | 98 | 130 | | TP-C |
| WSumCog | 32 | 99 | 135 | 99 | 135 | | WCog |
| SevCog | 3 | 98 | 131 | 98 | 131 | | Sev |
| FQ-% | 17% | 83 | 114 | 83 | 114 | | FQ-% |
| WD-% | 14% | 82 | 114 | 76 | 110 | | WD-% |
| FQo% | 43% | 11 | 82 | 8 | 79 | | FQo% |
| P | 5 | 39 | 96 | 45 | 98 | | P |
| **Stress and Distress** | | | | | | | |
| YTVC' | 4 | 49 | 100 | 37 | 95 | | YTVC' |
| m | 0 | 14 | 84 | 14 | 84 | | m |
| Y | 0 | 17 | 85 | 17 | 85 | | Y |
| MOR | 2 | 74 | 110 | 69 | 108 | | MOR |
| SC-Comp (Suicide Concern Comp.) | 3.7 | 26 | 90 | 20 | 87 | | SC-C |
| **Self and Other Representation** | | | | | | | |
| ODL% | 30% | 95 | 124 | 95 | 124 | | ODL% |
| SR (Space Reversal) | 2 | 82 | 113 | 82 | 113 | | SR |
| MAP/MAHP [0/0] | NA | | | | | | MAP Prp |
| PHR/GPHR [5/7] | 71% | 96 | 127 | 96 | 127 | | PHR Prp |
| M- | 1 | 81 | 113 | 81 | 113 | | M- |
| AGC | 1 | 17 | 86 | 13 | 83 | | AGC |
| H | 5 | 89 | 119 | 83 | 115 | | H |
| COP | 0 | 21 | 88 | 21 | 88 | | COP |
| MAH | 0 | 26 | 90 | 26 | 90 | | MAH |

© 2010-2016 R-PAS

C-ID: Nora   P-ID: 4   Age: 65   Gender: Female   Education: NA

| Domain/Variables | Raw Scores | Raw %ile | Raw SS | Cplx. Adj. %ile | Cplx. Adj. SS | Standard Score Profile R-Optimized | Abbr. |
|---|---|---|---|---|---|---|---|
| **Engagement and Cog. Processing** | | | | | | | |
| W% | 61% | 83 | 114 | 81 | 114 | | W% |
| Dd% | 9% | 32 | 93 | 37 | 95 | | Dd% |
| SI (Space Integration) | 4 | 77 | 111 | 80 | 113 | | SI |
| IntCont | 1 | 31 | 93 | 24 | 89 | | IntC |
| Vg% | 0% | 18 | 86 | 18 | 86 | | Vg% |
| V | 0 | 29 | 92 | 29 | 92 | | V |
| FD | 0 | 21 | 88 | 23 | 89 | | FD |
| R8910% | 35% | 72 | 109 | 73 | 109 | | R8910% |
| WSumC | 1.5 | 21 | 88 | 11 | 81 | | WSC |
| C | 0 | 36 | 95 | 36 | 95 | | C |
| Mp/(Ma+Mp) [2/3] | 67% | 81 | 113 | 81 | 113 | | Mp Prp |
| **Perception and Thinking Problems** | | | | | | | |
| FQu% | 39% | 76 | 110 | 76 | 110 | | FQu% |
| **Stress and Distress** | | | | | | | |
| PPD | 6 | 26 | 90 | 14 | 84 | | PPD |
| CBlend | 0 | 28 | 91 | 28 | 91 | | CBlnd |
| C' | 2 | 62 | 105 | 49 | 100 | | C' |
| V | 0 | 29 | 92 | 29 | 92 | | V |
| CritCont% (Critical Contents) | 74% | >99 | 140 | >99 | 140 | | CrCt |
| **Self and Other Representation** | | | | | | | |
| SumH | 7 | 65 | 106 | 57 | 102 | | SumH |
| NPH/SumH [2/7] | 29% | 10 | 81 | 10 | 81 | | NPH Prp |
| V-Comp (Vigilance Composite) | 3.6 | 63 | 105 | 53 | 101 | | V-C |
| r (Reflections) | 2 | 93 | 122 | 93 | 122 | | r |
| p/(a+p) [2/5] | 40% | 48 | 99 | 46 | 98 | | p Prp |
| AGM | 2 | 92 | 121 | 92 | 121 | | AGM |
| T | 2 | 89 | 118 | 89 | 118 | | T |
| PER | 2 | 89 | 118 | 89 | 118 | | PER |
| An | 5 | 97 | 128 | 97 | 128 | | An |

© 2010-2016 R-PAS

# PART III

## Using R-PAS in Forensic Evaluations

# CHAPTER 10

# Using R-PAS
# in a Criminal Responsibility Evaluation

## Marvin W. Acklin

Psychologists commonly provide psychological evaluation information concerning defendants' mental state at the time of an offense (MSO) to address issues of criminal responsibility (Melton, Petrila, Poythress, & Slobogin, 2007). Psychosis is typically implicated as a common MSO factor in determining criminal responsibility. The Rorschach Inkblot Test is peerless as a clinical measure for the assessment of psychosis (Acklin, 1999, 2008).

The case discussed in this chapter involved an MSO evaluation of an individual with a well-documented delusional belief that he was the "Son of God." He asserted, when charged with drug trafficking, that he had immunity from prosecution, given his divinity. He believed that the government had previously desisted from prosecuting him, because once it was revealed who he truly was, the "end times" would start, and the government would lose "all earthly authority." Following his prosecution for drug trafficking, a federal district judge ordered the evaluation to address issues of criminal responsibility and competency to stand trial.

### Mr. SOG's Background

"Mr. SOG" was born in a large Midwestern city in the 1940s. His developmental history was highly adverse. His biological father was unknown to him. He had a history of significant family disruption, abuse, and neglect, including foster placement. His mother was a sex worker, and his birth parents were proprietors of a wartime brothel. Despite these circumstances, he graduated from high school and college. After obtaining a bachelor's degree, he began teaching full-time in the public schools.

He fathered two children. His daughter was killed in a single-car accident as a small child. Soon afterward, he changed his name to ADB (pseudonym), a name with idiosyncratic religious significance. In the early 1980s, Mr. SOG was charged with drug possession; he accepted a deferred plea and a 3-month suspension from his teaching job. He was rearrested 3 months later on similar charges, but the case was dismissed. He was again arrested and convicted of drug possession, received a 2-year term of probation, and was referred to an outpatient drug treatment program. Several years later, at age 39, he was released from his teaching position in the public schools. He subsequently moved to Hawaii. His mother was a cocaine trafficker and he was designated to "learn the ropes" and take over for a nephew, who had been killed in a holdup. In a report to his parole officer, his therapist noted that Mr. SOG had a history of drug dependence with episodes of drug-induced depression and psychosis eventuating in repeated brief psychiatric hospitalizations. In the clinical history, his therapist stated, "It is apparent that SOG was becoming more psychotic during this period, likely because of the increasing cocaine use." This was about the time when he formed the delusional belief that he was the Son of God.

Mr. SOG believed that he had been under constant government surveillance for many years, and that he had his own dedicated government satellite that kept track of his every movement. He turned the TV against the wall when he was not using it, so it could not be used to spy on him in his apartment. The imagined surveillance was linked to his delusional divinity beliefs; its purpose was "to make sure I remain well behaved and not publicly known," out of concern that "the public would defer to me and no longer pay respect to civil authorities." The clinical record described repeated episodes of cocaine-induced psychosis, with prominent paranoid delusions, reflected in multiple hospital psychiatric admissions.

Since completing court-ordered drug rehabilitation, he had quit using cocaine. He did, however, continue to traffic the drug. Mr. SOG then went on to earn a doctorate in political science and to teach once more in public schools. In the 1990s he was again prosecuted for possession of cocaine and spent approximately 18 months in pretrial detention. He married while in detention. He was ultimately convicted and incarcerated at a federal prison, and later transferred to a low-security federal camp to complete his sentence. He changed his legal name to SOG (literal translation, "Jesus, Son of God") and developed his belief system that he was a "hidden messiah." He disclosed in treatment "[his] true identity as not the last but the next incarnation of Christ." He reported a history over the next several years of chronic delusions and cyclical depressive episodes.

## Mr. SOG's Criminal Prosecution

For the current offense, Mr. SOG was arrested for importing 500 g of cocaine through the U.S. mail. He was bewildered by the actions of the government. He protested, "No matter where I've gone, they've always known where I was; they hide in the shadows." He felt he was immune from prosecution. He fully assumed that what he was doing was visible to law enforcement and took no actions to conceal his actions. He believed the government was fully aware of his whereabouts and trafficking activities, but that the government granted him an exception based on "who

I am." He frequently referred to himself as "I am who I am," the words used by God when he revealed himself to Moses (Genesis 3:14). He believed that the government had reneged on the agreement. Now he ruefully faced his "Calvary." He was a depressed and reluctant messiah: "It ends in tragedy, and I am a coward. . . . This is my moment in Gethsemane. It's a bad joke on me . . . when they [police officers] came, it shattered that mythology . . . that I was the Christ, and had an exception." The events did not diminish his delusional belief, however; rather, they shattered only his preconceptions of immunity. He now faced the full weight of a federal criminal prosecution.

## Mr. SOG's Clinical and Forensic Evaluation

Given his well-documented delusions, his attorney filed a motion for mental examination. In spring 2015, Mr. SOG was examined in my office. Total face-to-face time for the evaluation was 15 hours. The examination included review of existing medical, psychiatric, and legal documents, and a multisession clinical and forensic evaluation. Included in the records were detailed clinical accounts from SOG's psychologist who had been seeing him for many years. A full battery of clinical and forensic assessment instruments was administered.

Specific clinical and forensic assessment measures included the Structured Interview of Reported Symptoms (SIRS); MacArthur Competence Assessment Tool—Criminal Adjudication (MacCAT-CA); Positive and Negative Syndrome Scale (PANSS); Rogers Criminal Responsibility Assessment Scales (RCRAS); Minnesota Multiphasic Personality Inventory–2 (MMPI-2); and Rorschach Performance Assessment System (R-PAS). He had previously been examined by a neuropsychologist, whose neurocognitive testing report was available.

Mr. SOG presented as a tall, well-built, neatly dressed and groomed man with short dreadlocks, wearing glasses. His manner was diffident but polite. His laconic manner was remarkable, since he showed almost no affect at all, avoided eye contact, and maintained an articulate but extremely flat rapport across the evaluation sessions. His tempo and body movements were stiff, slow, and mannered. The countertransference was one of almost complete absence, like there was nobody at home. Nevertheless, he was cooperative and demonstrated no evident cognitive impairment. He demonstrated a clear sensorium, denied auditory or visual hallucinations, but endorsed marked religious delusions and ideas of reference. His clinical presentation was entirely absent of loosened or disorganized thinking. He was profoundly demoralized about his existential predicament, facing the uncertainty of what he saw as a legal crucifixion.

### Distortion Analysis: SIRS

The SIRS (Rogers, Bagby, & Dickens, 1992)—considered the gold-standard measure for assessing feigning, simulation, and malingering of psychosis—was administered to assess the reliability of his symptomatic complaints. Overall, Mr. SOG endorsed symptoms and psychological problems in a manner that was consistent with individuals honestly reporting their difficulties.

## Current Psychopathology: PANSS

The PANSS (Kay, Fiszbein, & Opler, 1987) is a clinical rating scale for the assessment of positive and negative symptoms associated with schizophrenia and general psychopathology. Mr. SOG obtained ratings in the severe range for delusions, grandiosity, suspiciousness/persecution, blunted affect, emotional withdrawal, passive/apathetic social withdrawal, lack of spontaneity and flow of conversation, mannerisms and posturing, depression, motor retardation, unusual thought content, and preoccupation.

## Current Symptoms/Personality Function: MMPI-2

Results of his valid MMPI-2 profile (Welsh code: 07′6482+-1359/F-L/K#, mean profile elevation: 63.4) presented the picture of a distressed individual with notable thought problems, paranoid ideation, social withdrawal, and pronounced social and personal alienation. Code type analyses reflected a withdrawn person who was shy, worried, intropunitive, prone to rumination, and introverted to the point of nearly being mute. The picture indicated insomnia, preoccupation, and social withdrawal. He was continually apprehensive about being judged, evaluated, and attacked. He felt that he was under constant scrutiny or judgment. The Scale 7 elevation reflected anxiety, tension, indecision, and inability to concentrate. He displayed obsessive thoughts and ruminations, self-doubt, and associated depressive features. Item analysis revealed he was certain that others talked about him, looked at him critically, and he was afraid of losing his mind. He reported a number of symptoms suggestive of a psychotic process, including paranoid ideation and a paranoid character structure, tied to a generally suspicious, hostile, guarded, overly sensitive, and argumentative personality style. The Scale 8 elevation indicated significant thought problems, feelings of personal defectiveness, and difficulties in communication, which may reflect an actual psychotic thought disorder. Results suggested rigid moralism in his opinions and attitudes, which overemphasized rationality. Ancillary scales indicated feelings of distress, both dread and vulnerability. His anxiety was likely generalized; all events were seen as potentially disastrous and devastating.

## Evaluations of Criminal Responsibility

Mr. SOG's case differs from most insanity cases, where the criminal act itself is the direct result of a mental disorder, such as a case in which an individual kills someone because he delusionally believes the victim is an alien; or sets a house afire to "burn out the demons." Mr. SOG's activities were not delusional actions per se. Rather, it was Mr. SOG's delusional belief that, as the Son of God, he had a tacit immunity agreement previously struck with the government exempting him from prosecution. In a federal prosecution, the insanity standard is found in 18 U.S. Code, para. 17 ("It is an affirmative defense to a prosecution under any Federal statute that, at the time of the commission of the acts constituting the offense, the defendant, as a result of a severe mental disease or defect, was unable to appreciate the nature and quality or the wrongfulness of his acts"). In *U.S. v. Sullivan,*[1] it was ruled that a defendant lacks

---

[1] 544 F.2d 1052, United States Court of Appeals (9th Circuit, 1976).

substantial capacity to appreciate the wrongfulness of his conduct if he knows his act to be criminal but commits it because of a delusion that it is morally justified. The criminal act must be undertaken with a false belief that is the result of mental disease or defect. Provisionally, Mr. SOG lacked substantial capacity to appreciate the moral wrongfulness of the alleged offense because he delusionally believed he was the Son of God and immune from prosecution. The psychological evaluation was designed to test and validate these claims.

## Forensic Relevance of Psychosis

Melton et al. (2007) provide the best single reference of legal statutes and the conduct of MSO examinations. Acklin (2008) provides a complete review of psychosis, the insanity defense, and the Rorschach Inkblot Test. The major psychoses embrace a variety of clinical symptoms involving thinking (aberrant basic assumptions, illogical thinking, disorganization or confusion of thought or speech), perception (inaccurate input through auditory, visual, or other senses), and mood (extreme dampening or excitation of emotional responding). The term *psychotic* is reserved for when symptoms, particularly perception and thinking, cause *impaired reality testing* (Kleiger & Khadivi, 2015). In his classic text, Weiner (1966) referred to the centrally disturbed relation to reality observed in psychosis: impairment in the sense of reality and reality testing. The most common symptoms of psychosis include delusions (inaccurate but firmly held beliefs), auditory hallucinations, and ideas of reference.

Psychotic individuals may have a distorted sense of their personal importance. Their most intimate thoughts, feelings, and acts are often felt to be known to or shared by others, and explanatory delusions may develop, to the effect that natural or supernatural forces are at work to influence the afflicted individual's thoughts and actions in ways that are often bizarre. The individual may see him- or herself as the pivot of all that happens. The psychotic individual frequently feels caught up in mythic or predestined events: "Events seem to occur not by chance or at random, but because they are preordained" (Arieti, 1974, p. 31).

A key psychotic symptom is "thought disorder," a disturbance in the form and organization of thought and language (loosening of associations, incoherence, word salad, thought blocking), for which the Rorschach test has demonstrated unique sensitivity, even in the absence of obvious clinical disturbance (Acklin, 1999; Kleiger, 1999; Mihura, Meyer, Dumitrascu, & Bombel, 2013). Psychosis often involves a severe disturbance and impairment of self-awareness and self-reference. It is rare that psychotic individuals have "insight" into their nonsocially consensual perceptions and thoughts.

## Utility of the Rorschach Task in the Forensic Assessment of Psychosis

The Rorschach assessment of psychotic disorders rests on a robust behavioral science foundation, which has been largely exempt from attacks by Rorschach method critics (Acklin, 1999). The Rorschach is of particular value in relation to the problems with self-report where an individual may attempt to underreport, exacerbate, or malinger psychopathology. Hermann Rorschach noted the characteristic aspects of "schizophrenic" thinking in his seminal monograph (1942). He observed boundary disturbances and combinatory thinking frequently noted in psychotic records, including the Contamination response, observing that individuals with schizophrenia "give many interpretations in which confabulation, combination, and contamination are mixed in together." Rapaport referred to "deviant verbalizations" as indicative of thought disturbance (e.g., Fabulized Combinations, Confabulations, and Contaminations), the examination of which was "the highway for investigating disorders of thinking" (cited in Kleiger, 1999, p. 46).

Recent meta-analyses strongly support the Rorschach Comprehensive System (CS; Exner, 2003) Perceptual Thinking Index (PTI) as a discriminating variable in psychosis (Mihura et al., 2013). The Rorschach Performance Assessment System (R-PAS; Meyer, Viglione, Mihura, Erard, & Erdberg, 2011) was introduced to correct mounting criticism of CS psychometric problems. The Thought and Perception Composite (TP-Comp) was introduced in R-PAS as a fully dimensional refinement of the CS PTI that improved its reliability and validity (Viglione, Giromini, Gustafson, & Meyer, 2014). Independent teams of researchers in Serbia and Taiwan have also subsequently shown the TP-Comp to have incremental predictive validity over the CS in the detection of psychosis (Dzamonja-Ignjatovic, Smith, Jocic, & Milanovic, 2013; Su et al., 2015).

Acklin (1992, 1993, 1994) integrated innovations and developments in clinical psychoanalytic theory (object relations, defensive organization, and Kernberg's [1975, 1976, 1980, 1984] tripartite classification of personality organization: neurotic, borderline, and psychotic personality organization) with CS approaches to Rorschach psychodiagnosis. Translated into nomothetic and idiographic approaches, the psychodiagnostician examining an individual with suspected psychosis or psychotic personality organization might expect to find the following R-PAS[2] characteristics: (1) Loading up of Cognitive Codes, especially Level 2 Cognitive Codes; (2) a High to Very High WSumCog, with disturbances and oddities of syntax and representations indicative of thought disorder; (3) a High to Very High TP-Comp; (4) deterioration of form level, especially Human Movement percepts (M–); (5) disturbances in the structural features of percepts; (6) failure of defensive operations and utilization of primitive defenses; and (7) expression of raw, drive-laden, primary process material (e.g., Critical Contents).

## Rorschach Assessment of Paranoia

Rapaport, Gill, and Schafer (1968) delineated Rorschach structural features specifically indicative of clinical paranoia. They found that the emotional constriction and guardedness of the paranoid individual is reflected in (1) a low total number of responses, (2) a propensity to reject cards, (3) fewer color responses, and (4) a greater number of form-dominated and general form responses versus those that were dominated by color, suggesting heightened concern over emotional control. Rapaport et al. also indicated that a high number of Space responses would be characteristic of paranoid conditions, reflecting the individual's oppositionality and underlying hostility. They defined Space responses as objects residing in the white areas of the

---

[2]Acklin (1992) used CS variable names, which here are translated and updated to R-PAS variable names.

card, indicative of a reversal of the typical figure and ground and consistent with the R-PAS definition of the Space Reversal (SR) variable. Space responses, and most other responses, are accurately perceived because of the paranoid individual's rigidity and sharp attunement to external reality. Indicators of disordered thinking, namely pathological verbalizations, are minimized in paranoid states.

Rapaport et al. (1968) noted that patients with paranoid delusions remain exceedingly coherent, with great segments of their intellectual functioning unimpaired by delusional formation (p. 391). They noted that these patients are sparing in their use of pathological verbalizations (p. 435). Frosch (1983) noted that individuals with paranoid delusional disorders demonstrate a psychotic personality structure that "may be retained relatively intact with seemingly good adaptation to material reality" (p. 417). Systematized delusions appear to have a reality-adaptive value in terms of their integrative and unifying effect on the establishment of identity. As Kleiger (1999) notes, "The nonschizophrenic deluded subject may not reveal any formal disturbance in thought organization on the Rorschach" (p. 310). Schafer (1948) noted, "These cases are among the most difficult to diagnosis on the basis of test results. Many of them are indistinguishable from normals" (Kleiger, 1999, p. 91). However, a recent study suggests that the delusional nature of the paranoia is likely to be represented on the Rorschach by inaccurately perceived human activity (elevated M–; Biagiarelli et al., 2015).

## Mr. SOG's R-PAS Administration

Mr. SOG was presented the Rorschach task as the last clinical assessment measure in a 15-hour examination that took place over 3 weeks. Based on the rapport that had developed over several hours of interviews and face-to-face psychological testing, the situation created favorable circumstances for an in-depth and nondefensive response to the task. The administration was conducted according to instructions in the R-PAS Manual and required approximately 75 minutes. Mr. SOG had no questions and complied with task instructions.

## Summary of Mr. SOG's R-PAS Results

Mr. SOG was administered R-PAS in order to obtain a performance-based assessment to accompany the interview, clinician observational ratings, and self-report questionnaires. The Rorschach was administered by me, a senior clinical and forensic psychologist, with significant clinical and research experience in Rorschach coding and interpretation. (See Appendix 10.1 at the end of the chapter for Mr. SOG's R-PAS Responses, Location Sheet, Code Sequence, and Page 1 and 2 Profiles.)

### Test Validity

Mr. SOG indicated that he did not know anything about the inkblot task. He had never been previously administered the test, nor had he read about it on the Internet or elsewhere. Mr. SOG provided more than a sufficient number of responses, with the examiner overlooking the reminder to give two or three responses after obtaining a fourth (Prompts [Pr] SS[3] = 89 and Pulls [Pu] SS = 96). Generally, his responses were rich and indicative of engagement and ideational flexibility (Responses [R] = 30, SS = 117; Complexity SS = 107). Mr. SOG demonstrated an intact capacity to notice and articulate subtleties, nuances, and personally salient aspects of his experiential world (Complexity SS = 107), though with a low-average ability to engage in the synthesis and integration of concepts and ideas (Synthesis [Sy] SS = 91). Mr. SOG's above-average number of responses (R SS = 117) is also commonly found in individuals who are obsessive or highly vigilant.

## Coping

Mr. SOG's responses were characterized by a normal degree of enlivening thought and emotionally colored reactivity, which suggested generally above-average psychological resources and coping capacity (MC SS = 110), though other indicators in his protocol (discussed below) compromise these potential resources. Mr. SOG has a generally average capacity for stable, predictable, reliable, and resilient handling of stressful or upsetting situations (MC–PPD SS = 113). He tends to be the sort of person who copes through ideational means, with, as is seen below, strong passive, ruminative, and withdrawal trends (M SS = 118; M/MC SS = 115); in comparison, his level of emotional reactivity is rather low [(CF+C)/SumC SS = 91]. This is consistent with clinical observations of his reserved, vigilant manner and generally flat affect.

## Thinking and Cognition

Mr. SOG's responses reflect more general psychopathology than the average person (EII-3 SS = 113). However, he shows few instances of arbitrary perceptual inaccuracy or problems thinking clearly and logically (TP-Comp SS = 106). He does not demonstrate notable indications of formal thought disorder or infiltration of bizarre ideation (WSumCog SS = 100; SevCog SS = 94) and his general perceptual accuracy is intact and not arbitrary (FQ–% SS = 103; WD–% SS = 104; FQo% SS = 104; P SS = 96). These findings translate into accurate and generally adaptive reality judgments, which likely explain his general ability to function in society.

Mr. SOG is very likely to engage in thinking that is passive rather than active, effortful, and goal-directed, especially involving his perceptions of and attitudes toward people [Mp/(Ma+Mp) SS = 130; Mp = 7, FMp = 0, mp = 4]. This finding suggests a strong propensity for reflective imagination or passive fantasy, which can become maladaptive, escapist, or ruminative, and is an indicator of psychopathology. Despite his generally intact reality testing, the record contains significant ideational distortions associated with human representations (M– SS = 123, all passive movement), also indicating a potential proneness to delusional fantasies and projections.

## Self and Other

Mr. SOG exhibits an extreme, inflexible, and vigilant information-processing style that is accompanied by notable interpersonal distancing and wariness; he vigilantly scans

---

[3] Standard scores (SS) have a mean of 100 and an *SD* of 15.

others in the environment for signs of potential threat (V-Comp SS = 134). Associated with his hypervigilance, his responses indicate a highly unusual interest in and attentiveness to people, either real or imagined (SumH SS = 131), with a tendency to view humans fantastically or in part-object terms (NPH/SumH SS = 114). Mr. SOG demonstrates an above-average propensity for psychopathology rooted in malevolent schemas of self-and-other relationships (MAP/MAHP SS = 123), consistent with anticipations of attack and harm. Therefore, he likely experiences serious difficulty interacting with others in mature and mutually enhancing, supportive, and autonomous ways (also see COP = 0, SS = 88; MAH = 0, SS = 90). His inner experience is prone to be characterized by distorted, illogical or confused, damaged, malevolent, aggressive, personalized, partial, unrealistic, or vulnerable representations of people and interpersonal interactions (PHR/GPHR SS = 117, where 9 of 15 of his HR are poor).

As noted above, in addition to his wary distrust and expectation of malevolence, Mr. SOG demonstrates a strong tendency toward escapist, delusional fantasies regarding himself and others (M– SS = 123, all passive movement). Mr. SOG's responses also suggest a strong underlying oppositional interpersonal stance (Space Reversal [SR] SS = 132). He is stubborn, rigid, and resistant to changing his beliefs even in the face of disconfirming information. His tendencies to identify with fantastical characters are prone to be upsetting and persecutory. His internal objects are pervaded by preoccupations that interfere with the realistic appraisal and understanding of other people's thoughts and motives. Mr. SOG's interest in other people represents a vigilant preoccupation with tendencies to see others unrealistically, likely associated with deficient social skills and poor interpersonal relations (11 of Mr. SOG's 14 SumH responses were Hd or (Hd)). Mr. SOG's self and other perceptions indicate interpersonal aversion; his responses are more common in people who are alienated, guarded, and suspicious.

## Stress and Distress

Mr. SOG reported an above-average number of responses of objects moving without volitional control (m SS = 119). Thus, more than the average person, he experiences unwanted, distracting ideation that is associated with inner tension and environmental stressors. Mr. SOG also reported more than the average number of morbid images (MOR SS = 123), indicating concerns with damage, injury, or sadness. Mr. SOG likely sees himself as damaged, flawed, or somehow harmed by life and external events, and when linked to his high degree of vigilance, creates a perception of his environment as threatening, persecuting, or portending doom. Although he does not exhibit high levels of implicitly carried affective disturbance (YTVC' SS = 95, no V), he demonstrates higher than average implicit distress associated with risk for suicide or serious self-harm (SC-Comp SS = 114).

## Interpretive Summary

The R-PAS interpretation presents the vivid picture of an individual with extreme hypervigilance, proneness to passive rumination, with multiple indicators of delusional thinking. Mr. SOG's basic stance reflects an inflexible, hypervigilant cognitive style characterized by notable interpersonal distancing and wariness.

There are multiple, convergent indicators of impairments in his reality testing, in the absence of flagrant or bizarre content (absence of elevated WSumCog or SevCog or Level 2 codes) and in the absence of general deficits in perceptual accuracy (absence of elevated FQ–% or WD–%). Overall, the picture is consistent with a hypervigilant, ruminative, paranoid ideational style. In light of the clinical history, the differential diagnosis in the case would have to consider paranoid schizophrenia or delusional disorder, mixed grandiose and persecutory type. The DSM-5 (American Psychiatric Association, 2013) no longer requires that delusions be bizarre for the diagnosis of delusional disorder, though Mr. SOG's delusions were both bizarre (e.g., he is the divine Son of God exempt from criminal prosecution, he had a personal surveillance satellite) and nonbizarre (e.g., he is under government surveillance).

The etiology of delusional disorder is poorly understood. Mr. SOG's chronic paranoid delusions may have originated in his traumatic history or chronic cocaine dependence with associated episodes of substance-induced psychosis. It is well recognized that some individuals are prone to persistent or permanent psychosis resulting from chronic stimulant abuse or dependence, whether due to neurobiological sensitization mechanisms or underlying genetic predispositions.

Interpersonal and psychodynamic interpretations of paranoid delusions have great explanatory power. Mr. SOG's delusional resolution may be viewed as a comprehensive solution to an intolerably troubled and traumatic life history. This delusional resolution provides a clear linkage between his level of thought organization, struggle with internalized persecutory objects, and distorted human and human movement responses reflected in the R-PAS Perception and Thinking Problems and Self and Other clusters (Athey, 1974). Mr. SOG's special status, as God's only Son, having his own designated government surveillance satellite, with an exemption from prosecution—are all forms of psychotic insight (Arieti, 1974), and "seem to give the comfort of explaining how life has gone terribly wrong, while maintaining a sense of blamelessness and a powerful, if distorted, connection to one's fellow man. This is the paranoid development" (Blechner, 1995, p. 376). The paranoid, in contrast to the more serious, hebephrenic development, "hinged on whether the patient had enough of a decent human relationship some time in his life, so that he may be less willing to abandon hope of human contact altogether and prefer the organized and related, if delusional, protection of a paranoid system" (Blechner, 1995, p. 376).

## Contribution of R-PAS
## to the Referral Questions and Formulation of Findings

In forensic psychological evaluations of criminal responsibility, the methodological components (instruments, procedures, and methods of interpretation) are critical factors in developing theoretically and empirically grounded inferences. The primary utility of R-PAS in the current evaluation was its sensitive ability to validate the history, SOG's self-report, and clinician psychopathology ratings. Mr. SOG's Rorschach protocol demonstrates an absence of formal thought disorder indicators (WSumCog or SevCog) or bizarre content, highlighting the important role of R-PAS structural data (V-Comp, SR, FQ–, M–, SumH, Mp-, MAP, PHR, and NPH) in understanding Mr. SOG's experience. In combination with the clinical history and observation, self-report, and psychological evaluation data (PANSS, MMPI-2), the R-PAS findings provided significant convergent, incremental, and case validity (Teglasi, Nebbergall, & Newman, 2012). The integrated findings provided a sound evidentiary basis for the forensic opinion that Mr. SOG was not criminally responsible due to chronic delusional disorder. In this case, the R-PAS findings provide support for SOG's delusional thought processes, to the extent that he met criteria for the federal insanity statute.

## REFERENCES

Acklin, M. W. (1992). Psychodiagnosis of personality structure: Psychotic personality organization. *Journal of Personality Assessment, 58*, 454–63.

Acklin, M. W. (1993). Psychodiagnosis of personality structure II: Borderline personality organization. *Journal of Personality Assessment, 61*(2), 329–341.

Acklin, M. W. (1994). Psychodiagnosis of personality structure III: Neurotic personality organization. *Journal of Personality Assessment, 63*(1), 1–9.

Acklin, M. W. (1999). Behavioral science foundations of the Rorschach test: Research and clinical applications. *Assessment, 6*, 319–326.

Acklin, M. W. (2008). The Rorschach test and forensic psychological evaluation: Psychosis and the insanity defense. In C. B. Gacono & F. B. Evans (Eds.), *The handbook of forensic Rorschach assessment* (pp. 157–174). Mahwah, NJ: Erlbaum.

American Psychiatric Association. (2013). *Diagnostic and statistical manual of mental disorders* (5th ed.). Arlington, VA: Author.

Arieti, S. (1974). *Interpretation of schizophrenia* (2nd ed.). New York: Basic Books.

Athey, G. (1974). Schizophrenic thought organization, object relations, and the Rorschach test. *Bulletin of the Menninger Clinic, 38*, 406–429.

Biagiarelli, M., Roma, P., Comparelli, A., Andrados, M. P., Di Pomponio, I., Corigiliano, V., . . . Ferracuti, S. (2015). Relationship between the Rorschach Perceptual Thinking Index (PTI) and the Positive and Negative Syndrome Scale (PANSS) in psychotic patients: A validity study. *Psychiatry Research, 225*, 315–321.

Blechner, M. J. (1995). Schizophrenia. In M. Lionells, J. Fiscalini, C. H. Mann, & D. B. Stern (Eds.), *Handbook of interpersonal psychoanalysis* (pp. 375–396). Hillsdale, NJ: Analytic Press.

Dzamonja-Ignjatovic, T., Smith, B. L., Jocic, D., & Milanovic, M. (2013). A comparison of new and revised Rorschach measures of schizophrenic functioning in a Serbian clinical sample. *Journal of Personality Assessment, 95*, 471–478.

Exner, J. E. (2003). *The Rorschach: A comprehensive system* (Vol. 1, 4th ed.). New York: Wiley.

Frosch, J. (1983). *The psychotic process.* New York: International Universities Press.

Kay, S. R., Fiszbein, A., & Opler, L. A. (1987). The Positive and Negative Syndrome Scale (PANSS) for schizophrenia. *Schizophrenia Bulletin, 13*, 261–276.

Kernberg, O. (1975). *Borderline conditions and pathological narcissism.* New York: Aronson.

Kernberg, O. (1976). *Object relations theory and clinical psychoanalysis.* New York: Aronson.

Kernberg, O. (1980). Neurosis, psychosis, and the borderline states. In A. M. Freedman, H. I. Kaplan, & B. J. Sadock (Eds.). *Comprehensive textbook of psychiatry: Vol. III.* Baltimore: Williams & Wilkins.

Kernberg, O. (1984). *Severe personality disorders: Psychotherapeutic strategies.* New Haven, CT: Yale University Press.

Kleiger, J. H. (1999). *Disordered thinking and the Rorschach: Theory, research, and differential diagnosis.* New York: Routledge.

Kleiger, J. H., & Khadivi, A. (2015). *Assessing psychosis: A clinician's guide.* New York: Routledge.

Melton, G. G., Petrila, J., Poythress, N., & Slobogin, C. (2007). *Psychological evaluations for the courts: A handbook for mental health professionals and lawyers* (3rd ed.). New York: Guilford Press.

Meyer, G. J., Viglione, D. J., Mihura, J. L., Erard, R. E., & Erdberg, P. (2011). *Rorschach Performance Assessment System: Administration, coding, interpretation, and technical manual.* Toledo, OH: Rorschach Performance Assessment System.

Mihura, J. L., Meyer, G. J., Dumitrascu, N., & Bombel, G. (2013). The validity of individual Rorschach variables: Systematic reviews and meta-analyses of the comprehensive system. *Psychological Bulletin, 139,* 548–605.

Rapaport, D., Gill, M. M., & Schafer, R. (1968). *Diagnostic psychological testing* (rev. ed., R. R. Holt, Ed.). New York: International Universities Press.

Rogers, R., Bagby, R. M., & Dickens, S. E. (1992). *Structured Interview of Reported Symptoms (SIRS) and professional manual.* Odessa, FL: Psychological Assessment Resources.

Rorschach, H. (1942). *Psychodiagnostics.* New York: Grune & Stratton.

Schafer, R. (1948). *The clinical application of psychological tests.* New York: International Universities Press.

Su, W.-S., Viglione, D. J., Green, E. E., Tam, W. C., Su., J. A., & Chang, Y. T. (2015). Cultural and linguistic adaptability of the Rorschach Performance Assessment System as a measure of psychotic characteristics and severity of mental disturbance in Taiwan. *Psychological Assessment, 27,* 1273–1285.

Teglasi, H., Nebbergall, A. J., & Newman, D. (2012). Construct validity and case validity in assessment. *Psychological Assessment, 24,* 464–475.

Viglione, D. J., Giromini, L., Gustafson, M. L., & Meyer, G. J. (2014). Developing continuous variable composite for Rorschach measures of thought problems, vigilance, and suicide risk. *Assessment, 21,* 42–49.

Weiner, I. B. (1966). *Psychodiagnosis in schizophrenia.* Mahwah, NJ: Erlbaum.

### Rorschach Responses "Mr. SOG"

| Respondent ID: Son of God | Examiner: Marvin W. Acklin |
|---|---|
| Location: Examiner's Office | Date: **/**/**** |
| Start Time: 10:55 A.M. | End Time: 12:15 A.M. |

| Cd # | R # | Or | Response | Clarification | R-Opt |
|---|---|---|---|---|---|
| I | 1 | | Looks like a mask. (W) | E: (Examiner Repeats Response [ERR].)<br>R: Roundness of the cheeks, these look like—yes, this is the mouth, chin, ears. | |
| | 2 | | Also looks like a beetle or insect. (D4) | E: (ERR)<br>R: See these two pincers here—head, mouth, and two pincers. | |
| | 3 | | A carving, a pumpkin carving, a face, that's about it. (W) | E: (ERR)<br>R: Imagining the lines going around.<br>E: Face?<br>R: Looks like a person carved out the eyes and started carving out the mouth. [A query for "carved out the eyes" could have been appropriate for dimensionality.] | |
| II | 4 | | Looks like two people clasping hands. (W) | E: (ERR)<br>R: Here are the feet, torso, arms, hands, head, and hair, facing each other. | |
| | 5 | | Looks like a face. (W) | E: (ERR)<br>R: See the two eyes, nose, nostrils, mouth, and chin. | |
| | 6 | | Looks like he could be a Buddhist monk in prayer. (W) | E: (ERR)<br>R: Outline of body (points, outlines contour of D6 through D2 on both sides), hands like this in prayer (D4).<br>E: Buddhist monk?<br>R: The clothing, hanging loose like a robe. [E: Monk and robe are facing the viewer.] | |
| III | 7 | | Looks like a butterfly in the middle with two people standing over a bowl. (D1,3) | E: (ERR)<br>R: Here is the butterfly, and here's the two figures: head, nose, eyes, neck, torso, arms bent over the object (D7), legs with shoes. | |
| | 8 | | At the bottom looks like an alien face with big eyes. (D7) | E: (ERR)<br>R: Here's the alien face (D7), where the bowl was.<br>E: Alien face?<br>R: Big eyes, mouth is smiling upturned. | |
| | 9 | | Looks like a Cheshire cat with a big smile . . . could be a big jolly person with a big smile on their face. (W) | E: (ERR)<br>R: All together, nose, eyes, ears on side.<br>E: And you said it could be a big jolly person with a big smile on their face?<br>R: Reminds me of a Cheshire cat in *Alice in Wonderland*. [In the RP, E initially heard this as two responses but he resolved them as just being one in the CP.] | |
| IV | 10 | | Looks like roadkill, like a frog that has been squashed. (W) | E: (ERR)<br>R: Looks flat; somebody that has been squashed, flat, dead looking.<br>E: Dead looking?<br>R: The color is dark, lifeless. | |
| | 11 | | Could be a Kabuki dancer, one of those puppets; looks like a Japanese face. (W) | E: (ERR)<br>R: Headgear, ears, long nose, robe.<br>E: Robe?<br>R: The robe looks draped. | |

| Cd # | R # | Or | Response | Clarification | R-Opt |
|---|---|---|---|---|---|
| V | 12 | | This looks like an insect, a butterfly with antennae, a winged insect. (W) | E: (ERR)<br>R: Wings, antennae, here's the . . . I don't know what to call it—the thorax. | |
| | 13 | | Could get a winged alien out of that, with wings and head. (W) | E: (ERR)<br>R: Head, antennae, legs, and feet. | |
| VI | 14 | | Looks like a Stradivarius, a violin. (W) | E: (ERR)<br>R: Strings, neck, body of it, or a guitar as well. | |
| | 15 | | Again looks like a pelt that has been hung out to dry. (W) | E: (ERR)<br>R: Four legs of an animal that they killed, and head area.<br>E: Pelt?<br>R: The texture, the coloring. | |
| | 16 | | Looks like the hilt of a sword, in the sheath. (Dd99 = D2, rest of D5) | E: (ERR)<br>R: Hilt of the sword going into sheath. | |
| VII | 17 | | First glance, looks like two rabbits, facing each other. (D2) | E: (ERR)<br>R: Two rabbits (D2), ears, face, with tail.<br>E: Rabbits?<br>R: The overall shape, two bunnies. | |
| | 18 | | There's two gremlins in the midsection. (D3) | E: (ERR)<br>R: These faces, eyes, ears, snarly mouth. | |
| | 19 | | The bottom looks like a church with a cross coming out of the center of it. (Dd27) | E: (ERR)<br>R: Here's the building with the cross (Dd27). | |
| | 20 | | The very bottom looks like a courtyard with the sidewalk leading up to the building, with a steeple. (Dd28, 26) [E missed giving a Pull here.] | E: (ERR)<br>R: The light gray, the line is the sidewalk, the dark is a little door, here's a steeple going up (Dd28, Dd26) | |
| VIII | 21 | | Looks like something has been dissected and laid out: lungs, pelvis, rib cage. (W) | E: (ERR)<br>R: Looks like when you are in biology, rib cage, laid out, here's the throat area. | |
| | 22 | | The top looks like a figure with an elongated face, eyes, and nose. (DS3) | E: (ERR)<br>R: Here, eyes on either side, has some whiskers. | |
| | 23 | | I see a mask, a sad mask. (DS3) | E: (ERR)<br>R: Nose, eyes, turned-down mouth.<br>E: Sad?<br>R: The turned-down mouth. [E interpreted this as the mask experiencing a human emotion, scored Mp and INC1.] | |
| | 24 | | You can see some kind of animal, on four legs, walking towards the top of it. (D1) [E missed giving a Pull here.] | E: (ERR)<br>R: On the bottom sides, the animal with four legs. | |
| IX | 25 | | Looks like spillage; this one looks more random than anything—call it the palette, a painter's palette. I don't get anything out of it. (W) | E: (ERR)<br>R: Doesn't give me any distinct impression, mixing paints, bleed all over into each other. | |
| | 26 | | You can get a face if you tried hard enough: broad cheeks, nostrils, teeth, pointed ears. (W) | E: (ERR)<br>R: Face here, cheeks, nostrils, teeth, and ears. | |
| X | 27 | | On the sides you have two blue crabs, big green pinchers. (Dd99 = 1+12) | E: (ERR)<br>R: Crabs with multiple legs; here's the pinchers. | |
| | 28 | | In the very middle, you can get a face, maybe a helmet on. (Dd99 = 11, space between D8s) | E: (ERR)<br>R: Looks like one of those old German helmets. | |
| | 29 | | The pinkish looks like an ornament, a bell-shaped ornament. (Dd21) | E: (ERR)<br>R: Together they form the contours of a bell. | |
| | 30 | | Bottom looks like a guy with a mustache, two yellow eyes. (Dd99 = lower DdS30) [E did not give a Pull here.] | E: (ERR)<br>R: Here's the eyes, nose, mustache, like a bicycle mustache, turns up at the end. | |

# Rorschach Performance Assessment System (R-PAS)®

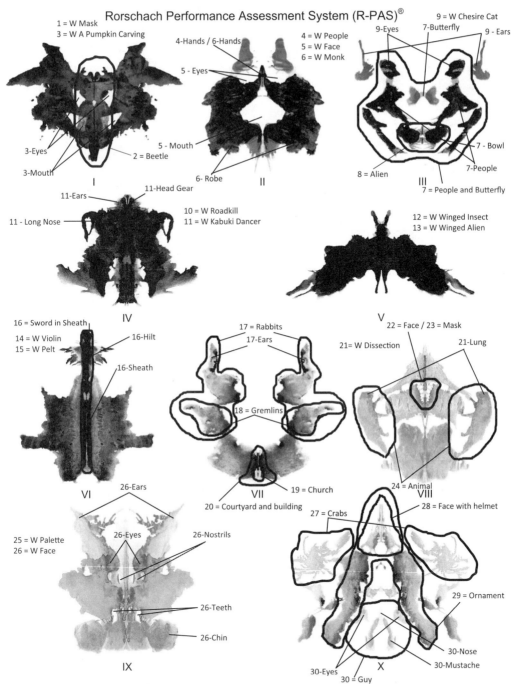

1 = W Mask
3 = W A Pumpkin Carving

4-Hands / 6-Hands
5 - Eyes

4 = W People
5 = W Face
6 = W Monk

9 = W Chesire Cat
9-Eyes    7-Butterfly    9 - Ears

3-Eyes
3-Mouth
2 = Beetle
5 - Mouth

6- Robe

8 = Alien

7 - Bowl
7-People
7 = People and Butterfly

I

II

III

11-Ears
11-Head Gear
11 - Long Nose

10 = W Roadkill
11 = W Kabuki Dancer

12 = W Winged Insect
13 = W Winged Alien

IV

V

16 = Sword in Sheath
14 = W Violin
15 = W Pelt
16-Hilt
16-Sheath

17 = Rabbits
17-Ears
18 = Gremlins

21= W Dissection
22 = Face / 23 = Mask
21-Lung

24 = Animal

19 = Church
20 = Courtyard and building

VI

VII

VIII

26-Ears
26-Eyes
26-Nostrils
25 = W Palette
26 = W Face
26-Teeth
26-Chin

27 = Crabs
28 = Face with helmet
29 = Ornament
30-Nose
30-Mustache
30-Eyes
30 = Guy

IX

X

# R-PAS Code Sequence: Mr. SOG

**C-ID**: Son of God    **P-ID**: 43    **Age**: 60s    **Gender**: Male    **Education**: 20

| Cd | # | Or | Loc | Loc # | SR | SI | Content | Sy | Vg | 2 | FQ | P | Determinants | Cognitive | Thematic | HR | ODL (RP) | R-Opt | Text |
|----|---|----|-----|-------|----|----|---------|----|----|---|----|---|--------------|-----------|----------|----|----------|-------|------|
| I | 1 | | W | | | SI | (Hd) | | | | o | | F | | | GH | | | |
| | 2 | | D | 4 | | | A | | | | o | | F | | AGC | | | | |
| | 3 | | W | | | SI | (Hd) | | | | o | | F | | MAP | GH | | | |
| Comment: A query for "carved out the eyes" could have been appropriate for dimensionality. | | | | | | | | | | | | | | | | | | | * |
| II | 4 | | W | | | | H | Sy | | 2 | o | | Mp | | | GH | | | |
| | 5 | | W | | | SI | Hd | | | | o | | F | | | PH | | | |
| | 6 | | W | | SR | SI | H,Ay,Cg | Sy | | | - | | Mp,mp | | | PH | ODL | | |
| III | 7 | | D | 1,3 | | | H,A,Cg,NC | Sy | | 2 | o | P | Mp | | | GH | | | |
| | 8 | | D | 7 | | | (Hd) | | | | o | | Mp | | | GH | | | |
| | 9 | | W | | | SI | (Ad) | | | | - | | Mp | | | PH | ODL | | |
| IV | 10 | | W | | | | A | | | | o | | C' | | MOR,MAP | | | | |
| | 11 | | W | | | | (H),Ay,Cg | | | | o | P | mp | | | GH | | | |
| V | 12 | | W | | | | A | | | | o | P | F | | | | | | |
| | 13 | | W | | | | (A) | | | | o | | F | | | | | | |
| VI | 14 | | W | | | | NC | | | | o | | F | | | | | | |
| | 15 | | W | | | | Ad | | | | o | P | mp,T | | MOR,MAP | | | | |
| | 16 | | Dd | 2,99 | | | NC | Sy | | | u | | F | | AGC | | | | |
| VII | 17 | | D | 2 | | | A | | | 2 | o | | F | | | | | | |
| | 18 | | D | 3 | | | (Hd) | | | 2 | o | | Mp | | AGM | PH | | | |
| | 19 | | Dd | 27 | | | NC | | | | - | | F | | | | | | |
| | 20 | | Dd | 26,28 | | | NC | | | | u | | FD | | | | | | |
| VIII | 21 | | W | | | | An | | | | u | | F | | MOR,MAP | | | | |
| | 22 | | D | 3 | SR | | Hd | | | | u | | F | | | PH | | | |
| | 23 | | D | 3 | SR | | (Hd) | | | | o | | Mp | INC1 | MOR | PH | | | |
| Comment: E interpreted this as the mask experiencing a human emotion, scored Mp and INC1. | | | | | | | | | | | | | | | | | | | * |
| | 24 | | D | 1 | | | A | | | 2 | o | P | FMa | | | | | | |
| IX | 25 | | W | | | | NC | | Vg | | n | | mp,C,Y | | | | | | |
| | 26 | | W | | SR | SI | Hd | | | | u | | F | | | PH | ODL | | |
| X | 27 | | Dd | 99 | | | A | | | 2 | o | | FC | INC1 | AGC | | | | |
| | 28 | | Dd | 99 | SR | SI | Hd,Ay,Cg | | | | u | | F | | AGC | PH | | | |
| | 29 | | Dd | 21 | | | NC | | | | u | | F | | | | | | |
| | 30 | | Dd | 99 | | SI | Hd | | | | o | | FC | INC1 | | PH | | | |

©2010-2016 R-PAS

## R-PAS Summary Scores and Profiles – Page 1

**C-ID:** Son of God  **P-ID:** 43  **Age:** 60s  **Gender:** Male  **Education:** 20

| Domain/Variables | Raw Scores | Raw %ile | Raw SS | Cplx. Adj. %ile | Cplx. Adj. SS | Standard Score Profile R-Optimized | Abbr. |
|---|---|---|---|---|---|---|---|
| **Admin. Behaviors and Obs.** | | | | | | | |
| Pr | 0 | 24 | 89 | | | | Pr |
| Pu | 0 | 40 | 96 | | | | Pu |
| CT (Card Turning) | 0 | 18 | 86 | | | | CT |
| **Engagement and Cog. Processing** | | | | | | | |
| Complexity | 84 | 69 | 107 | | | | Cmplx |
| R (Responses) | 30 | 87 | 117 | 78 | 112 | | R |
| F% [Lambda=1.00] (Simplicity) | 50% | 71 | 108 | 76 | 110 | | F% |
| Blend | 3 | 43 | 97 | 22 | 88 | | Bln |
| Sy | 4 | 27 | 91 | 15 | 85 | | Sy |
| MC | 9.5 | 75 | 110 | 60 | 104 | | MC |
| MC - PPD | 1.5 | 80 | 113 | 83 | 114 | | MC-PPD |
| M | 7 | 88 | 118 | 78 | 111 | | M |
| M/MC [7/9.5] | 74% | 84 | 115 | 84 | 115 | | M Prp |
| (CF+C)/SumC [1/3] | 33% | 28 | 91 | 28 | 91 | | CFC Prp |
| **Perception and Thinking Problems** | | | | | | | |
| EII-3 | 0.4 | 80 | 113 | 81 | 113 | | EII |
| TP-Comp (Thought & Percept. Com...) | 0.9 | 66 | 106 | 66 | 106 | | TP-C |
| WSumCog | 6 | 50 | 100 | 44 | 98 | | WCog |
| SevCog | 0 | 35 | 94 | 35 | 94 | | Sev |
| FQ-% | 10% | 57 | 103 | 58 | 103 | | FQ-% |
| WD-% | 9% | 61 | 104 | 53 | 101 | | WD-% |
| FQo% | 63% | 62 | 104 | 58 | 104 | | FQo% |
| P | 5 | 39 | 96 | 44 | 98 | | P |
| **Stress and Distress** | | | | | | | |
| YTVC' | 3 | 36 | 95 | 23 | 89 | | YTVC' |
| m | 4 | 90 | 119 | 82 | 114 | | m |
| Y | 1 | 48 | 99 | 36 | 94 | | Y |
| MOR | 4 | 94 | 123 | 92 | 122 | | MOR |
| SC-Comp (Suicide Concern Comp.) | 6.0 | 81 | 114 | 76 | 111 | | SC-C |
| **Self and Other Representation** | | | | | | | |
| ODL% | 10% | 52 | 101 | 46 | 98 | | ODL% |
| SR (Space Reversal) | 5 | 98 | 132 | 98 | 132 | | SR |
| MAP/MAHP [4/4] | 100% | 94 | 123 | 94 | 123 | | MAP Prp |
| PHR/GPHR [9/15] | 60% | 87 | 117 | 87 | 117 | | PHR Prp |
| M- | 2 | 94 | 123 | 94 | 123 | | M- |
| AGC | 4 | 70 | 108 | 64 | 106 | | AGC |
| H | 3 | 67 | 106 | 50 | 100 | | H |
| COP | 0 | 21 | 88 | 21 | 88 | | COP |
| MAH | 0 | 26 | 90 | 26 | 90 | | MAH |

## R-PAS Summary Scores and Profiles – Page 2

C-ID: Son of God     P-ID: 43     Age: 60s     Gender: Male     Education: 20

| Domain/Variables | Raw Scores | Raw %ile | Raw SS | Cplx. Adj. %ile | Cplx. Adj. SS | Standard Score Profile R-Optimized | Abbr. |
|---|---|---|---|---|---|---|---|
| **Engagement and Cog. Processing** | | | | | | | |
| W% | 50% | 67 | 107 | 64 | 105 | | W% |
| Dd% | 23% | 77 | 111 | 79 | 112 | | Dd% |
| SI (Space Integration) | 8 | 97 | 130 | 98 | 130 | | SI |
| IntCont | 3 | 67 | 107 | 61 | 104 | | IntC |
| Vg% | 3% | 39 | 96 | 37 | 95 | | Vg% |
| V | 0 | 29 | 92 | 29 | 92 | | V |
| FD | 1 | 60 | 104 | 60 | 104 | | FD |
| R8910% | 33% | 60 | 104 | 61 | 104 | | R8910% |
| WSumC | 2.5 | 40 | 96 | 26 | 90 | | WSC |
| C | 1 | 82 | 114 | 82 | 114 | | C |
| Mp/(Ma+Mp) [7/7] | 100% | 98 | 130 | 98 | 130 | | Mp Prp |
| **Perception and Thinking Problems** | | | | | | | |
| FQu% | 23% | 27 | 91 | 28 | 91 | | FQu% |
| **Stress and Distress** | | | | | | | |
| PPD | 8 | 42 | 97 | 29 | 92 | | PPD |
| CBlend | 1 | 69 | 107 | 43 | 97 | | CBlnd |
| C' | 1 | 41 | 97 | 23 | 88 | | C' |
| V | 0 | 29 | 92 | 29 | 92 | | V |
| CritCont% (Critical Contents) | 20% | 55 | 102 | 51 | 101 | | CrCt |
| **Self and Other Representation** | | | | | | | |
| SumH | 14 | 98 | 131 | 97 | 129 | | SumH |
| NPH/SumH [11/14] | 79% | 82 | 114 | 82 | 114 | | NPH Prp |
| V-Comp (Vigilance Composite) | 6.9 | 99 | 134 | 98 | 132 | | V-C |
| r (Reflections) | 0 | 36 | 95 | 36 | 95 | | r |
| p/(a+p) [11/12] | 92% | 99 | 133 | 98 | 132 | | p Prp |
| AGM | 1 | 75 | 110 | 75 | 110 | | AGM |
| T | 1 | 68 | 107 | 68 | 107 | | T |
| PER | 0 | 30 | 92 | 30 | 92 | | PER |
| An | 1 | 47 | 99 | 47 | 99 | | An |

Reproduced from the Rorschach Performance Assessment System® (R-PAS®) Scoring Program (© 2010–2016) and excerpted from the *Rorschach Performance Assessment System: Administration, Coding, Interpretation, and Technical Manual* (© 2011) with copyrights by Rorschach Performance Assessment System, LLC. All rights reserved. Used by permission of Rorschach Performance Assessment System, LLC. Further reproduction is prohibited without written permission from R-PAS.

CHAPTER 11

# Using R-PAS in Violence Risk Assessment

Saara Kaakinen
Emiliano Muzio
Hannu Säävälä

## Reason for Referral

"Max" was a 22-year-old Finnish single male outpatient who was evaluated as part of a voluntary violence risk assessment. The assessment was carried out at the Oulu University Hospital in Finland. Max was referred by a specialized outpatient mental health care unit, to which he had been taken by the police because of vague threats he had made against other students at the university. The students and teachers were worried he might harm someone or possibly himself. Prior to the evaluation he had not assaulted anyone in a school setting, but his appearance was aggressive and his behavior toward other students seemed impulsive and unpredictable. The outpatient unit determined that Max was not psychotic and did not meet criteria for involuntary treatment. Max was not interested in the psychotherapeutic treatment provided by the outpatient unit but reluctantly agreed to participate in the violence risk assessment. The referring outpatient clinic hoped to gain information about Max's aggressiveness and his violence risk in a school environment as well as his diagnosis and the severity of his psychopathology.

## Max's Background

Max was a visual arts student at the university. He had a sister who was 6 years younger. His parents had separated. Max had a difficult relationship with his father, who, according to Max, had never appreciated him and had been violent toward him once when he was a teenager (pressed him against a wall). His relationship with his mother was somewhat distant. Max had obtained average grades through high school. He enrolled at the university to study humanities, but soon found it to be too

205

theoretical and he dropped out. For the next 2 years he did short apprenticeships in schools and day care centers, until he was finally admitted to study visual arts, of which he had always dreamt. Max has had a few short relationships, mostly with girls several years his junior. He also has a few friends.

Since childhood, however, Max has had trouble relating to others. As a child, he had temper tantrums and was emotionally unstable. He remembered his childhood as bleak and agonizing, and himself as apathetic. He was bullied in primary school and had a tendency to end up in conflicts with other students. As a teenager he had dressed in an indifferent and careless way, which exposed him to ridicule and mockery as "a fag." During high school Max had struggled with his aggression, and he'd had to move to another school because of it. While separating from one girlfriend, he got so angry that he made serious threats to her. On a similar occasion with another girlfriend, he hit her in the face. In both cases the court issued a restraining order. In another instance, he threatened and attempted to strangle a man who had shouted insults at him. The police dismissed the case and referred him to reconciliation. Within the context of the present risk assessment, and regarding the vague threats he'd made to students at his university, no charges were pressed on the grounds that there had been no violence or direct threats against any particular individual.

Due to his lifelong emotional problems and aggressive behavior, Max had been evaluated in a psychiatric ward twice, at ages 10 and 17. He was suspected of suffering from Asperger syndrome, but diagnostic criteria were not met. He was diagnosed as suffering from depression and self-esteem problems, and later as having paranoid personality disorder. He was repeatedly in contact with outpatient mental health services, but creating a therapeutic alliance with him proved difficult. Psychiatric evaluations never found Max to be psychotic or in need of involuntary treatment. Max said he has always been misunderstood. He has been said to be scary, threatening, and aggressive; but he felt he was not. He interpreted these characterizations as false allegations, which made him furious.

## Violence Risk Assessment Research and Literature

Meta-analytic reviews of the predictive validity of the Historical Clinical Risk Management–20 (HCR-20) and the Psychopathy Checklist—Revised (PCL-R) show moderate predictive accuracy for both of these risk assessment tools (HCR-20, AUC = .71; PCL-R, AUC = .65; Yang, Wong, & Coid, 2010), although there is heterogeneity in their validity (Singh, Grann, & Fazel, 2011). Therefore, caution must be used when interpreting the results of these instruments.

At the present time, there are no meta-analyses about using the Rorschach in violence risk prediction, and meta-analyses by Wood et al. (2010) do not support the Rorschach as a measure of psychopathy. However, there is a growing body of literature about using the Rorschach in various other psycholegal contexts, including violence risk assessment as well as psychological injury, trial competency, and child custody evaluations (Erard, 2012; Erard, Meyer, & Viglione, 2014; Gacono, Evans, Kaser-Boyd, & Gacono, 2008), as well as using it to assess for heightened risk of antisocial and violent behavior (Benjestorf, Viglione, Lamb, & Giromini, 2013; Hartmann, Nørbech, & Grønnerød, 2006).

## Max's Other Assessment Results

Max was interviewed six times, including a summary/discussion session, which focused on his intrapsychic and interpersonal difficulties, particularly his violence and aggressiveness dynamics. Max's attitude toward the assessment was arrogant and verbally aggressive. He made every effort to emphasize that he was not interested in participating in the evaluation, but finally agreed to go through the process in order to "have something to do." Max refused to complete the Personality Assessment Inventory (PAI), stating that he was sick of filling out yet another questionnaire and threatened to tear up any self-report that contained questions about hearing voices. He also missed a couple of sessions. He was unwilling to discuss his own goals or assessment questions in an appropriate and nondefensive way. Finally, he stated, "I would really like to know why every time I try to express my artistic needs, someone is calling the police!"

When asked about his history of violence and the events that led to the violence risk assessment, Max easily lost his temper; however, his aggressive attitude could rapidly change into expressions of depression and hopelessness. When asked about these changes, he quickly switched back to a judgmental attitude and denied any possibility of being depressed. Max stated that he was not suffering from any kind of psychological problem. He thought that his interpersonal problems resulted from other people's stupidity and lack of comprehension. The countertransference feelings he provoked in the evaluating staff were frustration and anger, but also fearfulness, helplessness, and feelings of incompetence. It was as if Max needed to protect himself from the feelings of shame and humiliation that arose when someone was able to get too close to him. When confronted with these unbearable feelings, his need to gain back the feeling of being in control resulted in various attempts to make the interviewer feel uncomfortable.

As part of the violence risk assessment, a forensic psychiatrist met with Max six times. The forensic psychiatrist's evaluation focused on Max's history of violence, his anger management, the dynamics of his affective reactions, and his psychiatric diagnoses (using the Structured Clinical Interview for DSM-IV Disorders [SCID I and SCID II]).

### Summary of Non-R-PAS Assessment Findings

Max's efforts on intelligence testing (Wechsler Adult Intelligence Scale—Fourth Edition [WAIS-IV]) placed him just slightly above average (Full Scale IQ [FSIQ] = 110), which was consistent with his school performance and previous psychological evaluations. However, when completing Verbal Comprehension subtests, Max was overtly oppositional, arrogant, and sarcastic. His lack of effort made these subtest scores unreliable. For example, when asked why it was important to protect endangered species, he replied, "For the sake of PR image," or when asked about what animal was in Finland's coat of arms, his answer was, "A fly" (the correct answer being a lion, which almost every Finn knows). This response style was consistent with his behavior in social situations and throughout the assessment process, particularly in situations that presented a threat to his self-esteem. Congruent with his passion for the visual arts, however, he had a superior performance on Perceptual Reasoning (SS[1] = 126).

---

[1] Standard scores (SS) have a mean of 100 and an SD of 15.

Interestingly, in contrast to his externalizing behavior in the clinical interview, on the self-report questionnaires Max reported significant distress, internalization, and vulnerabilities, including feelings of inadequacy, weakness, and inferiority (Minnesota Multiphasic Personality Inventory [MMPI] 2–7–5 code-type; low Scale 4; Personality Diagnostic Questionnaire–4 [PDQ-4], Obsessive–Compulsive). The main externalizing personality characteristics he endorsed on the questionnaires were attention seeking and extreme emotionality (PDQ-4, Histrionic), and a passive resistance to social demands for performance (PDQ-4, Passive–Aggressive). Max endorsed some feminine attitudes (MMPI, Scale 5) similar to those expressed in the interview, which, in light of his aggressive behavior toward women, suggests inner conflict with regard to the feminine part of his identity. These results help better understand the dynamics of his behavior in school settings (e.g., making vague references to death and suicide as a way of attracting attention and provoking others). The self-report questionnaires seemed to have provided a less threatening way for Max to "open up" and describe himself, as opposed to revealing flaws and vulnerabilities in person and risking feelings of shame.

Max's responses to the Sentence Completion Test (SCT) showed a devaluing and arrogant attitude toward the task, but also slightly odd thinking (e.g., My nerves are "talking about stock exchange"). This was consistent with his behavior during interviews and in other social settings. Like he did on the WAIS, he also presented himself as witty and clever by playing with expressions and words, which is consistent with his self-reported histrionic features. Finally, the forensic psychiatrist's evaluation of Max's behaviors with the PCL-R resulted in scores far below the cut-off for psychopathy (PCL-R = 10/40 points: Factor 1 = 6/16 points; Factor 2 = 4/18 points). Based on a structured assessment with the HCR-20, including history of violent and aggressive behavior, Max's violence risk was considered to be moderate in a three-category scale of "low–moderate–high" (HCR-20 = 25/40 points).

## Why R-PAS for Max's Violence Risk Assessment?

By using a method such as the HCR-20, which is specifically for the structured assessment of violence risk, it is possible to draw conclusions about the person's violence potential. However, in order to understand the intrapsychic dynamics that trigger and aggravate the person's aggressive and violent behavior, other methods, such as the Rorschach, are needed. The Rorschach Performance Assessment System (R-PAS; Meyer, Viglione, Mihura, Erard, & Erdberg, 2011) provides an excellent means to observe how a person functions in a situation that is new, complex, and emotionally arousing. Being in a new, relatively unstructured situation typically causes some degree of anxiety in people. Observing how a person tolerates and copes with this anxiety can provide important information with regard to psycholegal questions, such as the potential for violent behavior. R-PAS cannot answer the question of whether or not a person is likely to act violently directly. However, it offers important information with regard to features of reality testing, thinking, judgment, impulse control and emotional regulation, internal representations of self and others, and other factors, all of which are essential in trying to understand the structure and intrapsychic dynamics of aggressive behavior (Gray, Meloy, & Jumes, 2008).

## The Introduction and Administration of R-PAS

The psychological evaluation took place in the Department of Psychiatry at the Oulu University Hospital in Finland, which offers specialized-level mental health care in both inpatient and outpatient settings. Max was assessed at the psychiatric emergency unit. Before entering the main premises, every visitor's belongings are checked in order to ensure the safety of the staff and other patients. Max found this cautionary measure extremely annoying and commented every time on how humiliated he felt during the inspection. This was also the case when it was time to begin the Rorschach. Before starting R-PAS, he refused to talk about how he had felt after our previous meeting, and simply stated in an annoyed tone that there was nothing new going on in his life. When asked about the Rorschach and whether he had read or heard anything about it before, Max took out his smartphone and started typing. When asked about this, he said he was on Wikipedia reading about the Rorschach. He read the page for a few minutes and didn't want to discuss it. Then he suddenly put away his phone and stated: "Just bring out Mr. Rorschach!"

After receiving the first card, Max became a different person. He cooperated well throughout the task and was very considerate of the examiner's writing pace, making sure that the examiner had written everything down before giving his next response. Despite his ability to work in a good alliance, Max seemed slightly annoyed with the examiner reminding him of the instructions to "give two, maybe three responses" and asking for the card back after the fourth response. Max's reaction prompted the examiner to adopt a somewhat more permissive approach to administration than what is standard in R-PAS. Max gave an extraordinarily lengthy protocol of 38 responses. R-PAS administration took approximately 2 hours.

After completing the task, there was a brief discussion concerning how Max felt about it. He stated, "For once you gave me a task that allowed me to use my intellect." Max appeared to have little awareness of the degree of psychological impairment and distress that was captured through his behavior on this task, which is described in the following section.

## Discussion of the R-PAS Results[2]

### Administration Behaviors and Observations

Max's behavior during the R-PAS administration was markedly different from his behavior during the interview sessions or the administration of other psychological tests. After receiving the first card and throughout the task, he was clearly interested, engaged, and accommodating. No prompting was necessary. Regular Card Turning (SS = 112) appeared to reflect a willingness to carefully examine the cards from different angles. Max's interest in art might have allowed him feel that his sense of creativity would serve him better on this task than on more structured methods, such as the WAIS-IV or self-report inventories, thus bringing his self-perceived strengths to the foreground.

---

[2]See Appendix 11.1 at the end of the chapter for Max's R-PAS Responses, Location Sheet, Code Sequence, and Page 1 and 2 Profiles.

However, the exceptionally elevated number of Pulls (SS = 144) throughout the task suggested a lack of willingness to follow the rules imposed on him by the testing situation, and could also be understood as an expression of his uninhibited "artistic needs." That is, in the microcosm of the R-PAS task, we see him play out his exclamation "I would really like to know why every time I try to express my artistic needs, someone is calling the police!" In this case, Max was doing something he felt he is good at—creatively and visually expressing himself in an unstructured task. The only problem was the task was not unstructured enough for him to satisfy these needs without restriction, which annoyed him. The extraordinarily high number of Responses (R = 38, SS = 143) and his regular Card Turning appeared to reflect Max's attempts to regulate his self-esteem and defend against his younger bullied and rejected self by ambitious and unrestricted overprocessing (suggested also by the PDQ-4 and MMPI). He is like no one else and proud of it, expressing his aggression toward those who reject him or attempt to impose boundaries on him, as further elaborated below.

## Engagement and Cognitive Processing

As a result of his unwillingness and inability to follow test-imposed boundaries, and apparently his desire to show off his strengths, Max produced an exceptionally long and complex protocol (Complexity SS = 130). Taking into account the reason for referral and the fact that his dramatic imagery (CritCont% SS = 113) was within normal limits,[3] the possibility of malingering or "faking bad" is highly unlikely. This is consistent with the fact that Max's MMPI validity scales also did not suggest overreporting. On the contrary, he appears to have a tendency to minimize psychological problems when describing himself to others, given the elevated psychopathology on this performance-based task (e.g., EII-3 SS = 126).

The above-average Complexity of Max's R-PAS protocol could, in theory, overestimate his psychological problems. In Max's case, however, it is important to note that the potentially problematic and uninhibited overproductivity of the protocol (R, Pulls) accounts for a significant part of this complexity. In fact, the number of responses remains elevated when Complexity is taken into account (Complexity Adjusted [CAdj] R SS = 119), indicating that his Complexity is elevated largely secondary to his high level of responding. Although Max's high level of responding might be (at least, in part) attributable to a more permissive than standard administration (the reminder of providing two or maybe three responses per card was given only two of the eight times Max gave four responses, and was worded in a way that may have implied giving four responses meant doing better), there are also indications of his psychological complexity being due to intrinsic factors (Det SS = 136; Cont SS = 129) and, even when adjusting for Complexity, his most pathological scores remain elevated (e.g., EII-3 SS = 120; SC-Comp SS = 127). Therefore, because this complex processing style seems to be Max's natural way of being, we focus mostly on his non-CAdj results.

---

[3]The R-PAS manual recommends interpreting Page 2 scores more tentatively than Page 1 scores; for instance, by using a deviation of SS > 15 from the mean in contrast to the Page 1 SS > 10 deviation from the mean (Meyer et al., 2011, p. 366).

Max's high number of Responses and protocol Complexity is consistent with his visual/perceptual intelligence, shown by his superior WAIS-IV Perceptual Reasoning score and his major in visual arts. The high number of Responses might also reflect Max's wish to be seen as productive, witty, and intelligent. This would be consistent with his performance on the SCT and his flamboyant remark, "Just bring out Mr. Rorschach!"

Max's Complexity also appears to be related to a hypervigilant processing style and emotional turmoil, rather than to psychological sophistication. This hypervigilant tendency to excessively attend to and articulate nuances and uncertainties in his environment appears to be both cognitively and emotionally overwhelming (F% SS = 87; V-Comp SS = 148; MC–PPD SS = 66; YTVC' SS = 139). In addition, it appears that when processing new, loosely structured, and emotionally arousing stimuli, Max's capacity to perceive things accurately and conventionally deteriorates significantly over time (FQ– responses start appearing on Card V; there are no Popular responses after Card V). He exhibits a significant tendency to process multiple features of his environment (Blend SS = 135), with a particular sensitivity to perceiving its dysphoric and distressful qualities (8 of 13 blends include C'; 7 of 13 include m and/or Y; Blend content: e.g., R3: "howling wolves. . . . Howling makes it shadow-like. Sorrow and shadow go together"; R6: "a screaming expression. . . . Fearful look but at the same time slightly panic-like"). However, despite his sensitivity to the nuances in his environment, he is significantly less likely to make connections, synthesize information, and "see the big picture," compared to other people with this level of complexity (CAdj Sy SS = 64; W% SS = 83).

As part of his complexity, Max has above-average psychological resources (MC SS = 125; M SS = 122), but they are hindered by significant affective disruption (MC–PPD SS = 66), difficulty understanding other people's thoughts and intentions, and a proneness to color experience excessively with fantasies and projections (M– SS = 123). Max shows a clear tendency to creatively process and integrate different aspects of his environment (SI SS = 132). However, in his case, this complex perceptual style appears to be more of a liability that may be better accounted for by his hypervigilant, negative, and oppositional way of relating to his environment (V-Comp SS = 148; SR SS = 141; five of seven SRs are also SI). Thus, one would expect him to be psychologically sensitive and easily overwhelmed by situational stress, distress, and feelings of helplessness (PPD SS = 140). These, in turn, lead to an increased risk for impulsive, poorly controlled, and unpredictable behavior.

Max's behavior appears to be guided by both thinking things through and more intuitive or immediate decision making (M/MC SS = 101). However, given the psychological liabilities described above, this apparent flexibility might further expose him to ambivalence, confusion, indecisiveness, and inefficiency in problem solving (Complexity in conjunction with low MC–PPD and high EII-3). In addition, Max tends to react to emotionally toned stimuli in his experiential environment in ways that are overly spontaneous, immediate, or poorly controlled [(CF+C)/SumC SS = 111]. At times he may become overwhelmed by explosive outbursts (Ex SS = 129; R33, ma,CF: "A sun. . . . Flaming colors, like a flaming sun. It's very close, like it's on fire. The colors of the sun are overwhelming, bursting into the air"; R34, ma,C,C': "An explosion. . . . It's so wide, those colors are spreading into the surroundings. I imagined that white area as a shock wave. Shock wave that begins to throw colors around. It's a really powerful explosion that can be seen at a distance of hundreds of kilometers"). These findings are consistent with his history: his occasional outbursts and rageful attacks on others when he feels rejected or shamed. Furthermore, as discussed in the next section, he might tend to inaccurately see his outbursts as justified, which increases his potential for violent and poorly controlled behavior.

## Perception and Thinking Problems

Max's risk for behavioral and coping difficulties is further increased by the severity of his psychopathology, poor ego functions, and distorted self- and other-representations (EII-3 SS = 126). His problems with perceptual accuracy, reality testing, and thinking suggest a potential vulnerability to psychotic levels of disturbance (TP-Comp SS = 117). At times, he has problems interpreting stimuli realistically (WD–% SS = 114; FQ–% SS = 112), perhaps particularly in cognitively demanding and emotionally arousing situations (three of six FQ– appear on the last three color cards), which are also when his previously described unmodulated and potentially frightening outbursts of explosiveness tend to occur. Furthermore, Max has a marked tendency to have an atypical perspective on internal and external events and experiences (FQu% SS = 127).

An analysis of the thematic imagery associated with Max's more likely projective responses (FQ–, cognitive codes, embellishments) suggests strange or paranoid thinking in connection with eyes in particular (R2: "Could be a fox with an unusual number of eyes [INC1]. . . . Here I saw the eyes; they stand out first. It feels like somebody is watching, there's that kind of reaction"; R17: "A slightly smiling face. Precisely because it could be the creasing of the eyes and forehead . . . a semi-surprised smiling face"; R32: "That head reminds me of creatures in the *Alien* movies. Except that the creature has eyes . . . I can't help but see the eyes; it bothers me a bit. I am forced to see them . . . it brought so much contrast that I couldn't help but to see them as eyes"). Max may also project his own physical vulnerabilities (An SS = 122), perhaps particularly in regard to the sexual objectification of female body parts and the vulnerability of femininity (R30: "Again parts of a body . . . brings to mind a feminine body. . . . Here's the triangular area, vulva, panties"; R35: "A woman. A hip bone there. . . . That looks like a bra. . . . The white area looks feminine because it appears to curve here"). He has a tendency to perceive devalued (R8: "disgusting teeth"; R14: "a hideous skull") or both devalued and idealized images (R29: "Some big fat dude . . . Michelangelo-like"; R32: "the queen of the aliens"), and perhaps also has needs to be helped and protected (ODL% SS = 114; also, R23: "Two open palms . . . two helpful hands"; R25: "A beetle . . . a strong, shell-like texture").

Max also tends to put things together in unrealistic ways (five of eight cognitive codes are INC1), which can lead to misunderstandings and further increase his risk for socially inappropriate behavior (WSumCog SS = 119). Further, as noted before, at times his preoccupations can result in significant misunderstandings of others (M– = 2, SS = 123).

The type of psychotic proneness described here, which includes unrealistic mental representations (INCs) and a modest propensity for distorted interpretations of the environment (FQ–%), would likely not be obvious in Max's speech during a clinical interview (absence of SevCog responses and neologisms [DV] and only modest elevation in FQ–%). This absence would tend to move diagnostic decisions away from psychotic disorders, which is consistent with Max's diagnostic history. The potential for psychotic-type lapses to detrimentally impact Max's capacity to exercise sound judgment and make it through the day without getting into trouble is elevated nonetheless (EII-3).

## Stress and Distress

Max is not only experientially sensitive, but also very likely to experience highly disruptive and implicitly irritating internal stimuli that are outside of his control (m SS = 119; YTVC' SS = 139). He may not always be fully aware of the degree of the latter and is likely to function in ways that significantly interfere with his capacity to cope and his overall level of adjustment. Max has significantly elevated levels of implicitly carried distress, which is particularly related to experiences of helplessness, dysphoria, irritation, and pessimistic and depressive ideation (YTVC' SS = 139; Y SS = 130; C' SS = 140; PPD SS = 140; MOR SS = 117, two of three MOR also include C'). Findings further suggest that Max's depression could be related to oral dependent needs (ODL% SS = 114; all three MOR include ODL). This marked sense of emotional neediness, and the anxiety and depression related to it, is probably best conveyed by the compelling thematic imagery found in these three responses: R3: "howling wolves. . . . Howling makes it shadow-like. Sorrow and shadow go together"; R6: "Somebody's eyes, nose. It's a screaming expression. . . . Fearful look but at the same time slightly panic-like"; R8: "A praying mantis from very close. . . . Here's the head, disgusting teeth. . . . It's so wide, like somebody has cut it in two and spread it out."

Max has a significantly elevated propensity for perspective taking that is likely accompanied by a sense of shame, which is aggressively defended against (V SS = 134; two Y,V blends, one with FQ– and AGC—a beetle with "a strong shell-like structure" and "barbs"; two C',V blends, one with INC1, MOR, and ODL— "a screaming expression"). This dynamic is consistent with Max's devaluation of others and with the psychological test results during the assessment. One might say that when he feels vulnerable, helpless, and ashamed, Max makes barbs at others and puts on his protective shell (R25).

Max's psychological functioning includes a collection of factors that, when considered together, significantly increases his risk for suicide or serious self-destructive behavior (SC-Comp SS = 143). This high implicit risk was not obvious during Max's interview or captured on his self-report measures. However, it was consistent with the concerns of the students and teachers at his school that he may harm himself (or others). Factors contributing the most to Max's risk for self-harm include potentially inescapable shame or self-criticism (V SS = 134), his tendency to have negative feelings spoil positive reactions and enjoyment (CBlend SS = 117), his dysphoria and propensity to view himself as damaged (MOR SS = 117), his inability to perceive the world as others do and his lack of connection with what is most obvious to others (FQo% SS = 72; P SS = 88), his excessive and burdensome mental complexity (SI SS = 132), his extremely individualistic and oppositional way of relating to his environment (SR SS = 141), and his overwhelming affective distress, which he does not have the mental resources to cope with and which significantly increases the risk for impulsive behavior (MC–PPD SS = 66). Furthermore, when considered in light of his misunderstandings of situations, problems in thinking, and hypervigilant style, the probability of Max acting out impulsively and in destructive and socially inappropriate ways is markedly elevated.

## Self and Other Representation

Max presents an interesting mix of implicit dependent needs (ODL% SS = 114) and preoccupation with aggressive images (AGC SS = 127). His dependency needs appear to be fraught with concerns related to helplessness, fear, vulnerability, and aggression (R3: "howling wolves"; R6: "a screaming expression"; R8: "A praying mantis"; R11: "A row of worshippers, people praying"; R14: "a hideous skull") and his aggressive preoccupations appear to occur in a context of—and might represent a reaction to—dysphoria, shame, helplessness, or loss of control (five of seven AGC come with C′, Y, m, or V).

Max's R-PAS results suggest a marked tendency for oppositional behavior and individualistic strivings, as well as a marked aversion to feeling controlled or pressured by others (SR SS = 141). Oppositional behavior appears to occur with people perceived as having limited or vaguely defined characteristics, at the expense of a more balanced and integrated view (six of seven SR responses are also Hd or [Hd]: R4: "Some kind of . . . very faint face, but it is not particularly obvious"; R6: "a screaming expression"; R9: "Upper part of a torso and neck"; R17: "A slightly smiling face . . . a semi-surprised smiling face"; R24: "an Aztec priest. Head and round headdress with protruding shoulders"; R35: "A woman. A hip bone there. [CP] That looks like a bra").

Max's self-assertive strivings (SR), as well as his suspicious and hypervigilant attitude towards others (V-Comp), are in conflict with his dependency needs (ODL). This conflict is probably contributing to his overall level of distress, ambivalent behavior, and confusion. On the one hand, Max appears to have strong interpersonal needs, but at the same time he feels threatened by others and feels the need to protect himself and keep others at arm's length. It is also likely that he tries to avoid experiencing these dependency needs because they are associated with fearful and sorrowful aversive feelings (descriptors such as R3 "sorrow," R6 "fearful . . . panic," R8 "disgusting," R14 "hideous"). Max also appears to have significant vulnerabilities regarding bodily and psychic integrity (An SS = 122). In response to interpersonal insecurity, he may bolster his sense of self with aggrandizing and self-justifying defensive reactions (PER SS = 118).

As previously noted, Max's views of self and others appear to be distorted and unrealistic, suggesting significant difficulties in relating to himself and others realistically and appropriately (PHR/GPHR SS = 118; M– SS = 123). Furthermore, Max tends to miss out on opportunities to identify and put into practice conventional forms of human interaction (no human Popular responses on Cards III and VII). Instead, in situations where such appropriate responses would be easy to identify and put to good use, he tends to feel hurt, devalued, victimized, and tends to distort what is happening and ultimately fails to interpret the situation realistically (first response on Card III is the "cut open," "praying mantis"; Card VII includes two FQ– responses).

Of note, all of Max's responses including depressive content (MOR) appear within the first quarter of the test, suggesting that both depressive ideation and a negatively colored self-image constitute important aspects of Max's immediate reaction to new, interpersonal, and emotionally arousing situations. Interpersonal stimuli and imagining human connection (COP and MAH on R21) appear to elicit in Max implicit shame and helplessness (R22: Y,V), a need for help (R23: "Two open palms. . . . Opening, two helpful hands") and protection (R25: "A beetle . . . a strong, shell-like texture"), and to fill a sense of emptiness (R25: "I filled the white space only in my head"). In reaction, he might cope with his dependency needs and vulnerability through the use of grandiose and idealized self-representations (R24: "an Aztec priest"; R26: "A decorative headdress. . . . It's really festive and luxurious"). The question also arises as to what extent shame and helplessness might be related to Max's problems in thinking and reality testing (EII-3; TP-Comp). This possibility might help explain his threat to tear up any self-report inventory that contained questions about hearing voices.

## Summary/Discussion Session

During the summary/discussion session, Max appeared to be depressed, apathetic, and submissive. He listened carefully to the summary of assessment results, but was reluctant to engage in a discussion concerning his psychological problems. Given his wish to be seen as creative, clever, and unique, he might have felt disappointed with this session, which put the emphasis on his psychological difficulties. However, during the summary/discussion session Max was able to recognize his depression to the extent that it ultimately resulted in the prescription of antidepressant medication. After the violence risk assessment, Max also agreed to start considering the possibility of engaging in psychotherapeutic treatment with the forensic psychiatrist. After a few months he decided to quit the psychotherapy assessment. When the forensic psychiatrist tried to reach him by the phone, Max answered with a text message: "No, I'm not going to come. No. It's always the same. Your mission is to prove that you are right and I'm wrong." This statement appeared to capture Max's difficulties tolerating the feelings of shame and humiliation that arise when someone gets too close to him. Not surprisingly, however, he later recontacted the forensic psychiatrist to receive more effective medication for his depression. The newly prescribed antidepressant/anxiolytic medication (Vortioxetine 20 mg; a selective serotonin reuptake inhibitor [SSRI]) alleviated his depressive symptoms and significantly moderated his aggression and paranoia. Antipsychotic medication was not recommended because of Max's strong need to believe that he was suffering exclusively from depression. Concurrently, signs of an emerging therapeutic alliance appeared.

## The Impact of the R-PAS Results on Max's Violence Risk Assessment

R-PAS provided valuable information regarding psychological difficulties that markedly influence Max's abilities to control his destructive impulses. According to the HCR-20 results, Max's violence risk potential was found to be moderate. However, R-PAS played a crucial role in understanding the psychodynamic factors underlying his potential to behave aggressively. According to the R-PAS results, the most notable features affecting Max's violence risk potential were his problems in reality testing—more specifically, his incapacity to read and interpret social situations conventionally and an occasional tendency to read them very inaccurately—and his paranoid guardedness and hypervigilance that tended to project aggressive impulses onto others.

R-PAS also brought to light the extent of Max's implicit distress that was difficult for him to fully acknowledge; his difficulties with emotional modulation; and the high likelihood of impulsive, self-destructive, and unpredictable behavior. Finally, R-PAS revealed Max's implicit dependency needs. With regard to his violence potential, it is possible that Max's problems accepting his dependency needs lead to aggression and provocative self-assertion as a way to defend against them. Moreover, R-PAS depicted Max's dysphoric and anxious inner reality in which helplessness, fear, and vulnerability are prominent, though often implicit and hidden behind his narcissistic defensiveness. Only glimpses of his underlying and overwhelming distress could be observed in interviews.

Although R-PAS is not a DSM or an International Classification of Diseases (ICD) diagnostic tool, it offered valuable insights into the structure and dynamics of Max's personality, which in turn allowed the forensic psychiatrist to formulate a reliable diagnosis as well as conclusions for the violence risk assessment and recommendations for future treatment. Max was diagnosed as suffering from a mixed personality disorder with paranoid and narcissistic features. Additionally, R-PAS allowed us to see how Max's personality structure presented many of the features typically associated with a borderline level of personality organization (Kernberg, 1975).

## REFERENCES

Benjestorf, S. T., Viglione, D. J., Lamb, J. D., & Giromini, L. (2013). Suppression of aggressive Rorschach responses among violent offenders and nonoffenders. *Journal of Interpersonal Violence, 28,* 2981–3003.

Erard, R. E. (2012). Expert testimony using the Rorschach Performance Assessment System in psychological injury cases. *Psychological Injury and Law, 5,* 122–134.

Erard, R. E., Meyer, G. J., & Viglione, D. J. (2014). Setting the record straight: Comment on Gurley, Piechowski, Sheehan, and Gray (2014) on the admissibility of the Rorschach Performance Assessment System (R-PAS) in court. *Psychological Injury and Law, 7,* 165–177.

Gacono, C. B., Evans, F. B., Kaser-Boyd, N., & Gacono, L. A. (Eds.). (2008). *The handbook of forensic Rorschach assessment.* New York: Routledge.

Gray, B. T., Meloy, J. R., & Jumes, M. T. (2008). Dangerousness risk assessment. In C. B. Gacono, F. B. Evans, N. Kaser-Boyd, & L. A. Gacono (Eds.), *The handbook of forensic Rorschach assessment* (pp. 175–194). New York: Routledge.

Hartmann, E., Nørbech, P. B., & Grønnerød, C. (2006). Psychopathic and nonpsychopathic violent offenders on the Rorschach: Discriminative features and comparisons with schizophrenic inpatient and university student samples. *Journal of Personality Assessment, 86,* 291–305.

Kernberg, O. F. (1975). *Borderline conditions and pathological narcissism.* New York: Aronson.

Meyer, G. J., Viglione, D. J., Mihura, J. L., Erard, R. E., & Erdberg, P. (2011). *Rorschach Performance Assessment System: Administration, coding, interpretation, and technical manual.* Toledo, OH: Rorschach Performance Assessment System.

Singh, J. P., Grann, M., & Fazel, S. (2011). A comparative study of violence risk assessment tools: A systematic review and metaregression analysis of 68 studies involving 25,980 participants. *Clinical Psychology Review, 31,* 499–513.

Wood, J. M., Lilienfeld, S. O., Nezworski, M. T., Garb, H. N., Allen, K. H., & Wildermuth, J. L. (2010). Validity of Rorschach inkblot scores for discriminating psychopaths from nonpsychopaths in forensic populations: A meta-analysis. *Psychological Assessment, 22,* 336–349.

Yang, M., Wong, S. P., & Coid, J. (2010). The efficacy of violence prediction: A meta-analytic comparison of nine risk assessment tools. *Psychological Bulletin, 136,* 740–767.

## Rorschach Responses "Max"

| Respondent ID: Max | Examiner: Saara Kaakinen |
|---|---|
| Location: Oulu University Hospital | Date: **/**/**** |
| Start Time: 14:45 P.M. | End Time: 16:55 P.M. |

| Cd # | R # | Or | Response | Clarification | R-Opt |
|---|---|---|---|---|---|
| I | 1 | | A bat comes to mind. (W) | E: (Examiner repeats response [ERR].)<br>R: Outspread wings (D2). I myself draw a lot, so bats are nice, that's why. This creature has open wings. And black color is associated with a bat. | |
| | 2 | | Could be a fox with an unusual number of eyes. (W) | E: (ERR)<br>R: Looks like the shape of a fox. The white spots simply resemble the eyes (Dd26). It could also have ears (D7). Here I saw the eyes; they stand out first. It feels like somebody is watching, there's that kind of reaction [i.e., fox's reaction]. [On the border between INC1 and INC2] | |
| | 3 | | Maybe some howling wolves are seen in these columns. Nothing else comes to mind. (Dd28) | E: (ERR)<br>R: Here is precisely the shape of a dog-creature's shadow. Looks like it's raising its head; one could imagine that there's also a sound associated with it.<br>E: What made it look like a shadow?<br>R: It's black. I can't imagine that the wolf would be totally black in nature. Howling makes it shadow-like. Sorrow and shadow go together. | |
| | 4 | | Some kind of . . . very faint face, but it is not particularly obvious. (Dd99 = Dd26+Dd27+portion of D4 between)<br>E: Thanks, that's good. Remember, you only need to give two or three responses to each card. [A standard reminder would more declaratively encourage the respondent to provide two, maybe three responses.] | E: (ERR)<br>R: Eyes (Dd30) and in the middle some kind of nose (Dd27). Grinning. I don't think this black area at all; I'm just thinking these figures here (Dd26). Gray shade looks like it could continue forward. [E could have clarified this for possible FD or V.] That gray starts to go to a smile (Dd29 and portion of D4 between). It looks like a Halloween mask. I think it's more like roguish than malicious. | Pu |
| II | 5 | | Two bears with their paws opposite each other and knees bent. (D6) | E: (ERR)<br>R: Shoulders, paws (D4) are touching each other. Two paws . . . they are crouching. I imagined them as bears, their features are so burly. Thick arms but small hands. One seems to have an ear even if not seen in the other. There are wrinkles in the snout, although it's such a small detail. The rest of the head looks flat, but it seems to be hilly in this one spot (the respondent shows the edges of the blot, thus not implying depth). Bears are mostly something other than black-colored, so I like to see these as shadows. Black color makes it shadowy. [E could have queried "wrinkles" for Y, T, or V.] | |
| | 6 | | Here comes somebody's eyes, nose. It's a screaming expression. Eyes (DdS30), hollow nose, and mouth (Dd99 = DS5 – Dd29). Yelling mouth, gaping look. (Dd99 = DS5+4+30) | E: (ERR)<br>R: The white areas resemble a face, visible features. Here's just a white hole, like a nose hole in a skull (DdS29). Couple of these shadows look exactly how those things above are seen in a skull . . . that little gray detail. The nostrils are showing and small furrows like shadows (D4 to DdS29). I associated that as nose; it was easy to imagine those furrows above. Finally, a white area makes it look like open, goes upward diagonally, which is a yelling look. Fearful look but at the same time slightly panic-like. | |

| Cd # | R # | Or | Response | Clarification | R-Opt |
|------|-----|----|----------|---------------|-------|
| | 7 | v | v Two dancing people, maybe Kabuki dancers. (D6) | E: (ERR)<br>R: Here's the tip of a leg (D4). The other leg is bending. The clothes are frilly and thick hands (D3) raised upward in the air. They are bouncing. These are somewhat exaggerated, so it brings Kabuki dancers to my mind.<br>E: What made it look like the clothes are frilly?<br>R: In humans it doesn't puff out like that; body shape of a human is portrayed in it. The shape is billowy, billowy figures. Humans are not this thickly drawn. There is space in the upper body, the sleeves are hanging. It's shadow-play, like silhouette.<br>E: What made it look like shadow-play?<br>R: The black color. | |
| III | 8 | | A praying mantis from very close. (D1) | E: (ERR)<br>R: Here's the head (D7), disgusting teeth. The appendages (D5) look like they could belong to some insect. It's so wide, like somebody has cut it in two and spread it out. [E could have asked what makes the teeth look "disgusting" as a "loaded" word.] | |
| | 9 | | A bow in the middle. Upper part of a torso and neck. It's a human's upper body. (DdS99 = 3, 24, 34s) | E: (ERR)<br>R: That resembles a bow (D3); it's shaped like that. Black-and white-colored suit, the white part is shirt (DdS24) and the surrounding part looks like a jacket. Wrinkles (Dd99 = protrusions just above D7 coming off of Dd30) in the cloth, those lines. I ignored the rest of the picture, because it didn't look like that. | |
| | 10 | | A hip bone. (Dd99 = lower half of W) | E: (ERR)<br>R: The formation brings to mind the bones that are found in the pelvis. Wide V-form brings a pelvis easily into mind. [R covered upper half of W with his hand] | |
| | 11 | v | v A row of worshippers, people praying. Hands on the sides, these persons are in the middle and two others are on the sides. (Dd35, D5)<br>E: Thanks, that's enough for this card. Do you remember, you only need to give two or three responses to each card. | E: (ERR)<br>R: Two dudes (Dd35) lifting their hands (Dd21), serving. Other people's hands (D5) on the sides, like serving in the same way. These people can't be seen, because the picture ends. Two rows of people, who lift their hands upward, like worshipping something. | Pu |
| IV | 12 | | A really big guy pictured from lower angle. (W) | E: (ERR)<br>R: Looks large-sized. Feet (D6) are really big and upper body is small. If you look at it like this, it makes sense (examinee tilts the card to point the top away from the viewer). | |
| | 13 | | Sea waves. (W) | E: (ERR)<br>R: Shades of gray with black color form alternating figures with each other. Surging sea texture. Comes to mind from that foot (referring to D6), like water bouncing, crashing on the sea bank. [E could have queried "alternating figures" for V.] | |
| | 14 | | In the middle looks like a hideous skull. I can't say what kind of skull it is. Looks tusky. (D1) | E: (ERR)<br>R: Looks like a pig animal. Eyes on the sides. Like bones protruding, brings fangs and a wild boar into mind. [E could have asked what makes it look "hideous" as a "loaded" word.] | |
| V | 15 | | This is pretty much a bat. (W) | E: (ERR)<br>R: Bat's tentacles-slash-ears (Dd34). There are feet (D9) or something tail-like below. Black color suits it. | |
| | 16 | | Or a moth. Two wide wings. (W) | E: (ERR)<br>R: It's a moth's form and silhouette. [The Finnish word for silhouette includes the idea of being black, not just outline.] | |
| | 17 | | A slightly smiling face. Precisely because it could be the creasing of the eyes and forehead. (DdS99 = white space beneath W, including DdS27) | E: (ERR)<br>R: The white area brings to mind a semi-surprised smiling face. It shows only from the nose upward, that creasing of the eyes and the corner of the eye. This in the middle (DdS27), looks like the nasal bridge. A little like a white silhouette. | |

| Cd # | R # | Or | Response | Clarification | R-Opt |
|------|-----|----|----------|---------------|-------|
| | 18 | | And a head of a crocodile. (D10) (E reaches out for the card and takes it back. A reminder of the instruction was not provided because the respondent seemed to understand the boundaries of the task and became slightly annoyed when the instruction was repeated.) | E: (ERR) <br> R: Those on the sides look like a smiling lizard which matches pretty much a crocodile. | Pu |
| VI | 19 | | A landscape, a tree on the top of that kind of hill. (W) | E: (ERR) <br> R: Here's a flat area (D1), a hill (Dd31), and on the top, a tree (D3). Two-dimensional rugged landscape . . . *eutrophicated* is the best word I can come up with. Sturdy and smooth tree trunk surrounded by eutrophicated vegetation, because that looks more colorful. <br> E: What do you mean by "more colorful"? <br> R: Because there is a lot of gray shades and not much black color. | |
| | 20 | < | < A spaceship. (W) | E: (ERR) <br> R: I played sci-fi games when I was a child. Looks like it would on a tactical map. Like watching my own ship. <br> E: What made it look like a spaceship? <br> R: Its shape. | |
| | 21 | v | v Two humans small in proportion and their shoulders touching each other. (D1) | E: (ERR) <br> R: Two dudes (D4s) with their other arm (Dd24) spread to the side and one dude takes another from the shoulder. Rejoining, dancing movement. | |
| | 22 | | ^ It's a canyon, a river below. (D1) (A reminder of the instruction was not provided.) | E: (ERR) <br> R: Shades of gray look like forming a deep canyon. Like a river (D12) glimmering below, especially when there is dark on the sides. Could be quite deep. It's lighter between the black shades, like water reflecting down below. | |
| VII | 23 | | Two open palms. (W) | E: (ERR) <br> R: Opening, two helpful hands. Come from inside, hands spreading to the sides (shows with his own hands). | |
| | 24 | v | v An Aztectic human. (D7) | E: (ERR) <br> R: Just the white area. I imagined it as an Aztec priest. Head and round headdress (D10) with protruding jags. Shoulders. | |
| | 25 | | A beetle. (W) | E: (ERR) <br> R: It seems a strong, shell-like texture. Barbs (D5) resemble the anatomy of a bug. I filled the white space only in my head. <br> E: What about the inkblot made it look like shell-like texture? <br> R: Changing of colors, in the middle darker and on the sides lighter, cup-like (shows dome with his own hands). A lot of lighter color, gives an impression of shining. | |
| | 26 | | A decorative headdress. (W) (E reaches out for the card and takes it back. A reminder of the instruction was not provided.) | E: (ERR) <br> R: Just the black part. Resembles a decorated headdress, with various embellishments on the sides. It's really festive and luxurious. [E could have queried "festive and luxurious" for Y or T.] | Pu |
| VIII | 27 | | Parts of a body. (D6) | E: (ERR) <br> R: This could be a neck (D4), lungs (D5). Pelvis (D2) curving, including intestines and other things, which are splashed into a single palette of color. A mixture of red and orange. I can't say what all it could include. I associated red with internal organs. [No reference was made to the D1 area.] | |
| | 28 | | Mountains, forest. (D8) | E: (ERR) <br> R: The gray and greenish shade, it's like a big mountain. The white part (between 4 and 5) is an artistic outline. The colors made me think, that it could be a mountain and a forest. And that shape, overall it's big and steep. | |

| Cd # | R # | Or | Response | Clarification | R-Opt |
|---|---|---|---|---|---|
| | 29 | | Some big fat dude. (D2) | E: (ERR)<br>R: A whole human. Star-shaped, Michelangelo-like [i.e., Vitruvian man]. Head, hands, and feet. I imagined straight away that it's a fatter human. | |
| | 30 | v | v Again parts of a body. (D6) (E reaches out for the card and takes it back. A reminder of the instruction was not provided.) | E: (ERR)<br>R: Sweeping, curved, brings to mind a feminine body. This is not a silhouette of a body. Hourglass-shaped, stops to the neck. Here's the triangular area, vulva, panties (D4). | Pu |
| IX | 31 | | A flower. (W) | E: (ERR)<br>R: Petals and flower on the top. Could be a chrysanthemum. Flat, doesn't look at all open. Those petals brought pretty much green into it. | |
| | 32 | | That head reminds me of creatures in the *Alien* movies. Except that the creature has eyes. (D8) | E: (ERR)<br>R: That in the middle resembles the queen of the aliens. Broader backside looks like a head. I can't help but to see the eyes (DdS22); it bothers me a bit. I am forced to see them, although I just try to see only the lighter green color.<br>E: Where do you see the eyes?<br>R: The eyes are the white spots; there's darker green shading them, so it brought so much contrast that I couldn't help but to see them as eyes. | |
| | 33 | | A sun. (Dd99 = D3, upper D8) | E: (ERR)<br>R: The circle here (upper half of D8), round shape. Flaming colors, like a flaming sun. It's very close, like it's on fire (D3). The colors of the sun are overwhelming, bursting into the air. | |
| | 34 | | An explosion. (W)<br>(E reaches out for the card and takes it back. A reminder of the instruction was not provided.) | E: (ERR)<br>R: It's so wide, those colors are spreading into surroundings. I imagined that white area as a shock wave (DS8). Shock wave that begins to throw colors (D3) around. It's a really powerful explosion that can be seen at a distance of hundreds of kilometers. | Pu |
| X | 35 | v | v A woman. A hip bone there. (Dd99 = D11 + white space between and slightly above D6) | E: (ERR)<br>R: That looks like a bra (D6). You can imagine that shape as a hip bone, wide V-form (D11). The white area looks feminine because it appears to curve here. [It is not clear that he saw the hip bone as internal anatomy so FAB2 was not coded.] | |
| | 36 | v | A fairy. (D10) | E: (ERR)<br>R: This green creature, looks like a human shape. Darker green wings (D4). Green brings a fairy into mind, forest-ish color. | |
| | 37 | | ^ Some coral. (D1) | E: (ERR)<br>R: Blue lumps (the examinee uses his own Finnish word which resembles "lumps"). The middle part is a big lump, some sharp branches. Looked like that, especially, because it's colorful. I wouldn't have thought it as a coral if it were black. | |
| | 38 | | Fleas. (D12) (E reaches out for the card and takes it back.) | E: (ERR)<br>R: These green splashes. Cute little balls with tentacles. Innocent and fragile, the shape is so simple. | Pu |

# Rorschach Performance Assessment System (R-PAS)®

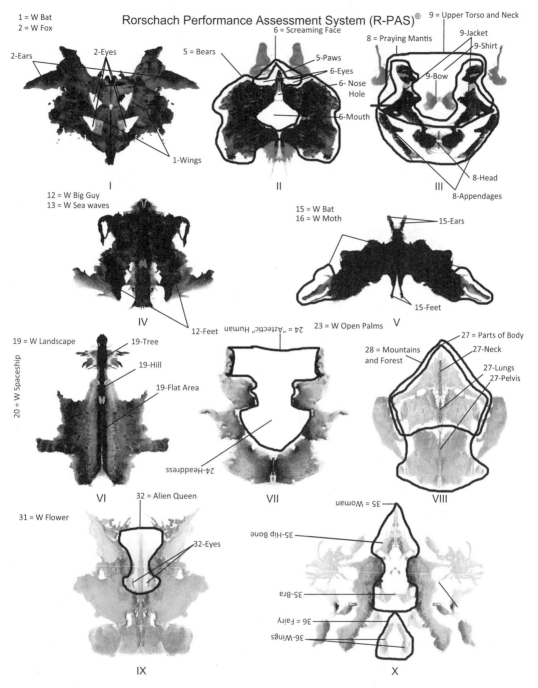

1 = W Bat
2 = W Fox

2-Ears
2-Eyes
1-Wings

I

5 = Bears
6 = Screaming Face
5-Paws
6-Eyes
6- Nose Hole
6-Mouth

II

9 = Upper Torso and Neck
8 = Praying Mantis
9-Jacket
9-Shirt
9-Bow
8-Head
8-Appendages

III

12 = W Big Guy
13 = W Sea waves

12-Feet

IV

15 = W Bat
16 = W Moth
15-Ears
15-Feet

V

19 = W Landscape
20 = W Spaceship
19-Tree
19-Hill
19-Flat Area

VI

24 = "Aztectic" Human
23 = W Open Palms
24-Headdress

VII

27 = Parts of Body
28 = Mountains and Forest
27-Neck
27-Lungs
27-Pelvis

VIII

31 = W Flower
32 = Alien Queen
32-Eyes

IX

35 = Woman
35-Hip Bone
35-Bra
36 = Fairy
36-Wings

X

© 2012 R-PAS; Rorschach® trademarks and images are used with permission of the trademark owner, Hogrefe AG, Berne, Switzerland

221

# Rorschach Performance Assessment System (R-PAS)®

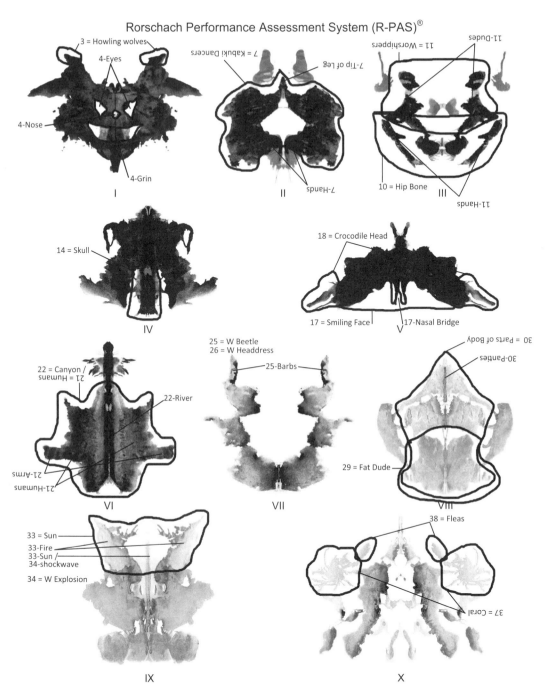

3 = Howling wolves
4-Eyes
4-Nose
4-Grin
I

7 = Kabuki Dancers
7-Tip of Leg
7-Hands
II

11 = Worshippers
11-Dudes
10 = Hip Bone
11-Hands
III

14 = Skull
IV

18 = Crocodile Head
17 = Smiling Face
17-Nasal Bridge
V

22 = Canyon
21 = Humans
22-River
21-Arms
21-Humans
VI

25 = W Beetle
26 = W Headdress
25-Barbs
VII

30 = Parts of Body
30-Panties
29 = Fat Dude
VIII

33 = Sun
33-Fire
33-Sun
34-shockwave
34 = W Explosion
IX

38 = Fleas
37 = Coral
X

# R-PAS Code Sequence: "Max"

**C-ID**: Max    **P-ID**: 4    **Age**: 22    **Gender**: Male    **Education**: NA

| Cd | # | Or | Loc | Loc # | SR | SI | Content | Sy | Vg | 2 | FQ | P | Determinants | Cognitive | Thematic | HR | ODL (RP) | R-Opt | Text |
|---|---|---|---|---|---|---|---|---|---|---|---|---|---|---|---|---|---|---|---|
| I | 1 | | W | | | | A | | | | o | P | FMp,C' | | | PER | | | |
| | 2 | | W | | | SI | Ad | | | | o | | FMp | INC1 | | | | | * |
| | | | | | | | | | | | | | | | | | | | |

Comment: On the border between INC1 and INC2

| Cd | # | Or | Loc | Loc # | SR | SI | Content | Sy | Vg | 2 | FQ | P | Determinants | Cognitive | Thematic | HR | ODL (RP) | R-Opt | Text |
|---|---|---|---|---|---|---|---|---|---|---|---|---|---|---|---|---|---|---|---|
| | 3 | | Dd | 28 | | | (Ad) | | | 2 | u | | FMa,C' | DR1 | AGC,MOR | | ODL | | |
| | 4 | | Dd | 99 | SR | SI | (Hd) | | | | o | | Mp | | | GH | | Pu | * |

Comment: E could have clarified this for possible FD or V.

| Cd | # | Or | Loc | Loc # | SR | SI | Content | Sy | Vg | 2 | FQ | P | Determinants | Cognitive | Thematic | HR | ODL (RP) | R-Opt | Text |
|---|---|---|---|---|---|---|---|---|---|---|---|---|---|---|---|---|---|---|---|
| II | 5 | | D | 6 | | | A | Sy | | | o | P | FMp,C' | INC1 | | | | | * |

Comment: E could have queried "wrinkles" for Y, T, or V.

| Cd | # | Or | Loc | Loc # | SR | SI | Content | Sy | Vg | 2 | FQ | P | Determinants | Cognitive | Thematic | HR | ODL (RP) | R-Opt | Text |
|---|---|---|---|---|---|---|---|---|---|---|---|---|---|---|---|---|---|---|---|
| | 6 | | Dd | 99 | SR | SI | Hd,An | | | | u | | Ma,C',V | INC1 | MOR | PH | ODL | | |
| | 7 | v | D | 6 | | | (H),Ay,Cg | Sy | | 2 | u | | Ma,mp,C' | | COP | GH | | | |
| III | 8 | | D | 1 | | | A | | | | u | | F | | MOR,MAP | | ODL | | * |

Comment: E could have asked what makes the teeth look 'disgusting' as a 'loaded' word.

| Cd | # | Or | Loc | Loc # | SR | SI | Content | Sy | Vg | 2 | FQ | P | Determinants | Cognitive | Thematic | HR | ODL (RP) | R-Opt | Text |
|---|---|---|---|---|---|---|---|---|---|---|---|---|---|---|---|---|---|---|---|
| | 9 | | Dd | 99 | SR | SI | Hd,Cg | | | | u | | C',V | | | PH | | | |
| | 10 | | Dd | 99 | | | An | | | | u | | F | | | | | | |
| | 11 | v | Dd | 35,5 | | | Hd | Sy | | 2 | u | | Ma | | COP | GH | ODL | Pu | |
| IV | 12 | | W | | | | H | | | | o | P | FD | | | GH | | | |
| | 13 | | W | | | | NC | | Vg | | u | | ma,Y | | | | | | * |

Comment: E could have queried "alternating figures" for V.

| Cd | # | Or | Loc | Loc # | SR | SI | Content | Sy | Vg | 2 | FQ | P | Determinants | Cognitive | Thematic | HR | ODL (RP) | R-Opt | Text |
|---|---|---|---|---|---|---|---|---|---|---|---|---|---|---|---|---|---|---|---|
| | 14 | | D | 1 | | | An | | | | u | | F | | AGC | | ODL | | * |

Comment: E could have asked what makes it look 'hideous' as a 'loaded' word.

| Cd | # | Or | Loc | Loc # | SR | SI | Content | Sy | Vg | 2 | FQ | P | Determinants | Cognitive | Thematic | HR | ODL (RP) | R-Opt | Text |
|---|---|---|---|---|---|---|---|---|---|---|---|---|---|---|---|---|---|---|---|
| V | 15 | | W | | | | A | | | | o | P | C' | DV1 | | | | | |
| | 16 | | W | | | | A | | | | o | | C' | | | | | | |
| | 17 | | Dd | 99 | SR | | Hd | | | | - | | Mp,C' | | | PH | ODL | | |
| | 18 | | D | 10 | | | Ad | | | 2 | o | | Mp | INC1 | AGC | PH | | Pu | |
| VI | 19 | | W | | | | NC | | | | u | | Y | | | | | | |
| | 20 | < | W | | | | NC | | | | u | | F | | PER | | | | |
| | 21 | v | D | 1 | | | H | Sy | | 2 | u | | Ma | | COP,MAH | GH | | | |
| | 22 | | D | 1 | | | NC | | | | o | | Y,V | | | | | | |
| VII | 23 | | W | | | | Hd | | | | - | | Mp | | | PH | | | |
| | 24 | v | D | 7 | SR | | Hd,Ay,Cg | Sy | | | u | | F | | | PH | | | |
| | 25 | | W | | | SI | A | | | | - | | Y,V | | AGC | | | | |
| | 26 | | W | | | | Art,Cg | | | | u | | F | | | | | Pu | * |

Comment: E could have queried 'festive and luxurious' for Y or T.

| Cd | # | Or | Loc | Loc # | SR | SI | Content | Sy | Vg | 2 | FQ | P | Determinants | Cognitive | Thematic | HR | ODL (RP) | R-Opt | Text |
|---|---|---|---|---|---|---|---|---|---|---|---|---|---|---|---|---|---|---|---|
| VIII | 27 | | D | 6 | | | An | | | | u | | CF,Y | | | | | | |
| | 28 | | D | 8 | | SI | NC | Sy | | | u | | CF | | | | | | |
| | 29 | | D | 2 | | | H,Ay | | | | - | | F | | | PH | ODL | | |
| | 30 | v | D | 6 | | | Hd,Cg,Sx | | | | - | | F | | | PH | | Pu | |
| IX | 31 | | W | | | | NC | | | | o | | FC | | | | | | |
| | 32 | | D | 8 | | SI | (Hd) | | | | u | | Y | DR1 | AGC | PH | | | |
| | 33 | | Dd | 99 | | | Ex,Fi | Sy | | | u | | ma,CF | | AGC | | | | |
| | 34 | | W | | SR | SI | Ex | | Vg | | o | | ma,C,C' | | AGC | | | Pu | |
| X | 35 | v | Dd | 99 | SR | SI | Hd,Cg,Sx | | | | - | | F | | | PH | | | * |

Comment: It is not clear that he saw the hipbone as internal anatomy so FAB2 was not coded.

| Cd | # | Or | Loc | Loc # | SR | SI | Content | Sy | Vg | 2 | FQ | P | Determinants | Cognitive | Thematic | HR | ODL (RP) | R-Opt | Text |
|---|---|---|---|---|---|---|---|---|---|---|---|---|---|---|---|---|---|---|---|
| | 36 | v | D | 10 | | | (H) | | | | u | | FC | | | GH | | | |
| | 37 | | D | 1 | | | NC | | | 2 | o | | CF | | | | | | |
| | 38 | | D | 12 | | | A | | | 2 | u | | F | INC1 | | | | Pu | |

©2010-2016 R-PAS

C-ID: Max                    P-ID: 4     Age: 22          Gender: Male          Education: NA

| Domain/Variables | Raw Scores | Raw %ile | Raw SS | Cplx. Adj. %ile | Cplx. Adj. SS | Standard Score Profile R-Optimized | Abbr. |
|---|---|---|---|---|---|---|---|
| **Admin. Behaviors and Obs.** | | | | | | | |
| Pr | 0 | 24 | 89 | | | | Pr |
| Pu | 7 | >99 | 144 | | | | Pu |
| CT (Card Turning) | 8 | 79 | 112 | | | | CT |
| **Engagement and Cog. Processing** | | | | | | | |
| Complexity | 130 | 98 | 130 | | | | Cmplx |
| R (Responses) | 38 | >99 | 143 | 89 | 119 | | R |
| F% [Lambda=0.36] (Simplicity) | 26% | 19 | 87 | 69 | 107 | | F% |
| Blend | 13 | 99 | 135 | 83 | 114 | | Bln |
| Sy | 7 | 55 | 102 | 1 | 64 | | Sy |
| MC | 14.5 | 95 | 125 | 53 | 101 | | MC |
| MC - PPD | -13.5 | 1 | 66 | 4 | 73 | | MC-PPD |
| M | 8 | 93 | 122 | 46 | 98 | | M |
| M/MC [8/14.5] | 55% | 52 | 101 | 47 | 99 | | M Prp |
| (CF+C)/SumC [5/7] | 71% | 76 | 111 | 76 | 111 | | CFC Prp |
| **Perception and Thinking Problems** | | | | | | | |
| EII-3 | 1.4 | 96 | 126 | 91 | 120 | | EII |
| TP-Comp (Thought & Percept. Com...) | 1.5 | 88 | 117 | 66 | 106 | | TP-C |
| WSumCog | 17 | 89 | 119 | 75 | 110 | | WCog |
| SevCog | 0 | 35 | 94 | 35 | 94 | | Sev |
| FQ-% | 16% | 79 | 112 | 71 | 108 | | FQ-% |
| WD-% | 14% | 82 | 114 | 61 | 104 | | WD-% |
| FQo% | 32% | 3 | 72 | 5 | 74 | | FQo% |
| P | 4 | 22 | 88 | 16 | 84 | | P |
| **Stress and Distress** | | | | | | | |
| YTVC' | 20 | >99 | 139 | 99 | 136 | | YTVC' |
| m | 4 | 90 | 119 | 50 | 100 | | m |
| Y | 6 | 98 | 130 | 93 | 123 | | Y |
| MOR | 3 | 87 | 117 | 74 | 110 | | MOR |
| SC-Comp (Suicide Concern Comp.) | 9.1 | >99 | 143 | 97 | 127 | | SC-C |
| **Self and Other Representation** | | | | | | | |
| ODL% | 18% | 82 | 114 | 64 | 105 | | ODL% |
| SR (Space Reversal) | 7 | 99 | 141 | 99 | 141 | | SR |
| MAP/MAHP [1/2] | NA | | | | | | MAP Prp |
| PHR/GPHR [10/16] | 62% | 89 | 118 | 89 | 118 | | PHR Prp |
| M- | 2 | 94 | 123 | 94 | 123 | | M- |
| AGC | 7 | 96 | 127 | 91 | 120 | | AGC |
| H | 3 | 67 | 106 | 10 | 79 | | H |
| COP | 3 | 91 | 120 | 70 | 108 | | COP |
| MAH | 1 | 64 | 105 | 26 | 90 | | MAH |

© 2010-2016 R-PAS

# R-PAS Summary Scores and Profiles – Page 2

C-ID: Max     P-ID: 4    Age: 22     Gender: Male     Education: NA

| Domain/Variables | Raw Scores | Raw %ile | Raw SS | Cplx. Adj. %ile | Cplx. Adj. SS | Standard Score Profile R-Optimized | Abbr. |
|---|---|---|---|---|---|---|---|
| **Engagement and Cog. Processing** | | | | | | | |
| W% | 34% | 41 | 97 | 13 | 83 | | W% |
| Dd% | 24% | 79 | 112 | 84 | 115 | | Dd% |
| SI (Space Integration) | 9 | 98 | 132 | 97 | 129 | | SI |
| IntCont | 4 | 79 | 112 | 49 | 99 | | IntC |
| Vg% | 5% | 55 | 102 | 60 | 104 | | Vg% |
| V | 4 | 99 | 134 | 97 | 127 | | V |
| FD | 1 | 60 | 104 | 24 | 89 | | FD |
| R8910% | 32% | 49 | 100 | 63 | 105 | | R8910% |
| WSumC | 6.5 | 90 | 119 | 52 | 100 | | WSC |
| C | 1 | 82 | 114 | 82 | 114 | | C |
| Mp/(Ma+Mp) [4/8] | 50% | 61 | 104 | 61 | 104 | | Mp Prp |
| **Perception and Thinking Problems** | | | | | | | |
| FQu% | 53% | 97 | 127 | 93 | 122 | | FQu% |
| **Stress and Distress** | | | | | | | |
| PPD | 28 | >99 | 140 | 96 | 126 | | PPD |
| CBlend | 2 | 88 | 117 | 51 | 100 | | CBlnd |
| C' | 10 | >99 | 140 | 99 | 135 | | C' |
| V | 4 | 99 | 134 | 97 | 127 | | V |
| CritCont% (Critical Contents) | 32% | 81 | 113 | 63 | 105 | | CrCt |
| **Self and Other Representation** | | | | | | | |
| SumH | 15 | 99 | 136 | 89 | 119 | | SumH |
| NPH/SumH [12/15] | 80% | 84 | 115 | 92 | 121 | | NPH Prp |
| V-Comp (Vigilance Composite) | 8.2 | >99 | 148 | 97 | 128 | | V-C |
| r (Reflections) | 0 | 36 | 95 | 36 | 95 | | r |
| p/(a+p) [8/16] | 50% | 66 | 106 | 72 | 109 | | p Prp |
| AGM | 0 | 31 | 93 | 31 | 93 | | AGM |
| T | 0 | 28 | 91 | 28 | 91 | | T |
| PER | 2 | 89 | 118 | 89 | 118 | | PER |
| An | 4 | 92 | 122 | 92 | 122 | | An |

© 2010-2016 R-PAS

# Using R-PAS in the Assessment of Possible Psychosis and Trauma Intrusions in a Psychopathic Female

Peder Chr. B. Nørbech
Ellen J. Hartmann
James H. Kleiger

Assessment of comorbid psychiatric symptoms in the psychopathic patient is challenging for a number of reasons. The psychopathic patient's ingrained distrust and hostility make it difficult not only to form a cooperative alliance around testing (McGauley, Adshead, & Sarkar, 2007), but the psychologist also must be cognizant of and prepared to deal with such patients' tendency to lie, deceive, and mislead the assessor at every turn (Gacono & Meloy, 2009). Psychiatric symptoms may be denied or exaggerated in order to skew the evaluation in a self-favorable manner. The validity of the evaluation thus depends upon a careful scrutiny and comparison of the assessment data and self-reported information with independent collateral information (Gacono & Meloy, 2009).

A less-acknowledged assessment concern when dealing with such a patient relates to the "diagnosis" of psychopathy in itself, as it often engenders serious skepticism, fear, and condemnation in clinicians. If such a countertransference reaction is allowed to progress, it may produce a salient pull within the assessor toward discrediting potentially "true symptoms" as "false." Enacting upon this pull, the assessor would paradoxically mimic the *psychopathic process of dismissal of the other,* and in doing so, likely also reinforce the patient's deep-rooted view of the world as an utterly corrupt and cruel place. Fruitful assessment encounters with such patients, therefore, depend on the assessor's ability to balance his or her necessary suspicion while maintaining an empathic, yet firm, attitude.

## Female Psychopathy

This chapter reports on the assessment and evaluation of a psychopathic female. Compared to the vast empirical (e.g., Patrick, 2006) and more clinically attuned (Gacono & Meloy, 1994) knowledge base on male psychopaths, relatively less is known about female psychopaths. Preliminary research suggests that, whereas male and female psychopaths share a comparable personality organization (borderline or psychotic: Cunliffe & Gacono, 2008; Smith, Gacono, Cunliffe, Kivisto, & Taylor, 2014), salient gender dissimilarities exist related to prevalence, phenotypic trait expression, and types of aggression (Dolan & Völlm, 2009; Verona & Vitale, 2006). Despite disagreements on how best to assess psychopathy in women and discern these gender-related differences (see Nicholls, Odgers, & Cooke, 2007), the Psychopathy Checklist—Revised (PCL-R; Hare, 2003) also shows good reliability and validity when applied to females (Beryl, Chou, & Völlm, 2014) and seems to be the instrument of choice.

A review of PCL-R-based studies on females is beyond the scope of this chapter and is thus only briefly touched upon here. The key takeaways from two fairly recent PCL-R reviews focusing on the forensic population (Beryl et al., 2014; Verona & Vitale, 2006) indicate a slightly lower prevalence of psychopathy among incarcerated females than for males when applying the standard cut-off criteria for "diagnosing" psychopathy (PCL-R $\geq$ 30). Evidence further suggests that although psychopathic females are less likely than psychopathic males to have had early behavior problems, they exhibit similar degrees of instrumental and manipulative behavior, lying, callousness, and criminal activity, but engage in sexual misbehavior such as prostitution more often (Verona & Vitale, 2006).

Differences in the manifestation of the core symptoms—the interpersonal and affective features of psychopathy—are also noteworthy. Compared to the overtly narcissistic, grandiose, and detached display of psychopathic males, female psychopaths often present with a coy, coquettish outlook, and are more prone to show emotion and pseudo-emotion. Psychopathic males and females also display disparate relational dominance patterns. Whereas the males often use threat and overt violence to obtain their goals, the females are more successful with sexual manipulation of men or displays of faux empathy and victim status designed to lure or charm unsuspecting and naïve victims (Beryl et al., 2014; Cunliffe & Gacono, 2008; Smith et al., 2014).

Although female psychopaths are less physically violent than their male counterparts, they evince more relational and covert aggression than antisocial females without psychopathy (Beryl et al., 2014; Gacono & Meloy, 1994). A typical scenario for female psychopaths would be to persuade an aggression-prone male ally to accomplish her criminal goals and to offend against those in her social milieu (intimates, children, and associates).

The psychodynamics of the female psychopath represents a further understudied area. Two Rorschach studies (Cunliffe & Gacono, 2008; Smith et al., 2014) have reported Comprehensive System (CS; Exner, 2003) descriptive data for psychopathic females. Because most of the CS variables reported in these studies are included in the Rorschach Performance Assessment System (R-PAS; Meyer, Viglione, Mihura, Erard & Erdberg, 2011), we use R-PAS instead of CS names for ease of comparing the results to the psychopathic female described in this chapter. Compared to the CS international norms (Meyer, Erdberg, & Shaffer, 2007), psychopathic antisocial females had a more negative self-image (Morbid; Vista), displayed less perspective taking (FD), and revealed significantly more thought disturbance (WSumCog; SevCog). In comparison, for the nonpsychopathic antisocial females, there were no statistically significant CS differences on these variables when compared to the CS international norms.

Compared to the aggressive narcissism noted in male psychopaths (Gacono & Meloy, 1994), Cunliffe and Gacono (2008) propose that the elevated interpersonal markers in female psychopaths' records constitute a malignant form of hysteria, reflecting a need to be the center of attention, while getting thrills out of manipulating those around them to hurt each other. Although the Cunliffe and Gacono Rorschach data on female psychopaths provides a valuable reference point for our clinical case study, their findings may not translate directly since our case is European, and comparative research on psychopathy has documented important cultural variations across the Atlantic (see Sullivan & Kosson, 2006). This is, as far as we know, the first Rorschach-based psychopathy case study of a European female.

## Case Description and History

"Toni" is a female in her late 40s serving a sentence for fraud and drug possession. After the trial, awaiting her incarceration, Toni had sought out a psychiatrist in private practice. Their meetings culminated in a medical letter to the prison officials in which the psychiatrist expressed concerns about Toni's mental health, recommending that she was unfit to serve time. The prison officials declined this recommendation, and Toni was imprisoned. A copy of the letter was sent to the prison's medical doctor, who then referred her to the prison psychiatric services for further evaluation. The referral was mostly based on the medical letter written by the psychiatrist, raising questions concerning a deteriorating mental health condition possibly related to early signs of dementia, a psychotic state, and/or trauma intrusions.

I (P. N.) was assigned to her case. A review of Toni's medical records revealed that a few years back, she had been evaluated for attention-deficit/hyperactivity disorder (ADHD). The assessment suggested that there was little evidence of ADHD, and at that time her mental status examination showed no signs of serious mental illness (psychosis), depression, or anxiety. Toni's criminal record pointed to an ingrained criminal lifestyle evinced by numerous previous offenses, including threats, violence, fraud, theft, drug possession and trafficking, and money laundering. She had also been involved in criminal debt collection and as a pimp managing underage girls. The psychologist who had conducted the ADHD assessment portrayed Toni as a tough, fairly successful, and unscrupulous gangster with no deep emotional ties or commitments. The psychologist also highlighted Toni's careless attitude toward her victims, expressing little hesitation toward breaking kneecaps if an indebted person did not pay his or her dues. In the prison, she was known for her cunningness, often placing other female prisoners in difficulties with fellow inmates or wardens. Toni was apparently also quite adept at gathering personal information about others, stating that "You know if someone has something on you, I'll be sure to have more on them." The overall character evaluation suggested a severe antisocial personality disorder

(ASPD) with paranoid and narcissistic features. The PCL-R assessment placed her in the higher range of psychopathy (PCL-R ≥ 30; Hare, 2003).

Toni's developmental history was difficult to establish. The available information indicated that she, like many other psychopathic women (Forouzan & Nicholls, 2015; Verona & Vitale, 2006), had been exposed to early and severe trauma and neglect. From what could be gathered, it appeared that her father had died early and her mother had remarried. Toni's stepfather was apparently a very paranoid individual who subjected Toni and her siblings to physical and sexual abuse (oral, then vaginal) over the course of several years. The abuse culminated in an intervention from social services with foster placement of Toni when she was about 10. The foster placement went well for a few years. Toni showed progress in school, albeit with some conduct problems. At 15 years of age, however, she was thrown out of her home due to escalating conflicts with her foster parents. She dropped out of school and started working in nightclubs while staying with different acquaintances. Turning 18, Toni moved to an Asian country. Here she became involved in the management of child prostitutes for some years before moving back to Norway. Her involvement in drug trafficking resulted in a 10-year stay at a correctional center. After her release, she was able to start a small import business despite her lack of formal education. Toni's work history has been interrupted by several shorter prison sentences and numerous brief periods of jail detention, often related to her business. She has had many short-term intimate relationships, mostly with men who had criminal records.

## Clinical Assessment

Toni's evaluation was conducted in the prison. She presented as a physically strong, tough, and engaging woman, wearing sports gear and a thick gold chain around her neck. She spoke effortlessly with rapid and fluctuating associations, which made it quite challenging to conduct a proper clinical assessment of her. During the first sessions she would typically start off by addressing the assessor's question, then swiftly wander off onto other topics with logic that was hard to follow—for example, complaining about being placed in a more secluded prion unit due to her alleged involvement in the drugging of a fellow prisoner, and providing a long-winded rationalization about her innocence. In the next turn she would suddenly engage the assessor with her own inquiries, asking about his other patients and his marital status, while making flirtatious and flattering comments. These professional boundary-testing behaviors were accompanied by her intense eye contact.

Initial interviews thus left a vague clinical impression. Her most overt difficulties seemed related to memory problems, particularly how often she forgot that she was heating food on the stove. She also complained about a constant tiredness and recurrent nightmares involving the physical and sexual abuse to which her stepfather had subjected her. The abuse was presented in different manners. The first time she spoke about it she appeared rather indifferent. In the next session, however, she started to cry. The assessor felt unmoved, understanding her display more as an appeal than reflecting true sadness and despair.

After these initial challenges, Toni became slightly more cooperative. She agreed to testing, though with an unconcealed curiosity as to whether positive test results for dementia or psychosis could get her released from prison. Asked why she had sought out a psychiatrist prior to her imprisonment, she explained that she had been harassed by the police for several years due to her status as top-priority criminal. After several unsuccessful conviction attempts, the police got Toni for drug possession. Toni knew about the drugs but denied involvement, claiming that the police had framed her. Desperation led her to seek out the psychiatrist for a statement that she was unfit to serve due to her mental condition.

## Assessment Methods

Cognitive testing indicated that Toni's measured intelligence was somewhat unevenly developed and below average. Her Wechsler Adult Intelligence Scale—Fourth Edition (WAIS-IV) showed a Full Scale IQ of 86, a Verbal IQ of 73, a Perceptual Reasoning IQ of 88, a Working Memory IQ of 88, and a Processing Speed IQ of 112. Toni's poor verbal concept formation may partly reflect her low formal education and long stays abroad, evinced via her notable difficulties with common proverbs and abstract thinking. Her short-term memory capacity, though below average, was not suggestive of significant difficulties. In contrast to her lower scores on composites of verbal expression and abstract thinking, nonverbal problem solving, and working memory, Toni demonstrated above-average visual–motor speed and fluency. The marked contrast between her borderline verbal abilities, on the one hand, and her high-average processing speed, on the other hand, suggests that she is an action-prone woman who is quick to execute behavioral responses that do not require previous knowledge or conceptual thought.

The Millon Clinical Multiaxial Inventory–III (MCMI-III), results showed elevations on Narcissistic and Paranoid Personality Disorder, and Anxiety and Delusional Disorder scales. During the Positive and Negative Syndrome Scale (PANSS) interview, Toni denied key positive and negative symptoms of psychosis. However, she reported both a sense that others were plotting against her and that she had an ability to foresee others' actions. Regarding both statements, Toni's ideas of reference and prescience must be considered in the context of a prison setting, where beliefs that others might be plotting revenge and heightened vigilance and anticipation of others' action may be neither unusual nor unrealistic. Ultimately, her statements regarding psychotic-sounding beliefs were considered to be characterologically based features, which fell below the threshold of psychosis.

The overall purpose of this evaluation was to discern whether Toni was suffering from a severe psychological condition, potentially related to psychosis, trauma intrusions, or dementia. Based on magnetic resonance imaging (MRI), initial clinical impressions, and information from prison coworkers, there was little indication of an acute psychotic state or severe mental deterioration (e.g., dementia). On the other hand, her serious distrust of official agencies and ideas about how they had conspired against her bordered on delusional paranoid thinking. Regardless of contextual issues, Toni remained convinced that her fellow inmates were plotting against her. Indeed, her second most elevated MCMI-III scale was Delusional Disorder. However, Toni's vague clinical presentation, history of deception, and expressed curiosity as to whether the evaluation could be used in her quest for a release from prison highlighted the need for a less transparent measurement of her psychological functioning.

## Why R-PAS for Toni's Assessment?

There were several reasons for selecting R-PAS as a supplementary instrument for Toni's evaluation. Compared to self-report instruments, the Rorschach method (Rorschach, 1921/1942) has been shown to be sensitive to less overt disturbances that may be hard to detect via interview and self-report methods (Meyer & Viglione, 2008; Mihura, 2012). More specifically, we used the Rorschach to help us address questions pertaining to Toni's reality testing, disturbed thought processes, and intrusive trauma content, keeping in mind her possible inclination toward malingering. Although the Rorschach can be faked, like any other psychological measure (Ganellen, 1996), it has a particular asset in that it contains dissimilar methods for evaluating malingering (Critical Contents) and the presence of psychosis (TP-Comp). In cases such as this, the greater independence of malingering and psychosis markers on the Rorschach relative to other self-report instruments should yield gains (Mihura, 2012; Mihura, Meyer, Dumitrascu, & Bombel, 2013). Finally, we were also curious to explore how Toni's protocol would compare to other female psychopaths' Rorschachs (Cunliffe & Gacono, 2008).

## The R-PAS Administration

### Behaviors and Engagement in the Task

Toni had never heard of the test. She became skeptical when she was told that the test contained different inkblots that would be presented to her. After being reassured that the test was part of the evaluation to better understand her presenting problems, she seemed less hesitant and had no further inquiries. The administration took 55 minutes.

### Pre-Interpretation Administration and Coding Considerations

Toni's record shows two places where coding could have benefited from additional clarification (see responses 9 and 11 [R9 & R11]). In each instance, the uncertain codes are Diffuse Shading, Achromatic Color, or Vista. Thus, with additional clarification, these scores as well as Complexity, Blends, YTVC', and PPD may have been a bit higher, and F% and MC–PPD a bit lower.

### Interpretation of Toni's R-PAS Results[1]

*Test Validity*

Before addressing Toni's R-PAS results, we need to consider the possibility that she attempted to malinger severe symptoms, given that she had revealed an interest in whether the test results could get her out of prison. Malingering psychopathology on the Rorschach is associated with a low number of responses, elevated dramatic

---

[1] See Appendix 12.1 at the end of the chapter for Toni's R-PAS Responses, Location Sheet, Code Sequence, and Page 1 and 2 Profiles.

content (assessed in R-PAS by Critical Contents), or via behavioral observations of the test taker's overdone emotional reactions "triggered" by the inkblot (Ganellen, 1996). None of these features seem particularly evident in the protocol. Toni's response production (R) and Critical Contents were in the average range (SSs[2] = 105 and 97), suggesting that overdramatization is most likely not the cause of the elevated psychopathology markers in her protocol. Although her remarks and expressions may have been manufactured, or could be viewed as a way of challenging the assessor, most of these reactions aligned with the content of her percepts. Thus, we understood these as genuine expressions of her discomfort, confusion, and suspicion.

### Administration Behaviors and Engagement in the Task

Toni's record yielded 25 responses, which is within the average range (R SS = 105). Note, however, that both Pr (SS = 119) and, in particular, Pu (SS = 131) were elevated. On more than half of the Rorschach cards, Toni had to be reminded of the instruction "Try to give two responses . . . or maybe three to each card" three times because of overproduction on Cards I, VII, and X and three times due to underproduction on Cards III, IV, and V. This is highly unusual but might reflect the weakness noted in her working memory due to difficulty holding the instructions in mind or to her general disregard of externally imposed boundaries.

Toni collaborated well on the first two cards, both in the Response and Clarification phases. However, during the Clarification Phase on Card II, she broke set after describing her response, "A snake with an open mouth." Abruptly she asked the assessor, "Why are you showing me these pictures?" To the subsequent two cards (III and IV), Toni gave only one spontaneous response and no second one, despite prompting. Furthermore, her only response to Card III (R8) had two Cognitive Codes (INC1 and FAB2), along with threatening imagery (AGC). Perhaps in response to this disturbing image and ideation, on the following response (Card IV R9), Toni seemed to become suddenly derailed, as she loosely inquired of the examiner, "Are you a psychologist or a psychiatrist?" The assessor considered halting the administration for fear that Toni had lost her grounding in the Rorschach task, but decided to continue after a brief check-in with her.

Though we cannot rule out that her erratic response style could reflect a malingering strategy, with Toni trying to appear less organized than she is, we understood these characteristics more in terms of her distractibility, working memory difficulties, and the disruptive effect of the disturbing images on her ability to think clearly. Similarly, her digressive question about the examiner's profession occurred in the context of R-PAS codes indicating bizarre, illogical combination of ideas (FAB2s) and dark (C's) and disturbing (AGC) imagery, as well as some rigidity or inflexible thinking (three Prompts in a row), perhaps suggesting that she was trying to keep it together by getting away from the images, as she finally was able to do on Card V.

Toni's average Complexity score (SS = 105) suggests that she was engaged and effortful during the task. Thus there was no need to complexity-adjust the results. Her scores on F% (SS = 99), Blends (SS = 102), and Sy (SS = 106) were also within average range. These findings are noteworthy and somewhat higher than we would

---

[2]Standard scores (SS) have a mean of 100 and an SD of 15.

expect, given her low-average WAIS score (Total IQ score = 86). Yet, Toni's ability to manipulate others in her environment while juggling several different schemes suggests that her R-PAS results may be more illustrative of her cognitive capacity than her IQ score, as it is not based on learned knowledge. In other words, given her very modest WAIS-IV findings, we were quite surprised to see indications of cognitive richness and complexity on her Rorschach.

## Coping

Although Toni's coping resources appear within the normal range (MC SS = 97), she might not have the coping capacity to manage the difficulties with which she is faced (MC–PPD SS = 85). Moreover, she has a scarcity of psychological resources to deal with distracting or discomforting experiences, especially those that involve upsetting or pressing needs or worries (MC–PPD again). Expressing such difficult affective states might also be an issue for her [(CF + C)/SumC could not be computed due to too few responses, though it is worth noting that both color responses were non-form-dominant]. Thus, she is more likely than others to be more influenced by situational stressors, leading to emotional upset, disruption of concentration, or impulsive behavior, all of which make her unstable. The results also denoted an equal affinity to be guided by both thinking and feelings (M/MC SS = 110). For mentally healthy people, this dual processing possibility may be an advantage. In the presence of psychopathology, however, there may be ambivalence and confusion about how to react, which may result in indecisive actions. This latter point converges with reports from prison officers highlighting Toni's inability to complete many of the projects she initiates on the ward.

## Perception and Cognition

A key assessment concern relates to whether Toni is psychotic or not. Although the interview data did not reveal psychotic symptomatology, and the reports of her from the ward suggested erratic and manipulative behavior as opposed to psychosis (bizarre and odd thinking and behavior), covert psychotic phenomena may be hard to detect via self-report and observation (Mihura, 2012). In reviewing Toni's Rorschach, the most striking feature of her protocol was the abundance of deviant scores on many of the codes in this domain (EII-3 SS = 121; WSumCog SS = 136; SevCog SS = 131; TP-Comp SS = 124; FQu% SS = 119; WD–% SS = 115; FQ–% SS = 112; and FQo% SS = 78). Toni's Ego Impairment Index (EII-3), a broadband measure of thinking disturbance and severity in psychopathology, was significantly elevated largely due to measures of disturbed and disordered thought (WSumCog), severe disruptions in thought processes (SevCog), and somewhat labile reality testing (FQ–). These findings are consistent with research that finds more thought disturbance and reality testing lapses in ASPD females with psychopathy than without psychopathy (Cunliffe & Gacono, 2008).

However, it is important to look more carefully at Toni's comments and Cognitive scores. Regarding her spontaneous comments while taking the Rorschach, Toni indicated during the Clarification on Card II that the inkblots were "not real pictures." Although she described them as "ugly," her comment about them not being real showed that she maintained an awareness of the "as if," interpretive nature of the task. Furthermore, with regard to the scores themselves, five of her nine Cognitive Codes were Level 1 INCs (e.g., "arms" on a wasp, R1). This and other benign INC1s are more indicative of Toni's low semantic knowledge and education than of deviant thinking. Additionally, a closer examination of two of her FAB responses, while meriting Level 2 scoring, thus reflecting boundary disturbance, were not all that peculiar, odd, or incomprehensible. For example, her FAB2 responses on R8 and R9 reflected a breech in boundaries, in which one animal was "sticking" or "sprouting" out of another. Two later responses (R11 and R21, another FAB2) repeated this theme of animals (in this case, snakes) "creeping" or "swimming out" of some amorphous mass. Each of these fabulized combinations involved boundary disruptions, symbolically reflecting merger–separation themes. Additionally, in each case, the implied separation was associated with negative, highly charged, and less modulated affect (C', CF, Fire, AGC). Such themes and Cognitive codes (FABs) are often associated with a borderline personality organization. Additionally, three of Toni's responses combined ODL and either AGC or AGM Thematic Codes (R8 "Snake with an open mouth," R9 "Animal is spitting out something," and R13 "Face screaming"), suggesting intense oral aggression. Again, thematically, "neediness made angry" suggests a borderline structural level.

Yet, a closer examination of her final FAB2 (R21) reveals a more pervasive boundary issue. Here, she gave two responses to the same areas of the inkblot. First, she saw animals standing on rocks and then mentioned an eye from another animal. The problem was that she was seeing the second animal (which she elaborated as a "snake swimming out from some green sediment") in the space occupied by the first animals, thus approaching a Contamination. This slippery response condensed two images into a single blot area. Toni provided little clarification or evinced little concern at her perceptual slippage. At best, this response suggests that, when she encounters intense affect, she perceives in an uncritical, careless manner, accepting contradictions and incompatibilities in how she is registering information. At worst, it may reflect a paranoid psychotic shift in her experience of the world. In either case, it seemed associated with affective complexity.

Thus, whereas her protocol shows more indicators of a borderline than a psychotic structure, she is prone to regressive thinking and may exhibit occasional magical ideation and ideas of reference. By and large, when left to structure and interpret her experience on her own, Toni conceives in an unusual and idiosyncratic manner (FQu% SS = 119), and may be susceptible to some misperceptions of her surroundings (FQ–% SS = 112). Nonetheless, she is as capable as others to pick up on the obvious and conventional cues of her surroundings (P SS = 96).

The elevated Cognitive codes also raise the question as to whether Toni's effortful processing might be a problem for her. Three of her Sy responses were assigned with a FAB code (R8, R9, and R21), suggesting that Toni's combinatory thinking is partly fused by unrealistic and threatening ideas. However, in each of these responses, the Form Quality was unusual, so there was no distortion of external reality per se.

Regarding the question of trauma, Toni's average CritCont% (SS = 97) does not indicate that traumatic experiences are of significant concern. Still, false negative scores often occur as trauma-related contents are frequently personalized in a manner that may not be caught by the more global Critical Content variables (Meyer et al.,

2011). Although we lack confirmative information on Toni's alleged childhood physical and sexual abuse, her acuity for identifying snakes on the Rorschach is conspicuous with a total of four snake percepts. Though Toni's Rorschach preoccupation with snakes likely reflects different aspects of her personality makeup, the likelihood that these identifications relate to her developmental history is difficult to refute. Three of the responses are unusually perceived and accompanied by disgust-signaling remarks and cognitive codes. Her fabulized response to Card IV (R9) of a spitting animal with snakes sprouting out and with a "black thing coming out of the bushes (its body)" culminated in an apparent loss of reality testing and highlights her confused immersion in frightening fantasy with underlying sexual connotations. Note also that this response is like R21 in that "the bushes" appear to be D7, which is the animal—much like the "green sediment" was also the animal in R21. Thus, the sheer frequency of these responses, their manner of presentation, and the salient symbolic nature of the snake as a possible distorted representation of the phallus, all align with her account of abuse. Her story is, as mentioned, also consistent with the developmental experiences of other psychopathic women (Forouzan & Nicholls, 2015).

## Stress and Distress

Although Toni's seeming absence of implicit stress and distress (m SS = 84; Y SS = 85; MOR SS = 100; SC-Comp SS = 91; CBlend; SS = 91; V SS = 92; CritCont% SS = 97; C' SS = 111; PPD SS = 112) is congruent with her rather detached, unworried clinical appearance, we would have expected some elevations in this section, given her complaints about recurrent and troubling nightmares involving her physical and sexual abuse. There may be several alternate explanations for this discrepancy. Although she may have fabricated or exaggerated the symptoms, their absence could be caused in part by clarification lapses. As noted earlier, additional questioning (R9 and R11) may have resulted in a more elevated C' and PPD. However, the queries for Y or V on R11 did not reveal a determinant. Thus, a more plausible explanation is that Toni did not have the capacity to recognize and articulate the subtle and nuanced nature of the pain and stress associated with her threatening and trauma-related imagery and ideas. This notion is consistent with the content of her responses, her low use of color determinants, her interactions with the assessor, and the manner of her complaints.

## Self and Other

Toni's interpersonal markers that suggest a needy and dependent, yet interpersonally attuned and cooperatively inclined individual (COP SS = 111; ODL% SS = 124; H SS = 98; PHR/GPHR SS = 105; MAH SS = 105), were unexpected given her shallow, deceptive, and unlawful presentation. However, the overall data in our case support the picture of female psychopaths painted by Cunliffe and Gacono (2008), in which there is a need for others, not for close relationships, but in order to be the center of attention and to exert interpersonal manipulative prowess. Information from prison coworkers indicated that Toni is always at the center of happenings. She is often entangled with fellow prisoners or wardens, and seems to find amusement in her ability to get co-felons in trouble. Now, this wicked knack likely requires some mentalizing skill, or at least an attunement to the interpersonal cues in her surroundings, perhaps reflected in her average and slightly elevated relational scores (COP, H, PHR/GPHR, MAH, and no M–).

Reviewing her protocol for indices that may elucidate the wicked element of Toni's character guides us to her significantly elevated AGC (SS = 136) and her many snake percepts, which we viewed as conveying idiosyncratic themes or symbols related to her past history with threat and danger. Assuming that these responses are indeed tied to her history of abuse, they would signal a strong identification with the aggressor, likely developed to master her painful, boundary-breaching experiences with abuse and her extreme interpersonal vulnerability. Consistent with this idea, Toni did not produce responses like many of Cunliffe and Gacono's (2008) psychopathic females, which indicated that they implicitly perceived themselves as damaged and flawed (MOR, V).

## Discussion

Toni's most explicit concerns were her difficulties with forgetting and feeling tired most of the time. The overall integration of Toni's R-PAS results with her history suggests that covert trauma intrusions coupled with interpersonal mistrust and boundary issues lay at the heart of her current problems, and that the amount of effort she is putting into holding troubling thoughts at bay is also tiring her out. Her dependency needs and interest in others (ODL%, H, COP) are in direct opposition to her emotional detachment (PCL-R), with the possibility of "snakes" or adversaries in every corner. Whereas the previous psychological report suggests that she probably mastered these conflicting themes better at earlier stages in her life, we proposed that the cumulative effect of age, an emotionally restrained character, lifestyle, and recent prolonged experiences with persecution from the police have led to a partial breakdown in her defensive armor. The pervasive repression of painful affective experience (low color and elevated C') and associated memories may, in itself, impair reality testing as much as other types of perceptual abnormality (McGauley et al., 2007). In this case, the R-PAS results suggest that these subtly pressing memories of torment may have affected her reality testing further, resulting in greater boundary disturbance and confusion, with further misperceptions of what is within and outside.

The manifestation of Toni's intrusive content merits some elaboration. Based on her presentation and inconspicuous CritCont% (SS = 97), we understood these symptoms more as muted fragmentations than as the elaborated, hyperactivating recollections seen in patients with posttraumatic stress disorder (PTSD). Although causing significant distress, Toni's reminiscences appeared more as forgotten relics from a distant past, affectively disconnected from her nonanxious character. We do, however, think that these images occasionally intruded in her present, disrupting her thinking and reality testing via dissociative fallouts, making her tired, forgetful, and suspicious.

## Impact of R-PAS Experience on Toni and Her Case

Toni returned for feedback on the results after the formal testing. She found the R-PAS experience very odd, yet expressed some curiosity about its purpose and about how these "pictures" could yield information about her problems. When told that the R-PAS results implied that her difficulties with memory and tiredness might be related to her past trauma becoming more prominent in her experience, tears appeared underneath her sunglass-covered eyes. Quietly she asked if there was any medication that could be of help. This time the assessor felt moved by her display, which perhaps reflected her intense dependency (ODL) and need for help at this point. The assessor explained that long-term psychotherapy could perhaps assist her somewhat with coping and containment, though this would require considerable effort on her own part. She was also offered a low dose of antipsychotic medication. Toni reappeared for a few more sessions. During these the assessor experienced her as slightly more attentive to his ideas. Attempts to make her connect somewhat with her feeling states, however, were unsuccessful, with Toni complaining about the polluted air in the therapy room. She was not willing to try out antipsychotic medications and also quite rejecting of the idea of changing her criminal lifestyle. Because Toni was soon to be released from prison and did not seem interested in further therapeutic work with her difficulties, the assessor ended the treatment. The assessor recommended that she should contact her medical doctor for a new referral to psychotherapy if her problems increased.

## Conclusion

This case study highlights the usefulness of R-PAS for picking up on the underlying dynamics and more covert disturbances of challenging patients. Before commencing with testing, we were worried that the validity of the protocol could be compromised by an insufficient number of responses. The R-Optimized R-PAS administration procedure not only ensured a sufficient number of responses, it provided a display for her erratic style, which would likely not have been so evident via other Rorschach administration procedures or tests. The solid empirical foundation of the R-PAS variables provided us with increased confidence in our interpretations. The most striking feature of Toni's protocol was the highly elevated markers of disturbed thought processes. Although these were also indicated by her MCMI, the R-PAS perceptual and cognitive scores gave us a much richer framework for assessing potential malingering and discerning her level of thought disturbance and her capacity for reality testing. R-PAS also helped elucidate the nature of her psychopathic disturbance, pointing, as well, to possible treatment implications.

## REFERENCES

Beryl, R., Chou, S., & Völlm, B. (2014). A systematic review of psychopathy in women within secure settings. *Personality and Individual Differences, 71*, 185–195.

Cunliffe, T. B., & Gacono, C. B. (2008). A Rorschach understanding of antisocial and psychopathic women. In C. B. Gacono, F. B. Evans, N. Kaser-Boyd, & L. A. Gacono (Eds.), *The handbook of forensic Rorschach assessment* (pp. 361–378). New York: Routledge.

Dolan, M., & Völlm, B. (2009). Antisocial personality disorder and psychopathy in women: A literature review on the reliability and validity of assessment instruments. *International Journal of Law and Psychiatry, 32*, 2–9.

Exner, J. E., Jr. (2003). *The Rorschach: A comprehensive system: Vol. 1. Basic foundations and principles of interpretation* (4th ed.). New York: Wiley.

Forouzan, E., & Nicholls, T. L. (2015). Childhood and adolescent characteristics of women with high versus low psychopathy scores: Examining developmental precursors to the malignant personality disorder. *Journal of Criminal Justice, 43*, 307–320.

Gacono, C. B., & Meloy, J. R. (1994). *The Rorschach assessment of aggressive and psychopathic personalities*. Hillsdale, NJ: Erlbaum.

Gacono, C. B., & Meloy, J. R. (2009). Assessing antisocial and psychopathic personalities. In J. N. Butcher (Ed.), *Oxford handbook of personality assessment* (pp. 567–581). New York: Oxford University Press.

Ganellen, R. J. (1996). Comparing the diagnostic efficiency of the MMPI, MCMI-II, and Rorschach: A review. *Journal of Personality Assessment, 67*, 219–243.

Hare, R. D. (2003). *Manual for the Hare Psychopathy Checklist—Revised* (2nd ed.). Toronto, ON: Multi-Health Systems.

McGauley, G., Adshead, G., & Sarkar, S. P. (2007). Psychotherapy of psychopathic disorders. In A. R. Felthous & H. Sass (Eds.), *International handbook of psychopathic disorders and the law: Vol. 1* (pp. 449–466). Chichester, UK: Wiley.

Meyer, G. J., Erdberg, P., & Shaffer, T. W. (2007). Towards international normative reference data for the Comprehensive System. *Journal of Personality Assessment, 89*(S1), S201–S216.

Meyer, G. J., & Viglione, D. J. (2008). An introduction to Rorschach assessment. In R. P. Archer & S. R. Smith (Eds.), *Personality assessment* (pp. 281–336). New York: Routledge.

Meyer, G. J., Viglione, D. J., Mihura, J., Erard, R. E., & Erdberg, P. (2011). *Rorschach Performance Assessment System: Administration, coding, interpretation, and technical manual*. Toledo, OH: Rorschach Performance Assessment System.

Mihura, J. L. (2012). The necessity of multiple test methods in conducting assessments: The role of the Rorschach and self-report. *Psychological Injury and Law, 5*, 97–106.

Mihura, J. L., Meyer, G. J., Dumitrascu, N., & Bombel, G. (2013). The validity of individual Rorschach variables: Systematic reviews and meta-analyses of the Comprehensive System. *Psychological Bulletin, 139*, 548–605.

Nicholls, T. L., Odgers, C. L., & Cooke, D. J. (2007). Women and girls with psychopathic characteristics. In A. R. Felthous & H. Sass (Eds.), *International handbook on psychopathic disorders and the law* (pp. 347–366). New York: Wiley.

Patrick, C. J. (Ed.). (2006). *Handbook of psychopathy*. New York: Guilford Press.

Rorschach, H. (1942). *Psychodiagnostics*. New York: Grune & Stratton. (Original work published 1921)

Smith, J. M., Gacono, C. B., Cunliffe, T. B., Kivisto, A. J., & Taylor, E. E. (2014). Psychodynamics in the female psychopath: A PCL-R/Rorschach investigation. *Violence and Gender, 1*, 176–187.

Sullivan, E. A., & Kosson, D. S. (2006). Ethnic and cultural variations in psychopathy. In C. J. Patrick (Ed.), *Handbook of psychopathy* (pp. 437–458). New York: Guilford Press.

Verona, E., & Vitale, J. (2006). Psychopathy in women: Assessment, manifestations, and etiology. In C. J. Patrick (Ed.), *Handbook of psychopathy* (pp. 415–436). New York: Guilford Press.

## Rorschach Responses "Toni"

| Respondent ID: Toni | Examiner: Peder Nørbech |
|---|---|
| Location: Prison | Date: **/**/**** |
| Start Time: 13:05 P.M. | End Time: 14:00 P.M. |

| Cd # | R # | Or | Response | Clarification | R-Opt |
|---|---|---|---|---|---|
| I | 1 | | The whole thing looks like a bug. (W) | E: (Examiner Repeats Response [ERR].) <br> R: Yes, a wasp. The body here (points to D4). They have this point at the back and mouth here (points, Dd22). Claws or arms here. (D1) | |
| | 2 | | Or bat. (W) | E: (ERR) <br> R: The whole thing. <br> E: What makes it look like a bat? <br> R: The wings. (D2) | |
| | 3 | | Hat here. Man, face, human there. Holding an animal. Humans on both sides. (W) | E: (ERR) <br> R: There you see the hat (upper portion of Dd28), face, and their outfit. Black outfit with wings (Dd34). They are holding the animal (points to D4). <br> E: What made it look like an animal? <br> R: Wings, mouth, and claws (D1), with a tail there (D3), the pointy thing. They're (the humans) wearing a ghost or angel outfit. | |
| | 4 | | R: Could be a Christmas tree on each side. (D2) <br> E: OK, thanks. Two, maybe three responses are sufficient. | E: (ERR) <br> R: Yes, here (respondent points to D2). <br> E: What made it look like a Christmas tree? <br> R: The shape of it. | Pu |
| II | 5 | | Two Santa Clauses (points). Hands, body. (W) | E: (ERR) <br> R: Yes. Sitting toward one another. Clapping their hands (D4) together. <br> E: What made it look like Santa? <br> R: Because of the Santa cap (D2) here (points to D2). Could also be two people that have dressed up in costumes. | |
| | 6 | | Heart here (points to D3). (D3) | E: (ERR) <br> R: Yes, here (points to D3). <br> E: What made it look like a heart? <br> R: The shape of it. | |
| | 7 | | Two animals hanging downward with their mouths open. (Dd99 = dark shapes in D3 outside Dd24 area) | E: (ERR) <br> R: Here (points). <br> E: What made it look like an animal? <br> R: Mouth here. A snake with an open mouth and long neck. Why are you showing me these pictures? | |
| III | 8 | | R: Two birds or humans holding onto something. Sick paintings. (D1) <br> E: OK. We would like two, maybe three responses to each card, so please try to give another one. <br> R: No, I can't see anything else. | E: (ERR) <br> R: Head (Dd32), beak, neck, chest, butt, body (Ddd22), with a pointed beak or claws. Claws on their feet (Dd33) as well. Holding their fingers over a fire. (D7) <br> E: What made it look like fire? <br> R: It's black. <br> E: Sick paintings? <br> R: Yes, they're not real pictures. They're ugly. And you see an animal head sticking out of their chest here (points to Dd27). | Pr |

239

| Cd # | R # | Or | Response | Clarification | R-Opt |
|------|-----|----|----------|---------------|-------|
| IV | 9 | | R: Big animal. Legs, head. Two snakes here. The animal is spitting out something. I can't stand looking at this picture. (W) (Hands the card to the examiner.)<br>E: Recall that we would like two, maybe three responses to each card; please look some more.<br>R: I don't see anything else. | E: (ERR)<br>R: Yes. The face (D3) is spitting out something (points below D3). Here you see the leg (D6) upward. Arms here. Pointed snake (D4) sticking out there (points to outer D4). They sprout out of the animal. Fits with the black thing (D1) coming out of the bushes (points to D1). Are you a psychologist or psychiatrist?<br>E: I'm a psychologist. Are you OK with this?<br>R: These are some weird pictures you are showing me. What is this test for?<br>E: We can talk more about these pictures when we are done with the test, OK?<br>R: OK.<br>E: Let's continue then. | Pr |
| V | 10 | | R: Bat. (W) (Hands the card back.)<br>E: Please look some more and try to see something else as well. Take your time.<br>R: It's a bat. I can't see anything else (looks at the card). | E: (ERR)<br>R: Yes, the whole thing.<br>E: What made it look like a bat?<br>R: Big wings (D4). | Pr |
| VI | 11 | | Serpent creeping out of mud. (W) | E: (ERR)<br>R: Yes. Something (D2) creeping out here (respondent points to D1). Creeping out the canal (D1) here. These are the tracks (D12) made by the snake.<br>E: What made it look like tracks?<br>R: You see here (points to D12).<br>E: OK. What about it made you think of tracks?<br>R: Snakes make such tracks. [E could have queried "mud" for C'.] | |
| | 12 | | A rug. I feel bad looking at it. (W) | E: (ERR)<br>R: Yes. The whole thing. One you would find lying on the floor.<br>E: What made it look like a rug?<br>R: Usually looks that way. The skin of a polar bear looks like that. [E could have queried "I feel bad looking at it" for MOR.] | |
| VII | 13 | @ | < v > ^ Face screaming. (D1) | E: (ERR)<br>R: Here. Eyes, nose, mouth screaming. Here's the head and the back of the head. Here is the neck. | |
| | 14 | | Face looking down. (D3) | E: (ERR)<br>R: Eye, nose, mouth, teeth, jaw, neck. | |
| | 15 | | Face looking up. (DdS23) | E: (ERR)<br>R: Yes. Animal, down here (points to Dd23). Looking up (turns card, >). Eye there (points), mouth (above Dd25), looking in that direction (points, toward D3). A spot here—the eye (points to light shading). | |
| | 16 | | R: Screwdriver. (Dd26)<br>E: OK, thanks. Two, maybe three responses are sufficient. | E: (ERR)<br>R: Yes, or small piece of wood.<br>E: What made it look like a screwdriver?<br>R: The shape of it. | Pu |
| VIII | 17 | | Animals there. Four legs. (D1) | E: (ERR)<br>R: (points to each D1) You see that, that's an animal. Both sides. Face, ears, and the body here. | |
| | 18 | | Fish (points). (Dd25). | E: (ERR)<br>R: Yes. The shape of a fish here (points to Dd25). | |
| | 19 | | Animal looking up there as well. (Dd99 = right half of D2). | E: (ERR)<br>R: Yes. It's looking upward. Eyes, mouth. The little spot there is a mouth. Maybe a dog or a bear. This part is the body. | |

| Cd # | R # | Or | Response | Clarification | R-Opt |
|---|---|---|---|---|---|
| IX | 20 | | Two animals with horns. Looking up. (D3) | E: (ERR) <br> R: Yes. You see it's very pointy above the front neck. Same on the other side (respondent falls asleep for 20 seconds, E wakes her). | |
| | 21 | | More animals. Standing on rocks. And an eye from an animal there. There's a post separating them. (Dd = 11, 6, 33, 5) | E: (ERR) <br> R: Yes. The whole green thing (D11) is the animals. The red beneath looks like rocks. (D6) <br> E: What made it look like rocks? <br> R: The shape of it. <br> E: You saw some eyes? <br> R: Here. Narrow eyes here (points to dark spot in Dd33), it looks like snake eyes. The snake (Dd33) is swimming out from some green sediment there. <br> E: A post? <br> R: The long one there (points to D5). | |
| X | 22 | | Animals butting their heads against a pole. (D11) | E: (ERR) <br> R: They're butting their heads against one another. [Animals = D8, pole = D14] | |
| | 23 | | Spider thing or animal with nose, arms, and eyes. (D1) | E: (ERR) <br> R: Yes a spider, or an animal in water. <br> E: What made it look like that? <br> R: It's got many legs. | |
| | 24 | | Animal with head, nose and mouth. Holding on to something. (D9s, D6) | E: (ERR) <br> R: Yes. Both sides. (D9s) They're looking toward one another. Deformed animals or humans. Face and head. | |
| | 25 | | R: Egg. (D13) <br> E: OK, thanks. Two, maybe three responses are sufficient. | E: (ERR) <br> R: The brown thing here. <br> E: What made it look like an egg? <br> R: Eggs may have brown shells as well. | Pu |

241

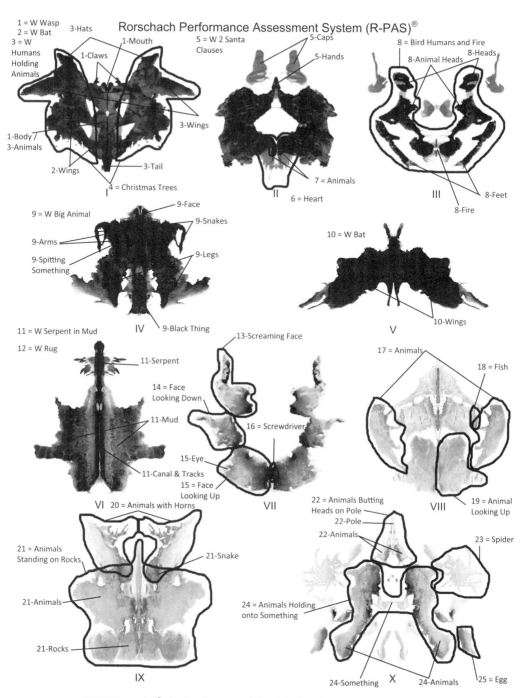

Rorschach Performance Assessment System (R-PAS)®

1 = W Wasp
2 = W Bat
3 = W Humans Holding Animals
3-Hats
1-Mouth
1-Claws
3-Wings
1-Body / 3-Animals
2-Wings
3-Tail
4 = Christmas Trees
I

5 = W 2 Santa Clauses
5-Caps
5-Hands
7 = Animals
6 = Heart
II

8 = Bird Humans and Fire
8-Animal Heads
8-Heads
8-Heads
8-Feet
8-Fire
III

9 = W Big Animal
9-Face
9-Snakes
9-Arms
9-Legs
9-Spitting Something
9-Black Thing
IV

10 = W Bat
10-Wings
V

11 = W Serpent in Mud
12 = W Rug
11-Serpent
11-Mud
11-Canal & Tracks
VI

13-Screaming Face
14 = Face Looking Down
16 = Screwdriver
15-Eye
15 = Face Looking Up
VII

17 = Animals
18 = FIsh
19 = Animal Looking Up
VIII

20 = Animals with Horns
21 = Animals Standing on Rocks
21-Snake
21-Animals
21-Rocks
IX

22 = Animals Butting Heads on Pole
22-Pole
22-Animals
23 = Spider
24 = Animals Holding onto Something
24-Something
24-Animals
25 = Egg
X

# R-PAS Code Sequence: "Toni"

**C-ID**: Toni    **P-ID**: 3    **Age**: 40s    **Gender**: Female    **Education**: NA

| Cd | # | Or | Loc | Loc # | SR | SI | Content | Sy | Vg | 2 | FQ | P | Determinants | Cognitive | Thematic | HR | ODL (RP) | R-Opt | Text |
|---|---|---|---|---|---|---|---|---|---|---|---|---|---|---|---|---|---|---|---|
| I | 1 | | W | | | | A | | | | - | | F | INC1 | AGC | | | | |
| | 2 | | W | | | | A | | | | o | P | F | | | | | | |
| | 3 | | W | | | | H,A,Cg | Sy | | 2 | u | | Ma,C' | INC1 | COP,AGC | GH | | | |
| | 4 | | D | 2 | | | NC | | | 2 | - | | F | | | | ODL | Pu | |
| II | 5 | | W | | | | H,Cg | Sy | | 2 | o | | Ma | | COP,MAH | GH | ODL | | |
| | 6 | | D | 3 | | | An | | | | o | | F | | | | | | |
| | 7 | | Dd | 99 | | | A | | | 2 | u | | FMp | | AGC | | ODL | | |
| III | 8 | | D | 1 | | | A,Ad,Fi,NC | Sy | | 2 | u | | FMp,C' | INC1,FAB2 | AGC | | | Pr | |
| IV | 9 | | W | | | | A,NC | Sy | | 2 | u | | FMa-p,C' | DR1,FAB2 | AGC | | ODL | Pr | |
| V | 10 | | W | | | | A | | | | o | P | F | | | | | Pr | |
| VI | 11 | | W | | | | A,NC | Sy | | | o | | FMa | | AGC | | | | * |

Comment: E could have queried 'mud' for C'.

| Cd | # | Or | Loc | Loc # | SR | SI | Content | Sy | Vg | 2 | FQ | P | Determinants | Cognitive | Thematic | HR | ODL (RP) | R-Opt | Text |
|---|---|---|---|---|---|---|---|---|---|---|---|---|---|---|---|---|---|---|---|
| | 12 | | W | | | | Ad | | | | o | P | F | | | | | | * |

Comment: E could have queried 'I feel bad looking at it' for MOR.

| Cd | # | Or | Loc | Loc # | SR | SI | Content | Sy | Vg | 2 | FQ | P | Determinants | Cognitive | Thematic | HR | ODL (RP) | R-Opt | Text |
|---|---|---|---|---|---|---|---|---|---|---|---|---|---|---|---|---|---|---|---|
| VII | 13 | @ | D | 1 | | | Hd | | | | o | P | Ma | | | GH | ODL | | |
| | 14 | | D | 3 | | | Hd | | | | o | | Mp | | | PH | | | |
| | 15 | | Dd | 23 | | | Ad | | | | u | | FMp | | | | | | |
| | 16 | | Dd | 26 | | | NC | | | | u | | F | | | | | Pu | |
| VIII | 17 | | D | 1 | | | A | | | 2 | o | P | F | | | | | | |
| | 18 | | Dd | 25 | | | A | | | | - | | F | | | | | | |
| | 19 | | Dd | 99 | | | A | | | | u | | FMp | | AGC | | | | |
| IX | 20 | | D | 3 | | | A | | | 2 | u | | FMp | | AGC | | | | |
| | 21 | | Dd | 5,6,11,33 | | | A,NC | Sy | | 2 | u | | FMa-p,CF | FAB2 | AGC | | | | |
| X | 22 | | D | 8,14 | | | A,NC | Sy | | 2 | o | | FMa | | AGM | PH | | | |
| | 23 | | D | 1 | | SI | A | | | | u | | F | INC1 | | | | | |
| | 24 | | D | 6,9 | | | A | Sy | | 2 | u | | FMp | | MOR | | ODL | | |
| | 25 | | D | 7 | | | NC | | | | - | | CF | INC1 | | | ODL | Pu | |

©2010-2016 R-PAS

# R-PAS Summary Scores and Profiles – Page 1

C-ID: Toni          P-ID: 3          Age: 40s          Gender: Female          Education:

| Domain/Variables | Raw Scores | Raw %ile | Raw SS | Cplx. Adj. %ile | Cplx. Adj. SS | Standard Score Profile R-Optimized | Abbr. |
|---|---|---|---|---|---|---|---|
| **Admin. Behaviors and Obs.** | | | | | | | |
| Pr | 3 | 90 | 119 | | | | Pr |
| Pu | 3 | 98 | 131 | | | | Pu |
| CT (Card Turning) | 1 | 38 | 95 | | | | CT |
| **Engagement and Cog. Processing** | | | | | | | |
| Complexity | 79 | 62 | 105 | | | | Cmplx |
| R (Responses) | 25 | 62 | 105 | 52 | 101 | | R |
| F% [Lambda=0.67] (Simplicity) | 40% | 48 | 99 | 50 | 100 | | F% |
| Blend | 4 | 56 | 102 | 44 | 98 | | Bln |
| Sy | 8 | 64 | 106 | 59 | 104 | | Sy |
| MC | 6.0 | 42 | 97 | 29 | 92 | | MC |
| MC - PPD | -7.0 | 15 | 85 | 16 | 85 | | MC-PPD |
| M | 4 | 58 | 103 | 43 | 97 | | M |
| M/MC [4/6.0] | 67% | 74 | 110 | 75 | 110 | | M Prp |
| (CF+C)/SumC [2/2] | NA | | | | | | CFC Prp |
| **Perception and Thinking Problems** | | | | | | | |
| EII-3 | 1.1 | 92 | 121 | 93 | 123 | | EII |
| TP-Comp (Thought & Percept. Com…) | 2.1 | 95 | 124 | 95 | 124 | | TP-C |
| WSumCog | 34 | 99 | 136 | 99 | 135 | | WCog |
| SevCog | 3 | 98 | 131 | 98 | 131 | | Sev |
| FQ-% | 16% | 79 | 112 | 81 | 113 | | FQ-% |
| WD-% | 16% | 85 | 115 | 83 | 114 | | WD-% |
| FQo% | 40% | 7 | 78 | 5 | 75 | | FQo% |
| P | 5 | 39 | 96 | 46 | 98 | | P |
| **Stress and Distress** | | | | | | | |
| YTVC' | 3 | 36 | 95 | 28 | 91 | | YTVC' |
| m | 0 | 14 | 84 | 14 | 84 | | m |
| Y | 0 | 17 | 85 | 17 | 85 | | Y |
| MOR | 1 | 51 | 100 | 46 | 98 | | MOR |
| SC-Comp (Suicide Concern Comp.) | 3.8 | 28 | 91 | 24 | 89 | | SC-C |
| **Self and Other Representation** | | | | | | | |
| ODL% | 28% | 94 | 124 | 94 | 123 | | ODL% |
| SR (Space Reversal) | 0 | 19 | 87 | 19 | 87 | | SR |
| MAP/MAHP [0/1] | NA | | | | | | MAP Prp |
| PHR/GPHR [2/5] | 40% | 62 | 105 | 62 | 105 | | PHR Prp |
| M- | 0 | 36 | 95 | 36 | 95 | | M- |
| AGC | 9 | 99 | 136 | 99 | 135 | | AGC |
| H | 2 | 45 | 98 | 32 | 92 | | H |
| COP | 2 | 78 | 111 | 78 | 111 | | COP |
| MAH | 1 | 64 | 105 | 40 | 95 | | MAH |

© 2010-2016 R-PAS

---

# R-PAS Summary Scores and Profiles – Page 2

C-ID: Toni    P-ID: 3    Age: 40s    Gender: Female    Education:

| Domain/Variables | Raw Scores | Raw %ile | Raw SS | Cplx. Adj. %ile | Cplx. Adj. SS | Standard Score Profile R-Optimized | Abbr. |
|---|---|---|---|---|---|---|---|
| **Engagement and Cog. Processing** | | | | | | 60 70 80 90 100 110 120 130 140 | |
| W% | 32% | 37 | 95 | 34 | 94 | | W% |
| Dd% | 24% | 79 | 112 | 80 | 113 | | Dd% |
| SI  (Space Integration) | 1 | 18 | 86 | 25 | 89 | | SI |
| IntCont | 0 | 11 | 81 | 11 | 81 | | IntC |
| Vg% | 0% | 18 | 86 | 18 | 86 | | Vg% |
| V | 0 | 29 | 92 | 29 | 92 | | V |
| FD | 0 | 21 | 88 | 26 | 90 | | FD |
| R8910% | 36% | 79 | 112 | 79 | 112 | | R8910% |
| WSumC | 2.0 | 31 | 92 | 22 | 88 | | WSC |
| C | 0 | 36 | 95 | 36 | 95 | | C |
| Mp/(Ma+Mp)          [1/4] | 25% | 23 | 89 | 23 | 89 | | Mp Prp |
| **Perception and Thinking Problems** | | | | | | 60 70 80 90 100 110 120 130 140 | |
| FQu% | 44% | 90 | 119 | 91 | 120 | | FQu% |
| **Stress and Distress** | | | | | | 60 70 80 90 100 110 120 130 140 | |
| PPD | 13 | 78 | 112 | 74 | 109 | | PPD |
| CBlend | 0 | 28 | 91 | 28 | 91 | | CBlnd |
| C' | 3 | 77 | 111 | 69 | 108 | | C' |
| V | 0 | 29 | 92 | 29 | 92 | | V |
| CritCont% (Critical Contents) | 16% | 43 | 97 | 42 | 97 | | CrCt |
| **Self and Other Representation** | | | | | | 60 70 80 90 100 110 120 130 140 | |
| SumH | 4 | 27 | 91 | 22 | 88 | | SumH |
| NPH/SumH            [2/4] | 50% | 31 | 92 | 29 | 91 | | NPH Prp |
| V-Comp (Vigilance Composite) | 2.3 | 24 | 90 | 20 | 87 | | V-C |
| r (Reflections) | 0 | 36 | 95 | 36 | 95 | | r |
| p/(a+p)             [9/16] | 56% | 76 | 110 | 74 | 110 | | p Prp |
| AGM | 1 | 75 | 110 | 75 | 110 | | AGM |
| T | 0 | 28 | 91 | 28 | 91 | | T |
| PER | 0 | 30 | 92 | 30 | 92 | | PER |
| An | 1 | 47 | 99 | 47 | 99 | | An |

© 2010-2016 R-PAS

# CHAPTER 13

# Using R-PAS in Family Law Cases
## *Child Custody Evaluations*

### S. Margaret Lee

One area of forensic assessment involves conducting child custody evaluations (CCEs). These evaluations are complex, necessitating assessment and understanding of both individual and family dynamics. Divorcing families requiring evaluation are those with the greatest conflict or most serious problems, as most parents are able to resolve their disputes through other mechanisms, such as mediation, attorney negotiation, or judicial hearings. Cases requiring evaluation involve parental behaviors that put the child's safety, well-being, or development at risk; these behaviors include problems such as substance abuse, mental illness, domestic violence, child abuse (physical, emotional, and/or sexual), enmeshed parent–child relationships, restrictive gate-keeping behaviors, alienation, poor parenting, and the allegation that one parent is generating the ongoing conflict (Gould & Martindale, 2007; Kuehnle & Drozd, 2012; Stahl, 2011).

Child custody disputes are "high-stakes" situations that affect control of the children's lives and the nature of the possible parent–child relationships. The evaluation process itself is high stakes, as judges tend to follow the evaluators' recommendations, largely because these evaluations are performed by neutral court-appointed experts who have gathered a broad range of data. The evaluator's role involves investigating for the court and explaining the results to the court. In many jurisdictions, evaluators are protected by court-based quasi-judicial immunity from malpractice suits. These factors place enormous pressure on the evaluator to "get it right."

Conducting CCEs is very challenging as enormous amounts of data are collected from multiple sources, and much of the data is of the "he said, she said" variety. Finding independent verification and corroborating data is vital as, without this information, the average psychologist is no better at assessing credibility than the average person on the street (Kassin, Meissner, & Norwick, 2005). The parents are assessed in conjoint and individual interviews and observations with their children in the evaluator's office and in their homes. These procedures allow an opportunity to behaviorally assess both the co-parenting relationship and the parent–child relationships. Children are also assessed through these observations and individual interviews. Independent data are primarily obtained through collateral informants (mostly professionals), document review (including the legal file, police reports, medical records, and child protective services [CPS] reports), and psychological assessment.

Nationally, child custody evaluators are aided by several guidelines. The American Psychological Association (APA) updated their Child Custody Evaluation Guidelines (APA, 2010) and the Association of Family and Conciliation Courts (AFCC) developed Model Standards for Conducting CCEs (AFCC, 2006). These guidelines are unenforceable in most of the United States (although frequently used in cross-examination); in California, however, there are Rules of Court (Rules of Court 5.220) that must be followed when conducting a CCE. All of these guidelines help the evaluator practice in an ethical manner that meets the standard of care.[1] The guidelines also stress the need for multiple methods of data gathering, establishing the scope of the evaluation, individually assessing each child, and focusing on the "best interest of the child" in making recommendations.

Challenges to evaluators center on the complexity of multiple, often dramatic, allegations; organizing and integrating data related to individuals, interpersonal dyads, and family dynamics; and the demands of the legal system—all while performing evaluations and writing reports that are helpful to families, facilitate settlement, and lead to effective interventions and child-centered parenting plans.

## Why R-PAS for This Custody Evaluation?

A formal psychological assessment can elucidate the interplay of individual and family dynamics, assess the parents' strengths and weaknesses and how these interact, and provide a measure of the child's development. Given the fact that self-report measures such as the Minnesota Multiphasic Personality Inventory—Second Edition (MMPI-2) and the Millon Clinical Multiaxial Inventory–III (MCMI-III) are often compromised by impression management, the performance-based assessment method of the Rorschach allows a unique opportunity to get underneath the defense system and illustrate one's personality dynamics, approach to problem solving, internalized object relationships, reality testing, cognitive functioning, and coping resources for a more complex analysis of a family. The Rorschach Performance Assessment System (R-PAS; Meyer, Viglione, Mihura, Erard, & Erdberg, 2011) administration and scoring system is currently being used in forensic evaluations and is being well received in the courts (Erard, 2012; Erard, Meyer, & Viglione, 2014).

## CCE Involving a 10-Year-Old Child

This case involves a family who was court-ordered to undergo a comprehensive CCE. My appointment was as the court's expert. I was informed that the parents had been

---

[1] Although not all states have Rules of Court regarding CCE, in my opinion, following California Rule of Court 5.220 would facilitate good practice.

separated for 4 years, yet the conflict continued despite the involvement of a co-parenting counselor, a parent coordinator (PC), and various therapists working with individual family members. At the time of referral, the parents had a shared parenting plan with equal parenting time of their only child, Ryan, age 10 years.

The referral from the court requested that the following areas of concern be investigated. The mother, "Julie," alleged that the father, "Peter," had engaged in domestic violence during the marriage and postseparation, was abusing illegal substances (primarily methamphetamines), had refused to follow orders made by the court and the PC, and had actively sabotaged her relationship with Ryan. Peter alleged that Julie was mentally ill, was violent toward him during the marriage and toward their son Ryan, and was attempting to severely curtail his time with Ryan. It was documented in police reports and by therapists that Ryan had been violent when in his mother's care; the police had been involved on numerous occasions and based on Julie's alleged violence, several reports to CPS had been made against Julie for physical abuse and negligence. Julie was requesting a domestic violence restraining order against Peter, as well as sole legal and sole physical custody. Peter was requesting joint legal and joint physical custody with the stipulation that if it were determined that there should be a primary parent with sole decision-making responsibilities, he should be that parent.

The evaluation commenced with a conjoint meeting with the parents to explain the evaluation process, to obtain a family and child history, and to observe the parents' communication, the consistency of their narratives, and their understandings of their child. Based on Peter's and Julie's report, their relationship was volatile from very early on, marked with yelling and poorly controlled emotional expression. Julie had difficulties with anxiety and a history of trauma. Peter was hedonistic, rebellious, anti-establishment, and engaged in significant substance use. Despite the volatility, it appears that their mutual insecurities led them to live together and Julie soon became pregnant. They decided to marry. After Ryan was born, Julie was somewhat depressed and continued to be volatile, whereas Peter withdrew. A cyclical dynamic emerged; Peter would withdraw, Julie would become anxious and upset, drawing him out, and then conflict would escalate between them. Each accused the other of becoming violent during the conflicts. Violence included Julie throwing objects such as her cellphone at Peter and scratching him. Peter would respond by restraining Julie. There were never serious injuries; however, both parents sustained bruises at times. Both parents acknowledged that Ryan had been exposed to their conflicts throughout his life. Despite what sounded like a chaotic home life, Ryan was described as doing well, adjusting to school, and developing as expected prior to his parents' separation.

After the separation and their agreement to co-parent with an equal timeshare, the volatility did not subside. Ryan often had difficulties at his mother's home, alleging that she hit and yelled at him. When this occurred, either Julie or Ryan called his father to help control the situation and intervene. At times this led to interparental conflict and alleged violence, culminating in police and CPS involvement. Peter became involved in more serious drug use, primarily methamphetamines. The court ordered interventions to help stabilize the family, including professionals assigned to monitor the family and help them make decisions, various therapeutic interventions, and drug treatments. However, the ordered services did not reduce the chaos or conflict.

Following the initial conjoint interview, a series of individual interviews were conducted to obtain personal histories from the parents, develop a more comprehensive understanding of their view of the problems, and to provide an opportunity for each parent to rebut the other parent's allegations. Detailed information was also collected regarding drug and alcohol use, alleged incidents of domestic violence, and detailed descriptions of the incidents when Ryan had alleged abusive behavior on the part of his mother.

Other data collection procedures included a full document review of police reports, CPS reports, PC reports and the court filings, and interviews with selected informants, mostly professionals involved with various family members. The parent–child relationships were assessed through questionnaires, parent interview data, observations of Ryan with each parent, and informant interviews. The final piece of the evaluation was formal assessment. Based on the results of the evaluation so far, I had formed a series of alternative hypotheses about alleged behaviors, possible dynamics in the family, and the underlying meaning of the parents' and child's behaviors, to be further confirmed or disconfirmed by subsequent testing.

## Evaluation of Ryan

Central to every CCE is a clear understanding of the child(ren), his or her psychological and developmental needs, and the impact of the pre- and postseparation events. Ryan was born after an unremarkable pregnancy and was healthy at birth. He was described as a generally happy and easy baby. Ryan attained his major developmental milestones as expected. He had had no significant illnesses or injuries. He was seen as a bright child who adjusted to and did well in school, reading several years above his chronological age. He had not participated in organized activities such as sports teams or after-school classes.

Both parents said Ryan was exposed to significant marital conflict starting early in his life. Since their separation when Ryan was 6 years old, he had engaged in violent interchanges with his mother and had become more withdrawn at her house, frequently disappearing into videogames. Peter described his son as a bright and funny child but also quite anxious, particularly when exposed to his mother's anger and loss of emotional control.

During the home visits Ryan had presented as very disturbed, regressed, withdrawn, and undersocialized but, surprisingly, in my individual office interviews, he was interactive and made good eye contact. In the initial interview he told me about being frightened of his mother's temper, having been hit and pushed by her, and wishing for more time with his father, who was nice to him and never hit him. Despite his engagement, Ryan's anxiety was notable, manifested by constant squirming and wandering around the office while being interviewed.

In a second interview, Ryan described the incidents of physical violence with his mother in significant detail and said they happened every few months. Asked about his own violence, Ryan explained that he usually became violent only after his mother was violent and then he would hit her or throw objects at her. He noted that most of his fights with her involved only yelling and screaming. Ryan expressed concern that his mother had frequently called the police when she couldn't control him or after his father came to help the situation. Ryan noted that when his parents were still together, they yelled and screamed at each other and occasionally his mother threw things during these fights.

School staff described Peter as the parent with more involvement at the school, and they described the father–son relationship as very close and loving. The staff had had little opportunity to observe Ryan's relationship with his mother. They noted that neither parent had involved the school in their family difficulties. Ryan is seen as a good student, and his difficulties at home did not appear to be interfering with his school performance. Ryan does well academically, always does his homework, and is a bright child. He is very engaged and loving with his teacher and enjoys communicating with adults. His peer relationships at school are quite limited.

## Parent–Child Observations

I observed the parent–child relationships separately in each parent's home during an unstructured after-school and dinner visit and in my office during a semistructured session. As I usually do, I asked the parent and child to play the Thinking, Feeling, Doing Game together during the office session.

I first evaluated the parent–child relationship between Ryan and his mother at her home. Ryan initially hid from me and then avoided significant engagement, lost in his iPad games. I attempted to interact, but he made little eye contact and only briefly answered a few questions. He was also unresponsive to his mother's requests for help. Over dinner, Ryan opened up about his friends and school, but his engagement remained limited. After dinner, Ryan had a negative reaction to his mother's setting a limit, stormed out of the room, slamming his door. He allowed me to enter the room to say goodbye. His room was chaotic.

In the office visit, Ryan rudely called his mother to join us but then snuggled up next to her. Ryan refused to follow the rules of the Thinking, Feeling, Doing Game, frequently hid the cards, and acted in a very regressed manner. Several times, he acted scared, which his mother took very seriously, although it seemed quite clear that he was intentionally being dramatic and not truly afraid. Throughout the session Julie was warm and accommodating but appeared manipulated by her son, perhaps afraid to set him off. She did not take an active, structuring role, nor did she use the game as a teaching activity, as many parents do. Julie had difficulty providing scaffolding both in terms of helping Ryan engage with me and in managing the home and office visits. In contrast the to the home visit, where there was no physical warmth between Ryan and Julie and little real engagement, in the office Ryan was like a much younger child seeking closeness with Julie. He alternated between being withdrawn and being regressive. Julie appeared passive and somewhat helpless in parenting her child.

At Peter's house, Ryan was also playing a videogame and did not acknowledge me. His father tried to get him to turn off the game and join in the visit, with limited success. At dinner, Ryan behaved in an "uncivilized" manner by immediately grabbing food and eating with his hands; Peter did not set any limits and allowed Ryan to behave as he wished.

The father–child office observation followed a testing session with Ryan. Ryan had wanted to rush through the testing so his father could join us. However, when I explained my need to gain reliable information, he became very cooperative and focused on the tasks presented. This suggested a level of self-control not previously observed in his behaviors with either parent.

When his father joined us, Ryan was very sweet and loving with him and appeared to be a completely different child than I had seen in the other evaluation contexts. He was relaxed, open, and animated. He followed directions and responded with mature and thoughtful answers. Peter set limits and was active in his parenting. In his own responses Peter was honest but shaped his answers to be useful to Ryan, making it a teaching experience. They appeared very comfortable with each other.

At times, Peter was a parent who did not establish structure or set limits. However, at other times he was engaged and facilitated mature functioning on Ryan's part, in an attuned and structuring way. Their comfort and closeness were evident in my office.

## Psychological Testing with Ryan

As is the case in almost all CCEs, I administered formal assessment measures to help determine the impact of the interparental conflict on Ryan; whether he has been traumatized by detrimental parental behavior; which of his behaviors were reactions to situational factors and which behaviors reflect internalized conflicts or ineffective defenses in response to family dysfunction; and, in particular, whether his apparent withdrawal was reflective of avoidance, depression, or was a reasonable survival strategy given his parents' difficulties with self-control. Ryan was administered R-PAS, the Roberts Apperception Test for Children–2 (Roberts-2), and selected subtests from the Wechsler Intelligence Scale for Children—Fourth Edition (WISC-IV). Cognitive testing was included due to Ryan's highly discrepant functioning, at times putting information together in a thoughtful, mature way, whereas at other times showing very immature thinking.

WISC-IV results indicated that Ryan is a bright child with good cognitive abilities (Full Scale IQ = 117). Ryan's cognitive strength is in verbally mediated thinking. He obtained scores in the average to high-average range on nonverbal, spatial reasoning. His performance on working memory tasks was variable (average to superior range), doing better on more demanding tasks. His processing speed was average. Ryan appeared to enjoy challenge; he showed very good concentration and weathered frustration well when he was fully engaged in a task.

## Ryan's R-PAS Results[2]

R-PAS was administered in my office during my second individual session with Ryan. I explained the task to Ryan and he had no questions about it. I had already developed a good alliance with him based on the home visits and interviews. As noted above, Ryan tended to respond quickly, as if rushing through the test; however, when I explained the need for his attention and effort, he responded appropriately.

Ryan appeared engaged in the task and utilized cognitive processing skills as expected for his age (Complexity SS[3] = 91). He had the capacity to view the environment flexibly from various viewpoints (R SS = 98), notice and articulate subtleties and nuances in a developmentally appropriate manner (F% SS = 110), and articulate multiple features of the environment (Blend SS = 92). He showed an adequate ability to synthesize and integrate his perceptions and ideas (Sy SS = 89). These are generally

---

[2]See Appendix 13.1 at the end of the chapter for Ryan's R-PAS Responses, Location Sheet, Code Sequence, and Page 1 and 2 Profiles.

[3]Standard scores (SS) have a mean of 100 and an *SD* of 15.

benign findings, yet are somewhat concerning when one considers his good cognitive abilities. These scores are in the low end of the average range and, given his WISC-IV scores (IQ = 117), one would expect more complexity and a better capacity for integration. This suggests that Ryan is currently not spontaneously using his strong cognitive skills to fully process and organize his everyday external and internal experiences. Similarly, although his F% (akin to Lambda in the Comprehensive System) was in the average range for his age, it was toward the upper end, suggesting he is at risk of relying on avoidant defenses if his difficult life situation does not improve.

Ryan appeared to have minimally adequate internal resources, given his age (MC SS = 86, the lowest score in the average range; M = 1, SumC = 1). The times when he did open himself to enlivening thinking or emotional reactivity were also associated with dependency needs (ODL), suggesting that when he allows himself access to a richer inner world, he is confronted with unmet needs. This was evidenced by the extremely dependent behaviors seen in the office visit with his mother. Ryan's apparent ability to manage his current stresses and internal conflicts (MC–PPD SS = 94), may be due in part to an underestimation of his stresses and conflicts in the R-PAS results, stemming from his difficulty noticing and articulating the nuances of his experience and his avoidant stance. As noted behaviorally in the evaluation, Ryan tended to avoid engagement and dealt with situations through disappearing into his screen games.

One major source of stress for Ryan is a sense that things are out of his control due to stressful external factors (m SS = 117). Changes in visitation, the involvement of police, CPS interviews, and periodic explosive incidents likely contribute to this perceived (and real) lack of self-determination. This sense of lack of control over his environment and experience can lead to distracting thoughts and difficulty with goal-directed behaviors.

Ryan's perceptual accuracy and reality testing appeared excellent. He had no clearly distorted perceptions of the environment (FQ–% SS = 71, WD–% SS = 73) and in fact demonstrated an above-average ability for someone of his age to view the environment in a conventional manner (FQo% SS = 118) without being overly conventional (P SS = 99). Thus, Ryan read the environment without distortion and with consensual understanding; furthermore, as he processed his perceptions, he did not distort them through illogical thinking, cognitive lapses, or ineffective thinking. Rather, his thinking appeared logical and effective (EII-3 SS = 79, TP-Comp SS = 71, WSumCog SS = 89, SevCog SS = 93). Generally, Ryan demonstrated no evidence of severe psychopathology (EII-3 SS = 79), and his psychological health is likely reflected in logical and accurate cognitive processing and a capacity to understand others and his environment at a developmentally appropriate level (EII-3 and TP-Comp = Low Average).

In terms of Ryan's representations of self and other, he did not show notable dependency needs (ODL% = Average for his age), although, as noted above, his engaging in more enlivening thinking and emotional reactivity was associated with the stimulation of such needs. Ryan generally appeared to be developing internal representations of others as expected, with some exceptions. He had normative social representations and therefore the potential for adequate social skills (PHR/GPHR SS = 99), and he did not evidence extreme distortions in his views of others (M– = 0, SS = 91). Like most children Ryan's age, he has not yet developed mature internal representations of human interactions reflecting autonomy (MAH = 0, SS = 92) or a propensity to see relationships with others as cooperative, collaborative, and reciprocal (COP = 0,

SS = 90). Given the nature of his family relationships, his interpersonal relationship development needs to be watched closely in the future to ascertain whether he takes these important developmental steps.

On the other hand, Ryan's protocol indicated that he has difficulties seeing people in a whole and integrated fashion (H = 0, SS = 84), suggesting that he is experiencing a developmental lag in terms of his understanding of people as complex and multifaceted. Rather, he appeared to see himself and others in more unrealistic or fragmented ways (NPH/SumH SS = 122). Ryan also showed very limited ability to mentalize human experiences or activities (M = 1), and the mentalization he achieved was not of a real human (Card I, R1 "a winged God summoning something") and was associated with dependency needs (ODL). Without an ability to see others in an integrated fashion, or to mentalize real human experiences, his relationships are likely to be superficial and lack real reciprocity. This finding is reflected in his rather limited peer interactions and lack of strong, meaningful friendships.

Ryan showed more oppositional or resistant qualities than most children his age, with a possible aversion to being controlled by others (SR SS = 128). Ryan was quite focused on dangerous, aggressive, powerful, and damaging images (AGC SS = 125). Given his history, this is not surprising, as he has been exposed to his parents' aggression throughout his life, and the relationship with his mother involves ongoing volatility and aggression. Ryan produced images that included both frightening beings that can be destructive as well as objects that can be hurtful (in particular, "monsters" and "claws" or "pincers" as on a bug or crab).

Ryan's R-PAS findings yielded important information for confirming or disconfirming the hypotheses that emerged from the other data collected. Ryan has not (yet) developed maladaptive defenses, nor are his defenses being overwhelmed by distressing underlying conflict or the effects of trauma. His sense of the world as dangerous is accurate, and his sense that things are outside of his control is accurate. What is concerning is that Ryan is not developing as well as one would hope, given his intelligence and generally adaptable temperament. Some areas of potential risk should be monitored and his therapy should be focused on these risks, such as helping him develop more adaptive coping mechanisms and internal resources instead of relying on avoidance, and helping him develop a more complex understanding of others. Ryan tends to withdraw into videogames; he is very intermittent in his willingness to engage; and he largely avoids peer relationships. The only significant disturbed or disturbing behavior identified in this evaluation is in Ryan's relationship with his mother. The above test findings suggest that the violence and chaos that occur is not reflective of psychopathology on Ryan's part. However, he is oppositional and may escalate situations, particularly if the situation is not handled well by his mother, which it is unlikely to be.

The findings from R-PAS were incorporated in the CCE report. They were used to support a recommendation that the court continue to order therapy for Ryan. The findings were also provided to Ryan's therapist to facilitate treatment planning.

## Evaluation of Julie

Highlights from Julie's interview provide a helpful context for test findings. Julie described her father as a very authoritarian man who used corporal punishment such as hitting her with a belt. She was very frightened of her father, and this fear generalized to all authority figures. She felt closer to her mother. Julie reported that, as a child, she was insecure, had trouble making friends, and was always seeking acceptance and approval. She said she was always a good student but never felt that she fit in with her peers. As an adolescent she had a brief, involuntary psychiatric hospitalization (for reasons that are not specified for confidentiality). Several years later she was sexually assaulted. After college, Julie found steady employment and has done well in her career.

Julie presented in a positive manner. She was articulate, engaged, well organized, and cooperative throughout the evaluation. I saw none of the alleged volatility or the self-described anxiety or fear. Her demeanor was unfailingly bland with a pleasant emotional tone regardless of the material being discussed. She presented herself as a "victim," stating that she was traumatized by the violence following the separation. She stated that in the marriage she would become angry, and Peter would provoke her by saying that she was crazy—and the conflict would escalate. In addition to being a victim of domestic violence, Julie complained about Peter's pattern of undermining her authority as a parent. This undermining dynamic escalated following their separation. Ryan would become violent, call his father alleging that his mother had hit him, and Julie would respond by calling for police intervention. According to Julie, Ryan had learned to lie about or exaggerate the events at her house, knowing that his father would believe whatever he said about Julie and would intervene. This dynamic resulted in Julie's feeling that she could not effectively parent Ryan. It should be noted that, early on, Julie, herself, had called Peter requesting that he manage the conflict.

Julie reported that, although the marriage was always quite volatile, problems escalated when Peter began using methamphetamines. As his drug use escalated, he became more provocative, leading her to become more agitated, which then led to more violent interchanges. She reported that it was after the separation that Ryan began to have significant difficulties with her, exhibiting violent behaviors that included hitting, biting, and kicking her. Julie said that in reaction to her son's aggression, she felt inadequate and helpless. She believed that Ryan couldn't allow himself a better relationship with her, as it would be seen as a betrayal of his loyalty with his father. There were several CPS reports of abuse made against Julie by Peter and mandated professionals, but none were substantiated as being child abuse.

Information from various mental health professional informants suggested concerns regarding Julie's emotional reactivity and her contribution to escalating situations. Several noted Julie's stable, competent presentation but suspected that she might be manipulative. A past couple's therapist indicated that Julie had acknowledged her violence toward Peter during the marriage. Professionals who had assessed Julie's parenting viewed her as passive and helpless. Julie's own therapist, however, saw her as insightful and open and reported that she had stabilized once appropriately medicated for anxiety.

There were several questions and hypotheses raised by the data collected that provide a context for framing the test results. Was Julie the instigator of the violence reported in the family, or the victim? What strengths and weaknesses did Julie bring to parenting? Was there evidence of Julie having a significant mental illness as alleged by Peter?

## Psychological Testing

The most common assessment tools used in CCEs include the Rorschach, MMPI-2, and MCMI-III (Ackerman & Pritzl, 2011). In my CCEs, I routinely administer selected subtests from the Wechsler scales to obtain a rough estimate of cognitive functioning. This is useful for interpreting other tests and is sometimes useful in understanding the interparental relationship. Given the scope of data collected during a CCE and the time required to perform such an evaluation, a complete battery is rarely administered. Julie was administered selected subtests from the WAIS-IV, MMPI-2, and R-PAS.

On the WAIS-IV, Julie obtained subtest scores ranging from Low Average to Very Superior, suggesting considerable variability in her functioning. Her strengths were related to an ability to make sense of social mores, respond to everyday events, and make sense of everyday interpersonal interactions. Julie had average abilities when asked to solve more abstract problems. Julie's estimated Full Scale IQ score was 100.

On the MMPI-2, Julie produced valid results with some tendency to present herself favorably. There was one significant elevation on the clinical scales, Scale 6. Rather than reporting explicit paranoid thoughts, Julie responded to items suggesting that she holds naïve views of others, sees herself as holding high moral values, and expects others to be honest and trustworthy. The difficulty with this view can occur when others do not live up to these standards, suggesting a judgmental attitude and difficulties with forgiveness. Julie seems vulnerable to criticism and will try to maintain self-control in order to present a public role as sociable and using correct etiquette. Julie endorsed other test items suggesting she may inhibit aggression and thus experience underlying hostility. She is likely not comfortable with her anger and may not always be aware of it. She likely gets upset when faced with others' aggression (Friedman, Lewak, Nichols, & Webb, 2001). On the positive side, Julie appears confident, well organized, and able to manage life effectively. She is likely to be outgoing and have a strong need for autonomy. Overall, however, the pattern of findings suggests a lack of insight.

## R-PAS Analysis[4]

R-PAS was explained to Julie in an office visit following several interview sessions. She was generally aware of the Rorschach task, had not researched it, and asked no questions. She approached the task in a cooperative manner and generally complied with the instructions—with the exception of Card X, where she provided five responses (I was unable to "pull" and ask for the card back before she gave the fifth response). As in interviews, Julie was engaged but tended to have an emotionally bland presentation.

Julie engaged in the R-PAS task with adequate resources and productivity, suggesting flexible thinking and effective coping (Complexity SS = 100). She generally complied with the instructions, saw the environment from multiple vantage points,

---

[4]See Appendix 13.2 at the end of the chapter for Julie's R-PAS Responses, Location Sheet, Code Sequence, and Page 1 and 2 Profiles.

and was reasonably able to articulate subtlety and nuances (R SS = 107, F% SS = 108), suggesting that she can engage with the more complex and nuanced aspects of both the environment and her internal world. Julie appeared reasonably able to attend to multiple facets of the environment and to synthesize aspects of situations (Blends SS = 91, Sy SS = 95).

Although Julie generally appeared to have sufficient internal resources to manage stress (MC SS = 92), she was limited in her capacity to mentalize human experiences (M = 1, SS = 83). This finding indicates a lack of reflectiveness and possible difficulties with taking others' perspectives and being empathic. Julie's approach to the world is to react emotionally and to process situations based on emotions, not by filtering her reactions through thoughtful deliberation (M/MC SS = 80). Although there were significant clinical and documented data suggesting that Julie can lack mature emotional modulation, this deficit was not reflected in the Color Dominance Proportion, an R-PAS index signifying little cognitive control over one's emotions [(CF+C)/SumC SS = 104], suggesting that her poor modulation is likely due to behaving provocatively in complex situations that stress her resources, rather than reflecting more characterological difficulties with emotion regulation.

On the positive side, there were no indications of significant psychopathology (EII-3 SS = 82). For example, Julie's scores suggested clear thinking, accurate reasoning, and no instances of cognitive distortions (TP-Comp SS = 80, WSumCog SS = 89, SevCog SS = 94). Julie can perceive the environment in a conventional manner when there is an obvious way to respond (P SS = 96). Julie did not tend to significantly misperceive situations (FQ–% SS = 85); however, she has a potential to frequently read situations idiosyncratically (FQu% SS = 121), which can lead to idiosyncratic understandings of herself, others, and the meaning of specific situations.

Julie has an average tendency to attend to inconsistencies, nuance, and uncertainties in the environment (YTVC' SS = 95) and did not appear to be experiencing the helplessness, distress, or unwanted distracting ideation that are often associated with external stressors (Y SS = 85, m SS = 106). In interviews Julie frequently described her feelings of helplessness, anxiety, and being traumatized, which somewhat contradicts her therapist's report of her lessened distress. Although self-reports of distress and discomfort are essentially uncorrelated with Rorschach indicators of these experiences, it may be that uncomfortable, distressing feelings are discharged quickly (M/MC SS = 80) through action rather than internalized with resulting internal pressure. It was noted that for Julie, primitive mental imagery and trauma were not salient concerns (CritCont% SS = 93); however, Critical Content images are more specifically associated with trauma that involves bodily damage, so these findings do not rule out the type of trauma that Julie described. However, Julie had described herself as traumatized, a victim, and very anxious—a narrative that is not supported by these data, clinical observations, or most of the collateral information obtained.

Regarding Julie's understanding of human interactions and what she brings to relationships, she showed significantly more opposition or resistant qualities than most adults (SR SS = 127). Although this can indicate independent strivings and creativity, at this high level it most likely indicates oppositional behavior. The combination of Julie's pervasive tendency to approach the world through her feelings, her reactivity, and a tendency toward oppositional behavior explains some of her difficulties engaging in effective co-parenting and in parenting Ryan. She has difficulty standing back when Ryan is provocative, appears to match his oppositional behavior, and when the situation becomes out of control, Julie calls the police, creating more chaos.

Although Julie did not have any instances of grossly misperceiving human activity (M– SS = 95), she did show some difficulty understanding herself and others as complex, multifaceted, and complete individuals (H SS = 88). Instead she is prone to see herself and others, and to mentally play out interpersonal interactions, in unrealistic and fanciful ways (NPH/SumH SS = 117). It was noted that Julie's only whole human movement response was a Popular response. This suggests that when there is an obvious human response, she can attend to and articulate it accurately, but one cannot assume that she would accurately read more ambiguous or subtle interactions. However, Julie appears to have an average ability to see relationships as cooperative and supportive and is likely to interact with others in an adaptive manner (COP SS = 102, PHR/GPHR SS = 100). Julie did not show affirmative evidence of the capacity to engage in mature, healthy relationships (MAH SS = 90); however, this is found in about 50% of nonpatients, so it is not a good predictor of problematic relationships. Julie did not appear to be driven by primitive dependency needs (ODL% SS = 96, T = 0, p/(a+p) SS = 91). Somewhat surprising was a lack of above-average focus on aggression (AGC SS = 94, AGM SS = 93). As noted in interview and collateral data and supported by the MMPI-2 findings, Julie is quite intent on being conventional, and the lack of aggressive themes could be due to impression management, a constant concern in CCEs.

Results suggest that Julie generally functions well and often has the capacity to interact with others in effective ways, although she is limited in her ability view others in integrated, complex ways, and her understanding of others is often idiosyncratic; other (non-R-PAS) assessment findings and clinical observations indicated that Julie is often conventional and follows social rules. Her ability to operate conventionally is a strength for her. However, she does not have sufficient backup resources to rely on, or an ability to delay, her reactions in more complex and stressful situations. In these situations, especially when faced with provocation, she has not developed ways to respond in a structured manner and likely lacks the resources to control her emotions, as seen in some of the situations with Ryan and with Peter. Julie's relationships are likely to be colored by her difficulty mentalizing others in complex, realistic, and integrated ways. She likely does well in clear, structured settings.

Julie does not bring a lot of resources to parenting Ryan, particularly in the complex and challenging situations that have occurred postseparation. Her limited resources, which contribute to situational lapses in control, support Ryan's descriptions of aggressive, chaotic incidents erupting from their conflicts (Julie's two "explosion" responses on Card II may also reflect anger that is poorly integrated and owned). A very important finding is that there was no evidence in the testing that Julie is mentally ill, as alleged by Peter.

## Evaluation of Peter

Peter reports growing up with an introverted father and an anxious mother. Peter saw himself as temperamentally like his father. He reports being a loner and gifted academically as a child and very intent on following the rules and acting in morally correct ways. Peter noted that after he left home to attend college, he rejected his obedient approach to life and began experimenting with drugs, frequently cut classes, and barely made it through college. He adopted a counterculture lifestyle, wherein the formerly rule-bound child became an anti-rule, anti-establishment young adult. Perhaps surprisingly, after college Peter was able to find and maintain good employment in the tech field until just before the marriage ended. Peter continued to use marijuana during the marriage, but for a number of years avoided other illegal drugs.

Peter presented as verbal, friendly, and he engaged easily. He dressed like a teenager and frequently noted that he liked being "Bohemian." He prided himself on having unconventional beliefs, interests, and perspectives. His stated attitude was that he refused to follow rules if they did not make sense to him. Rather, it was important to Peter that he adhere to morally correct actions in his own mind regardless of the rules (or court orders).

Peter's presentation was highly variable during the evaluation process. At his best Peter presented as a very bright, complex thinker, highly verbal, warm, thoughtful, and very open about his actions, his mistakes, and his drug use. At other times during the evaluation, Peter appeared hypomanic; for example, he rambled and evidenced pressured speech. He explained this state as arising from his anxiety about the evaluation, the lengthy legal process, and fear of being separated from his child. It was only toward the end of the evaluation that I discovered that Peter had continued to use methamphetamines. After the psychological testing was completed, Peter entered a rehab program that included random drug testing.

Peter described the relationship dynamic during the marriage as one whereby Julie was frequently violent toward him and afterward would fall apart emotionally. According to Peter, he was never violent toward Julie, although he had restrained her on occasion to stop her violence. He described her as being bipolar, emotionally volatile, and frequently losing control. Peter reported seeing his job as protecting his son from his mother's outbursts. He reported that his view of Ryan's extreme suffering had led him to stop setting limits with his son and to allow Ryan to be withdrawn and overuse videogames.

Peter described his use of drugs as an effort to self-medicate depressive and anxious feelings and as a way to withdraw from the chaos in the marriage. Peter appeared to have little understanding of the negative impact of his drug use, stating that he used drugs in a responsible, modulated manner. It was unclear whether Peter could really embrace the absolute need to stop using if he wanted to parent his son.

In interviews with mental health professionals, they noted that Peter was more attuned to his son's needs than Julie was, and when observed with his son, Peter was warm and engaged. Several professionals noted that Ryan was more mature and relaxed when interacting with his father than with his mother. It was confirmed by the couple's therapist that Julie talked in sessions about initiating aggressive incidents, such as pushing or hitting Peter, but the therapist also noted that Peter knew how to provoke her. A number of professionals noted Peter's occasional manic quality and his lack of adequate filtering, alternating with periods of withdrawal.

There were a number of questions and alternative hypotheses I developed prior to analyzing the psychological test findings. Is it more likely that Peter is the primary perpetrator of domestic violence as alleged by Julie, or that he is the victim of violence and the protector of his son? Is Peter's mood instability likely due to the influence of drug use, mental illness, or situational anxiety caused by the divorce and legal process? What difficulties does Peter bring to his parenting of Ryan, and what are his strengths and weaknesses as a parent?

## Psychological Testing

Peter was administered the same tests as Julie. Selected subtests from the WAIS-IV suggest that Peter is an intellectually gifted man with scores ranging from High Average to Very Superior. His estimated Full Scale IQ score was 136. His greatest strengths were seen in verbally mediated problem solving. He showed a very superior understanding of social mores and everyday interpersonal interactions.

Peter's MMPI-2 results indicate that he approached the test in an open manner. He obtained clinical elevations on Scale 6 and Scale 9. Regarding his elevation on the Scale 6 subscale of Persecutory ideas, Peter stated that he was thinking about Julie when answering a number of items. I inspected the items individually, and this test-taking attitude appears to account for that aspect of the scale elevation. The other possibility is that the methamphetamine use has, in fact, led to a more paranoid orientation, particularly aimed at Julie. The rest of the Scale 6 elevation was caused by an elevation in the Poignancy subscale. Thus, it suggests that he sees himself as more high strung and sensitive than others are, feels emotions more intensely than others, and feels misunderstood; there is a vulnerability for these individuals to seek risky or exciting activities to make them feel better. The Scale 9 elevation suggests accelerated thought processes, speech, and psychomotor activities. He is likely to be easily bored and to seek stimulation. Peter's results indicate an unrealistically high appraisal of his own abilities and self-worth.

## R-PAS Analysis[5]

R-PAS was explained to Peter in an office visit following several interview sessions. He was generally aware of the Rorschach task, had not researched it, and asked no questions. As in his interviews, Peter was engaged, expansive, and appeared eager to invite me into his thinking and perspective. His responses were confident, even when they appeared to include idiosyncratic and illogical material.

Overall, Peter provided a highly complex protocol with significant evidence of both personality strengths and serious psychopathology and compromised reality testing. In reviewing the findings, several factors that may have influenced the Rorschach were kept in mind. Peter had continued to use amphetamines during the evaluation process, and had been using for 2 years. Peter prided himself on being unconventional, having unique views, and being creative. He is also very bright.

Peter was very engaged in the task, evidencing complexity, flexibility in coping, integration of concepts, and sophistication of processing (Complexity SS = 112, Sy SS = 120, SI SS = 123). Although generally these abilities are associated with strengths, high Complexity can be associated with losing ideational control arising

---

[5]See Appendix 13.3 at the end of the chapter for Peter's R-PAS Responses, Location Sheet, Code Sequence, and Page 1 and 2 Profiles.

from trauma, anxiety, emerging psychosis, internal preoccupations, or drug use. He appears to have well-developed internal resources with the capacity to engage in the world with reflective thinking, emotional responsiveness, and sophisticated psychological activity (MC SS = 114). However, these resources may not always be used productively, and Peter evidences significant distortions in his perceptions (FQ–% SS = 129). Peter appears to have a good capacity to use his imagination, and to have the potential to be empathic and understand others' perspectives (M SS = 118), but his accuracy in understanding interpersonal situations can be severely compromised (M– = 3, SS = 129). Peter appears able to incorporate emotionality into his perceptions in a modulated manner [(CF+C)/SumC SS = 95, Pure C SS = 95] and to rely on both his feelings and thinking to process information and to guide his decisions and actions—an ability that can indicate flexibility in how he might approach different problems or challenges that arise (M/MC SS = 110). These positive findings are consistent with Peter's empathy and attunement with his son and much of the clinical presentation.

However, under certain circumstances, Peter's ability to use these strengths is compromised by significant difficulties with reality testing and perceptual accuracy. In looking at indicators of overall functioning, Peter has the resources to handle stress in challenging situations and will likely show resilience (MC–PPD SS = 102); however, other very elevated scores suggest that Peter is likely to have significant psychopathology and difficulties with reality testing (EII-3 SS = 121, TP-Comp SS = 128). Inspection of the elements that elevated these scores indicates that the dominant cause for the elevation was Peter's misreading of the environment (minus form quality). Peter rarely perceived the environment in a conventional manner (FQo% SS = 78, P SS = 80) and frequently reported perceptions that had little to do with the stimuli (FQ–% SS = 129, FQo% SS = 78, FQu% SS = 107, P SS = 80). It was noted that the majority of Peter's distortions occurred on cards with color (4/5), raising the probability that Peter is most likely to impose his own distorted interpretation in situations that are emotionally provocative. Close inspection of the findings did not suggest leakage of primitive material (CritCont% SS = 96) nor pervasive difficulties with clear thinking (WSumCog SS = 100). He did have one Level 2 Cognitive Code (INC2), suggesting some more notable cognitive slippage. This was his last Rorschach response: an "angry mouse soldier . . . with a frowning mouth, ready to bite." This response included aggressive movement and was minus form, but it seems more childish and a self-perception (his protective defense of Ryan) or perhaps a perception of other (Julie's dangerous aggression), rather than a psychotic perception.

As was true for Ryan and Julie, Peter showed significantly more oppositional and resistant qualities than most adults (SR SS = 127). The ways in which Peter understands himself and others is a combination of maturely developed capacities and effective social skills (MAP/MAPH SS = 99, MAH SS = 116, COP SS = 120) and the capacity for serious misunderstanding. He had an average ability to envision mutually enhancing interactions between people that respect autonomous functioning (MAP/MAPH SS = 99, MAH SS = 116). He had a propensity to view relationships as helpful and rewarding, so will likely seek relationships (COP SS = 120). He had a good ability to see people as complex, integrated beings and did not tend to view others as incomplete and in a fantasized manner (H SS = 119, NPH/SumH SS = 73). Although these findings could reflect efforts at impression management, common in

CCEs, throughout the evaluation Peter tended to not inhibit himself and, in fact, was quick to acknowledge "bad behavior" and responded openly on the MMPI-2. The findings suggest that Peter has the scaffolding for healthy and mature relationships and the building blocks for being interested in and understanding of himself and others. These attributes inform Peter's ability to respond to his child in an attuned manner and often with insight and depth. Despite these strengths, there were concerning findings regarding interpersonal functioning. He saw people in problematic and confused ways, which will likely lead to difficult interactions (PHR/GPHR SS = 111). Inspection of these PHR responses did not indicate a specific, consistent theme, although most (3/4) included distortions in reality testing and most occurred on cards with color (3/4). The propensity to have lapses in his understanding of others and to project his own beliefs was also noted in the number of human movement responses with poor form (M– SS = 129), and some tendency toward guardedness and interpersonal wariness (V-Comp SS = 113), which was consistent with the elevation on Scale 6 in the MMPI-2.

In some ways the R-PAS findings are confusing and contradictory, but in other regards they match the variability seen in Peter's clinical presentation. Peter can be a very complex, engaging man; he is quite attuned to his son and has the capacity to parent, at times, in a very effective manner, although at other times he disregards Ryan's need for structure and discipline. There is certainly instability in his functioning, some major difficulties in terms of his judgment, and he holds a quite distorted view of Julie. The view of her as seriously disturbed and his lack of awareness of his contributions to the difficulties they have experienced, suggest real distortions. In terms of his internalized object relationships, we see both the foundations and capacity for healthy, mature relationships as well as the notable propensity toward misreading others. Affect appears to dysregulate Peter, a finding consistent with the poor judgment he has shown in his interactions with Julie and in his exceedingly poor judgment in terms of disobeying court orders (both of which are emotionally provocative situations). Other possible factors contributing to Peter's R-PAS findings include increased dysfunction over the past few years, consistent with his increased use of amphetamines, and his drive to be unconventional, creative, different, and idiosyncratic. Until he is clean and sober for a period of time, the contribution of his drug use to his dysfunction cannot be determined.

## Integrating the R-PAS Findings

The R-PAS findings illuminate the manner in which both of these parents function best in situations that are not emotionally stimulating or provocative. In the marriage, the volatility combined Julie's reactivity and somewhat limited resources with Peter's distorted reactions to emotional stimuli—that is, misreading situations, resulting in incidents of very poor judgment. It is not surprising that their disputes escalated, oppositional behaviors emerged, and violent behaviors occurred. These R-PAS findings were very helpful in identifying the pattern of violence in the family as "situational couples violence" as opposed to a "coercive controlling" dynamic, with one partner as the perpetrator maintaining power and control through violence, threats, and more broadly controlling behaviors (Kelly & Johnston, 2008). In situational couples violence, conflict periodically gets out of control, escalates, and becomes physical. Identifying the type of domestic violence in a family is a critical aspect for determining parenting plans and interventions. With coercive and controlling violence, it is presumed that shared or joint parenting will not be in the child's best interest, whereas situational couples violence tends to cease once the partners separate (Jaffe, Johnston, Crooks, & Bala, 2008). The continued violence in this case is understood to have occurred when these parents were in proximity to each other, brought together by Ryan's out-of-control behavior or when Ryan called his father alleging violence by his mother.

Ryan is not emotionally provocative with his father, which allows Peter to bring his strengths to parenting. He is thoughtful, complex, and can provide an environment within which Ryan can often behave in a mature, engaged way. However, it is Peter's distorted view of Julie and his responses to her difficulties with Ryan that contribute to the chaos in this family. His reactions include withering criticism of Julie and discussions with Ryan about his mother's pathology and dangerousness, which serve to erode Julie's ability to parent more effectively. However, the greatest concern with Peter is his drug use. If he is unable to become sober, he will not be able to parent his child, which would be a huge loss to Ryan.

The R-PAS findings regarding Julie's lack of significant pathology were critical to this evaluation. Additionally, the pattern of Julie's strengths and liabilities identified in R-PAS illuminate her difficulties parenting, given her situation. Julie is aware that she feels helpless when confronted with Ryan's rebellious and provocative behavior, and aware that she conducts herself poorly. She has little ability to defuse, soothe, or repair the disruptions that occur with Ryan. Children whose parents feel helpless often feel insecure and react to the parent with contradictory and sometimes aggressive behavior, as was noted in these mother–child observations. Children are often quite frightened when a parent loses control of his or her emotions and physically act out, as Ryan has described to numerous professionals. For children to feel secure, they need their parents to be "older, wiser and kinder and in control" (Marvin, Cooper, Hoffman, & Powell, 2002, p. 109). Ryan becomes disorganized and regressed in his mother's care, but this does not appear due to his psychopathology (or hers) but rather reflects Julie's inability to manage more complex, emotionally stimulating situations and Peter's intrusions into their relationship, which heighten the instability.

## Recommendations

Once Peter can demonstrate his ability to maintain sobriety, other recommendations focused on creating structure, limiting unstructured contact between the parents, and providing a professional with sufficient power to monitor this family. That professional would help establish communication, debrief incidents, and avert crisis (the previous PC did not have these powers). Julie needs a parenting coach to build her repertoire for handling Ryan more effectively. One critical finding in this evaluation was that, postseparation, there had been continued violence. These parents should not be in proximity except in the most controlled environments; exchanges should be through school. Clearly, all family members need to continue their individual treatment, and hopefully having the feedback from this evaluation will promote less polarized, more effective services from involved mental health professionals. If Peter can demonstrate his ability to stay off drugs and Julie is willing to work with a coach, Ryan should remain in the shared care of his parents.

## REFERENCES

Ackerman, M. J., & Pritzl, T. B. (2011). Child custody evaluation practices: A 20-year follow-up. *Family Court Review, 49*, 618–628.

American Psychological Association. (2010). Guidelines for child custody evaluations in family law proceedings. *American Psychologist, 65*, 863–867.

Association of Family and Conciliation Courts. (2006). Model standards of practice for child custody evaluation. Available at *http://www.afccnet.org/Resource-Center/Practice-Guidelines-and-Standards.*

California Rules of Court. *www.courts.ca.gov/rules.htm.*

Erard, R. E. (2012). Expert testimony using the Rorschach Performance Assessment System in psychological injury cases. *Psychological Injury and Law, 5*, 122–134.

Erard, R. E., Meyer, G. J., & Viglione, D. J. (2014). Setting the record straight: Comment on Gurley, Piechowski, Sheehan, and Gray (2014) on the admissibility of the Rorschach Performance Assessment System (R-PAS) in court. *Psychological Injury and Law, 7*, 165–177.

Friedman, A. F., Lewak, R., Nichols, D. S., & Webb, J. T. (2001). *Psychological assessment with the MMPI-2.* Mahwah, NJ: Erlbaum.

Gould, J. W., & Martindale, D. A. (2007). *The art and science of child custody evaluations.* New York: Guilford Press.

Jaffe, P. G., Johnston, J. R., Crooks, C. V., & Bala, N. (2008). Custody disputes involving allegations of domestic violence: Toward a differentiated approach to parenting plans. *Family Court Review, 46*, 500–522.

Kassin, S. M., Meissner, C. A., & Norwick, R. J. (2005). "I'd know a false confession if I saw one": A comparative study of college students and police investigators. *Law and Human Behavior, 29*, 211–227.

Kelly, J. B., & Johnson, M. P. (2008). Differentiation among types of intimate partner violence: Research update and implications for interventions. *Family Court Review, 46*, 476–499.

Kuehnle, K., & Drozd, L. (Eds). (2012). *Parenting plan evaluations: Applied research for the family court.* New York: Oxford University Press.

Marvin, R., Cooper, G., Hoffman, K., & Powell, B. (2002). The circle of security project: Attachment-based intervention with caregiver-pre-school child dyads. *Attachment and Human Development, 4*, 107–124.

Meyer, G. J., Viglione, D. J., Mihura, J. L., Erard, R. E., & Erdberg, P. (2011). *Rorschach Performance Assessment System: Administration, coding, interpretation, and technical manual.* Toledo, OH: Rorschach Performance Assessment System.

Stahl, P. M. (2011). *Conducting child custody evaluations: From basic to complex issues.* Thousand Oaks, CA: SAGE.

**Ryan's R-PAS Responses, Location Sheet, Code Sequence, and Page 1 and 2 Profiles**

## Rorschach Responses "Ryan" (Child)

| Respondent ID: Ryan (Child) | Examiner: S. Margaret Lee, PhD |
|---|---|
| Location: Office | Date: **/**/**** |
| Start Time: 1:30 P.M. | End Time: 2:10 P.M. |

| Cd # | R # | Or | Response | Clarification | R-Opt |
|---|---|---|---|---|---|
| I | 1 | | Looks like maybe a winged God summoning something. (W) | E: (Examiner Repeats Response [ERR].) R: Head (Dd22), arms summoning (D1), wings (Dd34), and feet (D3). | |
| | 2 | v | v > v Or it looks like kind of a monster, almost a crab-ish monster. (W) | E: (ERR) R: Crab things (D1) and crab legs (Dd34). | |
| II | 3 | | It looks like a light in the darkness. (DS5,6) | E: (ERR) R: Black (D6). Light, a lamp (DS5). E: Lamp? R: Looks like it's hanging from the ceiling. | |
| | 4 | v | Right here looks like two feet. (D2) | E: (ERR) R: Toes (outer top when viewed in the v orientation) and the bottom, here. | |
| III | 5 | | Right here looks like a bow. (D3) | E: (ERR) R: All the things it would have. | |
| | 6 | | Looks like two faces. (Dd32) | E: (ERR) R: (subject outlines). The nose, almost an eye, the neck. | |
| | 7 | | And looks like a boot here and here. (Dd99 = upper portion of D5, from Dd26 up) | E: (ERR) R: Boots, the top, toe slips in. Kind of looks like a cowboy boot. | |
| IV | 8 | | It looks like—I don't know what it looks like. Only see one, kind of a monster. (W) E: I'd like you to give me two, maybe three responses to each card. Take your time and see what else it might be. | E: (ERR) R: Tiny head (D3), arms (D4), and feet (D2). | Pr |
| | 9 | @ | < v > Kind of maybe a giant foot right here. (D2) | E: (ERR) R: Giant foot, the toe. | |
| V | 10 | | Looks like a bat. (W) | E: (ERR) R: Antenna (Dd34), wings (D4), feet (D9). | |
| | 11 | @ | v ^And kind of a bat, crab. (W) (R changed from bat to crab quickly, and in CP he only reported crab parts.) | E: (ERR) R: Just a crab arm (D10). E: Crab arm? R: Has a space where it goes "clack, clack". | |
| VI | 12 | v | v > v Looks like a pincher bug, two pinchers, kind of. (Dd21) | E: (ERR) R: Pinchers, just the pinchers. | |
| | 13 | v | > v Kind of like the sun, a bit, here. (D3) | E: (ERR) R: Flare from the sun. E: Flare? R: Stuff (Dd22) coming out. | |
| VII | 14 | | Two child faces. (D9) | E: (ERR) R: Nose, mouth, and where the eye is. | |
| | 15 | | Another lamp. (DS7) | E: (ERR) R: Lamp. E: What makes it look like a lamp? R: I don't know. I've seen it somewhere before, a "vase-y" lamp, I've seen it. | |

| Cd # | R # | Or | Response | Clarification | R-Opt |
|------|-----|----|----------|---------------|-------|
| VIII | 16 | | Two leopards. (D1) | E: (ERR)<br>R: Feet and head and tail. | |
| | 17 | | And a mountain. (D4) | E: (ERR)<br>R: Top and steep sides. | |
| IX | 18 | @ | v ^ Looks like a fountain, kind of. (D8) | E: (ERR)<br>R: Water shooting up.<br>E: What makes it look like water?<br>R: Don't know. | |
| | 19 | | And maybe crab claws right here. (Dd25) | E: (ERR)<br>R: Crab claws, the pincer part. | |
| X | 20 | | Two creatures, plant creatures. (D8) | E: (ERR)<br>R: Plant creatures.<br>E: What makes them look like plant creatures?<br>R: Plants on their heads. | |
| | 21 | | Two creatures, mythical. (D1) | E: (ERR)<br>R: Tail, fire on them, arms, and two heads.<br>E: Fire?<br>R: Stuff coming off. | |
| | 22 | | Two banana creatures. (D2) | E: (ERR)<br>R: Banana, yellowish, and almost looks like bananas. | |
| | 23 | | Two just black-ish creatures. That was four things, and a grabber claw and that's all. (D7) [Because this was the last card, E did not provide a Pull with the reminder.] | E: (ERR)<br>R: Black and has a tail. [The "grabber claw" sounded like a quickly injected fifth response, so it was not clarified.] | |

# Rorschach Performance Assessment System (R-PAS)®

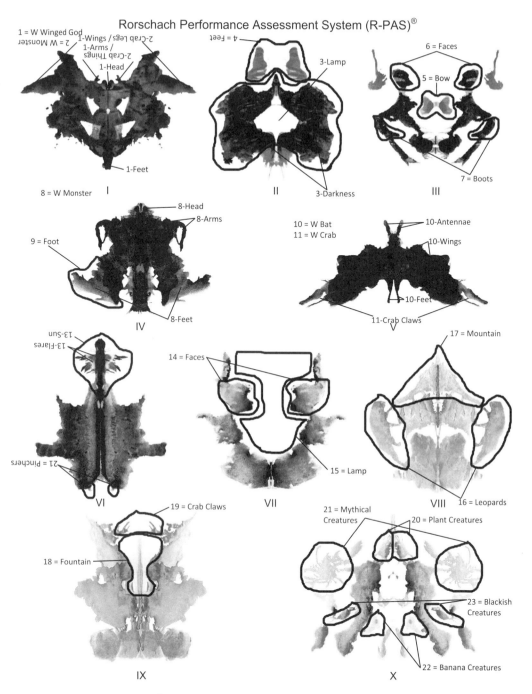

1 = W Winged God
2 = W Monster
1-Wings / 2-Crab Legs
1-Arms / 2-Crab Things
1-Head
1-Feet
8 = W Monster
I

4 = Feet
3-Lamp
3-Darkness
II

6 = Faces
5 = Bow
7 = Boots
III

8-Head
8-Arms
9 = Foot
8-Feet
IV

10 = W Bat
11 = W Crab
10-Antennae
10-Wings
10-Feet
11-Crab Claws
V

13-Sun
13-Flares
21 = Pinchers
VI

14 = Faces
15 = Lamp
VII

17 = Mountain
16 = Leopards
VIII

19 = Crab Claws
18 = Fountain
IX

21 = Mythical Creatures
20 = Plant Creatures
23 = Blackish Creatures
22 = Banana Creatures
X

© 2012 R-PAS; Rorschach® trademarks and images are used with permission of the trademark owner, Hogrefe AG, Berne, Switzerland

# R-PAS Code Sequence: "Ryan" (Child)

**C-ID**: Ryan (Child)   **P-ID**: 6   **Age**: 10   **Gender**: Male   **Education**: 4

| Cd | # | Or | Loc | Loc # | SR | SI | Content | Sy | Vg | 2 | FQ | P | Determinants | Cognitive | Thematic | HR | ODL (RP) | R-Opt |
|----|---|----|-----|-------|----|----|---------|----|----|---|----|---|--------------|-----------|----------|----|---------|-------|
| I | 1 | | W | | | | (H) | | | | o | | Ma | | | GH | ODL | |
| | 2 | v | W | | | | (A) | | | | u | | F | | AGC | | | |
| II | 3 | | D | 5,6 | SR | SI | NC | Sy | | | o | | mp,C' | | | | | |
| | 4 | v | D | 2 | | | Hd | | | | u | | F | | | PH | | |
| III | 5 | | D | 3 | | | Cg | | | | o | | F | | | | | |
| | 6 | | Dd | 32 | | | Hd | | | 2 | o | | F | | | PH | | |
| | 7 | | Dd | 99 | | | Cg | | | 2 | u | | F | | | | | |
| IV | 8 | | W | | | | (H) | | | | o | P | F | | AGC | GH | | Pr |
| | 9 | @ | D | 2 | | | Hd | | | | o | | F | | | PH | | |
| V | 10 | | W | | | | A | | | | o | P | F | INC1 | | | | |
| | 11 | @ | D | 10 | | | Ad | | | 2 | o | | F | | | | | |
| VI | 12 | v | Dd | 21 | | | Ad | | | | o | | F | | AGC | | | |
| | 13 | v | D | 3 | | | Fi | | | | u | | ma | | | | | |
| VII | 14 | | D | 9 | | | Hd | | | 2 | o | P | F | | | GH | | |
| | 15 | | D | 7 | SR | | NC | | | | o | | F | | PER | | | |
| VIII | 16 | | D | 1 | | | A | | | 2 | o | P | F | | AGC | | | |
| | 17 | | D | 4 | | | NC | | | | o | | F | | | | | |
| IX | 18 | @ | D | 8 | | | NC | | | | u | | ma | | | | | |
| | 19 | | Dd | 25 | | | Ad | | | | u | | F | | AGC | | | |
| X | 20 | | D | 8 | | | (A) | | | 2 | o | | F | | | | | |
| | 21 | | D | 1 | | | (A),Fi | Sy | | 2 | u | | FMa | | AGC | | | |
| | 22 | | D | 2 | | | (A) | | | 2 | u | | CF | | | | ODL | |
| | 23 | | D | 7 | | | (A) | | | 2 | u | | C' | | AGC | | | |

©2010-2016 R-PAS

# R-PAS Summary Scores and Profiles – Page 1

C-ID: Ryan (Child)  P-ID: 6  Age: 10  Gender: Male  Education: 4

| Domain/Variables | Raw Scores | Raw A-SS | Raw C-SS | Cplx. Adj. A-SS | Cplx. Adj. C-SS | Standard Score Profile R-Optimized | Abbr. |
|---|---|---|---|---|---|---|---|
| **Admin. Behaviors and Obs.** | | | | | | | |
| Pr | 1 | 104 | 105 | | | | Pr |
| Pu | 0 | 96 | 95 | | | | Pu |
| CT (Card Turning) | 7 | 110 | 111 | | | | CT |
| **Engagement and Cog. Processing** | | | | | | | |
| Complexity | 49 | 82 | 91 | | | | Cmplx |
| R (Responses) | 23 | 99 | 98 | 105 | 106 | | R |
| F% [Lambda=2.29] (Simplicity) | 70% | 122 | 110 | 114 | 102 | | F% |
| Blend | 1 | 84 | 92 | 98 | 104 | | Bln |
| Sy | 2 | 81 | 89 | 98 | 105 | | Sy |
| MC | 2.0 | 75 | 86 | 90 | 99 | | MC |
| MC - PPD | -4.0 | 93 | 94 | 93 | 93 | | MC-PPD |
| M | 1 | 83 | 90 | 92 | 98 | | M |
| M/MC [1/2.0] | NA | | | | | | M Prp |
| (CF+C)/SumC [1/1] | NA | | | | | | CFC Prp |
| **Perception and Thinking Problems** | | | | | | | |
| EII-3 | -0.9 | 86 | 79 | 93 | 85 | | EII |
| TP-Comp (Thought & Percept. Com...) | -0.6 | 74 | 71 | 85 | 77 | | TP-C |
| WSumCog | 2 | 89 | 89 | 96 | 93 | | WCog |
| SevCog | 0 | 94 | 93 | 94 | 93 | | Sev |
| FQ-% | 0% | 78 | 71 | 83 | 74 | | FQ-% |
| WD-% | 0% | 82 | 73 | 83 | 74 | | WD-% |
| FQo% | 61% | 103 | 118 | 96 | 111 | | FQo% |
| P | 4 | 88 | 99 | 95 | 106 | | P |
| **Stress and Distress** | | | | | | | |
| YTVC' | 2 | 89 | 98 | 98 | 108 | | YTVC' |
| m | 3 | 113 | 117 | 116 | 121 | | m |
| Y | 0 | 85 | 91 | 91 | 98 | | Y |
| MOR | 0 | 86 | 90 | 91 | 93 | | MOR |
| SC-Comp (Suicide Concern Comp.) | NA | | | | | | SC-C |
| **Self and Other Representation** | | | | | | | |
| ODL% | 9% | 98 | 110 | 104 | 116 | | ODL% |
| SR (Space Reversal) | 2 | 113 | 128 | 113 | 128 | | SR |
| MAP/MAHP [0/0] | NA | | | | | | MAP Prp |
| PHR/GPHR [3/6] | 50% | 111 | 99 | 111 | 99 | | PHR Prp |
| M- | 0 | 95 | 91 | 95 | 91 | | M- |
| AGC | 7 | 127 | 125 | 128 | 127 | | AGC |
| H | 0 | 75 | 84 | 84 | 90 | | H |
| COP | 0 | 88 | 90 | 99 | 101 | | COP |
| MAH | 0 | 90 | 92 | 90 | 89 | | MAH |

A-SS = Adult Standard Score; C-SS = Age-Based Child or Adolescent Standard Score

# R-PAS Summary Scores and Profiles – Page 2

C-ID: Ryan (Child)  P-ID: 6  Age: 10  Gender: Male  Education: 4

| Domain/Variables | Raw Scores | Raw A-SS | Raw C-SS | Cplx. Adj. A-SS | Cplx. Adj. C-SS | Standard Score Profile R-Optimized | Abbr. |
|---|---|---|---|---|---|---|---|
| **Engagement and Cog. Processing** | | | | | | | |
| W% | 17% | 84 | 88 | 90 | 94 | | W% |
| Dd% | 17% | 105 | 104 | 104 | 102 | | Dd% |
| SI (Space Integration) | 1 | 86 | 90 | 98 | 100 | | SI |
| IntCont | 0 | 81 | 90 | 92 | 102 | | IntC |
| Vg% | 0% | 86 | 90 | 86 | 87 | | Vg% |
| V | 0 | 92 | 94 | 92 | 94 | | V |
| FD | 0 | 88 | 91 | 100 | 100 | | FD |
| R8910% | 35% | 109 | 114 | 106 | 111 | | R8910% |
| WSumC | 1.0 | 83 | 90 | 94 | 100 | | WSC |
| C | 0 | 95 | 92 | 95 | 92 | | C |
| Mp/(Ma+Mp) [0/1] | NA | | | | | | Mp Prp |
| **Perception and Thinking Problems** | | | | | | | |
| FQu% | 39% | 110 | 109 | 119 | 116 | | FQu% |
| **Stress and Distress** | | | | | | | |
| PPD | 6 | 90 | 97 | 102 | 108 | | PPD |
| CBlend | 0 | 91 | 92 | 91 | 92 | | CBlnd |
| C' | 2 | 105 | 108 | 106 | 110 | | C' |
| V | 0 | 92 | 94 | 92 | 94 | | V |
| CritCont% (Critical Contents) | 9% | 87 | 93 | 95 | 99 | | CrCt |
| **Self and Other Representation** | | | | | | | |
| SumH | 6 | 101 | 102 | 110 | 113 | | SumH |
| NPH/SumH [6/6] | 100% | 127 | 122 | 124 | 118 | | NPH Prp |
| V-Comp (Vigilance Composite) | 3.7 | 106 | 109 | 116 | 121 | | V-C |
| r (Reflections) | 0 | 95 | 94 | 95 | 94 | | r |
| p/(a+p) [1/5] | 20% | 84 | 84 | 81 | 83 | | p Prp |
| AGM | 0 | 93 | 91 | 93 | 91 | | AGM |
| T | 0 | 91 | 92 | 91 | 92 | | T |
| PER | 1 | 109 | 104 | 109 | 104 | | PER |
| An | 0 | 85 | 88 | 85 | 88 | | An |

A-SS = Adult Standard Score; C-SS = Age-Based Child or Adolescent Standard Score

**Julie's R-PAS Responses, Location Sheet, Code Sequence, and Page 1 and 2 Profiles**

**Rorschach Responses "Julie" (Mother)**

| Respondent ID: Julie (Mother) | Examiner: S. Margaret Lee, PhD |
|---|---|
| Location: Office | Date: **/**/**** |
| Start Time: 11:00 A.M. | End Time: 11:35 A.M. |

| Cd # | R # | Or | Response | Clarification | R-Opt |
|---|---|---|---|---|---|
| I | 1 | | Insect. (W) | E: (Examiner Repeats Response [ERR].)<br>R: Shape of the wings (D2), body (D4), and head (Dd22). | |
| | 2 | | Bat. (Dd99: Upper 1/3 of card) | E: (ERR)<br>R: Shape of the wings (D7), head (Dd22). | |
| II | 3 | | Negative space looks like a spaceship (DS5) blasting off. (D3,5) | E: (ERR)<br>R: Shape.<br>E: Blasting off?<br>R: The downward streaks (D3) make it look like it's moving. | |
| | 4 | v | v ^ v Volcano. (D3) | E: (ERR)<br>R: It looks like it's erupting with streaks and red; looks like it's exploding up. | |
| III | 5 | | Two people cradling something. (D1) | E: (ERR)<br>R: Shape of the head (Dd32), torso (Dd22) of woman, legs (D5), and looks like supporting something (D7).<br>E: Something?<br>R: I don't know. | |
| | 6 | | Bow. (D3) | E: (ERR)<br>R: Shape. | |
| | 7 | < | < Two birds soaring. (DdS23) | E: (ERR)<br>R: Shape of the wings outstretched and the beak. | |
| IV | 8 | | Action figure, villain. (W) | E: (ERR)<br>R: Shape and bad guy.<br>E: You said a villain?<br>R: Head (D3) and large and dark; feet (D2). | |
| | 9 | | High heels. (D2) | E: (ERR)<br>R: Shape of the heels and sort of looks like shoes. | |
| | 10 | | A tree. (D1) | E: (ERR)<br>R: Top of the tree, branches out (top of D1), the shape and the roots, the trunk and roots on bottom. | |
| V | 11 | | Bat. (W) | E: (ERR)<br>R: Shape, wings (D4), and head (D6). | |
| | 12 | | Mouth of fish. (Dd34) | E: (ERR)<br>R: It's open (points).<br>E: What makes it look like it's open?<br>R: We took this trip to Minnesota when our son was. . . . And we all took our car and caught a fish.<br>E: What makes it look like a fish?<br>R: Just the shape of the open mouth. | |
| VI | 13 | | Canyon. (D1) | E: (ERR)<br>R: The dark line (D12) and the white makes it look like an opening; the lighter part looks like the bottom, and the sides of the mountain are darker; looks like if you are standing, looking down. | |
| | 14 | | Flying catfish-type animal. (D8) | E: (ERR)<br>R: Head of fish with whiskers (Dd26), wings (Dd22), catfish body (lower D8), shape of head with eye and mouth. | |
| | 15 | | Two sock puppets. (Dd31) | E: (ERR)<br>R: Shape. | |

| Cd # | R # | Or | Response | Clarification | R-Opt |
|------|-----|-----|----------|---------------|-------|
| VII | 16 | v | > ^ v Woman with curly hair, necklace, and shoulder pads. (DS7) | E: (ERR)<br>R: Shape of the head with curly hair (D10).<br>E: Curly?<br>R: Edges look rough. Necklace (space between D9s), shoulder pads (space between D5s). | |
| | 17 | | Crab legs. (D1) | E: (ERR)<br>R: Oh, I don't know, I'm hungry. Mostly the shape. | |
| VIII | 18 | | Pretty! Two iguanas climbing. (D1) | E: (ERR)<br>R: Just the shape of the head looks like lizard, legs, tail. | |
| | 19 | | Ribs. (D3) | E: (ERR)<br>R: Looks like a skeleton with ribs; lines in the center is the backbone, spine.<br>E: Ribs?<br>R: Just the lines (pointing to the white horizontal lines). | |
| IX | 20 | | Wizards. (D3) | E: (ERR)<br>R: Just the orange.<br>E: What makes it look like a wizard?<br>R: Shape of the caps on top, hands (Dd25), cloak (outer edge of D3). | |
| | 21 | | Feet, just toes (of one foot). (Dd99 = Dd30 plus the white spaces to either side) | E: (ERR)<br>R: The green.<br>E: What makes it look like toes?<br>R: Looks like five of them and long. | |
| | 22 | | Pink birds. (Dd35) | E: (ERR)<br>R: Like a beak (adjacent to Dd30), like a baby bird looking up, like waiting for Mom to come feed them and the shape of the body. | |
| X | 23 | | Eiffel Tower. (D11) | E: (ERR)<br>R: Gray and the shape. It's tall and triangular. [E could have queried "tall" for FD.] | |
| | 24 | | Seahorses. (D9) | E: (ERR)<br>R: The pink.<br>E: What makes it look like seahorses?<br>R: Snout and body and tail, and it's pink. | |
| | 25 | | Blue crabs. (D1) | E: (ERR)<br>R: The body, and it looks like the legs and it's blue. | |
| | 26 | | Coral reef. (D13,15,7) [E missed a Pull here.]<br>And leaves. (D10) | E: (ERR)<br>R: Just the colors and shapes. [The "leaves" were not clarified as they were a fifth response to the card.] | |

# Rorschach Performance Assessment System (R-PAS)®

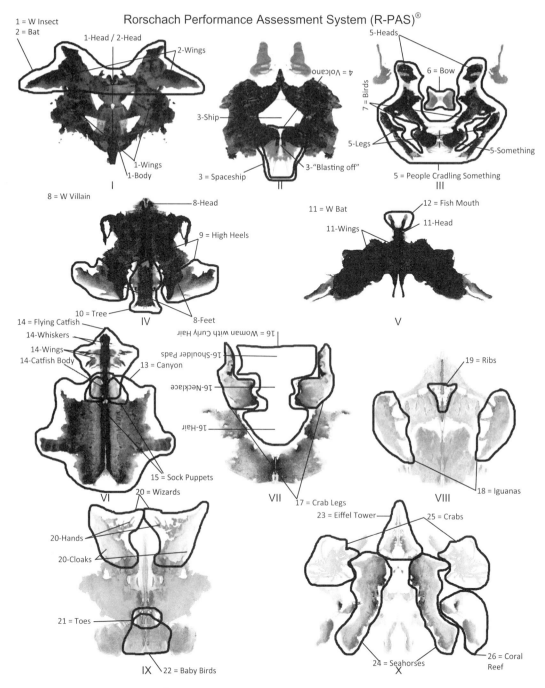

1 = W Insect
2 = Bat
1-Head / 2-Head
2-Wings
1-Wings
1-Body
I

4 = Volcano
3-Ship
3-"Blasting off"
3 = Spaceship
II

5-Heads
6 = Bow
7 = Birds
5-Legs
5-Something
5 = People Cradling Something
III

8 = W Villain
8-Head
9 = High Heels
10 = Tree
8-Feet
IV

11 = W Bat
12 = Fish Mouth
11-Head
11-Wings
V

14 = Flying Catfish
14-Whiskers
14-Wings
14-Catfish Body
13 = Canyon
15 = Sock Puppets
VI

16 = Woman with Curly Hair
16-Shoulder Pads
16-Necklace
16-Hair
17 = Crab Legs
VII

19 = Ribs
18 = Iguanas
VIII

20 = Wizards
20-Hands
20-Cloaks
21 = Toes
22 = Baby Birds
IX

23 = Eiffel Tower
25 = Crabs
24 = Seahorses
26 = Coral Reef
X

# R-PAS Code Sequence: "Julie" (Mother)

**C-ID**: Julie (Mother)    **P-ID**: 4    **Age**: **    **Gender**: Female    **Education**: NA

| Cd | # | Or | Loc | Loc # | SR | SI | Content | Sy | Vg | 2 | FQ | P | Determinants | Cognitive | Thematic | HR | ODL (RP) | R-Opt |
|----|---|----|-----|-------|----|----|---------|----|----|---|----|---|--------------|-----------|----------|----|----|----|
| I | 1 | | W | | | | A | | | | o | | F | | | | | |
| | 2 | | Dd | 99 | | | A | | | | u | | F | | | | | |
| II | 3 | | D | 3,5 | SR | SI | Ex,NC | Sy | | | o | | ma | | | | | |
| | 4 | v | D | 3 | | | Ex,NC | Sy | | | u | | ma,CF | | AGC | | | |
| III | 5 | | D | 1 | | | H,NC | Sy | | 2 | o | P | Ma | | COP | GH | | |
| | 6 | | D | 3 | | | Cg | | | | o | | F | | | | | |
| | 7 | < | Dd | 23 | SR | | A | | | 2 | u | | FMa | | | | | |
| IV | 8 | | W | | | | (H) | | | | o | P | C' | | AGC | GH | | |
| | 9 | | D | 2 | | | Cg | | | | u | | F | | | | | |
| | 10 | | D | 1 | | | NC | | | | u | | F | | | | | |
| V | 11 | | W | | | | A | | | | o | P | F | | | | | |
| | 12 | | Dd | 34 | | | Ad | | | | u | | FMp | | PER | | ODL | |
| VI | 13 | | D | 1 | | | NC | | | | o | | V | | | | | |
| | 14 | | D | 8 | | | A | | | | u | | F | | | | | |
| | 15 | | Dd | 31 | | | (Hd) | | | 2 | u | | F | | | GH | | |
| VII | 16 | v | D | 7 | SR | | Hd,Cg | Sy | | | u | | F | | | PH | | |
| | 17 | | D | 1 | | | NC | | | 2 | u | | F | | | | ODL | |
| VIII | 18 | | D | 1 | | | A | | | 2 | o | | FMa | | | | | |
| | 19 | | D | 3 | SR | | An | | | | o | | F | | | | | |
| IX | 20 | | D | 3 | | | (H),Cg | Sy | | 2 | o | P | F | | | GH | | |
| | 21 | | Dd | 99 | | | Hd | | | | - | | F | | | PH | | |
| | 22 | | Dd | 35 | | | A | | | 2 | u | | FMp,FC | | | | | |
| X | 23 | | D | 11 | | | Ay,NC | | | | o | | C' | | | | | |
| | 24 | | D | 9 | | | A | | | 2 | o | | FC | | | | | |
| | 25 | | D | 1 | | | A | | | 2 | o | P | CF | INC1 | | | | |
| | 26 | | D | 13,15,7 | | | NC | | | | u | | CF | | | | | |

©2010-2016 R-PAS

# R-PAS Summary Scores and Profiles – Page 1

C-ID: Julie (Mother)  P-ID: 4  Age: NA  Gender: Female  Education: NA

| Domain/Variables | Raw Scores | Raw %ile | Raw SS | Cplx. Adj. %ile | Cplx. Adj. SS | Standard Score Profile R-Optimized | Abbr. |
|---|---|---|---|---|---|---|---|
| **Admin. Behaviors and Obs.** | | | | | | | |
| Pr | 0 | 24 | 89 | | | | Pr |
| Pu | 0 | 40 | 96 | | | | Pu |
| CT (Card Turning) | 3 | 51 | 100 | | | | CT |
| **Engagement and Cog. Processing** | | | | | | | |
| Complexity | 70 | 49 | 100 | | | | Cmplx |
| R (Responses) | 26 | 69 | 107 | 67 | 106 | | R |
| F% [Lambda=1.00] (Simplicity) | 50% | 71 | 108 | 65 | 106 | | F% |
| Blend | 2 | 28 | 91 | 28 | 91 | | Bln |
| Sy | 5 | 37 | 95 | 43 | 97 | | Sy |
| MC | 5.0 | 31 | 92 | 31 | 92 | | MC |
| MC - PPD | -4.0 | 33 | 93 | 34 | 94 | | MC-PPD |
| M | 1 | 13 | 83 | 9 | 79 | | M |
| M/MC [1/5.0] | 20% | 9 | 80 | 10 | 80 | | M Prp |
| (CF+C)/SumC [3/5] | 60% | 61 | 104 | 61 | 104 | | CFC Prp |
| **Perception and Thinking Problems** | | | | | | | |
| EII-3 | -1.0 | 11 | 82 | 20 | 87 | | EII |
| TP-Comp (Thought & Percept. Com...) | -0.4 | 9 | 80 | 14 | 84 | | TP-C |
| WSumCog | 2 | 24 | 89 | 26 | 90 | | WCog |
| SevCog | 0 | 35 | 94 | 35 | 94 | | Sev |
| FQ-% | 4% | 16 | 85 | 27 | 91 | | FQ-% |
| WD-% | 0% | 11 | 82 | 11 | 82 | | WD-% |
| FQo% | 50% | 25 | 90 | 17 | 85 | | FQo% |
| P | 5 | 39 | 96 | 49 | 99 | | P |
| **Stress and Distress** | | | | | | | |
| YTVC' | 3 | 36 | 95 | 36 | 95 | | YTVC' |
| m | 2 | 66 | 106 | 58 | 103 | | m |
| Y | 0 | 17 | 85 | 17 | 85 | | Y |
| MOR | 0 | 18 | 86 | 18 | 86 | | MOR |
| SC-Comp (Suicide Concern Comp.) | 3.9 | 29 | 92 | 30 | 92 | | SC-C |
| **Self and Other Representation** | | | | | | | |
| ODL% | 8% | 40 | 96 | 43 | 97 | | ODL% |
| SR (Space Reversal) | 4 | 97 | 127 | 97 | 127 | | SR |
| MAP/MAHP [0/0] | NA | | | | | | MAP Prp |
| PHR/GPHR [2/6] | 33% | 50 | 100 | 50 | 100 | | PHR Prp |
| M- | 0 | 36 | 95 | 36 | 95 | | M- |
| AGC | 2 | 34 | 94 | 32 | 93 | | AGC |
| H | 1 | 21 | 88 | 18 | 86 | | H |
| COP | 1 | 54 | 102 | 60 | 104 | | COP |
| MAH | 0 | 26 | 90 | 26 | 90 | | MAH |

274

## R-PAS Summary Scores and Profiles – Page 2

C-ID: Julie (Mother)  P-ID: 4  Age: NA  Gender: Female  Education: NA

| Domain/Variables | Raw Scores | Raw %ile | Raw SS | Cplx. Adj. %ile | Cplx. Adj. SS | Standard Score Profile R-Optimized | Abbr. |
|---|---|---|---|---|---|---|---|
| **Engagement and Cog. Processing** | | | | | | 60 70 80 90 100 110 120 130 140 | |
| W% | 12% | 7 | 78 | 10 | 81 | | W% |
| Dd% | 23% | 77 | 111 | 78 | 111 | | Dd% |
| SI (Space Integration) | 1 | 18 | 86 | 30 | 92 | | SI |
| IntCont | 1 | 31 | 93 | 33 | 94 | | IntC |
| Vg% | 0% | 18 | 86 | 18 | 86 | | Vg% |
| V | 1 | 72 | 109 | 63 | 105 | | V |
| FD | 0 | 21 | 88 | 33 | 93 | | FD |
| R8910% | 35% | 72 | 109 | 71 | 108 | | R8910% |
| WSumC | 4.0 | 64 | 105 | 64 | 105 | | WSC |
| C | 0 | 36 | 95 | 36 | 95 | | C |
| Mp/(Ma+Mp) [0/1] | NA | | | | | | Mp Prp |
| **Perception and Thinking Problems** | | | | | | 60 70 80 90 100 110 120 130 140 | |
| FQu% | 46% | 92 | 121 | 94 | 123 | | FQu% |
| **Stress and Distress** | | | | | | 60 70 80 90 100 110 120 130 140 | |
| PPD | 9 | 51 | 101 | 55 | 102 | | PPD |
| CBlend | 0 | 28 | 91 | 28 | 91 | | CBlnd |
| C' | 2 | 62 | 105 | 55 | 102 | | C' |
| V | 1 | 72 | 109 | 63 | 105 | | V |
| CritCont% (Critical Contents) | 12% | 31 | 93 | 35 | 94 | | CrCt |
| **Self and Other Representation** | | | | | | 60 70 80 90 100 110 120 130 140 | |
| SumH | 6 | 53 | 101 | 58 | 103 | | SumH |
| NPH/SumH [5/6] | 83% | 88 | 117 | 84 | 115 | | NPH Prp |
| V-Comp (Vigilance Composite) | 3.7 | 66 | 106 | 70 | 108 | | V-C |
| r (Reflections) | 0 | 36 | 95 | 36 | 95 | | r |
| p/(a+p) [2/7] | 29% | 28 | 91 | 27 | 90 | | p Prp |
| AGM | 0 | 31 | 93 | 31 | 93 | | AGM |
| T | 0 | 28 | 91 | 28 | 91 | | T |
| PER | 1 | 72 | 109 | 72 | 109 | | PER |
| An | 1 | 47 | 99 | 47 | 99 | | An |

## Rorschach Responses "Peter" (Father)

| Respondent ID: Peter (Father) | Examiner: S. Margaret Lee, PhD |
|---|---|
| Location: Office | Date: **/**/**** |
| Start Time: 2:00 P.M. | End Time: 3:05 P.M. |

| Cd # | R # | Or | Response | Clarification | R-Opt |
|---|---|---|---|---|---|
| I | 1 | | Two birds flying. (D2) | E: (Examiner Repeats Response [ERR].) <br> R: Beak (Dd28), wings (Dd34). <br> E: Flying? <br> R: Wing-like structure, feathers sticking out. <br> E: Sticking out? <br> R: Triangular shape sticking out (extensions to Dd24). | |
| | 2 | | Person in the middle with two people dancing around her. (W) | E: (ERR) <br> R: Person in the middle (D4), female because it looks like she's wearing a dress, with hands raised (D1). <br> E: Other people? <br> R: Head (Dd28), arms outstretched (Dd34), bent knees (at Dd35) as though leaping, cape. <br> E: Cape? <br> R: Triangular. (Dd34) | |
| II | 3 | | Two men doing a high five. (W) | E: (ERR) <br> R: Shape of the bodies (D6), hands (D4) coming together in the middle, hat (D2), face (DdS30), with a little eye (small mark from the bottom of D2). | |
| | 4 | | Two guys doing a traditional Russian dance. (W) | E: (ERR) <br> R: Hat (D2), head (DdS30), bent knee (Dd28), like kicking out. <br> E: Russian dancing? <br> R: Similar with head, hat, hands (D4) together. | |
| III | 5 | | Cheshire cat face, smiling. (W) | E: (ERR) <br> R: Ears (D2), eyes (Dd32), nose (D3), smiling mouth (lower 1/3 of W) with mouth open (DdS23s) and smiling lips (ink around DdS23s). | |
| | 6 | | Red butterflies, flying around. (D2,3) | E: (ERR) <br> R: The center one (D3) looks like a butterfly because of the wings, and the others (D2) look like they could be turned to the side, all associated because of the red. | |
| IV | 7 | | Giant duck-billed platypus. (D7) | E: (ERR) <br> R: Shape of the head (D3) with a bill (Dd30), short stubby wings (D4). <br> E: Giant duck-billed platypus? <br> R: Big, long legs with big feet (D2). [E could have queried "long legs" for FD.] | |
| | 8 | | Guy riding a motorcycle towards me. (W) | E: (ERR) <br> R: Handlebars (D4), front tires (D1), head (D3), big, long legs with feet (D2) up. Looks like coming towards me because of the position of the legs and the front tire. | |
| V | 9 | | Two alligator heads, crawling out of the swamp. (D4) | E: (ERR) <br> R: Swamp (inner half of D4). <br> E: Swamp? <br> R: Muddy and black. Alligator heads (outer half of D4). <br> E: Alligator heads? <br> R: Long snouts with open jaws. | |
| | 10 | | Moth, flying. (Dd99 = W – D10) | E: (ERR) <br> R: (Outlined, excluding D10) Wing structures with two little legs (D9) and a head (Dd30) with antenna (Dd34). | |

276

| Cd # | R # | Or | Response | Clarification | R-Opt |
|------|-----|-----|----------|---------------|-------|
| VI | 11 | | Small, flattened animal, like road kill. (D1) | E: (ERR)<br>R: Back of the animal, shape of the legs (Dd24, 25), splayed. | |
| | 12 | | Native American doing a traditional dance, holding a totem above his head. (W) | E: (ERR)<br>R: Legs (Dd24), arms (Dd31) holding totem (D3), straight pole structure with feathers (Dd22).<br>E: Feathers?<br>R: Just the jagged shape. The guy looks like he's wearing an animal pelt.<br>E: Pelt?<br>R: Furry shape (respondent rubs card) and legs sticking out. | |
| VII | 13 | | Two squirrel-like figures, standing back to back with arms waving. (W) | E: (ERR)<br>R: Head (D9) with mouth open, arm (D5) sticking up, another arm (Dd21), mouth open, torso and back of body (D4+D3). [Client made arm movements consistent with what a squirrel would do.] | |
| | 14 | | Large, decorative necklace. (W) | E: (ERR)<br>R: Clasp (D5), the shape of the shells or some decorative material on each side. | |
| VIII | 15 | | Small animals climbing up the side of a cliff. (W) | E: (ERR)<br>R: Two animals (D1) with front legs, head, and looks furry.<br>E: Furry?<br>R: Because of jagged sides (respondent indicates edges). Rest looks like might be a cliff. (D6)<br>E: Cliff?<br>R: Just 'cause of outcropping and jagged. | |
| | 16 | | Underside of a tropical bird. (W) | E: (ERR)<br>R: Mostly different colors make it look tropical and the shape of the tail (D7), wings (D1). Beak and head (Dd24 area), wings, and looks like a tail. | |
| IX | 17 | | Building on fire. (D3,11,8) | E: (ERR)<br>R: Flames. (D3)<br>E: Flames?<br>R: Look like random shapes like flames licking, and the color. Billowing smoke (D11) looks like it's spreading out, and the grayish color. Center might be the general shape of the structure. (D8) | |
| | 18 | | Two old ladies, heads, facing away from each other. (W) | E: (ERR)<br>R: Head (D1) with nose, this (DdS29) is the eye, chin, part of the shoulders (D6). The orange would be hair (D3).<br>E: Hair?<br>R: On top and reddish color and crazy looking.<br>E: Old?<br>R: Cause the contour is not smooth. | |
| X | 19 | | Plaza around the Eiffel Tower. (DdS22) | E: (ERR)<br>R: (Respondent outlines). This (DdS30) is a white path with the red part on the sides (D9) would be the vendors and shops, not so defined but delineates the path.<br>E: Eiffel Tower?<br>R: Eiffel Tower (D11) because the gray color and triangular shape. I don't know what the yellow, blue, and green would be, maybe just more vendors and . . . I don't know. [E could have queried "the path" for FD.] | |
| | 20 | | Angry mouse soldier. (Dd22) | E: (ERR)<br>R: Helmet (D11), nose (top part of D3), eyes (Dd99 = inner lower protrusions of D8), mouth (the rest of D3), coat (D9), legs (D10). Same area, but half-open eyes make it look angry, and nose with frowning mouth, ready to bite. It would be a steel helmet because the color is metallic.<br>E: Metallic?<br>R: Grey. Red coat around his shoulders, blue looks like a breastplate (D6) across the chest. | |

277

# Rorschach Performance Assessment System (R-PAS)®

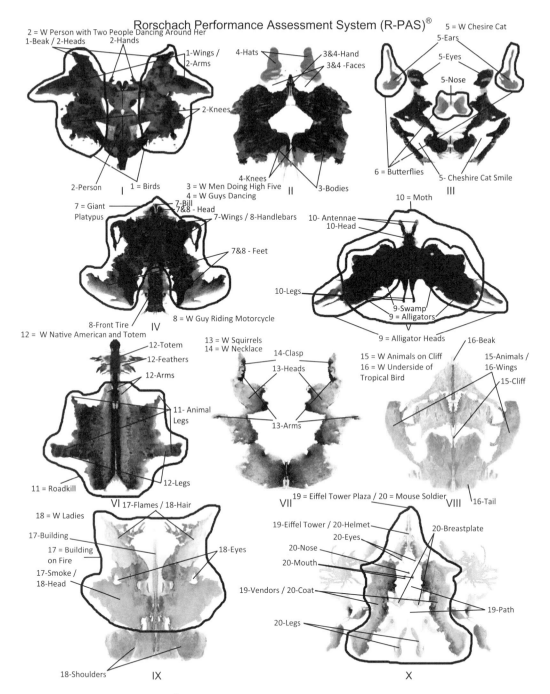

2 = W Person with Two People Dancing Around Her
1-Beak / 2-Heads
2-Hands
1-Wings / 2-Arms
4-Hats
3&4-Hand
3&4 -Faces
5 = W Chesire Cat
5-Ears
5-Eyes
5-Nose
2-Knees
2-Person
1 = Birds
4-Knees
3 = W Men Doing High Five
4 = W Guys Dancing
3-Bodies
6 = Butterflies
5- Cheshire Cat Smile
I
II
III

7 = Giant Platypus
7-Bill
7&8 - Head
7-Wings / 8-Handlebars
7&8 - Feet
8-Front Tire
8 = W Guy Riding Motorcycle
IV
10 = Moth
10- Antennae
10-Head
10-Legs
9-Swamp
9 = Alligators
9 = Alligator Heads

12 = W Native American and Totem
12-Totem
12-Feathers
12-Arms
11- Animal Legs
11 = Roadkill
12-Legs
VI

13 = W Squirrels
14 = W Necklace
14-Clasp
13-Heads
13-Arms
VII

15 = W Animals on Cliff
16 = W Underside of Tropical Bird
16-Beak
15-Animals / 16-Wings
15-Cliff
16-Tail
VIII

17-Flames / 18-Hair
18 = W Ladies
17-Building
17 = Building on Fire
17-Smoke / 18-Head
18-Eyes
18-Shoulders
IX

19 = Eiffel Tower Plaza / 20 = Mouse Soldier
19-Eiffel Tower / 20-Helmet
20-Eyes
20-Breastplate
20-Nose
20-Mouth
19-Vendors / 20-Coat
19-Path
20-Legs
X

# R-PAS Code Sequence: "Peter" (Father)

**C-ID**: Peter (Father)  **P-ID**: 5  **Age**: **  **Gender**: Male  **Education**:

| Cd | # | Or | Loc | Loc # | SR | SI | Content | Sy | Vg | 2 | FQ | P | Determinants | Cognitive | Thematic | HR | ODL (RP) | R-Opt | Text |
|---|---|---|---|---|---|---|---|---|---|---|---|---|---|---|---|---|---|---|---|
| I | 1 | | D | 2 | | | A | | | 2 | o | | FMa | | | | | | |
| | 2 | | W | | | | H,Cg | Sy | | 2 | o | | Ma-p | | COP | GH | | | |
| II | 3 | | W | | SR | SI | H,Cg | Sy | | 2 | o | | Ma | | COP,MAH | GH | | | |
| | 4 | | W | | SR | SI | H,Ay,Cg | Sy | | 2 | o | | Ma | | COP,MAH | GH | | | |
| III | 5 | | W | | | SI | (Ad) | | | | - | | Mp | | | PH | ODL | | |
| | 6 | | D | 2,3 | | | A | Sy | | 2 | - | | FMa,FC | | | | | | |
| IV | 7 | | D | 7 | | | A | | | | u | | F | INC1 | | | ODL | | * |

Comment: E could have queried 'long legs' for FD.

| | 8 | | W | | | | H,NC | Sy | | | o | | Ma,FD | | | GH | | | |
| V | 9 | | D | 4 | | | Ad,NC | Sy | | 2 | u | | FMa,C' | | AGC | | | | |
| | 10 | | Dd | 99 | | | A | | | | o | | FMa | | | | | | |
| VI | 11 | | D | 1 | | | A | | | | o | P | F | | MOR,MAP | | | | |
| | 12 | | W | | | | H,Ad,Ay | Sy | | | - | P | Ma,T | | | PH | ODL | | |
| VII | 13 | | W | | | | A | Sy | | 2 | u | | FMa | | | | | | |
| | 14 | | W | | | | Art,Cg | | | | u | | F | | | | | | |
| VIII | 15 | | W | | | | A,NC | Sy | | 2 | o | P | FMa | | | | | | |
| | 16 | | W | | | | A | | | | - | | CF | | | | | | |
| IX | 17 | | D | 3,8,11 | | | Fi,NC | Sy | | | u | | ma,CF,C' | | AGC,MAP | | | | |
| | 18 | | W | | | SI | Hd | | | 2 | u | | FC | | | PH | | | |
| X | 19 | | Dd | 22 | SR | SI | Ay,NC | Sy | | | u | | C' | | | | | | * |

Comment: E could have queried "the path" for FD.

| | 20 | | Dd | 22 | SR | SI | A,Cg,NC | Sy | | | - | | Ma,FC,C' | INC2 | AGM,AGC | PH | | | * |

Comment: This response contains elements of both an INC2 (angry mouse soldier) and FAB1 (mouse wearing a helmet and breastplate). They are intertwined in this response so only one was coded. They each have a weight of 4, so the more severe Level 2 code was assigned.

©2010-2016 R-PAS

**C-ID:** Peter (Father)    **P-ID:** 5    **Age:** NA    **Gender:** Male    **Education:** NA

| Domain/Variables | Raw Scores | Raw %ile | Raw SS | Cplx. Adj. %ile | Cplx. Adj. SS | Standard Score Profile R-Optimized | Abbr. |
|---|---|---|---|---|---|---|---|
| **Admin. Behaviors and Obs.** | | | | | | | |
| Pr | 0 | 24 | 89 | | | | Pr |
| Pu | 0 | 40 | 96 | | | | Pu |
| CT (Card Turning) | 0 | 18 | 86 | | | | CT |
| **Engagement and Cog. Processing** | | | | | | | |
| Complexity | 92 | 79 | 112 | | | | Cmplx |
| R (Responses) | 20 | 21 | 88 | 3 | 70 | | R |
| F% [Lambda=0.18] (Simplicity) | 15% | 5 | 75 | 13 | 83 | | F% |
| Blend | 6 | 75 | 110 | 53 | 101 | | Bln |
| Sy | 12 | 91 | 120 | 77 | 111 | | Sy |
| MC | 10.5 | 82 | 114 | 60 | 104 | | MC |
| MC - PPD | -1.5 | 56 | 102 | 60 | 104 | | MC-PPD |
| M | 7 | 88 | 118 | 72 | 109 | | M |
| M/MC [7/10.5] | 67% | 74 | 110 | 73 | 109 | | M Prp |
| (CF+C)/SumC [2/5] | 40% | 37 | 95 | 37 | 95 | | CFC Prp |
| **Perception and Thinking Problems** | | | | | | | |
| EII-3 | 1.1 | 92 | 121 | 91 | 121 | | EII |
| TP-Comp (Thought & Percept. Com...) | 2.5 | 97 | 128 | 96 | 126 | | TP-C |
| WSumCog | 6 | 50 | 100 | 39 | 96 | | WCog |
| SevCog | 1 | 80 | 113 | 80 | 113 | | Sev |
| FQ-% | 25% | 97 | 129 | 97 | 128 | | FQ-% |
| WD-% | 24% | 98 | 132 | 95 | 125 | | WD-% |
| FQo% | 40% | 7 | 78 | 6 | 77 | | FQo% |
| P | 3 | 9 | 80 | 11 | 81 | | P |
| **Stress and Distress** | | | | | | | |
| YTVC' | 5 | 61 | 104 | 42 | 97 | | YTVC' |
| m | 1 | 42 | 97 | 14 | 84 | | m |
| Y | 0 | 17 | 85 | 17 | 85 | | Y |
| MOR | 1 | 51 | 100 | 39 | 95 | | MOR |
| SC-Comp (Suicide Concern Comp.) | 6.1 | 82 | 114 | 74 | 110 | | SC-C |
| **Self and Other Representation** | | | | | | | |
| ODL% | 15% | 71 | 108 | 67 | 106 | | ODL% |
| SR (Space Reversal) | 4 | 97 | 127 | 97 | 127 | | SR |
| MAP/MAHP [2/4] | 50% | 48 | 99 | 49 | 99 | | MAP Prp |
| PHR/GPHR [4/8] | 50% | 76 | 111 | 76 | 111 | | PHR Prp |
| M- | 3 | 97 | 129 | 97 | 129 | | M- |
| AGC | 3 | 49 | 100 | 43 | 98 | | AGC |
| H | 5 | 89 | 119 | 79 | 112 | | H |
| COP | 3 | 91 | 120 | 87 | 117 | | COP |
| MAH | 2 | 86 | 116 | 68 | 107 | | MAH |

© 2010-2016 R-PAS

# R-PAS Summary Scores and Profiles – Page 2

C-ID: Peter (Father)  P-ID: 5  Age: NA  Gender: Male  Education: NA

| Domain/Variables | Raw Scores | Raw %ile | Raw SS | Cplx. Adj. %ile | Cplx. Adj. SS | Standard Score Profile R-Optimized | Abbr. |
|---|---|---|---|---|---|---|---|
| **Engagement and Cog. Processing** | | | | | | | |
| W% | 55% | 76 | 110 | 67 | 107 | | W% |
| Dd% | 15% | 56 | 102 | 61 | 104 | | Dd% |
| SI (Space Integration) | 6 | 94 | 123 | 94 | 123 | | SI |
| IntCont | 4 | 79 | 112 | 71 | 108 | | IntC |
| Vg% | 0% | 18 | 86 | 18 | 86 | | Vg% |
| V | 0 | 29 | 92 | 29 | 92 | | V |
| FD | 1 | 60 | 104 | 54 | 102 | | FD |
| R8910% | 30% | 37 | 95 | 40 | 96 | | R8910% |
| WSumC | 3.5 | 56 | 102 | 37 | 95 | | WSC |
| C | 0 | 36 | 95 | 36 | 95 | | C |
| Mp/(Ma+Mp) [2/8] | 25% | 23 | 89 | 23 | 89 | | Mp Prp |
| **Perception and Thinking Problems** | | | | | | | |
| FQu% | 35% | 69 | 107 | 65 | 106 | | FQu% |
| **Stress and Distress** | | | | | | | |
| PPD | 12 | 73 | 109 | 53 | 101 | | PPD |
| CBlend | 2 | 88 | 117 | 73 | 109 | | CBlnd |
| C' | 4 | 88 | 117 | 78 | 112 | | C' |
| V | 0 | 29 | 92 | 29 | 92 | | V |
| CritCont% (Critical Contents) | 15% | 40 | 96 | 32 | 93 | | CrCt |
| **Self and Other Representation** | | | | | | | |
| SumH | 6 | 53 | 101 | 34 | 94 | | SumH |
| NPH/SumH [1/6] | 17% | 4 | 73 | 4 | 74 | | NPH Prp |
| V-Comp (Vigilance Composite) | 4.3 | 80 | 113 | 63 | 105 | | V-C |
| r (Reflections) | 0 | 36 | 95 | 36 | 95 | | r |
| p/(a+p) [2/15] | 13% | 7 | 78 | 7 | 78 | | p Prp |
| AGM | 1 | 75 | 110 | 75 | 110 | | AGM |
| T | 1 | 68 | 107 | 68 | 107 | | T |
| PER | 0 | 30 | 92 | 30 | 92 | | PER |
| An | 0 | 16 | 85 | 16 | 85 | | An |

© 2010-2016 R-PAS

# CHAPTER 14

# Using R-PAS in the Assessment
# of Psychological Variables in Domestic Violence

Nancy Kaser-Boyd
Reneau Kennedy

Domestic violence is an ongoing and serious problem. Intimate partner violence, defined as physical, sexual, or psychological abuse by a current or former romantic partner, affects millions of women and men (Smith et al., 2017). In the United States, the lifetime prevalence of intimate partner violence—including rape, physical violence, and/or stalking—is 35.6% for women and 28.5% for men (Black et al., 2011). Some of these cases result in homicide. In the United States, 35% of murdered women were killed by a spouse or ex-spouse; males were responsible for 83% of spousal murderers and comprised 75% of the murderers who killed a boyfriend or girlfriend (Bureau of Justice Statistics, 2015).

The assessment clinician can receive referrals regarding domestic violence from many avenues. Individuals involved in domestic violence may be self-referred and come for therapy. They may be referred by the dependency courts after child protective services has intervened to protect the children. They may be referred by criminal court after the police have intervened in a domestic violence incident. Women claiming domestic violence may seek expert opinions to file tort claims in civil court against a violent husband or to invalidate a prenuptial agreement. Domestic violence may be raised in divorce cases, where "best interest" considerations for timesharing of the children are made by the court; in some states, allegations of domestic violence are lodged to avoid spousal support or to obtain full custody of children. (See Lee, Chapter 13, this volume, for a discussion of the use of the Rorschach in child custody cases.) The present chapter addresses how Rorschach Performance Assessment System (R-PAS; Meyer, Viglione, Mihura, Erard, & Erdberg, 2011) data can be useful when the question of domestic violence has been raised and how R-PAS can help us understand individuals and their functioning in the wake of such histories. This knowledge is applied to a forensic case wherein a mother has been charged with contempt of court for refusing the father visitation rights with their child.

## Domestic Violence

Domestic violence exists on a spectrum from mild to severe. At the mild end, there can be shoving, pushing, hitting, hair pulling, and psychological insults. At the more extreme end, there can be severe beating; choking; burning; threats against family, pets, and children; and lethal violence. Coercive control, sexual coercion, and economic abuse are often present and often occur without physical violence. In some domestic violence situations the threat and danger exist even after the partners separate, in the form of stalking, threats, or financial abuse. The perpetrator often has a great deal of anger, and the recipient, a great deal of fear.

A complicated picture has developed over years of domestic violence research that emphasizes that all domestic violence is not the same. Four patterns of domestic violence have emerged in the intimate partner violence (IPV) literature (Kelly & Johnson, 2008):

1. *Coercive controlling violence.* This is classic battering, characterized by a unilateral pattern of intimidation, coercion, control, and emotional abuse to dominate the other partner. This type of abuse usually does not stop with separation. It can continue with stalking, harassment, and attempts to win custody of children.
2. *Separation-instigated violence.* IPV incidents begin at the time of the separation, without a previous history of abusive power and control in the relationship.
3. *Situational couple violence.* Incidents emerge from conflict, but power and control are not central to the dynamic. Serious injuries are uncommon.
4. *Violent resistance.* The use of violence as self-defense against an abuser who is using violence or coercive control.

### The Victim

The general domestic violence research and clinical literature is overwhelmingly about women, as women are the predominant victims of domestic violence. The areas most researched are the personality dynamics of a battered woman and the *effects* of domestic violence, now referred to as the effects of IPV. There are certain myths about battered women. For example, a battered woman might be seen as unusually passive or dependent. Some authors (Walker, 1979) use the term "learned helplessness" to describe a passive, resigned quality. Bornstein (2006) asserts that economic dependency in women contributes to the risk of domestic violence. There is no one personality characteristic or set of characteristics that predisposes a woman to become abused, although risk factors include a history of childhood victimization (physical or sexual), knowledge of the mother's abuse, absent father, history of bullying, and severe health issues (Kaser-Boyd, 2007).

By the time a referral to a clinician is generated, effects of the abuse are likely to be seen. Living in a violent and threatening relationship creates strong emotions (e.g., fear or intense ambivalence) and dramatic methods of coping (denial, emotional numbing, avoidance, substance abuse). Because violent episodes can occur at any time, battered women have a high level of anticipatory anxiety punctuated by moments or hours of extreme fear or terror. The effects of such anxiety and fear can include impaired cognitive functions (attention, concentration), impaired sleep, anxiety-related somatic symptoms, and hypervigilance to danger. Fear and constant anxiety have a biological effect on the person (see Kaser-Boyd, 2007). Battered women often feel trapped. That is, although living with an abusive partner is frightening, leaving is often more frightening because of threats to kill the woman, pets, or her family. Battered women often feel profoundly devalued, worthless, and shameful. The experience of physical injury and violent sexual assault often results in feelings of fragmentation with permeable body boundaries.

Individuals who have experienced life-threatening abuse may have posttraumatic stress disorder (PTSD), and those for whom the threatening events have been prolonged may have the "associated features" of PTSD, including impaired affect modulation, self-destructive and impulsive behavior, dissociative experiences, damaged sense of self, and a loss in systems of meaning (Herman, 1992). Numerous clinical case and research studies have delineated the effects of being battered (Kaser-Boyd, 2007; Walker, 1979).

## The Perpetrator

There is no single personality characteristic, or set of personality characteristics, that constitute a "batterer." There are clinical descriptions of the "typical" batterer and studies that delineate typologies of batterers, which can inform the evaluator and generate hypotheses about potential Rorschach scores. The earliest studies of batterers (Walker, 1979), which consisted of clinical case studies, indicated that they came from homes where the male role model(s) used violence in family disputes and had little regard for women's needs or rights. Batterers were described as controlling, jealous, angry, blaming, suspicious, and markedly self-centered. They were said to have a poor tolerance for frustration of their needs and poor empathy for the distress they caused in others. Bornstein (2006) found that emotional dependency in a man increased the risk of domestic violence. A number of studies now indicate that batterers are not all the same and can be classified into subtypes. Holtzworth-Munroe and Stuart (1994) examined existing male batterer typologies to determine the subtypes that consistently appear across typological models and to identify underlying descriptive dimensions, including (1) severity and frequency of spousal physical violence, (2) generality of violence (i.e., family vs. extrafamilial violence), and (3) the batterer's psychopathology or personality disorder. On the basis of this review, they suggested three major subtypes of batterers, which were labeled "family only," "dysphoric/borderline," and "generally violent/antisocial." These three subtypes have been replicated by multiple studies, and a fourth subtype, "low level antisocial," emerges in samples derived from the general community versus those derived from clinical samples and extremely violent men (Holtzworth-Munroe, Meehan, Herron, Rehman, & Stuart, 2000).

## The Case Referral

"Jane," a 31-year-old woman, and "John," a 32-year-old man, were referred by the court after multiple cross-complaints of domestic violence. Jane was arrested after she refused to allow John to pick up their 8-year-old daughter for a court-ordered visitation. The two had been married for 4 years and were divorced at the time of the evaluations. Jane reported continuing threats and stalking by John to the police. She also alleged that their daughter was injured during the child's summer vacation stay with her father. Because of her fears, Jane refused to send their daughter on her court-ordered visitation. She had been charged with contempt of court and her attorney obtained a court order for the psychological evaluation of Jane. The evaluator requested that she be allowed to evaluate John as well, noting that this would be the best way to sort through the various cross-complaints, and his lawyer consented to this.

### Relevant History

*Jane*

Jane was a woman of above-average intelligence who was working toward a bachelor's degree. Her speech was fast-paced, quick-witted, and glib. Her mood was worried, anxious, upset, and sometimes overwhelmed. Her thought process was heavily affect-laden, but there was no sign of thought disorder. Trust of others was an issue, likely stemming from Jane's mother's departure from the family when Jane was 2. Jane's father remarried several years later, and Jane reports she was sexually molested by her stepbrother at age 8. As a preteen, she became suicidal and cut herself with scissors. Collateral records indicate that Jane was placed in a state psychiatric setting for 2 years as a preadolescent before she was returned to her father's custody. Within a short time after Jane returned to her father's care, she was charged as a teenager with an assault on her father. Because Jane's father claimed he could not adequately manage Jane's physical aggressiveness and frequent running away, the courts placed Jane in a juvenile detention facility followed by probation. Jane submitted documentation to become an emancipated child, and the courts granted her request. She reportedly lived out of a car from grades 10 through 12. Jane worked part-time to support herself. She graduated from high school with high marks and received a full-ride scholarship to college. Prior to her marriage to John, while still in college, she worked as an exotic dancer. She reported she was sexually and physically assaulted in the course of that work on two occasions.

Jane reported numerous incidents of domestic violence during her marriage to John. She claimed that when John returned from his second military deployment, he attempted to smother her with a pillow in her sleep. On another occasion, when their daughter was about 6 months old, she alleged that John pushed her down the stairs. In a separate domestic violence filing, Jane reported that John threw a knife at her, which landed in a door. She said that she made over 30 calls to the police about John, and the police had been to their home around 20 times. She claimed that she has had multiple hematomas noted by various doctors. She claimed that John was mandated to anger management classes by his military command.

When Jane tried to separate from John, she claimed that he would stalk her. She also claimed that John's friends assisted him in creating fictitious police reports against her. A criminal records search showed that none of Jane's arrests and charges resulted in a conviction. Because Jane and John shared custody of their daughter, they continued to have contact with one another. She reported that John continued to harass her by using her neighbors to spy on her, and that on one occasion John and his family followed her into a store and called her vulgar names.

Jane reported that she experienced a high level of anxiety about her daughter's safety when the child had visitations with John. Jane did not trust John and didn't want her daughter to spend time with him. She said that John has threatened to kill her if she tries to take their daughter from him.

### John

John appears to be of average to above-average intelligence. He enlisted in the military and was employed in a skilled position. He was easy to interview, proving to be logical and a good historian for dates and events. His stated he was worried about the legal proceedings between him and Jane. He was moderately guarded with the examiner about his emotions. John reported no childhood history of trauma and no history of domestic violence in his family of origin. He'd had no involvement with the juvenile court. John's father was a military officer. The family lived overseas during some of his father's deployments. John graduated from high school in the United States and attended a community college, after which he enlisted in the military. Although deployed, he did not see combat. There was no indication that he suffered trauma during his deployment.

John's marriage to Jane was his first. He denied perpetrating domestic violence in the marriage or after their separation and custody dispute. John claimed that Jane was making false allegations against him and she was systematically sabotaging his relationship with their daughter and his new wife. He claimed that Jane violated numerous court orders surrounding visitation and telephone contact. In one incident, he claimed that she refused to let their child get out of the car to go on visitation. The police became involved and threatened to arrest Jane if she did not allow the child to go with the father. According to John, former neighbors of the couple reported that Jane could become suddenly hostile with them. In one incident, John claimed that Jane spray-painted a neighbor's car after she and the neighbor had a disagreement.

## MMPI-2 and PAI Test Results for Jane and John

Both Jane and John were administered a battery of psychological tests that included the Minnesota Multiphasic Personality Inventory–2 (MMPI-2), Personality Assessment Inventory (PAI), and Rorschach Performance Assessment System (R-PAS) to elucidate their personality structure and psychological functioning. The findings from the psychological testing were used to address the credibility of each party's reports and formulate an intervention that might address each party's concerns. Before turning to the R-PAS findings, their MMPI-2 and PAI results are reviewed.

## Jane's Results

On the MMPI-2, Jane endorsed more disturbed items than the normative population (F = 85) and the psychiatric population (Fp = 89). Her profile type is associated with chronic maladjustment. Jane appears to harbor a significant amount of anger toward others, is resentful and mistrustful, sees the world as a dangerous place, and can be petulant and demanding (Scale 6 = 92). Jane appears to have many concerns about physical integrity and views her physical health as failing (Scale 1 = 80). She also has a potential for addiction (AAS = 73). Jane endorsed items reflecting a loss of control of thoughts and problems thinking clearly (Sc3 = 80). On the PAI, Jane appeared to have features of obsessive–compulsive disorder (ARD-O = 76), and a number of the physiological symptoms of depression (DEP-P = 67). She was not significantly elevated on symptoms of PTSD that are commonly seen in battered women (ARD-T = 60). However, she reports a predominance of unstable negative relationships (BOR-N = 65), a feature seen in those with borderline personality disorder. Given her report of being battered and threatened, it is interesting that she endorses statements consistent with having a dominant interpersonal style (DOM = 72) and inflated self-esteem (MAN-G = 79).

## John's Results

John completed the MMPI-2 without unusual defensiveness for a child custody dispute (K = 64). He reports that he has few psychological problems, and feels happy and in control of his life. Results suggest he has a low level of anxiety and is a risk taker (Scales 4 and 9 were the most elevated). He reported some problems with authority (Pd2 = 67) and appears to be somewhat impulsive (Scale 9 = 65). Despite these findings, he did not report traits of antisocial personality disorder (ASP1 = 40; ASP2 = 59). In interpersonal relationships, he is probably well liked, warm, and charming, but his relationships may be somewhat superficial and he may be somewhat manipulative (Scale 4 = 64). John's PAI was within normal limits, a finding probably influenced by a slight tendency toward positive impression management (PIM = 57). He is far less likely to have dominance as a personality trait than was Jane (DOM = 49). Given the referral question, it is important to note that his Violence Potential Index was not elevated (VPI = 43).

## Why R-PAS?

Self-report tests of personality may be unable to capture the personality dynamics of abusive partners or the effects of domestic violence. Years of research concerning what people say about themselves shows that it is often neither related to how they behave nor to how others see them (Mihura, 2012). As for the so-called "batterer," those referred by the court have a strong motivation to deny potentially problematic personality traits or behaviors. If the assessment referral is of a victim and survivor of domestic violence, the experience of trauma may result in greatly elevated self-report test profiles, which are likely situational, and do not accurately reflect the person's potential for coping and resilience.

R-PAS (Meyer et al., 2011) addresses both of these issues. For the defensive person, it has the potential to get underneath a person's psychological defenses, as the respondent usually does not know how Rorschach responses are coded, scored, or analyzed. For a perpetrator of domestic violence, the Rorschach provides data about variables such as aggressive ideation, reality testing, emotional control, self-focus, and capacity for insight. It is especially helpful in assessing the perception of human relationships. For a victim of domestic violence, the Rorschach can give valuable data about trauma, including one's sense of self (e.g., whole or fragmented, damaged), situational stress, depression, and feelings of helplessness. It can also provide helpful information about ego resilience. Importantly, R-PAS highlights the scores with the strongest meta-analytic support (e.g., Mihura, Meyer, Dumitrascu, & Bombel, 2013) by placing them on "Page 1" of the R-PAS Profile pages (Meyer et al., 2011).

## Expected Rorschach Results for Battered Women

What would we expect to find in the Rorschach protocols of battered women? We might think, first, of content. Looking for the effects of trauma, we might look at the R-PAS Critical Contents score. We might look at scores associated with anxiety, such as diffuse shading (Y) and inanimate movement (m). As for the damaged sense of self, we could look at the Morbid (MOR) score. The quality of human interactions will likely be important, as will whether human percepts are whole or part-human. With the Mutuality of Autonomy score (Urist, 1977), we might look at whether relationships are depicted as mutually enhancing and supportive, or negative and malevolent. We might look at the Oral Dependent Language score (Masling, Rabie, & Blondheim, 1967). Reality testing will likely be important, particularly whether the individual is inclined to misperceive reality.

There is currently no published Rorschach research on battered women or batterers using R-PAS. One Comprehensive System (CS) study (Kaser-Boyd, 1993) examined 28 battered women who killed their battering spouses and were awaiting trial. Subsequently, when the records were differentiated by complexity, signified by the CS Lambda score (F% in R-PAS), by dividing the sample into high-Lambda and low-Lambda groups, there were clear differences (Kaser-Boyd, 2007). Women with low-Lambda scores generated profiles that looked virtually psychotic. Their records were infused with morbid and aggressive images (e.g., bruised or bleeding bodies or body parts, threatening animals or malevolent creatures), images of entrapment, and a high level of inanimate movement. Those with high-Lambda records had an ambient and passive problem-solving style, intense and poorly modulated affect, poor scanning, and poor reality testing.

For survivors of severe trauma, the Rorschach research examining individuals with PTSD is important. A number of studies noted two types of records: those that were constricted or "coarctated," reflecting the avoidant symptoms of PTSD, and those that were "flooded," reflecting the reexperiencing symptoms of PTSD (Hartman et al., 1990; Swanson, Blount, & Bruno, 1990; van der Kolk, & Ducey, 1989). The flooded records in these studies were characterized by the extensive use of color and seemingly uncensored percepts of traumatic events, including numerous blood, anatomy, and morbid responses. The records, in general, in these studies exhibited perceptual distortion and ineffective coping strategies. Another common finding among these studies was an unusual number of inanimate movement responses, indicating the feeling of being the recipient of events caused by external forces.

## Expected Rorschach Results for Batterers

What might we expect in the Rorschach records of "batterers"? There are no published CS or R-PAS Rorschach studies of batterers. As noted, what exist are clinical descriptions of the dynamics of the subtypes of batterers. As previously noted, Holtzworth-Munroe and Stuart (1994) found three major subtypes of batterers—*family only, dysphoric/borderline,* and generally *violent/antisocial.* Due to overt antisocial and aggressive behaviors, the antisocial subtype is the easiest to identify. The family only and dysphoric/borderline batterers are hypothesized to have had chaotic or anxious early attachments (Dutton & Nicholls, 2005). These individuals may generate Rorschach responses that are unique in their depiction of human content: that is, a paucity of cooperative human movement and a greater number of aggressive human contents. They may deliver more scores associated with anxiety, and they may have higher Oral Dependent Language (ODL%) scores. A large number (80% or more) of batterers reportedly grew up in homes where there was domestic violence (Dutton & Nicholls, 2005; Walker, 1979), and they may have features of PTSD. The Rorschach protocols of this group of batterers may more closely resemble those of trauma survivors: that is, defensive and constricted, or with images of trauma and threat. In all three groups, the Mutuality of Autonomy Pathology (MAP) score, capturing the extent to which relationships are depicted as controlling, malevolent, hostile, or destructive, is likely to be a useful sample of how relationships are perceived. Aggressive Movement (AGM) and Aggressive Content (AGC) scores also can capture the extent to which such a person is mentally focused on aggression.

## R-PAS Findings for Jane and John[1]

### Test Administration and Scoring

The Rorschach was introduced to Jane and John as part of the overall test battery, with the explanation that psychological testing allows a forensic psychological evaluation to be based on more than just the evaluator's experience, broadening the scope to a larger data base. The Rorschach protocols were administered following standard R-PAS guidelines.

### Discussion of Jane's R-PAS Results

*Administration Behaviors and Observations*

Jane complied with the R-PAS instructions, with no Prompts or Pulls needed, by giving the minimal number of two responses per card for every card. She had a typical degree of willingness to interact with or manipulate the environment (CT SS[2] = 95).

---

[1]See Appendices 14.1 and 14.2, respectively, at the end of the chapter for Jane's and John's R-PAS Responses, Location Sheets, Code Sequences, and Page 1 and 2 Profiles.

[2]Standard scores (SS) have a mean of 100 and an *SD* of 15.

*Engagement and Cognitive Processing*

Jane's responses had an average level of Complexity, though she produced 20 responses, which was less than the average number of responses given by the typical adult (SS = 88). This may be due to defensiveness, a fearful inhibition to engage with the task, withdrawal secondary to depression or trauma, or cognitive rigidity secondary to anxiety. She had somewhat limited capacity to notice and articulate subtleties, nuances, and salient aspects of her perceptual environment (F% SS = 111), indicating that she may be less able than most to engage adequately with complex and subtle aspects of her experiences. However, she exhibited an average ability to process the experiential environment by simultaneously attending to its multiple features (Blend SS = 106). Seven of her responses were synthesized (Sy SS = 102). She had an average amount of enlivening thought and emotionally colored reactivity (MC SS = 101), which suggests average psychological resources and coping capacity to balance discomforting internal experiences. She had a slightly higher than average ability to envision human experiences and to reason and think before acting (M SS = 109), and she is somewhat more prone to reason and reflect than to react spontaneously to emotions or impulses (M/MC SS = 112). Emotional reactivity to stimuli appeared to be modulated by mental processing and cognitive control [(CF+C)/SumC SS = 91].

*Perception and Thinking Problems*

Jane appears to have logical and accurate cognitive processing and socially acceptable content of thought (EII-3 SS = 82). She is likely to see most things clearly and accurately, with organized thought processes (TP-Comp SS = 74), and logical and effective thinking and reasoning (WSumCog SS = 86). She displayed an average ability to see the external environment realistically (FQo% SS = 107), with a surprising absence of personalized distortion (FQ–% SS = 78), though at the same time tended not to attend to the most obvious and conventional features of the environment (P SS = 88).

*Stress and Distress*

Jane appears to have less sensitivity to the subtleties of her own internal experiences than most adults, or perhaps she suppresses her feelings (YTVC′ SS = 82). At the same time, a few potentially overlooked determinant-related queries may have contributed to a lower than expected YTVC′. Unlike other abuse survivors, she had no m responses, which occur following moderate to extreme stressors and can indicate unwanted, distracting ideation related to the trauma. She also does not appear to be experiencing implicit helplessness and distress (Y SS = 85). She does not display or report images of damage, injury, or sadness (MOR SS = 86). As with all variables in this domain, the relative absence of these markers on the Rorschach does not imply an absence of her having stressful experiences and discomforting emotion.

*Self and Other Representation*

Jane did not exhibit notable implicit dependency needs (ODL% SS = 108) or unusual needs for independence (SR SS = 102). She had an average number of images of whole human beings (H SS = 106) and did not display a tendency to misperceive human activity (M– SS = 95). Her one COP (SS = 102) indicates some potential to view rela-tionships as supportive and cooperative. Jane's representations of relationships did not fall on either the positive and healthy end of the spectrum or the pathological end (PHR/GPHR SS = 95; MAP Proportion was not computed because MAHP = 1). This finding suggests an average ability to understand herself and others and the potential for adequate interpersonal competence and skill in managing her relationships. This does not mean, however, that she maintains close and meaningful relationships or feels empathic toward others. Jane had aggressive images on her mind more than the typical person (AGC SS = 116), including a beetle with claws, a dragon, a boat with a military surface, a mountain lion, and "someone bad, wearing a mask." This eleva-tion suggests some concern about potential danger or harm, perhaps consistent with the hypervigilance of those who have experienced trauma.

### Other Variables

Although the R-PAS Page 2 variables have less empirical support, it is important to review these scores as a supplement to the Page 1 variables. Given the referral ques-tions, it is important to note that Jane gave an above-average number of Anatomy responses (SS = 116). On Card II, she saw a "pelvis bone." On Card VII, she saw an ultrasound of a uterus, and she referenced her pregnancy. On Cark VIII, she saw a "spine, like the x-ray of a back." These responses suggest vulnerability and a concern with physical wellness, which was also evident on the MMPI-2 Hs scale.

Jane was also slightly elevated on the scale of vigilance and guardedness (V-Comp SS = 114). She also gave an above-average number of Reflections (r = 2, SS = 122). On Card III she saw a "mirrored image of someone vacuuming the floor" and on Card VI she saw "a boat reflected in the water"). Although this response would not be seen in the typical battered woman, a heightened focus on or need for mirroring could reflect developmental arrest at a more childlike stage of development—a common finding in children who have been abused or neglected. Given her history of trauma in child-hood and adulthood, and her reports of domestic violence by John, it is important to note that her Critical Content Score is average (CritCont% SS = 102). However, research indicates that false negatives occur with this score, and it is most likely to be elevated when there has been severe trauma with dissociation (Meyer et al., 2011).

Additional idiographic content in Jane's responses reflect some of the inferences noted above. For instance, intersecting with her vigilance, a theme of hiding was evident, as there were two responses of masks and two instances where someone was hidden or obscured. Two responses also reflected highly polarized representations, with one being of a saint and the other of "someone bad." The percept of the "baby bat" with wings too big for its body is a representation of immaturity, though it may also reflect a vulnerability or insecurity. Finally, it is atypical to have two responses of gnomes, though it is not clear what significance that imagery may hold for her.

## Discussion of John's R-PAS Results

### Administration Behaviors and Observations

John needed three Prompts (SS = 119) while completing the task. This is unusual and, given his generally high intelligence, suggested a reluctance to spontaneously engage with the stimuli. However, he complied with the reminders and ultimately gave at least two responses per card. He never gave more than three responses to a card, resulting in no Pulls (SS = 96). He spontaneously turned the card twice, which is typical (CT SS = 98).

## Engagement and Cognitive Processing

John ultimately provided a 22-response protocol (SS = 96) that was average in Complexity (SS = 100). Again, given his high intelligence, a higher degree of Complexity would have been anticipated. He was slightly above average in his ability to articulate subtleties, nuances, and personally salient aspects of his experience (F% SS = 88), though average in terms of simultaneously attending to multiple features of his experiences (Blend SS = 102). His responses indicated that he has an average ability to meaningfully link together features of his experiences and identify relationships (Sy SS = 102). These responses were characterized by an average amount of enlivening thought and emotionally colored reactivity (MC SS = 103), which suggested average emotional resources and coping capacity, as well as the ability to balance his level of sensitivity to potentially distracting or discomforting internal experiences (MC–PPD SS = 92). He displayed an average ability to envision or imagine human experiences or activities and to think and reason before acting (M SS = 109), and his capacity to mentalize indicated that he is as able as most people to experience himself as the agent of his experiences and to take a cognitive perspective on the experiences of others. His responses indicated a roughly equivalent tendency to react spontaneously to emotions, impulses, or circumstances and to reflect and reason, with a tendency toward the latter (M/MC SS = 110).

## Perception and Thinking Problems

John's responses showed a low degree of general psychopathology that is similar to what is seen in the average person (EII-3 SS = 92). He displayed accurate thinking and reality testing (TP-Comp SS = 96) and did not produce any responses indicating significant lapses in conceptualization, reasoning, communication, or thought organization (SevCog SS = 94). In general, his perceptual accuracy was good. He had fewer instances of perceptual lapses or misperceptions than most people (FQ–% SS = 90), accompanied by an above-average proportion of responses that match the types of things seen regularly by others (FQo% SS = 118), and an average ability to recognize or identify the most conventional objects in his processing of events (P SS = 96).

## Stress and Distress

John showed an average sensitivity to the subtleties in one's internal or emotional life, but not to the degree that these sensitivities could interfere with adequate coping and adaptation (YTVC' SS = 108). At the same time, a few potentially overlooked determinant-related queries may have contributed to a lower than expected YTVC'. John's three C' responses suggested that he is drawn to dark stimuli more than most people; however, one C' was to the white parts of eyes, and two C' responses is within normal range (SS = 105). John had an above-average number of responses involving objects moving without volitional control (m = 3, SS = 113), suggesting that, at the time of testing, he was probably experiencing the kind of unwanted, distracting ideation that is associated with environmental stressors. At the same time, he did not appear to be experiencing increased implicit distress or helplessness (Y SS = 108) sometimes associated with environmental stress. His responses did not have notable themes or images of damage, injury, or sadness (MOR SS = 100).

### Self and Other Representation

John did not display noteworthy evidence of implicit dependency needs (ODL% SS = 89). He displayed an average capacity to perceive whole human beings (H SS = 106) and a much greater propensity to perceive images of cooperative and mutually beneficial interaction than most people (COP SS = 128, MAH SS = 134). His MAP Proportion (SS = 72) suggested an above-average capacity to envision relationships as mature and reciprocal as opposed to destructive or compromising. His PHR/GPHR is consistent (SS = 83), indicating that he is likely to envision people and relatedness in an adaptive or positive way. He may, on occasion, lapse into salient misunderstandings or misperceptions of people (M– = 113); his one M–, of a face "smiling at ya" on Card X, could indicate a particular context in which this lapse may occur. Given the referral question and Jane's depiction of John, it is important that he reported fewer aggressive images (AGC SS = 86) than is typical or than would be expected, given what was reported in the former couple's interpersonal history.

### Other Variables

In terms of Page 2 R-PAS variables, the most relevant to the referral question was pure color (C SS = 95). John's score indicated that there were no instances in which his response appeared to be based on unfettered reactivity to activating stimuli.

### Additional Considerations

Overall, John produced a relatively benign Rorschach protocol. In evaluating whether this is a true reflection of his personality functioning, we must consider that he required three prompts. His Card I responses of "camouflage" and "a mask" could similarly signal defensiveness. In addition, research indicates that it is possible to suppress aggressive content and replace it with positive content when the context supports doing so (Benjestorf, Viglione, Lamb, & Giromini, 2013).

## Summary of R-PAS Contributions

There is notable correspondence between the three tests given to each person. Jane's R-PAS converges with findings from the MMPI-2 and the PAI in describing her as somewhat vulnerable, concerned with physical integrity, and vigilant. R-PAS results indicate that she likely sees the world as a threatening place, and she is hypervigilant to danger, for herself and her daughter. The aggressive content of her Rorschach responses, scored AGC, could indicate the extent to which she scans the field for threat although having aggressive images on one's mind does not in itself indicate one's attitude toward it. Having aggressive images on her mind could stem from Jane's history of maternal neglect and sexual victimization, her report of domestic violence when married to John, or a combination of these experiences. Hypervigilance could cause her to overinterpret events, seeing them as more dangerous or malevolent than they are. Her elevated Anatomy score also indicates anxiety about physical integrity and perhaps harm. Her relatively significant self-focus may cause difficulty in understanding the needs and feelings of others. This might, for example, cause her to believe that her daughter has the same feelings as she has.

John's R-PAS scores indicate that he appears to be a person in generally good control, with enough resources to cope with stress. He may misperceive human motives and actions at times, but this does not appear to be a significant aspect of his functioning. He does not have the kind of Rorschach that might be seen in men who are habitually preoccupied with aggression, although research indicates that aggressive content can be suppressed in evaluative contexts like this and replaced with positive imagery, consistent with what was observed in his protocol.

John's test results (R-PAS, MMPI-2, and PAI) did not clearly indicate the type of pathology one would expect to see in either a man with poor emotional control or one who would plan ways to get Jane in trouble with the law (i.e., through false allegations). However, he may have been able to defend against revealing the pathological aspects of his personality. As with most allegations of domestic violence, it is best to try to substantiate them with evidence. Jane is a woman with multiple traumas across her lifespan. She has become hypervigilant to danger, and she is poised to respond in defense of her perceptions. This stance creates a provocative interpersonal environment where a former partner is viewed with suspicion. Empathy for the other person is weak. As for her legal troubles with violating court orders, a report might state that the actual allegations she makes against John cannot be verified with psychological testing, but that the test results do indicate that her traumatic life experiences have resulted in hypervigilance to potential dangers for her own safety as well as for her daughter. Her resistance to visitation could be addressed in a collaborative treatment plan developed by a court-appointed parenting coordinator or therapist. Specifically, treatment should address how to help Jane modulate her fears regarding her child's safety.

R-PAS provided information on these two individuals that was not colored by self-report. At the same time, it was quite consistent with the self-reports in each of their cases. R-PAS provided important information about Jane's worldview, especially her hypervigilance to aggression, her concerns about body integrity (V-Comp, AGC, An), and her self-absorption. As for John's R-PAS scores, his human percepts were generally cooperative, and his reality testing around human interaction was relatively good. However, there was some evidence that he may occasionally lapse into salient misunderstandings or misperceptions of people. John's Rorschach results, combined with the PAI's Violence Potential Index, suggested that he is unlikely to be a risk to their daughter.

The contempt-of-court charges against Jane were stayed and Jane was referred to a parenting coordinator regarding her concerns about the safety of her daughter when she is with John. Jane elected not to follow through. Subsequently, John was relocated by the military to a new duty station several thousand miles away from

Jane. The child, now age 9, travels between her parents' households, as ordered by the court, on designated school holiday breaks. At one such exchange, Jane sent the child to the airport in her pajamas, without luggage. There have been no new allegations by either parent. Although there is no direct tie to the psychological evaluations, the process of airing their concerns to a psychologist, as well as the experience of extensive psychological testing, seemed to serve as a deterrent to renewed allegations.

## REFERENCES

Benjestorf, S. T., Viglione, D. J., Lamb, J. D., & Giromini, L. (2013). Suppression of aggressive Rorschach responses among violent offenders and nonoffenders. *Journal of Interpersonal Violence, 28,* 2981–3003.

Black, M. C., Basile, K. C., Breiding, M. J., Smith, S. G., Walters, M. L., Merrick, M. T., . . . Stevens, M. R. (2011). *The National Intimate Partner and Sexual Violence Survey (NISVS): 2010 summary report.* Atlanta, GA: National Center for Injury Prevention and Control, Centers for Disease Control and Prevention.

Bornstein, R. F. (2006). The complex relationship between dependency and domestic violence: Converging psychological factors and social forces. *American Psychologist, 61,* 595–606.

Bureau of Justice Statistics. (2015). *Criminal victimization.* Washington, DC: U.S. Department of Justice.

Dutton, D. G., & Nicholls, T. L. (2005). The gender paradigm in domestic violence research and theory: Part 1. The conflict of theory and data. *Aggression and Violent Behavior, 10,* 680–714.

Hartman, W. L., Clark, M. E., Morgan, M. K., Dunn, V. K., Fine, A. D., Perry, G. G., & Winsch, D. L. (1990). Rorschach structure of a hospitalized sample of Vietnam veterans with PTSD. *Journal of Personality Assessment, 54,* 149–159.

Herman, J. L. (1992). Complex PTSD: A syndrome in survivors of prolonged and repeated trauma. *Journal of Traumatic Stress, 5,* 377–391.

Holtzworth-Munroe, A., Meehan, J. C., Herron, K., Rehman, U., & Stuart, G. L. (2000). Testing the Holtzworth-Munroe and Stuart (1994) batterer typology. *Journal of Consulting and Clinical Psychology, 68,* 1000–1019.

Holtzworth-Munroe, A., & Stuart, G. L. (1994). Typologies of male batterers: Three subtypes and the differences among them. *Psychological Bulletin, 116,* 476–497.

Kaser-Boyd, N. (1993). Rorschachs of women who commit homicide. *Journal of Personality Assessment, 60,* 458–470.

Kaser-Boyd, N. (2007). Battered woman syndrome: Assessment-based expert testimony. In C. B. Gacono, F. B. Evans, N. Kaser-Boyd, & L. A. Gacono (Eds.), *The handbook of forensic Rorschach assessment* (pp. 467–487). New York: Routledge.

Kelly, J. B., & Johnson, M. P. (2008). Differentiation among types of intimate partner violence: Research update and implications for interventions. *Family Court Review, 46,* 476–499.

Masling, J., Rabie, L., & Blondheim, S. H. (1967). Obesity, level of aspiration, and Rorschach and TAT measures of oral dependence. *Journal of Consulting Psychology, 31,* 233–239.

Meyer, G. J., Viglione, D. J., Mihura, J. L., Erard, R. E., & Erdberg, P. (2011). *Rorschach Performance Assessment System: Administration, coding, interpretation, and technical manual.* Toledo, OH: Rorschach Performance Assessment System.

Mihura, J. L. (2012). The necessity of multiple test methods in conducting assessments: The role of the Rorschach and self-report. *Psychological Injury and Law, 5,* 97–106.

Mihura, J. L., Meyer, G. J., Dumitrascu, N., & Bombel, G. (2013). The validity of individual Rorschach variables: Systematic reviews and meta-analyses of the comprehensive system. *Psychological Bulletin, 139,* 548–605.

Smith, S. G., Chen, J., Basile, K. C., Gilbert, L. K., Merrick, M. T., Patel, N., . . . Jain, A. (2017). *The National Intimate Partner and Sexual Violence Survey (NISVS): 2010–2012 state report.* Atlanta, GA: National Center for Injury Prevention and Control, Centers for Disease Control and Prevention.

Swanson, G. S., Blount, J., & Bruno, R. (1990). Comprehensive System Rorschach data on Vietnam combat veterans. *Journal of Personality Assessment, 54,* 160–169.

Urist, J. (1977). The Rorschach test and the assessment of object relations. *Journal of Personality Assessment, 41,* 3–9.

van der Kolk, B. A., & Ducey, C. (1989). The psychological processing of traumatic experiences: Rorschach patterns in PTSD. *Journal of Traumatic Stress, 2,* 259–274.

Walker, L. (1979). *The battered woman.* New York: Harper & Row.

**Rorschach Responses "Jane"**

| Respondent ID: Jane Doe | Examiner: Reneau Kennedy |
|---|---|
| Location: Outpatient | Date: **/**/**** |
| Start Time: 9:30 A.M. | End Time: 10:20 A.M. |

| 99 | R # | Or | Response | Clarification | R-Opt |
|---|---|---|---|---|---|
| I | 1 | | This looks like a masquerade mask of an animal. Some sort of an animal. (W) | E: (Examiner Repeats Response [ERR].)<br>R: All of it. The nose (D3) is large, antlers here (Dd28), ears (Dd34), and definite spaces for the eyes (DdS30) and mouth (DdS29). | |
| | 2 | | Kind of looks like a face of a cow or goat. (W) | E: (ERR)<br>R: All of it. Cow face. [E could have queried for a determinant.] | |
| II | 3 | | It looks like a pelvis bone. (D6) | E: (ERR)<br>R: Here. Just the anatomy.<br>E: What makes it looks like that to you?<br>R: The shape of it. | |
| | 4 | | Or . . . two garden gnomes high-fiving one another with little red hats (D2). (W) | E: (ERR)<br>R: Their hands (D4) are touching, and see (respondent points), they are facing each other. | |
| III | 5 | | It looks like a mirrored image of someone vacuuming the floor. (D1) | E: (ERR)<br>R: Kind of like a butler, a professional of some sort. Here's the person (D9) and the vacuum (D7).<br>E: You said *mirrored image*?<br>R: Yes, one person, reflected here. [E could have queried "butler" for C'.] | |
| | 6 | | Kind of looks like the eyes of a beetle. (D7) | E: (ERR)<br>R: Eyes (Dd31), mouth (lower portion of D8), and the front claws. | |
| IV | 7 | | It looks like a man who is lying down. (W) | E: (ERR)<br>R: All of it.<br>E: You said he is lying down?<br>R: He is in a supine position; see his feet (D6) and arms (points to D4). [E could have queried "lying down" for FD.] | |
| | 8 | | Or it could be a dragon. (W) | E: (ERR)<br>R: The whole thing. There's the head (D1) and there's the wings (D6). | |
| V | 9 | | This looks like a butterfly moth. (W) | E: (ERR)<br>R: All of it. The wings (D4) and the antennae (Dd34). | |
| | 10 | | Or a baby bat; wings are too big for the body size, therefore it is not full grown. (W) | E: (ERR)<br>R: All of it. Feet (D9) and ears (Dd34) and the wings (D4). | |
| VI | 11 | > | > Could be a boat reflected in the water. (W) | E: (ERR)<br>R: Whole thing. I can see the mast (Dd24) of it and I can see the front and the sides and a crow's nest (Dd25). Looks like a military surface.<br>E: Military surface?<br>R: On the boat. Grayish tone, like a flat mat. | |
| | 12 | | Could be a saint standing on top of a mountain. (Dd; 3, 31s) | E: (ERR)<br>R: Position of the arms and looking upward in a stoic position. (head = Dd23, mountain = Dd31s, arms = upper portion of Dd22) | |

| 99 | R # | Or | Response | Clarification | R-Opt |
|---|---|---|---|---|---|
| VII | 13 | | This looks like two gnomes facing each other. (W) | E: (ERR)<br>R: All of it. Lady gnomes. Skirts (D4) and a feather (D5), a fancy feather on top of the hat. [A query about "fancy feather" would have been appropriate.] | |
| | 14 | | Or it could be a uterus, like a diagram. (DS7) | E: (ERR)<br>R: This is the negative space.<br>E: Diagram?<br>R: Like an ultrasound. It is the shape and the curve of where a cervix would be (portion of DS7 adjacent to Dd25). I've had these for both of my pregnancies. | |
| VIII | 15 | | This looks like a mountain lion (points to one on each side) climbing up a mountain. (W) | E: (ERR)<br>R: All of it. (lion = D1, mountain = D6) | |
| | 16 | | Or, it could be a spine. (W) | E: (ERR)<br>R: The whole thing. Like the x-ray of a back. [What it is and where it is are clear; a query is indicated for why it looks the way it does.] | |
| IX | 17 | | It looks like someone bad who is wearing a mask. (Dd = 99, 11, 28) | E: (ERR)<br>R: Part of it. Right in here. (Dd22)<br>E: In here?<br>R: Behind the orange (Dd28) and the green (D11). The red part would be the arms. (D6) [A query for "someone bad" would have been appropriate.] | |
| | 18 | | Or, it could be someone hiding behind something. (W) | E: (ERR)<br>R: All of it. Chest (D6), and the face area (D8) is behind. [unstated object = D12s.] | |
| X | 19 | | This looks like two seahorses. (D9) | E: (ERR)<br>R: Yes here, just their shape. | |
| | 20 | | A large underwater scene. Looks like art. (W) | E: (ERR)<br>R: The whole thing, very tropical.<br>E: Tropical?<br>R: Colorful . . . very sea-like, shrimp and crayfish. | |

# Rorschach Performance Assessment System (R-PAS)®

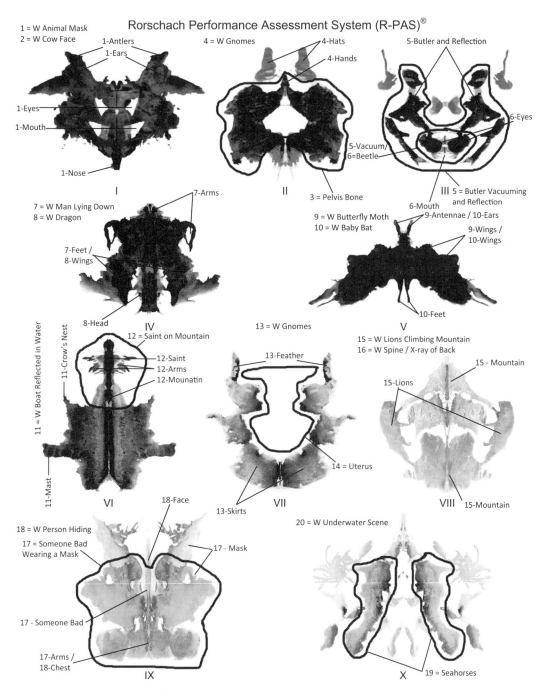

1 = W Animal Mask
2 = W Cow Face
1-Antlers
1-Ears
1-Eyes
1-Mouth
1-Nose
I

4 = W Gnomes
4-Hats
4-Hands
II
3 = Pelvis Bone

5-Butler and Reflection
6-Eyes
5-Vacuum/
6=Beetle
6-Mouth
III  5 = Butler Vacuuming and Reflection

7 = W Man Lying Down
8 = W Dragon
7-Arms
7-Feet /
8-Wings
8-Head
IV

9 = W Butterfly Moth
10 = W Baby Bat
9-Antennae / 10-Ears
9-Wings /
10-Wings
10-Feet
V

11 = W Boat Reflected in Water
11-Crow's Nest
12 = Saint on Mountain
12-Saint
12-Arms
12-Mounatin
11-Mast
VI

13 = W Gnomes
13-Feather
14 = Uterus
13-Skirts
VII

15 = W Lions Climbing Mountain
16 = W Spine / X-ray of Back
15 - Mountain
15-Lions
VIII  15-Mountain

18 = W Person Hiding
17 = Someone Bad Wearing a Mask
18-Face
17 - Mask
17 - Someone Bad
17-Arms /
18-Chest
IX

20 = W Underwater Scene
19 = Seahorses
X

# R-PAS Code Sequence: "Jane"

**C-ID**: Jane Doe    **P-ID**: 1    **Age**: 31    **Gender**: Female    **Education**: 16

| Cd | # | Or | Loc | Loc # | SR | SI | Content | Sy | Vg | 2 | FQ | P | Determinants | Cognitive | Thematic | HR | ODL (RP) | R-Opt | Text |
|----|---|----|----|-------|----|----|---------|----|----|---|----|---|--------------|-----------|----------|----|----------|-------|------|
| I | 1 | | W | | | SI | (Ad) | | | | o | | F | | | | | | |
| | 2 | | W | | | | Ad | | | | u | | F | | | | | | * |
| Comment: E could have queried for a determinant. |||||||||||||||||||
| II | 3 | | D | 6 | | | An | | | | o | | F | | | | | | |
| | 4 | | W | | | | (H),Cg | Sy | | 2 | o | | Ma,FC | | COP,MAH | GH | | | |
| III | 5 | | D | 1 | | | H,NC | Sy | | | o | P | Ma,r | | | GH | | | * |
| Comment: E could have queried "butler" for C'. |||||||||||||||||||
| | 6 | | D | 7 | | | Ad | | | | u | | F | | AGC | | | | |
| IV | 7 | | W | | | | H | | | | o | P | Mp | | | GH | | | |
| Comment: E could have queried "lying down" for FD. |||||||||||||||||||
| | 8 | | W | | | | (A) | | | | o | | F | | AGC | | | | |
| V | 9 | | W | | | | A | | | | o | | F | DV1 | | | | | |
| | 10 | | W | | | | A | | | | o | P | F | | | | | ODL | |
| VI | 11 | > | W | | | | NC | | | | o | | C',r | | AGC | | | | |
| | 12 | | Dd | 3,99 | | | H | Sy | | | u | | Mp | | | GH | ODL | | |
| VII | 13 | | W | | | | (H),Cg | Sy | | 2 | o | | F | | | GH | | | * |
| Comment: A query about 'fancy' feather would have been appropriate. |||||||||||||||||||
| | 14 | | D | 7 | SR | | An,Sx | | | | u | | F | | PER | | ODL | | |
| VIII | 15 | | W | | | | A,NC | Sy | | 2 | o | P | FMa | | AGC | | | | |
| | 16 | | W | | | | An | | | | u | | F | | | | | | * |
| Comment: What it is and where it is are clear; a query is indicated for why it looks the way it does. |||||||||||||||||||
| IX | 17 | | Dd | 99,11,28 | | | Hd,(Hd) | Sy | | | u | | FC,FD | | AGC | PH | | | * |
| | 18 | | W | | | | Hd,NC | Sy | | | u | | Mp,FD | | | PH | | | |
| X | 19 | | D | 9 | | | A | | | 2 | o | | F | | | | | | |
| | 20 | | W | | | | A,Art | | | | o | | CF | | | | | | |

©2010-2016 R-PAS

# R-PAS Summary Scores and Profiles – Page 1

C-ID: Jane Doe     P-ID: 1     Age: 31     Gender: Female     Education: 16

| Domain/Variables | Raw Scores | Raw %ile | Raw SS | Cplx. Adj. %ile | Cplx. Adj. SS | Standard Score Profile R-Optimized | Abbr. |
|---|---|---|---|---|---|---|---|
| **Admin. Behaviors and Obs.** | | | | | | | |
| Pr | 0 | 24 | 89 | | | | Pr |
| Pu | 0 | 40 | 96 | | | | Pu |
| CT (Card Turning) | 1 | 38 | 95 | | | | CT |
| **Engagement and Cog. Processing** | | | | | | | |
| Complexity | 66 | 40 | 96 | | | | Cmplx |
| R (Responses) | 20 | 21 | 88 | 22 | 89 | | R |
| F% [Lambda=1.22] (Simplicity) | 55% | 78 | 111 | 72 | 109 | | F% |
| Blend | 5 | 66 | 106 | 70 | 108 | | Bln |
| Sy | 7 | 55 | 102 | 67 | 107 | | Sy |
| MC | 7.0 | 53 | 101 | 57 | 103 | | MC |
| MC - PPD | 5.0 | 95 | 124 | 95 | 124 | | MC-PPD |
| M | 5 | 72 | 109 | 71 | 109 | | M |
| M/MC [5/7.0] | 71% | 80 | 112 | 82 | 114 | | M Prp |
| (CF+C)/SumC [1/3] | 33% | 28 | 91 | 28 | 91 | | CFC Prp |
| **Perception and Thinking Problems** | | | | | | | |
| EII-3 | -1.0 | 11 | 82 | 22 | 88 | | EII |
| TP-Comp (Thought & Percept. Com...) | -0.6 | 4 | 74 | 10 | 81 | | TP-C |
| WSumCog | 1 | 18 | 86 | 23 | 88 | | WCog |
| SevCog | 0 | 35 | 94 | 35 | 94 | | Sev |
| FQ-% | 0% | 7 | 78 | 10 | 80 | | FQ-% |
| WD-% | 0% | 11 | 82 | 11 | 82 | | WD-% |
| FQo% | 65% | 67 | 107 | 56 | 103 | | FQo% |
| P | 4 | 22 | 88 | 31 | 92 | | P |
| **Stress and Distress** | | | | | | | |
| YTVC' | 1 | 12 | 82 | 15 | 84 | | YTVC' |
| m | 0 | 14 | 84 | 14 | 84 | | m |
| Y | 0 | 17 | 85 | 18 | 86 | | Y |
| MOR | 0 | 18 | 86 | 20 | 87 | | MOR |
| SC-Comp (Suicide Concern Comp.) | 3.2 | 13 | 83 | 18 | 86 | | SC-C |
| **Self and Other Representation** | | | | | | | |
| ODL% | 15% | 71 | 108 | 75 | 110 | | ODL% |
| SR (Space Reversal) | 1 | 56 | 102 | 56 | 102 | | SR |
| MAP/MAHP [0/1] | NA | | | | | | MAP Prp |
| PHR/GPHR [2/7] | 29% | 36 | 95 | 36 | 95 | | PHR Prp |
| M- | 0 | 36 | 95 | 36 | 95 | | M- |
| AGC | 5 | 85 | 116 | 85 | 116 | | AGC |
| H | 3 | 67 | 106 | 66 | 106 | | H |
| COP | 1 | 54 | 102 | 62 | 105 | | COP |
| MAH | 1 | 64 | 105 | 48 | 99 | | MAH |

C-ID: Jane Doe        P-ID: 1        Age: 31        Gender: Female        Education: 16

| Domain/Variables | Raw Scores | Raw %ile | Raw SS | Cplx. Adj. %ile | Cplx. Adj. SS | Standard Score Profile R-Optimized | Abbr. |
|---|---|---|---|---|---|---|---|
| **Engagement and Cog. Processing** | | | | | | 60  70  80  90  100  110  120  130  140 | |
| W% | 65% | 87 | 117 | 89 | 119 | | W% |
| Dd% | 10% | 37 | 95 | 37 | 95 | | Dd% |
| SI (Space Integration) | 1 | 18 | 86 | 33 | 93 | | SI |
| IntCont | 1 | 31 | 93 | 36 | 95 | | IntC |
| Vg% | 0% | 18 | 86 | 18 | 86 | | Vg% |
| V | 0 | 29 | 92 | 29 | 92 | | V |
| FD | 2 | 84 | 115 | 87 | 118 | | FD |
| R8910% | 30% | 37 | 95 | 34 | 94 | | R8910% |
| WSumC | 2.0 | 31 | 92 | 36 | 94 | | WSC |
| C | 0 | 36 | 95 | 36 | 95 | | C |
| Mp/(Ma+Mp) [3/5] | 60% | 72 | 109 | 72 | 109 | | Mp Prp |
| **Perception and Thinking Problems** | | | | | | 60  70  80  90  100  110  120  130  140 | |
| FQu% | 35% | 69 | 107 | 74 | 110 | | FQu% |
| **Stress and Distress** | | | | | | 60  70  80  90  100  110  120  130  140 | |
| PPD | 2 | 3 | 73 | 7 | 77 | | PPD |
| CBlend | 0 | 28 | 91 | 28 | 91 | | CBlnd |
| C' | 1 | 41 | 97 | 35 | 94 | | C' |
| V | 0 | 29 | 92 | 29 | 92 | | V |
| CritCont% (Critical Contents) | 20% | 55 | 102 | 62 | 104 | | CrCt |
| **Self and Other Representation** | | | | | | 60  70  80  90  100  110  120  130  140 | |
| SumH | 8 | 74 | 109 | 79 | 112 | | SumH |
| NPH/SumH [5/8] | 62% | 51 | 100 | 45 | 98 | | NPH Prp |
| V-Comp (Vigilance Composite) | 4.5 | 83 | 114 | 87 | 117 | | V-C |
| r (Reflections) | 2 | 93 | 122 | 93 | 122 | | r |
| p/(a+p) [3/6] | 50% | 66 | 106 | 63 | 105 | | p Prp |
| AGM | 0 | 31 | 93 | 31 | 93 | | AGM |
| T | 0 | 28 | 91 | 28 | 91 | | T |
| PER | 1 | 72 | 109 | 72 | 109 | | PER |
| An | 3 | 85 | 116 | 85 | 116 | | An |

© 2010-2016 R-PAS

## Rorschach Responses "John"

| Respondent ID: John Doe | Examiner: Reneau Kennedy |
|---|---|
| Location: Outpatient | Date: **/**/**** |
| Start Time: 1:00 P.M. | End Time: 2:05 P.M. |

| Cd # | R # | Or | Response | Clarification | R-Opt |
|---|---|---|---|---|---|
| I | 1 | | Looks like it could be a moth. (W) | E: (Examiner Repeats Response [ERR].)<br>R: All of it. The wings (D2), the shading, and the shape. The empty spots are like a camouflage pattern (DdS26) to blend in. | |
| | 2 | | Or a mask. (W) | E: (ERR)<br>R: The entire thing. There are the ears (Dd34), eye holes (DdS30), mouth holes (DdS29). [E could have queried "holes" for FD or V.] | |
| II | 3 | | Looks like two gnomes playing patty cake. (W) | E: (ERR)<br>R: Red caps (D2), the black spots (D6) are where they are sitting at an angle playing patty cake. There's their hands. (D4) | |
| | 4 | | This could be a butterfly. (D3) | E: (ERR)<br>R: Just the shape. Wings here, bottom of the wings. | |
| III | 5 | | That looks like two people bowing toward one another before they dance. (W)<br>E. Please remember to try to give two responses, maybe three. | E: (ERR)<br>R: Just the black. Heads (Dd32), bodies, and legs (D5), which are coming out in a bowing position.<br>E: Dance?<br>R: Oh, the red (D3, D2) looks like they are getting ready to party. So I guess all of it. | Pr |
| | 6 | | This could be a butterfly in the center. (D3) | E: (ERR)<br>R: Just the shape. | |
| IV | 7 | v | > v This looks like a boar. That's all I see. (D1)<br>E: Remember to try to find two maybe three responses on each card. | E: (ERR)<br>R: All of it. Snout (D1) and tusks (Dd28) and eyes and these are the ears (upper middle protrusions). The eyes are the white part (in D1).<br>E: I'm not sure I am seeing it the same as you.<br>R: Just the face of a boar. | Pr |
| | 8 | | This could be the head of a penguin. (D4) | E: (ERR)<br>R: Here is the beak, and the shape of the head looks like the shape of a penguin. [E could have queried "penguin" for C'.] | |
| V | 9 | | That looks like a moth. (W) | E: (ERR)<br>R: All of it. Just the shape | |
| | 10 | | Or a bat. (W) | E: (ERR)<br>R: All of it. The shape and the color. | |
| VI | 11 | | I don't see anything here . . .<br>E: Take your time.<br>R: Maybe a fur skin laying on the floor. (W) | E: (ERR)<br>R: All of it. Like a deer pelt. There are lines that are light and dark that bunch up. Mentally, to me, it is always how I see them. | Pr |
| | 12 | | This could be an Indian headdress at the top. (D3) | E: (ERR)<br>R: Just the shape of it. The outside part looks like fur of some kind. [E could have clarified "fur" for Y or T.] | |
| VII | 13 | | Looks like two girls walking away from one another but looking back at one another and staring. Does that make sense? (W) | E: (ERR)<br>R: All of it. This looks like their hair (D5) is up in a knot and looks like they are wearing dresses or a coat, and the heads (D9) are turned toward one another and their bodies are heading the other way.<br>E: I'm not sure what you mean by "staring."<br>R: Well, it looks more catty than friendly. | |
| | 14 | | These could be stones or boulders down here. (D4) | E: (ERR)<br>R: Just the shape of them; also the gray color. | |

| Cd # | R # | Or | Response | Clarification | R-Opt |
|---|---|---|---|---|---|
| VIII | 15 | | That looks like a ship sailing through the fog. (D6) | E: (ERR)<br>R: Just this center. Here's the fog (D7) and the pink is the keel (Dd33) coming through the fog with the two sails (D5, D4) up. [A query about "coming through the fog" could have been asked for dimensionality.] | |
| | 16 | v | > v This looks like a CT scan of the brain. (W) | E: (ERR)<br>R: All of it. Looks like when they show on TV with the missing parts of the brain.<br>E: What makes it looks like a brain CT scan?<br>R: All the colors. | |
| | 17 | | Looks like two animals climbing something. (D1) | E: (ERR)<br>R: Just here on the side. [A query about "something" would have clarified if W and Sy were appropriate to code.] | |
| IX | 18 | | Looks like a waterfall. (W) | E: (ERR)<br>R: All of it. The center is the waterfall (center of W, width of and including D8) and the top part is a peak (upper portion of D8) where the sun is hitting it. The dark part is where there is no sun. The bottom part is the water billowing (D6) from the fall. | |
| | 19 | | Looks like a horse or a bull which is blowing steam out of their nose. (DS8, D11) | E: (ERR)<br>R: The white strip in the center is the main part of the long face; these are the nostrils (DdS23). And this looks like steam (D11) coming out from the nostrils, like breath on a cold day. | |
| X | 20 | | I see a face (points to center white section). (D99 = 29+6+2+S99) | E: (ERR)<br>R: Yes, here, these are the two eyes (D6) and a mouth (white space between D2) smiling at ya. | |
| | 21 | | These looks like some insects pushing something up. (D11) | E: (ERR)<br>R: Looks like two insects (D8) that are trying to push something (D14) skyward.<br>E: I'm not sure I understand "pushing skyward."<br>R: Looks like they are working together to get this object in the middle to go up. | |
| | 22 | | This looks like two guys climbing up a wall and pushing off. I can't see anything else. (D6, D9) | E: (ERR)<br>R: Looks like their foot is pressed against another's foot and they are each trying to climb up a rock wall. | |

# Rorschach Performance Assessment System (R-PAS)®

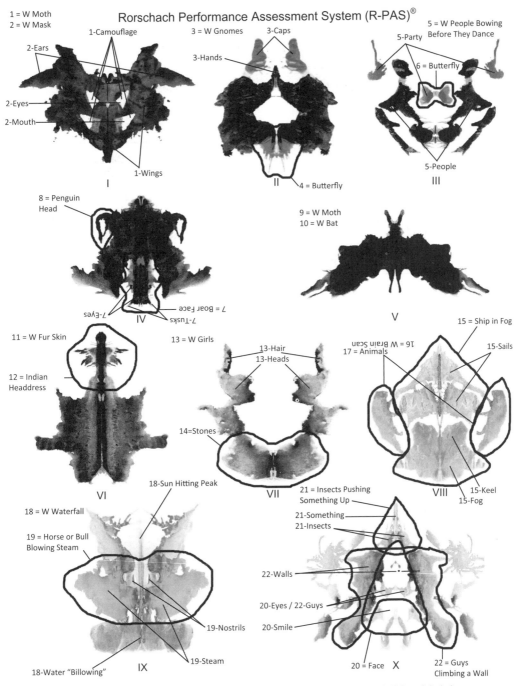

1 = W Moth
2 = W Mask
1-Camouflage
2-Ears
2-Eyes
2-Mouth
1-Wings
I

3 = W Gnomes
3-Caps
3-Hands
II
4 = Butterfly

5 = W People Bowing
Before They Dance
5-Party
6 = Butterfly
5-People
III

8 = Penguin Head
7-Eyes
7 = Boar Face
7-Tusks
IV

9 = W Moth
10 = W Bat
V

11 = W Fur Skin
12 = Indian Headdress
VI

13 = W Girls
13-Hair
13-Heads
14=Stones
VII

16 = W Brain Scan
17 = Animals
15 = Ship in Fog
15-Sails
15-Keel
15-Fog
VIII

18-Sun Hitting Peak
18 = W Waterfall
19 = Horse or Bull Blowing Steam
19-Nostrils
19-Steam
18-Water "Billowing"
IX

21 = Insects Pushing Something Up
21-Something
21-Insects
22-Walls
20-Eyes / 22-Guys
20-Smile
20 = Face
X
22 = Guys Climbing a Wall

# R-PAS Code Sequence: "John"

**C-ID**: John Doe    **P-ID**: 3    **Age**: 32    **Gender**: Male    **Education**: 12

| Cd | # | Or | Loc | Loc # | SR | SI | Content | Sy | Vg | 2 | FQ | P | Determinants | Cognitive | Thematic | HR | ODL (RP) | R-Opt | Text |
|----|---|----|----|----|----|----|---------|----|----|---|----|---|--------------|-----------|----------|----|----|----|----|
| I | 1 | | W | | | SI | A | | | | o | | Y | | | | | | |
| | 2 | | W | | | SI | (Hd) | | | | o | | F | | | GH | | | * |
| _Comment_: E could have queried "holes" for FD or V. | | | | | | | | | | | | | | | | | | | |
| II | 3 | | W | | | | (H),Cg | Sy | | 2 | o | | Ma,FC | | COP,MAH | GH | ODL | | |
| | 4 | | D | 3 | | | A | | | | o | | F | | | | | | |
| III | 5 | | W | | | | H,NC | Sy | | 2 | o | P | Ma,CF | | COP,MAH | GH | | Pr | |
| | 6 | | D | 3 | | | A | | | | o | | F | | | | | | |
| IV | 7 | v | D | 1 | | SI | Ad | | | | u | | C' | | AGC | | | Pr | |
| | 8 | | D | 4 | | | Ad | | | | o | | F | | | | | | * |
| _Comment_: E could have queried "penguin" for C'. | | | | | | | | | | | | | | | | | | | |
| V | 9 | | W | | | | A | | | | o | | F | | | | | | |
| | 10 | | W | | | | A | | | | o | P | C' | | | | | | |
| VI | 11 | | W | | | | Ad | | | | o | P | T | | | | | Pr | |
| | 12 | | D | 3 | | | Ay | | | | o | | F | | | | | | * |
| _Comment_: E could have clarified "fur" for Y or T. | | | | | | | | | | | | | | | | | | | |
| VII | 13 | | W | | | | H,Cg | Sy | | 2 | o | P | Mp | | | GH | | | |
| | 14 | | D | 4 | | | NC | | | | o | | C' | | | | | | |
| VIII | 15 | | D | 2,7 | | | NC | Sy | | | o | | ma | | | | | | * |
| _Comment_: A query about 'coming through the fog' could have been asked for dimensionality. | | | | | | | | | | | | | | | | | | | |
| | 16 | v | W | | | | An | | | | u | | CF | | MOR | | | | |
| | 17 | | D | 1 | | | A | | | 2 | o | P | FMa | | | | | | * |
| Comment: A query about 'something' would have clarified if W and Sy were appropriate to code. | | | | | | | | | | | | | | | | | | | |
| IX | 18 | | W | | | | NC | | | | u | | ma,Y | | | | | | |
| | 19 | | D | 8,1 | | | Ad,NC | Sy | | | o | | FMa,mp | | | | | | |
| X | 20 | | Dd | 99 | | SI | Hd | | | | - | | Mp | | | PH | | | |
| | 21 | | D | 1 | | | A,NC | Sy | | 2 | o | | FMa | FAB1 | COP,MAH | GH | | | |
| | 22 | | D | 6,9 | | | H,NC | Sy | | 2 | u | | Ma | | COP,MAH | GH | | | |

©2010-2016 R-PAS

# R-PAS Summary Scores and Profiles – Page 1

C-ID: John Doe     P-ID: 3     Age: 32     Gender: Male     Education: 12

| Domain/Variables | Raw Scores | Raw %ile | Raw SS | Cplx. Adj. %ile | Cplx. Adj. SS | Standard Score Profile R-Optimized | Abbr. |
|---|---|---|---|---|---|---|---|
| **Admin. Behaviors and Obs.** | | | | | | | |
| Pr | 3 | 90 | 119 | | | | Pr |
| Pu | 0 | 40 | 96 | | | | Pu |
| CT (Card Turning) | 2 | 44 | 98 | | | | CT |
| **Engagement and Cog. Processing** | | | | | | | |
| Complexity | 71 | 51 | 100 | | | | Cmplx |
| R (Responses) | 22 | 38 | 96 | 35 | 94 | | R |
| F% [Lambda=0.38] (Simplicity) | 27% | 20 | 88 | 17 | 86 | | F% |
| Blend | 4 | 56 | 102 | 54 | 102 | | Bln |
| Sy | 7 | 55 | 102 | 61 | 105 | | Sy |
| MC | 7.5 | 57 | 103 | 56 | 102 | | MC |
| MC - PPD | -4.5 | 29 | 92 | 31 | 92 | | MC-PPD |
| M | 5 | 72 | 109 | 66 | 107 | | M |
| M/MC [5/7.5] | 67% | 74 | 110 | 76 | 111 | | M Prp |
| (CF+C)/SumC [2/3] | 67% | 70 | 108 | 70 | 108 | | CFC Prp |
| **Perception and Thinking Problems** | | | | | | | |
| EII-3 | -0.6 | 29 | 92 | 39 | 96 | | EII |
| TP-Comp (Thought & Percept. Com...) | 0.2 | 40 | 96 | 45 | 98 | | TP-C |
| WSumCog | 4 | 37 | 95 | 39 | 96 | | WCog |
| SevCog | 0 | 35 | 94 | 35 | 94 | | Sev |
| FQ-% | 5% | 25 | 90 | 39 | 96 | | FQ-% |
| WD-% | 0% | 11 | 82 | 11 | 82 | | WD-% |
| FQo% | 77% | 89 | 118 | 81 | 113 | | FQo% |
| P | 5 | 39 | 96 | 48 | 99 | | P |
| **Stress and Distress** | | | | | | | |
| YTVC' | 6 | 70 | 108 | 69 | 108 | | YTVC' |
| m | 3 | 81 | 113 | 75 | 110 | | m |
| Y | 2 | 70 | 108 | 68 | 107 | | Y |
| MOR | 1 | 51 | 100 | 50 | 100 | | MOR |
| SC-Comp (Suicide Concern Comp.) | 3.7 | 26 | 90 | 26 | 90 | | SC-C |
| **Self and Other Representation** | | | | | | | |
| ODL% | 5% | 23 | 89 | 27 | 91 | | ODL% |
| SR (Space Reversal) | 0 | 19 | 87 | 19 | 87 | | SR |
| MAP/MAHP [0/4] | 0% | 3 | 72 | 3 | 72 | | MAP Prp |
| PHR/GPHR [1/7] | 14% | 12 | 83 | 12 | 83 | | PHR Prp |
| M- | 1 | 81 | 113 | 81 | 113 | | M- |
| AGC | 1 | 17 | 86 | 16 | 85 | | AGC |
| H | 3 | 67 | 106 | 62 | 104 | | H |
| COP | 4 | 97 | 128 | 97 | 129 | | COP |
| MAH | 4 | 99 | 134 | 98 | 130 | | MAH |

© 2010-2016 R-PAS

# R-PAS Summary Scores and Profiles – Page 2

C-ID: John Doe     P-ID: 3     Age: 32     Gender: Male     Education: 12

| Domain/Variables | Raw Scores | Raw %ile | Raw SS | Cplx. Adj. %ile | Cplx. Adj. SS | Standard Score Profile R-Optimized | Abbr. |
|---|---|---|---|---|---|---|---|
| **Engagement and Cog. Processing** | | | | | | | |
| W% | 45% | 61 | 104 | 63 | 105 | | W% |
| Dd% | 5% | 16 | 85 | 17 | 86 | | Dd% |
| SI  (Space Integration) | 4 | 77 | 111 | 84 | 115 | | SI |
| IntCont | 1 | 31 | 93 | 33 | 94 | | IntC |
| Vg% | 0% | 18 | 86 | 18 | 86 | | Vg% |
| V | 0 | 29 | 92 | 29 | 92 | | V |
| FD | 0 | 21 | 88 | 32 | 93 | | FD |
| R8910% | 36% | 79 | 112 | 78 | 111 | | R8910% |
| WSumC | 2.5 | 40 | 96 | 40 | 96 | | WSC |
| C | 0 | 36 | 95 | 36 | 95 | | C |
| Mp/(Ma+Mp)   [2/5] | 40% | 47 | 99 | 47 | 99 | | Mp Prp |
| **Perception and Thinking Problems** | | | | | | | |
| FQu% | 18% | 19 | 87 | 24 | 90 | | FQu% |
| **Stress and Distress** | | | | | | | |
| PPD | 12 | 73 | 109 | 75 | 110 | | PPD |
| CBlend | 0 | 28 | 91 | 28 | 91 | | CBlnd |
| C' | 3 | 77 | 111 | 72 | 109 | | C' |
| V | 0 | 29 | 92 | 29 | 92 | | V |
| CritCont% (Critical Contents) | 9% | 20 | 87 | 25 | 89 | | CrCt |
| **Self and Other Representation** | | | | | | | |
| SumH | 6 | 53 | 101 | 57 | 103 | | SumH |
| NPH/SumH   [3/6] | 50% | 31 | 92 | 27 | 90 | | NPH Prp |
| V-Comp (Vigilance Composite) | 3.7 | 66 | 106 | 69 | 107 | | V-C |
| r (Reflections) | 0 | 36 | 95 | 36 | 95 | | r |
| p/(a+p)   [3/11] | 27% | 26 | 90 | 24 | 89 | | p Prp |
| AGM | 0 | 31 | 93 | 31 | 93 | | AGM |
| T | 1 | 68 | 107 | 68 | 107 | | T |
| PER | 0 | 30 | 92 | 30 | 92 | | PER |
| An | 1 | 47 | 99 | 47 | 99 | | An |

© 2010-2016 R-PAS

# Using R-PAS in Pre-Employment, Neuropsychological, and Educational Evaluations

# CHAPTER 15

# Using R-PAS in the Pre-Employment Evaluation of a Candidate for a Roman Catholic Seminary

Philip Keddy

## Identifying Information and Referral Question

"Luke" was 22 when I assessed him as a candidate for the Roman Catholic diocesan priesthood. Diocesan priests are typically assigned to work in a parish by the bishop who oversees the geographical area known as a *diocese*. In contrast, order priests and brothers live in communities that usually have a specific mission, such as serving the poor or working in education.

Luke was referred by the vocation director of a diocese without any specific questions or concerns being raised. If a diocese decides to accept a candidate, they then sponsor his education at the seminary. Although assessing a seminary candidate fits under the rubric of pre-employment screening, it is important to remember how long it takes before a priest aspirant is ordained. For a diocesan priest, ordination may take place 6–8 years after entering the college-level seminary. For order priests or brothers, it may take even longer—perhaps as many as 12 years for a Jesuit. The period of education and training prior to ordination is known as *formation*. To draw a parallel with the training of psychologists, I was not assessing Luke's *readiness* to be a priest any more than I would be assessing a 22-year-old's readiness to be a psychologist when he or she is just deciding to major in psychology.

In the pre-employment context, the focus of the psychological assessment is typically on *screening out* potentially problematic candidates rather than *selecting in* the most promising candidates (e.g., see Spilberg & Corey, 2014). However, in my experience, vocation directors want not only information to help them decide whether or not to accept a candidate, but also recommendations for the candidate's continued growth and development in formation. Plante and Boccaccini (1998) found the same. With this secondary purpose, the assessment of priest candidates may differ from pre-employment screening for other job candidates.

## Candidate Background

Luke is white and the eldest male in a Catholic family of more than six children. He grew up in urban and suburban communities in the Midwestern United States as the family moved a few times. Luke had completed 2 years at a Catholic liberal arts college before approaching the vocation director.

Luke had thought of becoming a priest since he was a child serving as an altar boy and helping the priests. He liked that the priest celebrated Mass and he was drawn to the idea of giving himself to God for service to others. Luke noted that he had learned a sense of responsibility being the eldest male child in a large family. He said that although it had been fun growing up in his family, he had learned that he "wasn't the only person on the face of the earth" and that "there are other people one has to think about and care for as one gets older."

Luke felt safe everywhere growing up and denied any experience of physical, sexual, or emotional abuse. He had not suffered any head injuries or major medical illnesses. The family struggled financially at times. When Luke visited the seminary he saw that the students all had their own rooms—something he didn't have growing up. Luke learned about sex from talks with his parents. He dated very little in high school but had a girlfriend for a year in college. They did not have intercourse because they both wanted to wait for marriage. That relationship ended when Luke left to pursue the priesthood.

Luke denied any behavioral problems in school or in the various summer jobs he had held. He thought his best characteristic was his positive attitude and his ability to get along with people. Luke described his mood as typically calm. He acknowledged that growing up in a large family with members "bumping up against each other" could be irritating; he said he had a bit of a temper at times.

Luke's height and weight were average, and he was exercising several times a week. He reported drinking moderately (one drink with dinner, once a week on average) and denied any use of street drugs.

## Discussion of Methods Used and Selection of Tests

Barry (2013) provided clinicians with a very helpful review of personality assessment measures for screening seminary applicants and concluded with proposals for the components of a comprehensive multimethod test battery. Barry's conclusions were consistent with Mihura's (2012) arguments for the value of multiple test methods—encompassing both self-report and performance-based tests—in doing assessments. Barry recommended the following: one broadband self-report measure of psychopathology (the Minnesota Multiphasic Personality Inventory–2 [MMPI-2] because of its history of use with seminary students); one broadband self-report measure of normal-range personality (the Sixteen Personality Factor Questionnaire [16PF] or NEO Personality Inventory [NEO-PI]); one empirically supported performance-based measure (the Rorschach or Thematic Apperception Test [TAT]); and one measure of cognitive functioning (the Wechsler Adult Intelligence Scale–IV [WAIS-IV] or the Wechsler Abbreviated Scale of Intelligence—Second Edition [WASI-II]). The assessment I conducted with Luke was consistent with Barry's recommendations, with the exception of the self-report measure of normal-range personality. Although

including such an instrument could be helpful, normal-range personality character-
istics can also be gleaned from both the MMPI-2 (e.g., see Levak, Siegel, Nichols, &
Stolberg, 2011) and the Rorschach without the time and expense of another test. The
Rorschach Performance Assessment System (R-PAS; Meyer, Viglione, Mihura, Erard,
& Erdberg, 2011) can also be used to identify strengths and is not inherently biased
toward psychopathology.

I was thankful Barry suggested using the Rorschach or the TAT as an empirically supported
performance-based measure. I only used the Rorschach and considered the TAT as a
supplemental test rather than a substitute for the Rorschach. As Mihura (2012) noted,
"The TAT has some scales with research support; however, these are not accompanied by norms, and clinicians are not typically trained in their use. [The Rorschach,
in contrast, offers] (a) standard administration, (b) at least some scales with reliability
and validity support, and (c) the availability of norms" (p. 99).

I also asked Luke to complete the Penn Inventory of Scrupulosity (PIOS–Revised)
(Olatunji, Abramowitz, Williams, Connolly, & Lohr, 2007), a 15-item questionnaire.
Candidates are asked how often they have the experiences described by the items on
a scale from 0 (Never) to 4 (Constantly). Scrupulosity has been defined as a religious
variant of obsessive–compulsive disorder. For example, a person suffering from scrupulosity may fear that they have committed a sin when a religious authority would
not concur. The corresponding compulsion might be excessive praying or seeking
reassurance from clergy (see Olatunji et al., 2007, p 772.)

In the course of my work, I have obtained a copy of "Psychological Evaluation
Guidelines: Information for Vocation Directors and Evaluating Psychologists" from
the Pontifical North American College at the Vatican.[1] The MMPI-2 and the Rorschach were both notably described as "preferred" tests. These guidelines requested
any appropriate psychiatric diagnoses but not a "suitable vs. unsuitable" determina-
tion. This is consistent with my practice too.

Plante and Boccaccini (1998) deserve credit for first proposing a standardized
protocol to assess applicants to religious life in the Roman Catholic Church, as stan-
dardization enables clinicians and researchers to compare findings. However, as Barry
(2013) pointed out, Plante and Boccaccini offered little rationale for their selection
of tests beyond mentioning "the availability of relevant research, clinical utility, and
affordability" (p. 4). Plante and Boccaccini recommended two self-report measures:
the MMPI-2 (traditionally used to screen for psychopathology) and the 16PF (a measure of normal personality differences). The only performance-based measure they
recommended was the Forer Structured Sentence Completion Test. Holaday, Smith,
and Sherry (2000) noted that the Forer manual does not provide norms or reliability
and validity information. In contrast, R-PAS has test variables with either excellent or
good reliability and validity support and internationally generalizable norms (Meyer
et al., 2011; Mihura, Meyer, Dumitrascu, & Bombel, 2013). It provides a much more
powerful representative of performance-based testing than a sentence completion
test.

Furthermore, Plante and Boccaccini (1998) did not include a measure of cognitive capacity (intelligence). Luke's case proved to be a strong example of the value of
adding a standard IQ test for a more comprehensive understanding of how a candidate is functioning in the world.

---

[1] I thank Monsignor James Checchio, Rector, for permission to describe these undated guidelines.

## Methods Used in Luke's Assessment

For Luke's assessment, I used the (1) Client Information Form (developed for my practice and completed by aspirant); (2) clinical interview (1.5 hours), drawing on questions recommended by Levo (2004) for the psychosexual interview; (3) MMPI-2; (d) R-PAS; (4) WASI-II; and the (5) Penn Inventory of Scrupulosity (PIOS–R).

## Literature Relevant to Luke's Case

When we first met, I told Luke that I would not be discussing the results of the assessment with him or giving him a report. According to the American Psychological Association's "Ethical Principles of Psychologists," pre-employment screening is a context in which candidates may be asked to waive access to assessment results (Standard 9.10, Explaining Assessment Results; American Psychological Association, 2010). Promising to discuss results with candidates places the psychologist in a dual relationship and can compromise objectivity when the psychologist is drawn to simultaneously serve the interests of the hiring agency (in this case, the diocese) and the candidate (Spilberg & Corey, 2014, p. 100). Furthermore, in the case of rejected candidates, psychologists who agree to give feedback may find themselves in the awkward position of trying to explain the decision of the hiring agency or the role that the assessment played in that decision when the candidate is not accepted.

Psychologists have an ethical responsibility to be aware of and respect cultural differences, including those based on religion (APA Ethics, General Principle E; American Psychological Association, 2010). As Plante (2015) has emphasized, members of this worldwide church come from a variety of races, ethnicities, cultures, and national origins that influence their expression of Roman Catholicism. Because many psychologists do not come from the Roman Catholic religious traditions, they may know fairly little about the influence of those traditions on their clients. My own work assessing priest candidates has been informed by the experience of having priests, brothers, and sisters as psychotherapy clients for many years, and study of the literature (Ciarrocchi & Wicks, 2000; Plante, 2015; Shafranske, 2000).

The interpretation of the MMPI-2 L scale for priest aspirants is complicated by the fact that elevations on this scale have been found in Christian samples even outside of the pre-employment screening context (e.g., Bridges & Baum, 2013; Keddy, Erdberg, & Sammon, 1996). Duris, Bjorck, and Gorsuch (2007) presented preliminary evidence that the responses of Christian subjects to a subset of L Scale items may be shaped by a religious motivation response characteristic. This may make traditional interpretations of L scale elevations as reflecting naïve defensiveness or lack of insight inappropriate, and is another reason why the performance-based R-PAS is a helpful addition in the assessment of priest aspirants.

## Brief Summary of Luke's Non-R-PAS Findings

On the WASI-II, Luke's Verbal IQ was 129 and his Performance IQ was 114. This resulted in a Full Scale IQ of 124, in the Superior Range. Luke's IQ score was as high as or higher than 95% of the population in his age range.

On the MMPI-2, Luke produced a within-normal-limits profile with no elevations above 65T on either the Validity or Clinical Scales. Luke obtained moderate elevations on Validity Scales L (raw = 6, T = 61), K (T = 60), and S (T = 63). Scale F was low (T = 45). This pattern could be taken to suggest he was describing himself in a somewhat self-favorable manner. Priest aspirants are likely to obtain L Scale elevations in particular as a function of both the context (pre-employment screening) and of their membership in a particular group (Christian religious), as described above. Luke's modest elevation on the K Scale suggests that he was either being somewhat careful about reporting any type of psychological distress or was a self-reliant person capable of dealing with everyday problems, or some combination of these characteristics (Greene, 2011, p. 84). Elevations on the S Scale in the range of 60–70 T have been described as suggesting some limited self-awareness (Nichols, 2011, p. 79).

Luke's MMPI-2 profile did not deviate substantially from the mean profile of a group of 962 seminary students (Protestant and Catholic) provided in the Seminary Students Interpretive Report (Butcher, 2002). This interpretive report concluded that he would probably have little trouble adapting to a wide range of work environments. Luke's score on Scale 2 (T = 59) suggests that he might have been slightly dissatisfied about something or with himself, but he would probably not consider this to be depression (Greene, 2011, p. 114). Levak et al. (2011, p. 84) noted that sometimes people with similar semi-elevations on Scale 2 grew up with more responsibilities than is normal for a young child. This may well have applied to Luke as the eldest male in a large family. Finally, Luke's scores on the PIOS–R did not suggest significant issues with scrupulosity.

## Why R-PAS?

Finn (1996) nicely outlined the four combinations of high–low elevations seen when integrating MMPI-2 and Rorschach results for individual clients: Both tests can indicate a high level of disturbance, both tests can indicate a low level of disturbance, or one test can suggest a higher level of disturbance than the other. Finn noted that the situation where both tests suggest a low level of disturbance is common in the pre-employment context (1996, p. 547). However, he also noted that the combination of less disturbance on the MMPI-2 and more disturbance on the Rorschach is common in "those settings where clients have been preselected for a certain level of adaptive functioning" (p. 546). In my experience, this description often applies to the screening of priest aspirants. They have been "preselected" by the time they are referred for the psychological assessment, and a greater degree of disturbance is frequently seen from the results of the Rorschach than from the more obvious self-report items of the MMPI-2. The Rorschach may circumvent some of the defensiveness seen on the MMPI-2, and can also provide important information about how the candidate might function in less structured situations in everyday life.

Because the vocation director had not raised any specific concerns about Luke, I examined the overall R-PAS data for information about both potential problems and strengths. I looked at the data in terms of all the dimensions the test measures: problem-solving and coping styles, perception and thinking problems (including reality testing), indicators of stress and distress, interpersonal behavior, and representations of self and others. I also examined the data for information as to what Luke might focus on in his further growth and development, the secondary purpose in the screening of priest aspirants.

## Introducing R-PAS to Luke

I told Luke I was going to give him the Rorschach inkblot test when we first sat down together and went over the agenda for the assessment. Luke said he had heard of the Rorschach, but had not taken it before and had not learned about it online or elsewhere. After the interview and a short break, we started the Rorschach promptly, as he did not have any questions. Luke's approach was calm and matter-of-fact, as it was with other parts of the assessment.

## Luke's R-PAS Administration

I administered R-PAS to Luke in my private office where I also see psychotherapy clients. While I had been sitting across from him for the interview, I sat beside him for the R-PAS administration, with an end table between us on which I had stacked the cards. I used a rolling desk cart to hold the laptop computer on which I typed his responses. Luke was overtly cooperative in taking the Rorschach, although, as we shall see in the discussion of his results, it can be argued that he limited his self-disclosure. Although I allowed 90 minutes for Luke to take the test, we were finished in only 42 minutes.

### Discussion of Luke's R-PAS Results[2]

Like his MMPI-2 profile, Luke's R-PAS results were mostly within normal limits; he had very few Standard Scores[3] (SS) less than 80 or greater than 120. There were, however, some scores outside of both the 90–110 range on Page 1 and the 85–115 range on Page 2,[4] suggesting that the R-PAS results might add to his assessment, keeping in mind strengths that might be indicated by average scores as well.

### Administrative Behaviors and Cognitive Processing

Luke was overtly cooperative in his approach to taking the Rorschach, requiring no Prompts or Pulls (Pr SS = 89, Pu SS = 96). He showed some hesitancy to interact with the environment or perhaps more a compliant willingness to accept circumstances as they are, with no Card Turns (CT SS = 86).

---

[2] See Appendix 15.1 at the end of the chapter for Luke's R-PAS Responses, Location Sheet, Code Sequence, and Page 1 and 2 Profiles.

[3] Standard scores (SS) have a mean of 100 and an SD of 15.

[4] The R-PAS manual recommends interpreting Page 2 scores more tentatively than Page 1 scores; for instance, by using a deviation of SS > 15 from the mean in contrast to the Page 1 SS > 10 deviation from the mean (Meyer et al., 2011, p. 366).

## Engagement and Cognitive Processing

While the complexity of Luke's responses was not so low at to call for the use of Complexity Adjusted scores, he was still in the low-average range (Complexity SS = 87)— which was a surprise given his Superior Range results on the IQ test. Although this combination could suggest a limited engagement with the test that was defensively motivated, I suspect it represented a more pervasive characterological style of responding. Luke likely limited his self-disclosure in most settings. Parishioners expect their priests to exemplify moral virtue, and young men called to the priesthood don't usually "let their hair down" easily. Luke's low Complexity score further suggested he would do well with the structure provided by life in the church, but might have some difficulty coping with the occasional chaotic problems that can arise in parish ministry.

Luke showed an average capability for perceiving the environment from different perspectives (R SS = 105) but a preference for "keeping it simple" (F% SS = 112). His ability to attend to multiple features of either his own internal experiences or the experiences of others (or the general environment) was at the low end of the average range (Blends SS = 91).

Luke appeared to focus on the common, straightforward elements of situations or problems as opposed to the combinatory, relational, and synthetic (Sy SS = 74). He might have difficulty finding alternative solutions to cause-and-effect problems. Luke might not take into account the whole situation and use all available information as much as the average person (Complexity SS = 87, W% SS = 71). This finding points to an area for further growth of which he should be capable, given his high IQ score.

Luke demonstrated an average internal capacity to cope effectively with the day-to-day events of life. He appeared likely to be stable, predictable, reliable, and resilient in handling typical stressful or upsetting situations (MC SS = 90, MC–PPD SS = 99). The Seminary Students Interpretive Report for the MMPI-2 also noted that individuals with similar profiles "typically consider themselves able to manage their lives well" and that "they generally show resiliency in dealing with problems when they occur" (Butcher, 2002, p. 5).

Luke displayed an average ability on the Rorschach to reason and think before acting. He showed a moderate preference for a coping style characterized by deliberation and thoughtful strategy, as opposed to spontaneous reactivity, and his decisions did not appear to be strongly impacted by immediate and strong reactions, emotionality, or interplay with external stimuli (M/MC SS = 110). However, his score was just at the high end of the average range, suggesting that he can let himself be guided by some affective reactions and feelings too.

Luke's reactions to emotionally toned situations tended to be modulated and even muted by mental processing and cognitive control. Although this tendency could reflect emotional development and maturity, it more likely meant that Luke was relying excessively on logic and emotional constriction in response to emotional situations and strong environmental stimuli. Again, there was the suggestion that he might not be able to "let go" and enjoy life very easily [(CF+C)/Sum C SS = 75].

## Perception and Thinking Problems

Luke showed no more evidence of general psychopathology than is true for the average person (EII-3 SS = 94). He did not appear to have trouble thinking clearly or seeing things accurately (TP-Comp SS = 82) and did not exhibit problems in accurate, logical, and effective thinking and reasoning (WSumCog SS = 95, SevCog SS = 94). This finding was consistent with his low-to-average scores on the MMPI-2, particularly on Scales 6, 8, and 9. A caveat here, though, is that Luke may have limited his self-disclosure in a way that kept some thinking problems out of view, given his low Complexity score. However, Complexity has only a modest impact on R-PAS perception and thinking problem scores (Meyer et al., 2011, p. 466, Table 15.3).

Luke gave some mixed evidence on the Rorschach as to how conventional his perceptions were. He saw the kinds of things regularly seen by others (FQo% SS = 102), but he was slightly less likely than the average person to report conventional and widely accepted interpretations of the environment (P SS = 88). The latter may be due to his tendency not to take on the whole situation (W% SS = 71), since most of the cards on which he did not report the conventional response would have required a response to the whole card. However, Luke showed an above-average capacity to see the external environment without mistaken or distorted perceptions (FQ–% SS = 85, WD–% SS = 82). This suggested he had the ability to navigate day-to-day challenges.

Luke did not show a tendency to detach himself from everyday life by intellectualizing emotional situations (IntCont SS = 81). This was consistent with his MMPI-2, which suggested that he preferred traditional, action-oriented activities to artistic and literary pursuits or introspective experiences (Mf T = 42). He also did not generally use a vague or impressionistic processing style (Vg% SS = 86), and he seemed to be as responsive as most people when confronted with provocative situations in everyday life, be they interpersonal or internal (R8910% SS = 89).

## Stress and Distress

Based on Rorschach indicators, Luke did not appear to be struggling with significant implicit stress or distress, as he had no significant elevations on his scores in this domain. (The adjective *implicit* refers here to stress or distress that the test taker may not be consciously experiencing or prepared to report.) This was consistent with the absence of any elevations above 65T on his MMPI-2 profile.

Luke's Rorschach responses suggested that he was as likely as the average person to attend to and articulate the inconsistencies, uncertainties, and nuances in the environment. This finding likely represents an average sensitivity to subtleties in his internal or emotional life, or to those occurring within interpersonal experiences (YTVC' SS = 100). He did not evidence the generally unwanted, distracting ideation that interferes with goal-directed thought and is often associated with environmental stressors (m SS = 97). Luke also did not appear to be experiencing the implicit helplessness and distress often associated with external stressors (Y SS = 99), and there was no evidence that he had themes of damage, injury, or sadness on his mind (MOR SS = 86). As might be expected, then, he did not score in the risk range on the implicit measure of risk for suicide or serious self-harm (SC-Comp SS = 89).

Luke was no more likely than the average person to be subject to disquieting, disruptive, or irritating internal demands (PPD SS = 94). His positive and enlivening reactions were not spoiled by an uncomfortable, distressing state (CBlend SS = 91). Luke did not seem especially drawn to dreary or gloomy stimuli (C' SS = 105).

Primitive mental imagery and traumatic experiences were not salient concerns (Crit-Cont% SS = 97).

There was some chance that Luke's Stress and Distress scores might be underestimated due to his generally limited engagement and elaboration of his responses (low Complexity score and high F% score). Furthermore, there were three instances during the Clarification when a question would have been appropriate, two for C′ versus Y and one for V versus FD (responses 13, 17, and 21). Further clarification might have led to higher scores on these variables. However, as noted above, Luke's moderate elevation on Scale 2 of the MMPI-2 (T = 59) suggested a mild degree of dissatisfaction with something or with himself, but not something he would consider depression.

## Self and Other Representation

Luke did not give evidence of potential interpersonal problems such as notable implicit dependency needs (ODL% SS = 96), oppositionality (SR SS = 87), distorted perception of others (M– SS= 95), aggressive preoccupations (AGC SS = 100), or defensive self-assertion (PER SS = 92). At the same time, the data suggested he was having more-than-average difficulty in understanding people as complex, complete, or multifaceted individuals (H SS = 88). His understanding of himself and others and his ability to be effective in his interactions appeared to be slightly limited (PHR/GHR SS = 111). Luke also showed a slight tendency to view himself and others in unrealistic or fanciful ways more often than in full and complete ways (NPH/Sum H SS = 111). In the interview, Luke told me how he enjoyed talking with older priests. He seemed to have a longing for closer relationships with priests who could function as role models and mentors. Perhaps this longing was his way of seeking to further develop those personal areas described in this paragraph.

Finally, Luke's Rorschach responses suggested that he had some bodily concerns on his mind (An SS = 116). This pattern might have been due to actual physical illness or other bodily concerns, or to more psychologically based concerns about vulnerability and psychic integrity. On the MMPI-2, Luke had an elevated score on the Health Concerns Subscales, Gastrointestinal Symptoms (T = 70), suggesting he might have been having stomachaches or other issues. I recommended that Luke review any physical symptoms or concerns with a physician.

## Integration of Luke's R-PAS Results with Other Methods

The R-PAS results added support to the findings from the interview and MMPI-2 as to the absence of major problems. It was possible to draw that conclusion with more confidence because it did not come from the self-report measure (the MMPI-2) or the interview alone.

I described what I had learned about Luke's strengths and weaknesses in the report to the vocation director, attempting to use everyday language and give examples as much as possible. I wrote that Luke was capable of graduate work, given his IQ test results. I noted that Luke did not manifest any serious thinking problems and did not seem to be experiencing any significant stress or distress. I concluded that

Luke did not manifest any major psychiatric illness, referencing the current edition of the *Diagnostic and Statistical Manual of Mental Disorders, Fifth Edition* (DSM-5; American Psychiatric Association, 2013).

The R-PAS findings provided further help with the second goal of this type of assessment: identifying areas for further growth and development while in seminary formation. I noted that Luke's cognitive processing style showed a preference for "keeping it simple," focusing on the common, straightforward components of a situation. Similarly, it was a noteworthy finding that Luke seemed less inclined than average to challenge himself by taking on the whole situation, to "see the big picture" or "put it all together" (W% SS = 71). The potential problem with this approach would be that Luke might have trouble recognizing the complexity of a situation and identifying alternative solutions to problems (Complexity SS = 87, Sy SS = 74). To help with this area, an exercise was suggested. Luke could be asked to propose a few *different* solutions to problems that typically arise in parish life. Small-group discussion might help him to generate alternative solutions and so promote his ability to synthesize and integrate different concepts and ideas.

The combined R-PAS finding related to affect modulation [(CF+C)/Sum C SS = 75] and the MMPI-2 Scale 2 score (T = 59) suggested that Luke was a serious-minded person who might have trouble letting go and enjoying life. Luke seemed to have developed a very responsible attitude as the eldest male child in a large family. Hopefully, Luke would become more relaxed as he went on in his training and education.

The R-PAS data suggested that Luke might have a limited and less adaptive understanding of himself and others that could result in more difficult or less effective interactions (PHR/GPHR SS = 111, H SS = 88). This finding could be seen as corresponding to the Validity Scale configuration on the MMPI-2 (low F, moderately elevated L, K, & S). By mentioning this in the report, I hoped to alert the vocation director that this was another area to help Luke develop during his education and training. Although Luke might benefit from some formal social skills training, more life experience with different relationship situations would likely promote his growth. As noted, he was just 22 at the time of the assessment.

## How Did the R-PAS Results
## Help Answer the Assessment Questions and Help Luke?

The primary question from the referral source, the vocation director, was whether the diocese should accept Luke into training for the priesthood. Having the performance-based R-PAS results meant that I could describe Luke's strengths and weaknesses with greater confidence. I did not have to rely on a self-report measure (the MMPI-2, in this case) and interview alone. This is the multimethod approach (Erdberg, 2008).

R-PAS provided further information to help with the secondary purpose of this kind of assessment: making recommendations for Luke's further growth and development. Here the R-PAS results went beyond corroborating the MMPI-2 and interview findings to identify some specific potential concerns. For example, despite his high intelligence, when left to his own predilections on a task with few demands, Luke tended to take a simplistic approach to problem solving that could lead to difficulty recognizing the total complexity of a situation and to trouble seeing alternative solutions to problems. R-PAS also provided some data in the domain of Self and Other Representation that was unique to the assessment: Luke's understanding of himself and others and his ability to be effective in his interactions appeared to be slightly limited at the point in his life (PHR/GHR SS = 111). Becoming more aware of these issues could help Luke to further his growth and development.

## Impact of the R-PAS Experience on Luke

Luke was accepted into the seminary. The vocation director did not have any questions about the report and did not ask Luke to come back and discuss any parts of it with me.

A couple of years later I received a call from the same vocation director saying that Luke was struggling with something and asking to meet with me again. I was pleased Luke felt comfortable enough with the assessment process that he asked to return to me, even though he had not learned anything about the results of that assessment from me. Although I think it is best to not promise candidates feedback in the pre-employment screening context, I am also a practitioner of collaborative/therapeutic assessment (Finn, 2007; Finn, Fischer, & Handler, 2012; Fischer, 2006). Consequently, I sometimes wish I could discuss the assessment results with priest aspirants. (I try to bring the spirit of collaborative assessment to the writing of the report.)

When Luke came in, he told me that he had been assigned to work in a high school setting and was troubled by the attraction he felt to some of the teenage girls. He had received some reassurance that such attractions were normal from priests with whom he had consulted, but he had also been encouraged to discuss the issue further with a psychotherapist. Luke was bothered by the fact of being attracted to teenage girls because they were underage. He was mindful of the child abuse scandal in the church and uncertain as to what these attractions meant. Luke said he was not thinking about any one girl in particular and was also attracted to young women who were in their 20s, the same age as he was. Luke still felt called to the priesthood and was not thinking he wanted to marry. After exploring these various points, I reassured Luke that attractions were normal, much as the priests he had spoken to had done. I also emphasized that psychologically, it was crucial to keep in mind the distinction between *feelings* of attraction and *behaviors*. His feelings were internal and private. I suggested that if he were not preoccupied with these thoughts or having trouble maintaining appropriate conduct, he need not worry. Luke clearly stated he was not thinking of any one girl in particular and he was not having trouble maintaining appropriate conduct. As the hour drew to a close, I offered to meet with him again, but Luke felt satisfied with this one discussion.

The problem that Luke was presenting reminded me of the R-PAS finding that he might have been relying excessively on logic and constricting affect in response to emotional situations and strong environmental stimuli [(CF+C)/Sum C SS = 75]. Luke's attraction to teenage girls challenged him to acknowledge these feelings within himself while maintaining appropriate behavior. The issue Luke was struggling with was also reminiscent of some of the scores he obtained in the Self and Other Representation domain. Specifically, the data had suggested that Luke was struggling to understand people in their totality (H SS = 88), and that he might have a limited and less adaptive understanding of himself and others that could result in more difficult or less effective interactions (PHR/GPHR SS = 111). Accordingly, we might say that Luke was struggling with where to "place" his attraction to the teenage girls in his mind.

I praised Luke for seeking consultation about the issue. Moderate elevations on the MMPI-2 K scale are clinically associated with self-reliance: A person scoring in this range may be unwilling to seek help when under stress (Greene, 2011, p. 84). To the extent that was true for Luke, I wanted to commend him for reaching out to both priests and to me.

Luke's return to my office meant not only that I was able to do a little work with him in a more collaborative mode, but that I could hear how his life had gone since the assessment. Those of us who do pre-employment evaluations do not always get that opportunity.

## ACKNOWLEDGMENT

I would like to thank Philip Erdberg for his helpful feedback on this case study.

## REFERENCES

American Psychiatric Association. (2013). *Diagnostic and statistical manual of mental disorders* (5th ed.). Arlington, VA: Author.

American Psychological Association. (2010). Ethical principles of psychologists and code of conduct (2002, Amended June 1, 2010). Retrieved from *http://www.apa.org/ethics/code/index. aspx.*

Barry, J. R. (2013). *Finding a good candidate: The use of personality assessment measures in the screening of religious and seminary applicants.* Unpublished doctoral dissertation, Widener University, Chester, PA.

Bridges, S. A., & Baum, L. J. (2013). An examination of the MMPI-2-RF L-r Scale in an outpatient Protestant sample. *Journal of Psychology and Spirituality, 32,* 115–123.

Butcher, J. N. (2002). *User's guide to the Minnesota Report: Revised personnel report* (3rd ed.). Minneapolis, MN: National Computer Systems.

Ciarrocchi, J. W., & Wicks, R. J. (2000). *Psychotherapy with priests, Protestant clergy, and Catholic religious: A practical guide.* Madison, CT: Psychosocial Press.

Duris, M., Bjorck, J. P., & Gorsuch, R. L. (2007). Christian subcultural differences in item perceptions of the MMPI-2 Lie Scale. *Journal of Psychology and Christianity, 26,* 356–366.

Erdberg, P. S. (2008). Multimethod assessment as a forensic standard. In C. B. Gacono & F. B. Evans (Eds.), *The handbook of forensic Rorschach assessment* (pp. 561–566). New York: Routledge.

Finn, S. E. (1996). Assessment feedback integrating MMPI-2 and Rorschach findings. *Journal of Personality Assessment, 67,* 543–557.

Finn, S. E. (2007). *In our clients' shoes: Theory and techniques of therapeutic assessment.* Mahwah, NJ: Erlbaum.

Finn, S. E., Fischer, C. T., & Handler, L. (Eds.). (2012). *Collaborative/therapeutic assessment: A casebook and guide.* Hoboken, NJ: Wiley.

Fischer, C. T. (2006). Phenomenology, Bruno Klopfer, and individualized/collaborative psychological assessment. *Journal of Personality Assessment, 87,* 229–233.

Greene, R. L. (2011). *The MMPI-2/MMPI-2-RF: An interpretive manual* (3rd ed.). Boston: Allyn & Bacon.

Holaday, M., Smith, D. A., & Sherry, A. (2000). Sentence completion tests: A review of the literature and results of a survey of members of the Society for Personality Assessment. *Journal of Personality Assessment, 74,* 371–383.

Keddy, P. J., Erdberg, P., & Sammon, S. D. (1996). The psychological assessment of Catholic clergy and religious referred for residential treatment. In L. J. Francis & S. H. Jones (Eds.), *Psychological perspectives on Christian ministry: A reader* (pp. 166–174). Herefordshire, UK: Gracewing. (Reprinted from *Pastoral Psychology*, 1990, *38,* 147–159)

Levak, R. W., Siegel, L., Nichols, D. S., & Stolberg, R. A. (2011). *Therapeutic feedback with the MMPI-2: A positive psychology approach.* New York: Routledge.

Levo, L. M. (2004). Taking a sexual history. *Horizon, 4,* 13–20.

Meyer, G. J., Viglione, D. J., Mihura, J. L., Erard, R. E., & Erdberg, P. (2011). *Rorschach Performance Assessment System: Administration, coding, interpretation, and technical manual.* Toledo, OH: Rorschach Performance Assessment System.

Mihura, J. L. (2012). The necessity of multiple test methods in conducting assessments: The role of the Rorschach and self-report. *Psychological Injury and Law, 5,* 97–106.

Mihura, J. L., Meyer, G. J., Dumitrascu, N., & Bombel, G. (2013). The validity of individual Rorschach variables: Systematic reviews and meta-analyses of the Comprehensive System. *Psychological Bulletin, 139,* 548–605.

Nichols, D. S. (2011). *Essentials of MMPI-2 assessment* (2nd ed.). Hoboken, NJ: Wiley.

Olatunji, B. O., Abramowitz, J. S., Williams, N. L., Connolly, K. M., & Lohr, J. M. (2007). Scrupulosity and obsessive–compulsive symptoms: Confirmatory factor analysis and validity of the Penn Inventory of Scrupulosity. *Journal of Anxiety Disorders, 21,* 771–787.

Plante, T. G. (2015). Six principles to consider when working with Roman Catholic clients. *Spirituality in Clinical Practice, 2,* 233–237.

Plante, T. G., & Boccaccini, M. T. (1998). A proposed psychological assessment protocol for applicants to religious life in the Roman Catholic Church. *Pastoral Psychology, 46,* 363–372.

Shafranske, E. (2000). Psychotherapy with Roman Catholics. In P. S. Richards & A. E. Bergin (Eds.), *Handbook of psychotherapy and religious diversity* (pp. 59–88). Washington, DC: American Psychological Association.

Spilberg, S. W., & Corey, D. M. (2014). *Peace officer psychological screening manual.* Sacramento, CA: California Commission on Peace Officer Standards and Training.

# APPENDIX 15.1. Luke's R-PAS Responses, Location Sheet, Code Sequence, and Page 1 and 2 Profiles

## Rorschach Responses "Luke"

| Respondent ID: Priest Aspirant "Luke" | Examiner: Philip Keddy, PhD |
|---|---|
| Location: Examiner's Office | Date: **/**/**** |
| Start Time: 11:35 A.M. | End Time: 12:17 P.M. |

| Cd # | R # | Or | Response | Clarification | R-Opt |
|---|---|---|---|---|---|
| I | 1 | | I am reminded of the face of an animal, possibly a rabbit. I can see two eyes, two ears (D7), not entirely distinct, just what I am reminded of. (W) | E: (Examiner Repeats Response [ERR].)<br>R: Face here, two eyes (DdS30), can't pinpoint kind of animal, maybe a deer or rabbit. | |
| | 2 | | Can maybe sense anger or dark malicious quality. (W) | E: (ERR)<br>R: Image is dark, sense of dark clouds, dark sky, angry or malicious face if these were eyes (DdS30), slanted and if this was a mouth here (DdS29).<br>E: Face?<br>R: Dark, evil kind of face. | |
| II | 3 | | I can see the head of two different cows. (D6) | E: (ERR)<br>R: Head (Dd21), ears (Dd31), reason why they are cows maybe because of spots, red spots; could have said dogs, too. | |
| | 4 | | I can see a heart. (D3) | E: (ERR)<br>R: Right here, more of the realistic heart, the typical image of a heart.<br>E: What is there that makes it look like that?<br>R: Symmetrical and curves that come together, red, joins together. | |
| | 5 | | I can see two hands coming together (respondent nods and hands card back). (D4) | E: (ERR)<br>R: Here, hands are flat and facing each other. Two thumbs.<br>E: Thumbs?<br>R: Maybe because it is darker, maybe you could see sleeves of someone's clothes.<br>E: Sleeves?<br>R: Oh, yeah. | |
| III | 6 | | I can see two people facing each other. (D9) | E: (ERR)<br>R: Heads (Dd32), chin, definitely exaggerated, maybe the breasts right here (Dd27), hard to tell whether woman or man, but definitely more female breasts, arms sloping downwards. Kneecaps, pointed shoes (Dd33).<br>E: Facing each other?<br>R: Yes. | |
| | 7 | | I can see two stomachs, if that makes any sense, [and] the esophagus that leads into the stomach. (D2) | E: (ERR)<br>R: More in terms of inner, stomach, the sack, esophagus leading up. | |
| | 8 | | I can also see a butterfly. (D3) | E: (ERR)<br>R: Right in the middle, you can see two wings and body that joins the two wings. | |
| IV | 9 | | I can see the head or heads of three different birds. (Dd99 = Dd30 + surrounding area within D3) | E: (ERR)<br>R: Mostly what I can see is sharpness of beak and roundness of the head, more silhouettes (points to outer parts of D3, excluding Dd30).<br>E: And the third?<br>R: At the top, outline of the beak (Dd30), feathers right here.<br>E: Beak?<br>R: Pointed, white there, delineates. Maybe the fact that you have these two images here. | |
| | 10 | | I can see two boots. (D6) | E: (ERR)<br>R: Top, heel and then back up. | |
| | 11 | | And too, maybe the texture, part of the image looks like feathers or fur. (D3) | E: (ERR)<br>R: Reminded of that towards the top, can be seen as feathers, darker gray on top of lighter gray, feathers or fur. | |

| Cd # | R # | Or | Response | Clarification | R-Opt |
|---|---|---|---|---|---|
| V | 12 | | I can see, ah, an insect, with two antennae. (D6) | E: (ERR)<br>R: Antennae here, head, maybe caterpillar or butterfly.<br>E: Just the head?<br>R: Yeah, just the head. | |
| | 13 | | Maybe mountains or hills. That's all I can make up. (Dd35) | E: (ERR)<br>R: I saw those maybe here, the silhouettes. [E could have queried "silhouettes" for C' or Y.] | |
| VI | 14 | | I can see the head of an instrument, possibly a guitar. (D3) | E: (ERR)<br>R: Head, nodes for tuning, don't know what they are called. Straight up and down, kind of rectangular. Triangular shapes on the sides, reminds me of where those screws would go. | |
| | 15 | | Two different, I would say, shelves. (Dd24) | E: (ERR)<br>R: Protrudes and is attached to the wall. | |
| VII | 16 | | I can see the face of women facing each other. (D1) | E: (ERR)<br>R: Hair on top (D5), maybe eyes, nose, chin, neck. | |
| | 17 | | I can see tall ears. (D5) | E: (ERR)<br>R: Maybe rabbit's ears, the silhouettes of rabbit's ears. [E could have queried "silhouettes" for C' or Y.] | |
| | 18 | | Maybe two different handlebars to a bicycle. (Dd21) | E: (ERR)<br>R: One right here and one right here. | |
| VIII | 19 | | I can see two (respondent smiles) hyenas I am reminded of. (D1) | E: (ERR)<br>R: Legs, and paws, somewhat crouching, have the back here, kind of lunging. Face isn't very distinct. Picked hyenas because snouts are shorter. | |
| | 20 | | When ah, when we try to visualize sound, those vibrations. (Dd99 = Dd21 extended to bottom of image + D3 and equivalent width of D4) | E: (ERR)<br>R: I don't know if you have ever seen *Fantasia*; they are playing different instruments, line going straight up and down, and almost triangle here (D3), gives sense of a vibration almost. | |
| IX | 21 | | I can see the face of a horse. (D8) | E: (ERR)<br>R: Nostrils (Dd23) with nose at the bottom. The snout, the top would be where the head is.<br>E: Nostrils?<br>R: Two open spaces like nostrils. [An additional query here for dimensionality would have been helpful.] | |
| | 22 | | I can see the breasts of a man, or the chest of a man. (D6) | E: (ERR)<br>R: The two breasts (D4), and maybe the chest in between.<br>E: What is there that makes it looks like that?<br>R: Two circles on the side and space in between, pinkish color, images beneath the skin. [E could have queried "images beneath the skin" to more confidently code An over Hd.] | |
| X. | 23 | | I can see maybe two different crabs. (D1) | E: (ERR)<br>R: Right here and here (D1). Different kind of pointing legs that surround this image here. | |
| | 24 | | Two frogs. (D7) | E: (ERR)<br>R: Here is body, legs, so maybe jumping, in the air. | |
| | 25 | | I am also reminded of the boundaries of Vietnam. Outlining of the country. (D9) | E: (ERR)<br>R: Here (respondent points to both sides), not exact.<br>E: Two of them?<br>R: Symmetrical and mirror each other.<br>E: Vietnam twice, then. Am I understanding you correctly?<br>R: (Respondent smiles.) Yes. | |

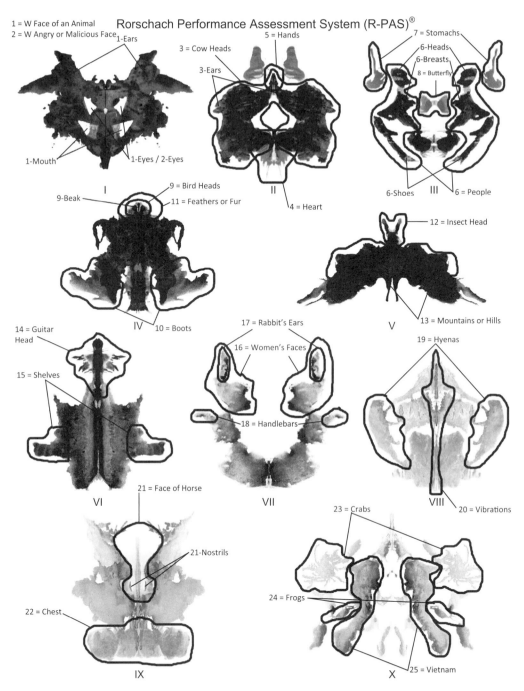

Rorschach Performance Assessment System (R-PAS)®

1 = W Face of an Animal
2 = W Angry or Malicious Face
1-Ears
3 = Cow Heads
3-Ears
5 = Hands
7 = Stomachs
6-Heads
6-Breasts
8 = Butterfly
1-Mouth
1-Eyes / 2-Eyes
6-Shoes
6 = People
I
II
III
4 = Heart
9 = Bird Heads
9-Beak
11 = Feathers or Fur
12 = Insect Head
IV
10 = Boots
13 = Mountains or Hills
V
14 = Guitar Head
15 = Shelves
17 = Rabbit's Ears
16 = Women's Faces
18 = Handlebars
19 = Hyenas
VI
21 = Face of Horse
VII
VIII
20 = Vibrations
21-Nostrils
23 = Crabs
24 = Frogs
22 = Chest
25 = Vietnam
IX
X

# R-PAS Code Sequence: "Luke"

**C-ID**: Priest Aspirant "Luke"    **P-ID**: 6    **Age**: 22    **Gender**: Male    **Education**: 16

| Cd | # | Or | Loc | Loc # | SR | SI | Content | Sy | Vg | 2 | FQ | P | Determinants | Cognitive | Thematic | HR | ODL (RP) | R-Opt | Text |
|----|---|----|----|----|----|----|----|----|----|----|----|----|----|----|----|----|----|----|----|
| I | 1 | | W | | | SI | Ad | | | | u | | F | | | | | | |
| | 2 | | W | | | SI | (Hd) | | | | o | | Ma,C' | | AGM,AGC | PH | | | |
| II | 3 | | D | 6 | | | Ad | | | 2 | u | | FC | INC1 | | | | | |
| | 4 | | D | 3 | | | An | | | | o | | FC | | | | | | |
| | 5 | | D | 4 | | | Hd,Cg | Sy | | 2 | o | | Mp,Y | | | PH | | | |
| III | 6 | | D | 9 | | | H,Cg | | | 2 | o | P | Mp | | | GH | | | |
| | 7 | | D | 2 | | | An | | | | o | | F | | | | ODL | | |
| | 8 | | D | 3 | | | A | | | | o | | F | | | | | | |
| IV | 9 | | Dd | 99 | | | Ad | | | 2 | u | | C' | | AGC | | | | |
| | 10 | | D | 6 | | | Cg | | | 2 | o | | F | | | | | | |
| | 11 | | D | 3 | | | Ad | | | | n | | T | | | | | | |
| V | 12 | | D | 6 | | | Ad | | | | o | | F | | | | | | |
| | 13 | | Dd | 35 | | | NC | | | | o | | F | | | | | | * |
| Comment: E could have queried 'silhouettes' for C' or Y. ||||||||||||||||||| |
| VI | 14 | | D | 3 | | | NC | | | | u | | F | | | | | | |
| | 15 | | Dd | 24 | | | NC | | | 2 | u | | F | | | | | | |
| VII | 16 | | D | 1 | | | Hd | | | 2 | o | P | F | | | GH | | | |
| | 17 | | D | 5 | | | Ad | | | 2 | o | | F | | | | | | * |
| Comment: E could have queried 'silhouettes' for C' or Y. ||||||||||||||||||| |
| | 18 | | Dd | 21 | | | NC | | | 2 | u | | F | | | | | | |
| VIII | 19 | | D | 1 | | | A | | | 2 | o | P | FMa | | AGC | | | | |
| | 20 | | Dd | 99 | | | NC | | | | - | | ma | | | | | | |
| IX | 21 | | D | 8 | | SI | Ad | | | | o | | F | | | | | | * |
| Comment: An additional query for dimensionality would have been helpful. ||||||||||||||||||| |
| | 22 | | D | 6 | | | An | | | | u | | FC | INC1 | | | ODL | | * |
| Comment: E could have queried "images beneath the skin" to more confidently code An over Hd. ||||||||||||||||||| |
| X | 23 | | D | 1 | | | A | | | 2 | o | P | F | | | | | | |
| | 24 | | D | 7 | | | A | | | 2 | o | | FMa | | | | | | |
| | 25 | | D | 9 | | | NC | | | 2 | u | | F | | | | | | |

©2010-2016 R-PAS

C-ID: Priest Aspirant "Luke"    P-ID: 6    Age: 22    Gender: Male    Education: 16

| Domain/Variables | Raw Scores | Raw %ile | Raw SS | Cplx. Adj. %ile | Cplx. Adj. SS | Standard Score Profile R-Optimized | Abbr. |
|---|---|---|---|---|---|---|---|
| **Admin. Behaviors and Obs.** | | | | | | 60 70 80 90 100 110 120 130 140 | |
| Pr | 0 | 24 | 89 | | | | Pr |
| Pu | 0 | 40 | 96 | | | | Pu |
| CT (Card Turning) | 0 | 18 | 86 | | | | CT |
| **Engagement and Cog. Processing** | | | | | | 60 70 80 90 100 110 120 130 140 | |
| Complexity | 55 | 19 | 87 | | | | Cmplx |
| R (Responses) | 25 | 62 | 105 | 71 | 109 | | R |
| F% [Lambda=1.27] (Simplicity) | 56% | 79 | 112 | 64 | 106 | | F% |
| Blend | 2 | 28 | 91 | 49 | 100 | | Bln |
| Sy | 1 | 4 | 74 | 27 | 91 | | Sy |
| MC | 4.5 | 25 | 90 | 46 | 98 | | MC |
| MC - PPD | -2.5 | 46 | 99 | 45 | 99 | | MC-PPD |
| M | 3 | 43 | 97 | 55 | 102 | | M |
| M/MC [3/4.5] | 67% | 74 | 110 | 78 | 112 | | M Prp |
| (CF+C)/SumC [0/3] | 0% | 5 | 75 | 5 | 75 | | CFC Prp |
| **Perception and Thinking Problems** | | | | | | 60 70 80 90 100 110 120 130 140 | |
| EII-3 | -0.5 | 35 | 94 | 49 | 99 | | EII |
| TP-Comp (Thought & Percept. Com…) | -0.3 | 12 | 82 | 30 | 92 | | TP-C |
| WSumCog | 4 | 37 | 95 | 49 | 100 | | WCog |
| SevCog | 0 | 35 | 94 | 35 | 94 | | Sev |
| FQ-% | 4% | 16 | 85 | 40 | 97 | | FQ-% |
| WD-% | 0% | 11 | 82 | 11 | 82 | | WD-% |
| FQo% | 60% | 55 | 102 | 39 | 96 | | FQo% |
| P | 4 | 22 | 88 | 35 | 94 | | P |
| **Stress and Distress** | | | | | | 60 70 80 90 100 110 120 130 140 | |
| YTVC' | 4 | 49 | 100 | 61 | 104 | | YTVC' |
| m | 1 | 42 | 97 | 48 | 99 | | m |
| Y | 1 | 48 | 99 | 55 | 102 | | Y |
| MOR | 0 | 18 | 86 | 26 | 89 | | MOR |
| SC-Comp (Suicide Concern Comp.) | 3.6 | 24 | 89 | 33 | 94 | | SC-C |
| **Self and Other Representation** | | | | | | 60 70 80 90 100 110 120 130 140 | |
| ODL% | 8% | 40 | 96 | 52 | 101 | | ODL% |
| SR (Space Reversal) | 0 | 19 | 87 | 19 | 87 | | SR |
| MAP/MAHP [0/0] | NA | | | | | | MAP Prp |
| PHR/GPHR [2/4] | 50% | 76 | 111 | 76 | 111 | | PHR Prp |
| M- | 0 | 36 | 95 | 36 | 95 | | M- |
| AGC | 3 | 49 | 100 | 52 | 101 | | AGC |
| H | 1 | 21 | 88 | 32 | 93 | | H |
| COP | 0 | 21 | 88 | 42 | 97 | | COP |
| MAH | 0 | 26 | 90 | 26 | 90 | | MAH |

© 2010-2016 R-PAS

# R-PAS Summary Scores and Profiles – Page 2

C-ID: Priest Aspirant "Luke"  P-ID: 6  Age: 22  Gender: Male  Education: 16

| Domain/Variables | Raw Scores | Raw %ile | Raw SS | Cplx. Adj. %ile | Cplx. Adj. SS | Standard Score Profile R-Optimized | Abbr. |
|---|---|---|---|---|---|---|---|
| **Engagement and Cog. Processing** | | | | | | | |
| W% | 8% | 3 | 71 | 11 | 82 | | W% |
| Dd% | 20% | 70 | 108 | 69 | 107 | | Dd% |
| SI (Space Integration) | 3 | 60 | 104 | 78 | 111 | | SI |
| IntCont | 0 | 11 | 81 | 24 | 89 | | IntC |
| Vg% | 0% | 18 | 86 | 18 | 86 | | Vg% |
| V | 0 | 29 | 92 | 29 | 92 | | V |
| FD | 0 | 21 | 88 | 45 | 98 | | FD |
| R8910% | 28% | 22 | 89 | 19 | 87 | | R8910% |
| WSumC | 1.5 | 21 | 88 | 38 | 95 | | WSC |
| C | 0 | 36 | 95 | 36 | 95 | | C |
| Mp/(Ma+Mp) [2/3] | 67% | 81 | 113 | 81 | 113 | | Mp Prp |
| **Perception and Thinking Problems** | | | | | | | |
| FQu% | 32% | 53 | 101 | 73 | 109 | | FQu% |
| **Stress and Distress** | | | | | | | |
| PPD | 7 | 34 | 94 | 57 | 102 | | PPD |
| CBlend | 0 | 28 | 91 | 28 | 91 | | CBlnd |
| C' | 2 | 62 | 105 | 63 | 105 | | C' |
| V | 0 | 29 | 92 | 29 | 92 | | V |
| CritCont% (Critical Contents) | 16% | 43 | 97 | 55 | 102 | | CrCt |
| **Self and Other Representation** | | | | | | | |
| SumH | 4 | 27 | 91 | 49 | 99 | | SumH |
| NPH/SumH [3/4] | 75% | 76 | 111 | 69 | 107 | | NPH Prp |
| V-Comp (Vigilance Composite) | 2.8 | 38 | 95 | 61 | 104 | | V-C |
| r (Reflections) | 0 | 36 | 95 | 36 | 95 | | r |
| p/(a+p) [2/6] | 33% | 36 | 95 | 33 | 93 | | p Prp |
| AGM | 1 | 75 | 110 | 75 | 110 | | AGM |
| T | 1 | 68 | 107 | 68 | 107 | | T |
| PER | 0 | 30 | 92 | 30 | 92 | | PER |
| An | 3 | 85 | 116 | 85 | 116 | | An |

© 2010-2016 R-PAS

# Using R-PAS in a Neuropsychological Evaluation of a High-Functioning Adult Patient with Depression, Anxiety, and a Relational Trauma History

Nicolae Dumitrascu

It is well established today that people who were exposed in childhood to relational trauma (i.e., interpersonal traumatic events, such as abuse, loss, neglect, or witnessing violence) are at lifelong risk to exhibit impairment in multiple domains of psychological functioning. Studies with traumatized children and adults show changes in brain structure and chemistry (Nemeroff, 2004), which can result in neuropsychological deficits (Gabowitz, Zucker, & Cook, 2008). Adverse childhood experiences can negatively impact self-esteem (Kim & Cichetti, 2006); mood and emotion regulation (Spertus, Yehuda, Wong, Halligan, & Seremetis, 2003); thinking, memory and learning, and executive functioning (Twamley, Hami, & Stein, 2004; Wolfe & Charney, 1991); and social adjustment (Malinosky-Rummell & Hansen, 1993).

There is a rich Rorschach literature on trauma, though there have been very few published studies on relational trauma other than sexual abuse. After reviewing the literature, Viglione, Towns, and Lindshield (2012) identified five qualities that characterize the Rorschach protocols of people exposed to trauma: (1) simplistic and shorter records suggestive of cognitive constriction and rigidity as a defense against traumatic memories; (2) increased trauma-related and damage imagery; (3) signs of perceptual and ideational disturbance; (4) responses suggesting "anxious sensitivity"; and (5) emotional distancing and affective numbing (e.g., less responsiveness to emotionally triggering aspects of the inkblot stimuli such as color).

## Basic Client Information and Referral Questions

"Lisa" is a 24-year-old unmarried female college student living in a small urban area. She has a history of relational trauma, depression, anxiety, executive functioning problems, and social adjustment difficulties. She was referred by her therapist for a neuropsychological evaluation in order to (1) determine the nature (e.g., developmental) and severity of her reported dysexecutive, emotional, and social difficulties; (2) gain information about her psychological strengths and weaknesses and about her interpersonal functioning; (3) make recommendations for treatment (i.e., suitability for an insight-based therapy); and (4) determine if Lisa is at high risk for developing a psychotic disorder, since she has a family history of schizophrenia.

## Lisa's Neuropsychological Evaluation: The Interview

### Behavioral Observations

Lisa was appropriately dressed and well groomed. She was alert and oriented to person, time, and location. Eye contact was appropriately maintained. Spontaneous speech was normal for rate and prosody, but she spoke in a soft voice. Thought processes were goal-oriented. The examiner noted Lisa's ability to describe nuanced aspects of her internal processes associated with her social difficulties. Affect was somewhat restricted. Lisa was very cooperative with the testing process and engaged well with the tasks. However, she was anxious, low in self-confidence, and a little reserved and awkward interpersonally. She had mild delay in understanding and responding to humor, but no major difficulties with social pragmatics were noticed.

### Clinical Interview

#### Presenting Concerns

Lisa's own presenting concerns included (1) *difficulty managing stress and being dysregulated by negative emotions,* leading to outbursts of crying or anger; (2) *executive functioning difficulties* (initiating, organizing, keeping track of, and completing tasks), which left her forgetful about deadlines and assignments and often feeling overwhelmed when both school and daily tasks piled up; and (3) *social adjustment difficulties and social anxiety.* Lisa reported difficulty forming and maintaining relationships, feeling uneasy in social situations, having difficulty grasping subtle social cues, and sometimes talking at the wrong time. She also reported difficulty expressing her feelings to people, which included her significant others.

#### Psychosocial History

Lisa was born and raised in a small town, mostly by her mother and grandfather. Her childhood was marked by poverty and significant psychosocial stress. Her parents separated when she was very young and she witnessed her father being physically violent with her mother. Lisa reported that later she was physically and emotionally abused by one of her mother's partners. As an adolescent, she was involved in a relationship with an emotionally abusive boyfriend, at the end of which she became seriously depressed and emotionally dysregulated.

Academically, Lisa denied an early history of learning difficulties. However, she noted that her difficulties with organization impacted her academic effectiveness and that she would often forget to complete or turn in her homework as a young student.

## *Medical, Psychiatric, and Substance Use History*

In high school Lisa struggled with anxiety, depression, and obsessive–compulsive symptoms. She was treated with psychotherapy for more than 2 years and with antidepressant medication (Sertraline, Zoloft, and Wellbutrin), but the antidepressants were not helpful. In college Lisa continued to struggle with depression and anxiety. She received cognitive-behavioral therapy for obsessive–compulsive disorder (OCD) 1 year before the current evaluation, which was helpful in controlling this disorder. However, at the date of the evaluation she was still reporting residual symptoms (e.g., worrying about dirt and germs, overchecking if she turned off appliances). Lisa was also recovering from a recent depressive episode that significantly impacted her functioning (e.g., disruption in daily and self-care routines). She was currently treated with counseling at an outpatient mental health clinic and with Abilify (an antipsychotic used when antidepressant treatment has failed) by her psychiatrist for depression. There was no reported history of hallucinations, delusions, or hypomanic symptoms. There was a family history of autism spectrum disorder and schizophrenia (on father's side), depression (grandfather), and anxiety (grandmother).

Lisa denied current suicidal ideation, intention, or plan. Problems with appetite and sleep were also denied. Medical history was unremarkable. There was no history of problematic alcohol use. She reported using marijuana occasionally in college and experimenting a few times with "club drugs."

## Neuropsychological and Other Non-R-PAS Measures and Test Results

Lisa's comprehensive neuropsychological assessment included measures of cognitive and executive functioning, as well as self-report and performance measures of emotional, social, and personality functioning. The following sections summarize Lisa's non-R-PAS test results, focusing particularly on her therapist's referral questions and her own presenting concerns that she wanted addressed by the assessment.

### Cognitive Functioning

Lisa's general cognitive abilities (Wechsler Adult Intelligence Scale—Fourth Edition [WAIS-IV], Full Scale IQ) were above average, with relative strengths in perceptual reasoning skills (PRI = superior range). Her VCI was in the high-average range, indicating solid verbal comprehension abilities.

Lisa's performance on tests of processing speed (WAIS-IV PSI; Delis–Kaplan Executive Function System [D-KEFS] Trail Making) was good. On a test of visual sustained attention and concentration (Conners Continuous Performance Test—Second Edition [CPT-II]) Lisa had mild difficulty maintaining her vigilance for the entire duration of the test, but otherwise she performed well. Also, her auditory attention and ability to hold in and operate with information in short-term memory (WAIS-IV WMI) was intact. Taken together, these findings indicated that Lisa's reported academic and daily functioning difficulties were not related to neurocognitive deficits in attention/concentration, working memory, or processing speed.

However, Lisa struggled on tests measuring aspects of executive functioning (organization, planning, strategic processing of information, self-monitoring, and shifting mental set). Illustrative of her organizational difficulties, on a test of constructional praxis and planning (copying a complex figure; Rey Complex Figure Test [RCFT] Copy), she exhibited a very piecemeal approach and did not adequately use the stimulus configuration to guide her execution (although her copy was still within normal limits for accuracy). This was unexpected given her very good performance on tests of visual spatial processing (WAIS-IV PRI, particularly the Block Design subtest). A potential explanation of this discrepancy is that the RCFT Copy may be more sensitive to weaknesses in organization than the WAIS-IV PRI subtests, where her organizational deficits may have been compensated and masked by her strong visual–spatial reasoning abilities.

Her performance on tests of auditory verbal memory (California Verbal Learning Test, Second Edition [CVLT-II], a word list) and visual memory (RCFT Immediate Recall, reproducing a complex figure) was below average, which likely reflected weaknesses in organizing information that impacted encoding of new information, leading to the loss of some of that information or to difficulty accessing it later. Finally, she demonstrated weaknesses on some measures of mental set shifting (D-KEFS Color-Word; Wisconsin Card Sorting Test [WCST] Perseverative Errors; D-KEFS Category Fluency).

In the light of these data, there was little doubt that Lisa presented with executive functioning difficulties that impacted her effectiveness in daily life activities, including studying, keeping track of tasks, monitoring her own performance, organizing her environment, adjusting to changes, and approaching problems in a flexible way. These findings were overall consistent with a meta-analytic review by Scott et al. (2015) reporting medium size deficits in verbal learning, delayed memory, attention/working memory, and executive functioning in people with a history of trauma (although Lisa did not show impairment in information-processing speed).

## Emotional Functioning

### Developmental History Questionnaire (Completed by Mother)

To gain more information about a potential neurodevelopmental disorder, Lisa's mother completed a questionnaire covering many aspects of her daughter's childhood history (medical, social, emotional, educational). According to her mother, Lisa had mildly delayed speech. She reported that Lisa was easily distressed as a young child and had a tendency to flap or rock when excited or distressed. She indicated that Lisa was socially passive and did not like to participate in competitive games with her peers. No other behavioral, cognitive, or communication peculiarities were reported. Academically, her mother noted that Lisa was a perfectionistic student, spent hours on school assignments, and had long-standing difficulties with organization.

Based on Lisa's clinical history, it was suspected that her emotional difficulties were an important contributing factor to her dysexecutive difficulties. Thus, measures of emotional, social, and personality functioning were used to (1) determine the severity of her emotional difficulties and their impact on her functioning, (2) assess for a thought disorder, (3) understand her coping strategies, and (4) suggest treatment recommendations.

### Self-Report Tests

Regarding the broadband self-report measure of psychopathology used in the assessment, Lisa's Minnesota Multiphasic Personality Inventory–2 (MMPI-2) was valid for interpretation. Although not an invalidating elevation, she reported experiencing a very high number of psychological symptoms (Scale F T[1] = 82). This was interpreted as a "cry for help" and as suggesting that her self-image was marked by a sense of vulnerability or damage.

Overall, Lisa's self-report results suggested that she was in significant distress (e.g., Scale 7 = 90). She was feeling very demoralized and depressed and viewed herself, the world, and her future in a highly negative manner (Scale 2 = 75; $DEP_3$ = 68). Lisa often overreacted to situations with intense anxiety (A = 74; ANX = 84), had low stress tolerance, and was very vulnerable to emotional dysregulation (Es = 30), all of which were likely deleterious to her attention/concentration and executive functioning. Lisa's MMPI-2 results also suggested low self-confidence (LSE = 68) and a tendency to ruminate or obsess over her problems (Scale 7 = 90). Interpersonally, Lisa felt shy and self-conscious ($Si_1$ = 74); she had difficulty trusting people or engaging in social interactions for fear of being hurt, rejected, or criticized ($Pa_2$ = 84).

In regard to Lisa's assessment question as to whether her family history of schizophrenia had left her vulnerable to schizophrenia, the MMPI-2 scale that targets psychosis was not elevated ($BIZ_1$ = 54), consistent with the interview of no reported history of delusions and hallucinations. Also, a scale targeting schizotypal thinking was not significantly elevated ($BIZ_2$ = 60). However, Lisa did endorse MMPI-2 items that were suggestive of disturbances in her thought processes (e.g., having strange and peculiar thoughts; feeling as if things were not real), which is not uncommon for people with a history of abuse and severe emotional difficulties. To rule out severe reality testing impairment, a more direct assessment of her perceptual–cognitive processes was deemed necessary.

In order to determine if Lisa's reported social difficulties stemmed from difficulties with processing emotions and grasping social cues, she took the Toronto Alexithymia Scale–20 (TAS-20), Cambridge Behaviour Scale—Empathy Quotient (EQ), and WAIS-IV Social Cognition tests. Her responses on the TAS-20 indicated difficulties primarily with describing emotions, but less so with identifying emotional experiences or overinvesting in external reality (TAS-20 raw = 68). Difficulty describing emotions is not unusual for people who have a history of disruptive emotional and attachment experiences (Bagby & Taylor, 1997; Hund & Espelage, 2006). On the EQ, Lisa's responses suggested that she viewed herself as having significant difficulty understanding how others feel and using people's expressed emotions as cues in social exchanges (EQ T = 27). This finding was consistent with Lisa's reported interpersonal awkwardness and difficulties grasping social cues.

### Performance Tests

Unlike the self-report results on the EQ, Lisa performed much better (average to high-average range) on *performance* measures of social cognition (Social Perception subtests from the WAIS-IV Advanced Clinical Solutions) that assess components of social cognition such as affect labeling and recognition, identification of sarcasm,

---

[1]T scores (T) have a mean of 50 and an *SD* of 10.

and ability to verbalize a speaker's intent. These findings suggested that Lisa's ability to grasp and process social–emotional cues was comparable to that of her peers and better than what she thought. This finding further suggested that, to a large extent, her reported difficulties understanding emotional cues likely reflected her social inhibitions and low self-confidence.

## Implications of Neuropsychological and Other Non-R-PAS Findings

In conclusion, neuropsychological and personality testing suggested that Lisa's difficulties with cognitive, executive, and social functioning were related, to a large extent, to her depression, anxiety, emotional dysregulation, and low self-confidence. However, more information was needed about a potential thought disorder, stress coping strategies, self- and interpersonal perceptions, and psychological resources.

## Why R-PAS for Lisa?

Although some of the referral questions were already addressed by her neuropsychological and self-report findings, the Rorschach Performance Assessment System (R-PAS; Meyer, Viglione, Mihura, Erard, & Erdberg, 2011) was deemed suitable to gain valuable information about Lisa's (1) reality testing and potential psychotic processes, (2) coping style and emotional functioning, (3) interpersonal style and difficulties, (4) self-perception, and (5) personality strengths and resources. R-PAS is a privileged assessment instrument to explore these issues, given its robust empirical foundations (Meyer et al., 2011; also see Mihura, Meyer, Dumitrascu, & Bombel, 2013) and its relatively unstructured and quasi-ambiguous nature that can trigger responses relevant for the accuracy and quality of how people view the world and themselves, how they respond to emotional stimuli, and the complexity and coherency of their ideation. Along these lines, Arnon, Maoz, Gazit, and Klein (2011) stated: "The Rorschach test makes it possible to analyze the client's complex response to the trauma, taking into account cognition, emotion, defenses, sense of self, interpersonal issues, perception, and content" (p. 7). Armstrong and Kaser-Boyd (2004) indicated that performance personality testing such as the Rorschach has an important role in trauma assessment because it can access psychological layers that are not readily available to self-reflection and self-sharing, and thus can reveal covert trauma signs. Also, it can reveal psychological resources that may be needed to tolerate specific forms of trauma treatment.

## The R-PAS Administration

The R-PAS administration took place in the examiner's office in a mental health outpatient setting. Lisa took the test in the third assessment session, when she was already familiarized with the examiner and with the setting. She was informed that she was taking this test to explore her psychological functioning in more depth. As with the other tests, Lisa easily understood the instructions and did not ask clarifying questions. Upon inquiry, she indicated that she had never seen the inkblots before and did not know anything about this test.

The administration took about 1 hour. Despite the good effort that she put forth on the Rorschach, it was evident even from the first card that this task was not easy for her. Lisa often appeared hesitant, low in self-assurance, and took long pauses before responding, during which she turned the card searching for responses. Interestingly, in the semistructured and somewhat ambiguous interpersonal context that defines the Rorschach situation, Lisa replicated *in vivo* her reported cognitive and emotional inhibitions in social settings.

## Lisa's R-PAS Results[2]

Despite her hesitations and slowness in taking this test, Lisa was persistent and provided sufficient data for a valid protocol (R = 27, SS[3] = 110; Complexity SS = 107). As her Complexity score was in the average range, the results did not need to be Complexity Adjusted. However, she was somewhat more prone to give responses with a concrete, emotionally neutral, and simplistic quality than the average adult; in particular, Lisa was somewhat less likely to notice and articulate subtleties and nuances of her environment (F% SS = 112). These R-PAS findings were consistent with Lisa's report that she has difficulty grasping subtle social cues and noticing and articulating her emotional experiences. They also suggested that Lisa approaches the world in a manner that is somewhat disengaged, distant, and uninvolved, which is consistent with the examiner's observations that she was hesitant, reserved, and somewhat interpersonally awkward. Lisa also showed a preference for using a cerebral versus emotional problem-solving style, whereby she prefers to "live in her head" and use thoughtful deliberation with little room left for spontaneity and emotional expressivity (M/MC SS = 118). These findings are consistent with her behaviors during the interview and during the R-PAS administration.

In the emotional domain, none of the R-PAS variables indicative of implicit dysphoric emotions (e.g., YTVC′, MOR, CBlend) were elevated, which was not consistent with Lisa's reported clinical history and her self-report test results. Rather, this finding reflected her emotional and cognitive inhibitions that prevented her from attending to or articulating Rorschach stimulus characteristics associated with negative emotions (i.e., shadings). As mentioned above, almost all of her responses had an emotionally neutral quality both in tone and content. Along with other R-PAS data (quasi-absence of color responses; high F%) and self-report data (TAS-20), this finding suggested that Lisa uses emotional avoidance or shutting down of painful emotions as a main strategy to deal with them. However, occasional flashes of anxiety or fear penetrated this "defensive armor," as suggested by the contents of two of her responses (e.g., R3: "Some kind of monster, like an alien; and R4: "A person trapped in something"). In line with the research findings already mentioned on the Rorschach trauma assessment (Viglione et al., 2012), this avoidance coping style is not uncommon for people who were exposed to significant psychosocial stress or traumatic experiences and could account for Lisa's reported difficulty with processing and expressing her emotions socially.

---

[2] See Appendix 16.1 at the end of the chapter for Lisa's R-PAS Responses, Location Sheet, Code Sequence, and Page 1 and 2 Profiles.

[3] Standard scores (SS) have a mean of 100 and an *SD* of 15.

All five of Lisa's representations of human activity had a passive quality [Mp/(Ma+Mp) SS = 130], suggesting that she often used "flight into fantasy" as a coping strategy (i.e., daydreaming and withdrawing as a way to compensate for her frustrations and difficulties). This coping style is thought to promote a passive interpersonal style and to contribute to her loneliness and social adjustment difficulties. Lisa's interpersonal R-PAS data indeed suggested passivity and hesitance to engage in meaningful social exchanges, which were also consistent with her mother's observations. Lisa reported no perceptions of cooperative or collaborative interactions between people or animals (COP = 0, SS = 88). A very timid allusion to closeness was articulated in only one response (R7; "Two people with their hands against each other").

There was some evidence that Lisa may tend to be interpersonally resistive at times to exert a sense of control or autonomy (SR SS = 113). She is also prone to be vigilant for threats and to be guarded in interpersonal situations (V-Comp SS = 120), indicating that Lisa's hesitancy and inhibition are not fueled simply by low self-confidence and difficulty noticing subtle emotional cues, but also by interpersonal wariness. This constant search for threats may further help explain the significantly high anxiety she reported on the MMPI-2 and lead to a depletion of her coping abilities. This combination of test findings suggested that instead of asserting her needs and feelings, she is prone to use a passive–resistant and vigilant interpersonal style in which she "bottles up" her resentments rather than dealing with them in a more appropriate way—a pattern of response that can increase the risk for emotional dysregulation and lead to periodic unmodulated discharges of anger.[4]

On a more positive side, other R-PAS data suggested that Lisa was able to have whole, integrated representations of other people and herself (H SS = 119), with no evidence of significant interpersonal misperceptions (M– = 0), and to envision human images and activity with the same degree of positive and negative characteristics as most people (PHR/GPHR SS = 103). Although, as noted above, Lisa did not show evidence of mental representations of cooperative human interactions, she did show a good ability to mentalize representations of others, which is essential for empathy (M = 5, SS = 109). These were considered healthy features of her interpersonal perception and were associated with some ability for empathy and with some level of social competence (at least for routine social exchanges). Interestingly, although this finding was not congruent with her self-report data, it was consistent with Lisa's good performance on the WAIS-IV test of social cognition.

Lisa's R-PAS results also showed some positive signs of openness to imagination (M SS = 109), particularly in the context of her otherwise "dry" and concrete protocol. This was important because it suggested that Lisa had some ability to put in words and images her internal experiences. From a therapeutic viewpoint, this finding was judged to reflect some ability to do insight-based work. Lisa presented with average psychological resources (MC SS = 99), although this score was relatively lower than her above-average cognitive abilities because it was likely impacted by her inhibited approach to the task. The R-PAS variable that assesses the balance between internal resources and discomforting or distracting experiences (MC–PPD) was in the average range. However, in the light of Lisa's tendency to not articulate the subtle

---

[4]Although Lisa provided responses suggesting that failures of mirroring could feel devastating to her (Reflections = 2, SS = 122), based on research by Horn, Meyer, and Mihura (2009), Card Turning must be considered when interpreting this score since, frequently turning the card significantly increases this score, and Lisa turned the cards significantly more than most people (CT SS = 127).

negative or inconsistent aspect of the test stimulus (YTVC′ was below average), this score would be an overestimate of her current stress tolerance.

From a cognitive perspective, there was very little indication of distorted communication or illogical and bizarre ideation in Lisa's R-PAS profile (the EII-3, TP-Comp, WSumCog, and SevCog were not elevated), and the rate of her perceptual distortions was only slightly above average (FQ–% SS = 111), suggesting that at times Lisa misinterpreted events, situations, or people's intentions or behaviors. However, this mild elevation is not uncommon for people who have emotional and social adjustment difficulties and, in itself, is not enough to indicate major impairment in reality testing. A qualitative analysis of her four FQ– responses revealed that three occurred while responding to the multicolor cards. These findings suggested that Lisa's lapses in judgment may occur when she approaches things from a simplistic perspective in affect-laden situations. Lisa gave only four Popular responses in her protocol (SS = 88), which was interpreted as evidence of limited shared cultural conventions, perhaps due to her reported social isolation/withdrawal. Nevertheless, all in all there was very little indication that Lisa had a thought disorder or impaired reality testing.

## Using R-PAS to Answer the Referral Questions

The R-PAS data provided useful information to answer the referral questions. First, they helped rule out a psychotic process, which was one of Lisa's concerns. Second, the R-PAS results suggested that, as a way to cope with emotional distress, Lisa often tried to suppress or avoid her emotional experience and exerted a rigid emotional control by "shutting down" affectively. Very likely, the neurotic-level rigid defensive mechanisms that she employed to protect herself from processing painful material made her very vulnerable to emotional dysregulation and acting out in daily life. Additionally, the R-PAS data suggested that she often "flew into fantasy" as a coping strategy, which promotes a passive problem-solving style, perhaps contributing to her social isolation and feelings of helplessness. Third, the R-PAS data revealed that Lisa may use a passive–resistant and vigilant interpersonal coping style, likely in response to the broken trust engendered from her past interpersonal traumas.

R-PAS data also revealed some of Lisa's strengths and resources. Despite her somewhat constricted Rorschach protocol and self-reported alexithymic features, there were data that suggested some openness for imagination and some ability to put her internal experiences into words and images. This was consistent with the examiner's observations during the interview. Also, her R-PAS performance spoke of some cognitive ability for empathy and competence for routine social exchanges.

## Conclusions and Recommendations

In conclusion, the current evaluation provided little evidence of a pervasive developmental disorder, despite Lisa's difficulty with social adjustment, understanding social cues, and with social–emotional reciprocity. However, it was judged that her history of significant psychosocial stress and relational trauma constituted an important factor impacting her cognitive, social, and emotional development from an early age. Therefore, it was considered that a diagnosis of other specified neurodevelopmental disorder captured these developmental issues. There was also much evidence of depression and anxiety in her test profile. Finally, a diagnosis of obsessive-compulsive disorder was added as a rule-out diagnosis, given her reported residual symptoms.

Four main recommendations were given: First, following up with her psychiatrist for an appropriate medication regimen for depression and anxiety was suggested. Second, continuing psychotherapy to improve depression, anxiety, emotional regulation, self-image, coping with stress, social skills, and organization was recommended. The test results suggested that Lisa needed much emotional support and reassurance. Given her vulnerability to dysregulation under intense affect and her tendency to ruminate, it was judged that a supportive and structured approach, focused on skill building, response prevention, and empathic listening, would work better in the first stages of the therapy than an insight-based approach. However, the R-PAS data suggested that, after becoming more stable emotionally, an insight-based component may be added to the treatment to help her build a meaningful narrative of her past disruptive experiences. Additionally, given the dissociation from emotions that was revealed by the R-PAS and other test findings, it was judged that Lisa could benefit from practicing mindfulness meditation to help her be more aware and accepting of her emotional experience. Third, dialectical behavior therapy in a group format was recommended to help with emotional regulation. Fourth, executive functioning coaching was recommended to help improve her organization difficulties.

## Discussing the Assessment Findings and Recommendations with Lisa

The results of this evaluation were discussed with Lisa in the interpretive conference. She expressed relief that she did not have "schizophrenia" symptoms and that there was very little evidence of psychotic processes in her test results. She also appeared comforted to hear that she presented with a high level of cognitive abilities. The session included psychoeducation on the impact of relational trauma on her psychological functioning (including thinking, organization, emotional well-being, difficulty understanding and expressing her emotions, attachment and social adjustment problems, low self-confidence), in reference to her history of past disruptive attachment experiences. At the same time, her strengths and internal resources were emphasized and it was noted that Lisa tended to underestimate her abilities, including her ability to read social cues. Her pervasive fear of being judged by people was mentioned as a factor contributing to her mental blocking in social settings, leading to social inhibitions and awkwardness.

With the patient's permission, her therapist and psychiatrist were informed about the testing results and provided with a copy of the report. Lisa continued outpatient therapy for a few weeks after the evaluation, and then relocated to another area, as she had planned.

## Closing Remarks

As a closing remark, the general goal of the current material was to highlight the important role that R-PAS can play, along with more structured measures of cognitive and emotional functioning, in the neuropsychological assessment of patients who have complex psychiatric and developmental problems associated with a history of traumatic experiences. It is my opinion that these patients can benefit from such a multifaceted approach for an in-depth understanding of their difficulties and for appropriate treatment recommendations.

## REFERENCES

Armstrong, J., & Kaser-Boyd, N. (2004). Projective assessment of psychological trauma. In M. J. Hilsenroth & D. L. Segal (Eds.), *Comprehensive handbook of psychological assessment: Vol. 2. Personality assessment* (pp. 500–512). New York: Wiley.

Arnon, Z., Maoz, G., Gazit, T., & Klein, E. (2011). Rorschach indicators of PTSD: A retrospective study. *Rorschachiana, 32,* 5–26.

Bagby, R. M., & Taylor, G. J. (1997). Affect dysregulation and alexithymia. In G. J. Taylor, R. M. Bagby, & J. D. A. Parker (Eds.), *Disorders of affect regulation: Alexithymia in medical and psychiatric illness* (pp. 26–45). Cambridge, UK: Cambridge University Press.

Gabowitz, D., Zucker, M., & Cook, A. (2008). Neuropsychological assessment in clinical evaluation of children and adolescents with complex trauma. *Journal of Child & Adolescent Trauma, 1,* 163–178.

Horn, S. L., Meyer, G. J., & Mihura, J. L. (2009). Impact of card rotation on the frequency of Rorschach reflection responses. *Journal of Personality Assessment, 91,* 346–356.

Hund, A. R., & Espelage, D. L. (2006). Childhood emotional abuse and disordered eating among undergraduate females: Mediating influence of alexithymia and distress. *Child Abuse & Neglect, 30,* 393–407.

Kim, J., & Cicchetti, D. (2006). Longitudinal trajectories of self-system processes and depressive symptoms among maltreated and nonmaltreated children. *Child Development, 77,* 624–639.

Malinosky-Rummell, R., & Hansen, D. J. (1993). Long-term consequences of childhood physical abuse. *Psychological Bulletin, 114,* 68–79.

Meyer, G. J., Viglione, D. J., Mihura, J. L., Erard, R. E., & Erdberg, P. (2011). *Rorschach Performance Assessment System: Administration, coding, interpretation, and technical manual.* Toledo, OH: Rorschach Performance Assessment System.

Mihura, J. L., Meyer, G. J., Dumitrascu, N., & Bombel, G. (2013). The validity of individual Rorschach variables: Systematic reviews and meta-analyses of the comprehensive system. *Psychological Bulletin, 139,* 548–605.

Nemeroff, C. B. (2004). Neurobiological consequences of childhood trauma. *Journal of Clinical Psychiatry, 65*(Suppl.), 18–28.

Scott, J. C., Matt, G. E., Wrocklage, K. M., Crnich, C., Jordan, J., Southwick, S. M., . . . Schweinsburg, B. C. (2015). A quantitative meta-analysis of neurocognitive functioning in posttraumatic stress disorder. *Psychological Bulletin, 141,* 105–140.

Spertus, I. L., Yehuda, R., Wong, C. M., Halligan, S., & Seremetis, S. V. (2003). Childhood emotional abuse and neglect as predictors of psychological and physical symptoms in women presenting to a primary care practice. *Child Abuse & Neglect, 27,* 1247–1258.

Twamley, E. W., Hami, S., & Stein, M. B. (2004). Neuropsychological function in college students with and without posttraumatic stress disorder. *Psychiatry Research, 126,* 265–274.

Viglione, D. J., Towns, B., & Lindshield, D. (2012). Understanding and using the Rorschach inkblot test to assess post-traumatic conditions. *Psychological Injury and Law, 5,* 135–144.

Wolfe, J., & Charney, D. S. (1991). Use of neuropsychological assessment in posttraumatic stress disorder. *Psychological Assessment, 3,* 573–580.

# APPENDIX 16.1.  Lisa's R-PAS Responses, Location Sheet, Code Sequence, and Page 1 and 2 Profiles

## Rorschach Responses "Lisa"

| Respondent ID: Lisa (fictive name) | Examiner: Nicolae Dumitrascu, PhD |
|---|---|
| Location: Mental Health Clinic | Date: **/**/**** |
| Start Time: 2:00 P.M. | End Time: 3:10 P.M. |

| Cd # | R # | Or | Response | Clarification | R-Opt |
|---|---|---|---|---|---|
| I | 1 | | A butterfly. (W) | E: (Examiner Repeats Response [ERR].)<br>R: Yeah, here are the wings (D2) and . . . the body (D4). | |
| | 2 | @ | (@, long pause) Maybe . . . like dogs. (D7) | E: (ERR)<br>R: This is the ear (Dd28), snout (Dd34) . . . two of them (points to D7). | |
| | 3 | v | (v, @, v) Some kind of monster, like an alien. (W) Should I say more?<br>E: Remember? I'm asking you to give two or possibly three responses to each card.<br>R: Then I'm done (subject hands card back to E). (W) | E: (ERR)<br>R: Two sets of eyes (DdS26) . . . and a strange face shape (points to the contour of the entire blot) and little pinchers (D1).<br>E: Not sure where you saw the little pinchers.<br>R: Here. | |
| | 4 | | No, I'd say one more. Like a person trapped in something. (W) I'm done. (Examinee hands card back.)* | E: (ERR)<br>R: Yeah, the legs (D3), arms (D1), the rest is some kind of a sludge . . . like a black sludge (D2), I guess; like being trapped in something.<br>E: Not sure I see the sludge. Can you show me?<br>R: Its shape is undefined . . . like I was thinking of a person trapped. | |
| II | 5 | v | (>, v, <, v) I see . . . can I see parts?<br>E: It's up to you.<br>R: I see legs here. (D2) | E: (ERR)<br>R: Here. (D2)<br>E: What makes it look like legs?<br>R: The shape and the thigh . . . and now I see a body on top . . . maybe. . . . [This was said with a tentative voice and added in CP, so it was not coded.] | |
| | 6 | v | (@, v) Some kind of a bug. (D3) | E: (ERR)<br>R: Antennae and just . . . the head. (D3) | |
| | 7 | | Two people with their hands against each other. (W) | E: (ERR)<br>R: Their feet are crouched; here are their knees, holding their hands up like this (subject demonstrates with hands), and here are their heads. (D2) | |
| III | 8 | | I see two people again, sitting and looking at each other. (D9) | E: (ERR)<br>R: Legs, arms, here are the two faces. (Dd32) | |
| | 9 | v | (v) Still seeing another bug. (D1) (^, v, >, v, subject pauses for a long time.) That's it. | E: (ERR)<br>R: Two eyes (Dd31) and arms (D5) and body. Now I also see a butterfly here. | |
| IV | 10 | @ | (@) Two penguins. (DS4) | E: (ERR)<br>R: Just the heads, here and here. (DS4).<br>E: What makes it look like penguins?<br>R: They are white and black and have that shape of a penguin. | |
| | 11 | | Two large feet. (D6) | E: (ERR)<br>R: Almost Bigfoot feet.<br>E: Not sure I see them like you do.<br>R: They are hairy and . . . their shape is not exactly human.<br>E: You said hairy?<br>R: Yes, see these little lines around . . . like jagged (subject points to the contour). | |
| V | 12 | | A bat. (W) | E: (ERR)<br>R: The legs (D9), wings (D4), ears (subject points to Dd34). | |
| | 13 | < | (>, V, <) A bird. (W) (<, ^, v, ^) Yeah, I'm done. | E: (ERR)<br>R: The beak (D6); looks like it is flying this way (points to left side). | |

*This protocol was administered when the manual had somewhat conflicting guidelines for Pulls. The guidelines now make it clear that even if the card is spontaneously handed back, the examiner is to give a reminder every time a fourth response is given to a card, except on Card X, and to code a Pull.

341

| Cd # | R # | Or | Response | Clarification | R-Opt |
|------|-----|-----|----------|---------------|-------|
| VI | 14 | @ | (v, ^, @, v, <, ^) Like a totem pole. (Dd99) | E: (ERR)<br>R: It looks like a pole going up this way (D5) and the design up here (D3).<br>E: Not sure how you see the design.<br>R: Like a bird design, the wings (Dd22) are here. | |
| | 15 | < | (><) Some kind of a fish. (W) (Examinee hands card back.) | E: (ERR)<br>R: This looks like its mouth (Dd33); here is a fin (Dd22), and fins here too (Dd24, Dd25). | |
| VII | 16 | | Some two people again. (W) | E: (ERR)<br>R: Looks like two girls to me. Faces, pony tails (D5), arms, legs, sitting down, facing each other. | |
| | 17 | < | (@, <) An arrow. (DS7) | E: (ERR)<br>R: I just saw an arrow in the middle here. (DS7)<br>E: What makes it look like an arrow?<br>R: There's a point here (subject points) and then an opening here (subject points). | |
| | 18 | | Fingers. (D5, Dd21) | E: (ERR)<br>R: Just looking at these lines (subject points to D5 and Dd21), [they] look like fingers.<br>E: Can you tell me how you see them?<br>R: See their shapes? This one (D5) looks like a thumb (subject demonstrates pointing her thumb upward). | |
| VIII | 19 | | It looks like two lizards climbing something. (W) | E: (ERR)<br>R: The lizards (D1) could be here and here. And here is a tree (D6) or something.<br>E: What makes it look like a tree?<br>R: Because they are climbing something and a tree was the first thing that came to my mind. | |
| | 20 | < | (<) Or a lizard (D1) climbing and its reflection on the other side, like a hill or mountain. (W) | E: (ERR)<br>R: And when I turned it this way (<), it looks like rocks (D6) . . . like climbing something, and the reflection in the water is underneath.<br>E: What makes it look like rocks?<br>R: Because they are small, just parts of a mountain. | |
| | 21 | v | (v) Or a face. (W) | E: (ERR)<br>R: The eyes (Dd33), ears (D1), mouth. (DdS99 = the space between D4 and D5) | |
| IX | 22 | < | (<) A reflection again; a baby and some kind of an animal. (W) | E: (ERR)<br>R: I saw a baby here (half of D6); the head (D4) and a little arm. And some kind of an animal (D1) walking up some kind of a hill or something (D3); the baby is behind it. And the reflection is everything underneath.<br>E: You said the baby is behind the animal?<br>R: Yes, the animal is here and the baby is here (points to D1 and then ½ D6) [positional description, no depth implied].<br>E: I'm not sure I see the animal as you did.<br>R: Its arm is here, the body, head (Dd24), and it's going up on this incline (D3).<br>E: You said it's a hill or something?<br>R: Yeah, something inclined. | |
| | 23 | v | (v) Or the face of an animal. (W) | E: (ERR)<br>R: Looks like . . . the skeleton or skull of an animal; here are the eye sockets (D4), the nose (DdS22) . . . so it's . . . like the head. | |

| Cd # | R # | Or | Response | Clarification | R-Opt |
|---|---|---|---|---|---|
| X | 24 | | Looks like . . . the Eiffel Tower. (D8) | E: (ERR)<br>R: Just this part up here (points).<br>E: I'm not sure how you see it. Can you help me?<br>R: Sure . . . it's pointed; these are its legs and it's like . . . broad here at the bottom. | |
| | 25 | | Some bugs. (D1, D12) | E: (ERR)<br>R: They are two (D1) . . . have like a leaf (D12) or something. . . . Here are their eyes and horns.<br>E: What makes it look like a leaf?<br>R: It's green and its shape. And it looks like they are holding it. | |
| | 26 | v | Another . . . some kind of a face . . . I don't know (subject seems unsure) (Dd99 = top 3/4 of Dd29). | E: (ERR)<br>R: Two eyes here (D6), a little mouth (D3).<br>E: I'm not sure where you saw that. Please, can you show me?<br>R: Here (subject circles the area). | |
| | 27 | | Some flowers. (D7, D15, D13) (Examinee hands card back.) | E: (ERR)<br>R: Here (D15) and here (D7) look like little buds with green stems. And here is another flower (D13) attached to them.<br>E: I'm not sure what makes it look like a flower.<br>R: Here (subject points), like . . . it's attached to them (subject points to D7). | |

343

# Rorschach Performance Assessment System (R-PAS)®

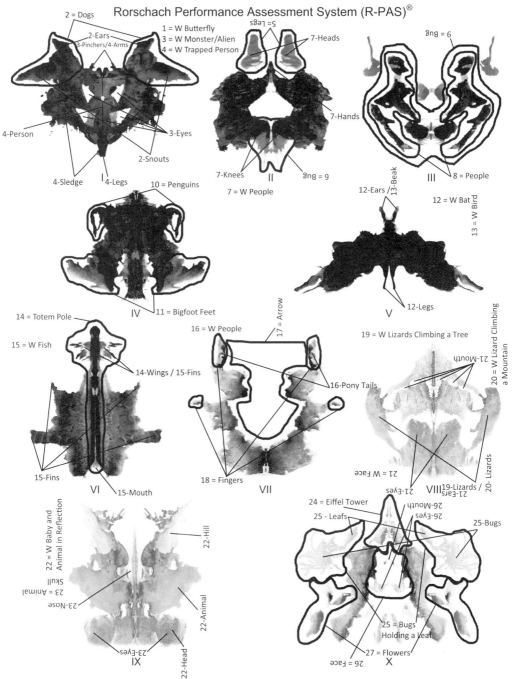

2 = Dogs
2-Ears
3-Pinchers/4-Arms
4-Person
3-Eyes
2-Snouts
4-Sledge
4-Legs

1 = W Butterfly
3 = W Monster/Alien
4 = W Trapped Person

5 = Legs
7-Heads
7-Hands
7-Knees
6 = Bug
7 = W People
II

8 = Bug
8 = People
13-Beak
12-Ears
12 = W Bat
13 = W Bird
III

10 = Penguins
11 = Bigfoot Feet
IV

12-Legs
V

14 = Totem Pole
15 = W Fish
14-Wings / 15-Fins
15-Fins
15-Mouth
VI

16 = W People
17 = Arrow
16-Pony Tails
18 = Fingers
VII

19 = W Lizards Climbing a Tree
20 = W Lizard Climbing a Mountain
21-Mouth
21 = W Face
21-Ears
21-Eyes
19-Lizards / 20-Lizards
VIII

22 = W Baby and Animal in Reflection
23 = Animal Skull
23-Nose
23-Eyes
22-Head
22-Animal
22-Hill
XI

24 = Eiffel Tower
25 - Leafs
26-Mouth
26-Eyes
25-Bugs
25 = Bugs Holding a Leaf
27 = Flowers
26 = Face
X

# R-PAS Code Sequence: "Lisa"

**C-ID**: Lisa (fictive name)  **P-ID**: 849  **Age**: 24  **Gender**: Female  **Education**: 14

| Cd | # | Or | Loc | Loc # | SR | SI | Content | Sy | Vg | 2 | FQ | P | Determinants | Cognitive | Thematic | HR | ODL (RP) | R-Opt |
|----|---|----|-----|-------|----|----|---------|----|----|---|----|---|-------------|-----------|----------|----|---------|-------|
| I | 1 | | W | | | | A | | | | o | P | F | | | | | |
| | 2 | @ | D | 7 | | | Ad | | | 2 | o | | F | | | | | |
| | 3 | v | W | | | SI | (Hd) | | | | o | | F | | AGC | GH | | |
| | 4 | | W | | | | H,NC | Sy | | | o | | Mp,C' | | MAP | GH | ODL | |
| II | 5 | v | D | 2 | | | Hd | | | | - | | F | | | PH | | |
| | 6 | v | D | 3 | | | Ad | | | | u | | F | | | | | |
| | 7 | | W | | | | H | Sy | | 2 | o | | Mp | | | GH | | |
| III | 8 | | D | 9 | | | H | Sy | | 2 | o | P | Mp | | | GH | | |
| | 9 | v | D | 1 | | | A | | | | o | | F | INC1 | | | | |
| IV | 10 | @ | D | 4 | SR | SI | Ad | | | 2 | o | | C' | | | | | |
| | 11 | | D | 6 | | | (Hd) | | | | o | | F | | | GH | | |
| V | 12 | | W | | | | A | | | | o | P | F | | | | | |
| | 13 | < | W | | | | A | | | | o | | FMa | | | | | |
| VI | 14 | @ | Dd | 99 | | | (A),Ay | | | | u | | F | | | | ODL | |
| | 15 | < | W | | | | A | | | | u | | F | | | | | |
| VII | 16 | | W | | | | H | | | 2 | o | P | Mp | | | GH | | |
| | 17 | < | D | 7 | SR | | NC | | | | o | | F | | AGC | | | |
| | 18 | | Dd | 5, 21 | | | Hd | | | | o | | Mp | | | PH | | |
| VIII | 19 | | W | | | | A,NC | Sy | | 2 | o | | FMa | | | | | |
| | 20 | < | W | | | | A,NC | Sy | | | o | | FMa,r | | | | | |
| | 21 | v | W | | | SI | Hd | | | | - | | F | | | PH | | |
| IX | 22 | < | W | | | | H,A,NC | Sy | | | u | | FMa,r | | | GH | | |
| | 23 | v | W | | | SI | An | | | | - | | F | | | | | |
| X | 24 | | D | 11 | | | NC | | | | o | | F | | | | | |
| | 25 | | D | 1, 12 | | SI | A,NC | Sy | | 2 | o | | FMp,CF | | | | | |
| | 26 | v | Dd | 99 | | | Hd | | | | o | | F | | | PH | | |
| | 27 | | Dd | 13, 99 | | | NC | Sy | | 2 | - | | FC | | | | | |

©2010-2016 R-PAS

# R-PAS Summary Scores and Profiles – Page 1

C-ID: Lisa (fictive name)   P-ID: 849   Age: 24   Gender: Female   Education: 14

| Domain/Variables | Raw Scores | Raw %ile | Raw SS | Cplx. Adj. %ile | Cplx. Adj. SS | Standard Score Profile R-Optimized | Abbr. |
|---|---|---|---|---|---|---|---|
| **Admin. Behaviors and Obs.** | | | | | | | |
| Pr | 0 | 24 | 89 | | | | Pr |
| Pu | 0 | 40 | 96 | | | | Pu |
| CT (Card Turning) | 15 | 97 | 129 | | | | CT |
| **Engagement and Cog. Processing** | | | | | | | |
| Complexity | 83 | 68 | 107 | | | | Cmplx |
| R (Responses) | 27 | 74 | 110 | 63 | 105 | | R |
| F% [Lambda=1.25] (Simplicity) | 56% | 79 | 112 | 84 | 115 | | F% |
| Blend | 4 | 56 | 102 | 38 | 95 | | Bln |
| Sy | 8 | 64 | 106 | 53 | 101 | | Sy |
| MC | 6.5 | 47 | 99 | 29 | 92 | | MC |
| MC - PPD | -0.5 | 64 | 105 | 67 | 107 | | MC-PPD |
| M | 5 | 72 | 109 | 54 | 101 | | M |
| M/MC [5/6.5] | 77% | 88 | 118 | 88 | 118 | | M Prp |
| (CF+C)/SumC [1/2] | NA | | | | | | CFC Prp |
| **Perception and Thinking Problems** | | | | | | | |
| EII-3 | -0.7 | 25 | 90 | 27 | 91 | | EII |
| TP-Comp (Thought & Percept. Com...) | 0.7 | 58 | 103 | 58 | 103 | | TP-C |
| WSumCog | 3 | 30 | 92 | 24 | 89 | | WCog |
| SevCog | 0 | 35 | 94 | 35 | 94 | | Sev |
| FQ-% | 15% | 77 | 111 | 77 | 111 | | FQ-% |
| WD-% | 13% | 79 | 112 | 72 | 108 | | WD-% |
| FQo% | 70% | 77 | 111 | 76 | 110 | | FQo% |
| P | 4 | 22 | 88 | 27 | 90 | | P |
| **Stress and Distress** | | | | | | | |
| YTVC' | 2 | 23 | 89 | 13 | 83 | | YTVC' |
| m | 0 | 14 | 84 | 14 | 84 | | m |
| Y | 0 | 17 | 85 | 17 | 85 | | Y |
| MOR | 0 | 18 | 86 | 18 | 86 | | MOR |
| SC-Comp (Suicide Concern Comp.) | 3.7 | 26 | 90 | 20 | 87 | | SC-C |
| **Self and Other Representation** | | | | | | | |
| ODL% | 7% | 37 | 95 | 34 | 93 | | ODL% |
| SR (Space Reversal) | 2 | 82 | 113 | 82 | 113 | | SR |
| MAP/MAHP [1/1] | NA | | | | | | MAP Prp |
| PHR/GPHR [4/11] | 36% | 58 | 103 | 58 | 103 | | PHR Prp |
| M- | 0 | 36 | 95 | 36 | 95 | | M- |
| AGC | 2 | 34 | 94 | 29 | 92 | | AGC |
| H | 5 | 89 | 119 | 83 | 115 | | H |
| COP | 0 | 21 | 88 | 21 | 88 | | COP |
| MAH | 0 | 26 | 90 | 26 | 90 | | MAH |

© 2010-2016 R-PAS

346

## R-PAS Summary Scores and Profiles – Page 2

C-ID: Lisa (fictive name)  P-ID: 849  Age: 24  Gender: Female  Education: 14

| Domain/Variables | Raw Scores | Raw %ile | Raw SS | Cplx. Adj. %ile | Cplx. Adj. SS | Standard Score Profile R-Optimized | Abbr. |
|---|---|---|---|---|---|---|---|
| **Engagement and Cog. Processing** | | | | | | 60 70 80 90 100 110 120 130 140 | |
| W% | 48% | 65 | 106 | 62 | 105 | | W% |
| Dd% | 15% | 56 | 102 | 59 | 104 | | Dd% |
| SI (Space Integration) | 5 | 89 | 118 | 90 | 119 | | SI |
| IntCont | 1 | 31 | 93 | 24 | 89 | | IntC |
| Vg% | 0% | 18 | 86 | 18 | 86 | | Vg% |
| V | 0 | 29 | 92 | 29 | 92 | | V |
| FD | 0 | 21 | 88 | 23 | 89 | | FD |
| R8910% | 33% | 60 | 104 | 60 | 104 | | R8910% |
| WSumC | 1.5 | 21 | 88 | 11 | 81 | | WSC |
| C | 0 | 36 | 95 | 36 | 95 | | C |
| Mp/(Ma+Mp) [5/5] | 100% | 98 | 130 | 98 | 130 | | Mp Prp |
| **Perception and Thinking Problems** | | | | | | 60 70 80 90 100 110 120 130 140 | |
| FQu% | 15% | 13 | 83 | 13 | 83 | | FQu% |
| **Stress and Distress** | | | | | | 60 70 80 90 100 110 120 130 140 | |
| PPD | 7 | 34 | 94 | 22 | 88 | | PPD |
| CBlend | 0 | 28 | 91 | 28 | 91 | | CBlnd |
| C' | 2 | 62 | 105 | 49 | 100 | | C' |
| V | 0 | 29 | 92 | 29 | 92 | | V |
| CritCont% (Critical Contents) | 4% | 7 | 78 | 5 | 75 | | CrCt |
| **Self and Other Representation** | | | | | | 60 70 80 90 100 110 120 130 140 | |
| SumH | 11 | 93 | 122 | 89 | 118 | | SumH |
| NPH/SumH [6/11] | 55% | 38 | 95 | 38 | 95 | | NPH Prp |
| V-Comp (Vigilance Composite) | 5.2 | 91 | 120 | 88 | 118 | | V-C |
| r (Reflections) | 2 | 93 | 122 | 93 | 122 | | r |
| p/(a+p) [6/10] | 60% | 81 | 113 | 80 | 112 | | p Prp |
| AGM | 0 | 31 | 93 | 31 | 93 | | AGM |
| T | 0 | 28 | 91 | 28 | 91 | | T |
| PER | 0 | 30 | 92 | 30 | 92 | | PER |
| An | 1 | 47 | 99 | 47 | 99 | | An |

© 2010–2016 R-PAS

# CHAPTER 17

# Using R-PAS in the Neuropsychological Assessment of an 8-Year-Old Boy

Jessica Lipkind
Jack Fahy

In this chapter, we present a complex, multimethod assessment of a young boy by exploring his cognitive, neuropsychological, academic, and social–emotional functioning. Although all of his results are reviewed, our primary emphasis is on the interpretation of his Rorschach Performance Assessment System (R-PAS; Meyer, Viglione, Mihura, Erard, & Erdberg, 2011) results.

## Client Background

"Luis" was an 8-year, 11-month-old boy of Mexican American descent who was referred by his adoptive father, "Martin," for a psychological assessment. The assessment occurred at an outpatient psychological center that provides assessment and therapy for children, adolescents, and families. Prior to participating in the assessment, a treatment manager, who is a licensed clinical social worker, conducted an intake with Luis and Martin. Martin shared that, at home, Luis easily became angry and frequently argued with family members; the arguments with his siblings typically escalated into pushing and shoving. Martin expressed frustration that, when he set a limit, Luis often became agitated and insulted him.

Luis was born to a mother with a history of polysubstance abuse. She was incarcerated during her pregnancy with him but released in her third trimester. According to court documentation, Luis was delivered at a hospital and the toxicology screen was positive for methamphetamines. He was removed from his mother's care at the age of 2 days and placed in an emergency foster home, where he remained for 3 months, and subsequently was reunified with his mother in a drug treatment facility. Court documents stated that the treatment staff contacted child protective services due to concerns that his mother did not supervise him adequately. For instance, he was left in the care of various residents and was bitten several times by another child. When Luis was 8 months old, his mother abandoned him at the facility. He again was placed in emergency foster care, but removed from this home after a few weeks due to the foster parents' report that he was agitated and inconsolable. Luis spent some time in another foster home before moving in with his adoptive fathers, Martin and Carlos, at the age of 1 year, 3 months. His older half-brother and half-sister were already in the home. Court documents indicated that Luis walked by the time he entered his adoptive home, and Martin reported that Luis was making vocal sounds but not yet speaking words. Martin and Carlos separated when Luis was 2½ years old and Carlos moved out. Luis had weekend visits with Carlos and, at the time of the assessment, Carlos often took him to school.

Luis started kindergarten in a public school prior to age 5 at the recommendation of staff in his preschool. Martin explained that it was a very difficult year because Luis was often inattentive and oppositional. He repeated kindergarten in a different public school, which Martin recalled as a positive experience. In first grade, Luis had few behavioral disruptions, but he struggled in second grade. His second-grade teacher expressed concern about Luis's difficulty sitting still and completing tasks. Luis's current third-grade teacher had similar concerns.

At the age of 2, Luis was diagnosed with neurofibromatosis type 1 (NF1). NF1 is a genetic disorder with a variety of clinical manifestations involving various organs and the nervous system. Common symptoms include neurofibromas—mostly benign tumors that grow on the nerves—and cutaneous anomalies. Fifty percent of people with NF1 have a neurodevelopmental disorder such as attention-deficit/hyperactivity disorder (ADHD) and/or a learning disability (see Hachon, Iannuzzi, & Chaix, 2011, for review). Luis had café au lait spots on his skin, freckles in his armpits, and Lisch nodules in his eyes. Since his diagnosis, he has been evaluated annually by a geneticist and twice per year by an endocrinologist to monitor his growth. At the time of the assessment, he was not taking any medication, but his physician was considering growth hormone injections because Luis was below the third percentile in height for his age.

## Referral Questions

Martin requested an assessment to evaluate Luis's cognitive, academic, neuropsychological, and emotional functioning, as well as to determine causes for his behavioral disruptions at home and at school. He specifically asked, "How can I help him be independent?" and "Do you think he's hyper?" It is important to note that, when these questions were explored, Martin clarified that he did not believe that Luis was hyper. Martin also inquired about the need for individual therapy. Luis did not have any questions about himself during the assessment process.

## Behavioral Observations

At the time of testing, Luis was in third grade and appeared much younger than his stated age due to his extremely short stature. He made good eye contact and related well with the assessor. Sometimes he was excitable and loud, but most of the time his speech volume was appropriate. His speech was notable for minor articulation difficulties (e.g., "bool" for bowl).

Luis was motivated to do well on tests, but struggled to stay focused; he frequently stared off and needed redirection to the task. He was easily distracted by extraneous sounds and objects in the room. He needed frequent breaks to help sustain the mental energy needed for testing. Moreover, he often required repetition of instructions and had great difficulty controlling impulsivity. Luis demonstrated hyperactive behaviors, such as tapping the table with his fingers, kicking his feet back and forth vigorously, and walking around the room during testing. He struggled to keep multistep instructions in mind and often repeated them under his breath. He was highly anxious about his performance and stated he was worried the tests would be "too hard." Luis also had difficulty with motor tasks, specifically fine motor activities. He had an atypical pencil grip and displayed weak graphomotor control.

## Collateral Reports

The treatment manager contacted three of Luis's teachers: his current after-school teacher, his teacher in a combined kindergarten and first-grade classroom, and his second-grade teacher. All three teachers described him as a bright student who seemed to learn easily when he applied himself. He was also described as socially adept and a leader among his peers. Concerns included difficulty staying focused and impulsivity in the classroom, such as calling out answers and other hyperactive behaviors. The teachers noted challenges with writing due to poor fine motor control. During his second-grade year, a behavioral plan was implemented to address disruptive behaviors and improve his participation. The plan helped somewhat, but his teacher also remarked that, at times, Luis struggled to take responsibility for his behaviors.

## Cognitive and Neuropsychological Measures

Performance-based measures were administered to Luis that covered a wide range of cognitive and neuropsychological functions, as well as areas of academic achievement.[1]

### General Cognitive Ability

Luis's performance on the Differential Ability Scales—Second Edition (DAS-II; Elliott, 2007) verbal measures revealed personal strengths in above-average verbal conceptual reasoning and knowledge of word meanings (Verbal Cluster SS = 115; Similarities T = 60; Word Definitions T = 58). In comparison, his visual–spatial abilities were weaker and less sophisticated, with scores falling within the low-average range (Spatial Cluster SS = 83; Recall of Designs T = 38; Pattern Construction T = 42). His ability to reason with nonverbal, visual material was in the average range

---

[1]Standard Score (SS) mean = 100, $SD$ = 15; scaled score (ss) mean = 10, $SD$ = 3; T score (T) mean = 50, $SD$ = 10.

(Nonverbal Reasoning Cluster SS = 93; Matrices T = 43; Sequential and Quantitative Reasoning T = 48). Luis's primary challenge with visual–spatial tasks was that they required the integration of both visual-perceptual and graphomotor skills (i.e., Recall of Designs, Pattern Construction). His DAS-II results were consistent with other findings that indicated struggles on tasks of visual–motor integration and graphomotor functions (Beery–Buktenica Developmental Test of Visual–Motor Integration [VMI] SS = 76; Beery & Beery, 2010).

## Attention

To address the presenting questions regarding difficulties with schoolwork and the possibility of ADHD, we used a standard neuropsychological conceptualization of attention to assess its three subdomains: selective, sustained, and divided attention (Baron, 2004). Luis showed a personal strength in selective attention (Test of Everyday Attention for Children [TEA-Ch; Manly, Robertson, Anderson, & Nimmo-Smith, 1998] Score! ss = 10; Delis–Kaplan Executive Function System [D-KEFS; Delis, Kaplan, & Kramer, 2001] Trail Making Test Visual Scanning ss = 14; Conners Continuous Performance Test—Second Edition [CPT-II; Conners & MHS Staff, 2004] Number of Omission errors T = 51; and he was in the average range on measures of divided attention (TEA-Ch [Manly et al., 1998] Sky Search Dual Task ss = 8, TEA-Ch Score! Dual Task ss = 11). He showed deficits in his ability to put forth extra mental effort on repetitive and less interesting tasks (DAS-II Digit Span–Forward T = 29; NEPSY-II [Korkman, Kirk, & Kemp, 2007] Auditory Attention ss = 5; TEA-Ch Code Transmission ss = 5).

Behaviorally, Luis needed reminders and verbal prompts to stay on task, which indicated that he not only had trouble attending to details but also sustaining attention. Luis often approached timed tasks in a hasty manner; thus, his completion times were fast, but he missed critical details and his accuracy was low (TEA-Ch Sky Search Time per Target ss = 15, # Targets Identified ss = 6). An exception was his performance on the CPT-II, on which he adopted a more cautious approach, resulting in a slow reaction time for the task (CPT-II Mean Hit Reaction Time T = 68). However, the number of times he missed a target was within the average range (Omission errors T = 51), and he made a few impulsive errors (Commission errors T = 29).

## Executive Functions

Both prenatal methamphetamine exposure and NF1 increased Luis's risk for executive functioning difficulties (Gilboa, Rosenblum, Fattal-Valevski, Toledano-Alhadef, & Josman, 2014; Smith et al., 2015). We assessed three key components of executive functioning via performance-based methods: response inhibition, cognitive flexibility, and verbal fluency. Luis's performance revealed strengths in cognitive flexibility and inhibition (D-KEFS Trail Making Test Number–Letter Switching ss = 8, D-KEFS Color–Word Interference Inhibition ss = 11). He was at a superior level when the task increased in complexity and involved both response inhibition and cognitive flexibility (Inhibition/Switching ss = 15).

Luis also showed strengths in verbal fluency, scoring in the superior range in his ability to fluidly generate verbal thoughts and ideas under the structured condition of a categorical cue (D-KEFS Verbal Fluency Test Category Fluency ss = 14; Category Switching Total Correct ss = 17). In contrast, he had significant difficulty generating verbal responses under the less structured condition (Letter Fluency ss = 6). These results suggest that, verbally, he will have difficulty in unstructured conditions, but when given scaffolding and structure, his verbal fluency will be excellent. These results have important implications for his verbal problem-solving abilities.

### Academic Achievement

Select measures of academic achievement were administered in order to gauge the impact of his neuropsychological difficulties on basic academic skills. Luis's performance on measures of reading was at age level. However, his attention and executive functioning problems impacted his performance on math tasks. He made a number of careless, inattentive errors while solving simple pencil-and-paper math problems (Wechsler Individual Achievement Test—Third Edition [WIAT-III; Wechsler, 2009] Numerical Operations SS = 101, Math Fluency–Subtraction ss = 87) and had mild difficulty figuring out which math operations to use (Math Problem Solving SS = 91). On measures of writing, Luis performed at an average, age-appropriate level in spelling but was low average in his ability to compose sentences (Spelling SS =106; Sentence Composition SS = 83). He generated a sentence to nearly every item on the Sentence Composition subtest, but he showed problems with grammar and handwriting.

## Emotional and Behavioral Measures

Several measures were administered to assess Luis's emotional functioning. His scores on the Revised Children's Manifest Anxiety Scale—Second Edition (RCMAS-2; Reynolds & Richmond, 2008) and the Piers–Harris Children's Self-Concept Scale—Second Edition (Piers–Harris 2; Piers & Herzberg, 2002) validity scales indicated that he approached most items in a straightforward and consistent manner (RCMAS-2 Inconsistent Index = 3 [cut-off = 6], Defensiveness Scale T = 49; Piers–Harris 2 Inconsistent T = 43, Response Bias T = 43). However, his score on the Piers–Harris 2 Happy Domain subscale (T = 59) was judged to be somewhat elevated, given the various stressors he was experiencing, and suggested that he engaged in slight minimization or avoidance of negative affect.

Luis's main self-reported concerns were his physical appearance and conflicted feelings about his biological parents. On the Piers–Harris 2 (Physical Appearance and Attributes T = 42), he endorsed items indicating concerns with both physical strength and appearance (i.e., short stature). On the Sentence Completion test he said (his words are in *italics*): "I don't like people who *be mean to me because of my height*," "The thing that hurts my feelings most *is people making fun of my height*," "I sure wish my father *would come back, my real father*," "My mother *took drugs*," and "I like my mother, but *I got mad that she took drugs, because I really miss her*."

On the Behavior Assessment System for Children, Second Edition (BASC-2; Reynolds & Kamphaus, 2004), both Martin and Luis's teacher indicated that he was argumentative and showed more externalizing than internalizing behaviors. However, his teacher identified more problems with attention, hyperactivity, and impulsivity. These results indicated that either Martin did not fully appreciate the intensity of Luis's distractibility and hyperactivity or that these problems mainly manifest at school.

## Rationale for R-PAS

R-PAS was administered to more fully understand Luis's emotional functioning. The reports by his father and his teacher were helpful, but there were indications that they did not have a deep understanding of what he was feeling and how he coped with his anger and anxiety. As is common with children this age, Luis's insight into his own emotional experiences was limited. There were also indications from his behavior and results on self-report measures that he sometimes minimized concerns and avoided negative affect. We have found that the R-Optimized method of administration helps generate a more accurate and useful set of responses regarding the nature of a youth's internal distress and the difficulties he or she may be experiencing.

## R-PAS Administration

R-PAS was conducted with Luis on the second of three consecutive days of testing. The administration occurred halfway through the 3-hour testing session and took approximately 45 minutes to complete. Prior to the R-PAS administration, Luis took a break, had a snack, and played briefly with a board game in the testing room (which doubles as a child therapy space). He was willing to settle back into the testing, but needed a few prompts to do so. He struggled to transition from play breaks throughout the assessment.

Luis appeared to clearly understand the R-Optimized administration instructions and did not have any questions. He was initially very excited to see the inkblots, which he recalled making with paint in his kindergarten classroom. However, as the administration progressed, Luis complained of fatigue and yawned frequently; at times, he complained that his "eyes hurt" and pushed the card back toward the examiner and refused to look at the blot further. Consistent with his behavior throughout the testing sessions, Luis also fidgeted frequently, made noises with his mouth, and impulsively grabbed at the cards. However, with support and encouragement, Luis was able to complete the R-PAS administration and provide a valid protocol.

## Discussion of R-PAS Results[2]

When interpreting Luis's R-PAS profile, we began by considering how the variables plotted on the Summary Scores and Profiles pages were different than those for adults. As discussed in Meyer and Erdberg (Chapter 3, this volume), in a child's profile, the expected mean score for each variable is designated with an "X"; a dotted line whisker extends one standard deviation (15 SS) above and below each mean value. Thus, the child and adolescent standard scores (C-SS) indicate how far a score is from the

---

[2]See Appendix 17.1 at the end of the chapter for Luis's R-PAS Responses, Location Sheet, Code Sequence, and Page 1 and 2 Profiles.

mean (i.e., the X). For example, for Card Turning, the expected mean value for an 8-year-old is approximately four times. Luis turned the card six times, which is in the average range (SS = 109). Similarly, the number of Prompts (1) and Pulls (0) were in the average range (Pr SS = 105; Pu SS = 96), suggesting that he understood and complied with the instructions.

## Engagement and Cognitive Processing

Luis provided a protocol with high Complexity (SS = 141) and an average number of responses (R = 26, SS = 109), which suggests a variety of strengths. The high Complexity score indicates that Luis was very engaged and, compared to other 8-year-olds, demonstrated sophisticated processing.

Luis was much more likely to synthesize and integrate his ideas and perceptions (Sy) and to articulate multiple features (Blends) compared to other children his age, even compared to those with his level of complexity. Unfortunately, most of the ways that Luis synthesized information included aggression (e.g., Fi, Ex, AGM, AGC) due to internal presses (m, FM), not due to actual features of his external environment. These distracting, aggressively tinged ideas and internal presses severely compromised (MC–PPD SS = 71) what otherwise would be above-average psychological resources (MC SS = 129), such as the ability to reflect on his and others' experiences (M SS = 119). He struggled to control and modulate his reactions to the environment when emotionally provoked [(CF+C)/SumC SS = 128], such that he generally tries to avoid affective stimulation (e.g., R8910% SS = 67; pushing the card away and complaining of eye pain during the administration), but his inability to avoid such stimulation in everyday life could account for his episodic outbursts.

## Perception and Thinking Problems

Luis was highly elevated on a measure of general psychopathology, which was indicative of thought disturbance, problematic interpersonal representations, and intrusive thought content (EII-3 SS = 147). Luis perceived illogical and implausible relationships, as well as struggled with linguistics and effective communication (WSumCog SS > 150). In addition, he evidenced psychotic-like processes in reasoning, conceptualization, communication, and thought organization (SevCog SS = 142). Despite these areas of concern, his perceptual accuracy was age-appropriate, and he was able to attend to common and obvious aspects of the environment (WD–% SS = 101; FQo% SS = 94), with some tendency, however, to have lapses in perceiving his environment (FQ–% SS = 111). Almost all of these lapses were associated with internal press (FM, m) and themes of implicit anger and aggression (AGM, AGC, MOR). However, he was much more able than most children his age to identify the most conventional and obvious elements of his perceptual environment (Populars SS = 131).

## Stress and Distress

Luis was elevated on an aggregated measure of implicit stress (PPD SS = 145). In particular, he was experiencing a high degree of unwanted ideation and felt a loss of control associated with a history of moderate to severe environmental stressors (m SS > 150). In general, he was troubled by disquieting, irritating internal stimuli, likely due to early childhood maltreatment and loss. An exceedingly large number of his responses involved aggression, fire, explosions, and damaged objects (CritCont% SS > 150, MOR SS = 139).[3] It is also worth noting that his Complexity was elevated in part because of variables in the Stress and Distress domain. That is, his highly elevated number of Blends, and thus his Determinant Complexity, was driven by variables that spoke to disruptive and irritating internal stimuli. Specifically, each of his 12 Blends was formed from PPD variables, most notably m (in eight Blends), FM (in four Blends), and C′ (in four Blends).

## Self and Other Representation

This domain was of particular interest in the assessment, given Luis's history of early attachment disruptions and his father's concerns regarding their interactions. Luis demonstrated that he can envision people in intact, multifaceted, and integrated ways (H SS = 123). Moreover, there was evidence that he internalized the potential for healthy emotional closeness (MAH = 1, SS = 119). These findings represent valuable interpersonal strengths for Luis. At the same time, despite his desire for closeness (T SS = 123), Luis was preoccupied with dangerous, aggressive, and threatening imagery (AGC SS = 137), and imagining relationships were marked by aggression and combativeness (AGM SS > 150). At times, this preoccupation with aggression contributed to emotional dysregulation, particularly in the context of interpersonal conflict (four out of five CFs associated with aggressiveness and destruction: AGMs, AGCs, and MORs ["erupting volcano"; people who "ripped out [their] hearts"; robot whose "head blew up"; "lions wrestling"]).

Luis evidenced a less adaptive understanding of himself and others relative to same-age peers, along with a tendency to experience difficult and problematic interactions (PHR/GPHR SS = 117). Some of his Morbid responses, particularly on Card III (R8), indicated a damaged sense of self, which may be related to his NF1 diagnosis and feeling rejected by his biological parents, "Persons took out both their hearts, connected together" and RP: "Ripped out their own hearts." Consistent with his intermittent struggle with reality testing, Luis was at significant risk for misunderstanding other people's thoughts and intentions (M– SS = 146), with each instance of significant misunderstanding associated with aggressive imagery (AGM, AGC). Taken together, Luis's preoccupation with aggression, emotional dysregulation, and sense of having his "heart ripped out" could explain his outbursts toward family members.

## The Feedback and R-PAS Impact on the Case

Findings were discussed with Luis, both parents in separate meetings, and his newly assigned individual psychotherapist. The treatment manager also participated in each of the feedback sessions with Martin and Carlos. Feedback was approached utilizing tenets of Finn's (2007) Therapeutic Assessment model, which provides a framework

---

[3] His SC-Composite was not interpreted because it is only interpreted for those above 15 years of age.

for presenting information according to the client's and each parent's readiness to hear the findings. Finn describes Level 1 information as validating the ways that clients see themselves and others in their lives. Level 2 data provide a reframe that helps clients think about themselves or their relationships in a new way. Level 3 information conflicts with clients' view of themselves or their relationships, which may result in defensiveness or rejection of the findings.

In the parent sessions, Luis's strengths in verbal reasoning and reading fundamentals were emphasized. His challenges with spatial reasoning and visual–motor integration and his deficits in attention and impulse control were discussed. This seemed to be Level 2 information, as both parents indicated that they had not noted his challenges with attention previously, but now understood that, much of the time, Luis was not willfully restless and hyperactive. The results of the emotional testing were summarized, and both Martin and Carlos were presented with examples of Luis's tendency to constrict his feelings and then become flooded and emotionally overwhelmed. We discussed how this difficulty with flexibly regulating affect is common in children who have experienced neglect and attachment disruptions. We briefly discussed research identifying the neurological underpinnings of these struggles (Cook et al., 2005; Schore, 2001).

There was discussion around the implications of Luis's NF1 diagnosis, as his short stature left him feeling vulnerable and fragile, which is a particular struggle for a boy entering preadolescence. Again, this appeared to be Level 2 information initially, but both parents seemed to integrate it easily into their conceptualization of Luis's difficulties. We also discussed Luis's unresolved feelings of loss, sadness, and anger related to his early history. This feedback appeared to fall between Level 2 and Level 3, and both Martin and Carlos were thoughtful and open to the information and asked appropriate questions about the best ways to support Luis. His DSM-IV-TR diagnoses were reviewed, which included ADHD–combined type, developmental coordination disorder, and mood disorder not otherwise specified.

We discussed a variety of recommendations, including Luis participating in individual therapy, getting an evaluation for medication, and engaging in occupational therapy to address his graphomotor struggles. We also suggested that he would benefit from an individualized education plan (IEP) for ADHD. Martin raised questions about Luis's treatment for NF1 and how medication that targets attention may impact his growth and contribute further to his short stature. The team members agreed it would be important for all professionals to be in close collaboration, and the treatment manager planned to support Martin with this process as the referrals were arranged.

Feedback was also conducted with Luis; due to scheduling issues, it occurred shortly after he began individual therapy. Luis was energetic and hyperactive in the session. He was told that he was bright and capable, and strong at thinking with words and reading, to which he responded, "I know." His challenges with attention and hyperactivity were also discussed, and Luis agreed that it was often difficult to stay focused and slow down so as to avoid mistakes in his schoolwork. Luis's strong feelings were also addressed and how, when he keeps them inside, they become very powerful and lead him to act out. This area was linked to his NF1 condition and to how Luis may worry often about his health or his small stature. It was clear when this specific component of feedback was given that it was Level 3 information, as Luis rejected it wholeheartedly by stating, "I forgot I had NF1 until you said that; I don't even think about it." At this point, Luis got out of his chair and grabbed a noisy electronic toy, indicating that he no longer wanted to stay on this topic and hear further results. The assessor joined Luis in play briefly, and as the session ended, encouraged him to bring his "big, strong feelings" to his therapist.

## R-PAS Impact on the Therapy Relationship

Luis began weekly, psychoanalytically informed, individual treatment after the assessment ended. Prior to initiating treatment, the assessor met with his therapist to review the assessment findings and thereby inform Luis's treatment. In preparation for this chapter, contact was made with his therapist to obtain information about treatment progress. The therapist had worked with Luis for 18 months. He reported that the overarching issues were Luis's struggles with self-esteem, depressive symptoms, and a sense of vulnerability and fragility. For instance, he described Luis's identification with superheroes as a representation of his need to feel strong and invulnerable. Fear of rejection and abandonment were also present, as Luis expressed worry about the clinician's age and that he may suddenly "die of a heart attack." They explored the projection of Luis's own anger toward those no longer in his life, such as his biological parents. For example, sessions focused on Luis telling "Yo Momma" jokes, which permitted them to explore feelings of contempt toward the mother who had left him. Over time, Martin reported to the therapist that Luis's academic skills and self-esteem had improved. He also described a willingness to try new activities and be less fearful. Luis was able to develop an attachment to a female teacher, which was a new experience for him. He continues to participate in weekly treatment.

## Conclusion

In conclusion, R-PAS has enabled us to shift our lens when interpreting results from a child's neuropsychological assessment. Traditionally, neuropsychological assessments emphasize cognitive tests, along with self-report measures and behavior rating scales. Incorporating R-PAS into a neuropsychological assessment allows for a fuller and richer conceptualization of a child's experience, with clear practical implications to improve the child's life.

### REFERENCES

Baron, I. S. (2004). *Neuropsychological evaluation of the child.* New York: Oxford University Press.

Beery, K. E., & Beery, N. A. (2010). *The Beery–Buktenica Developmental Test of Visual–Motor Integration (VMI), with supplemental developmental tests of visual perception and motor coordination* (6th ed.). Bloomington, MN: NCS Pearson.

Conners, C. K., & MHS Staff. (Eds.). (2004). *Conners Continuous Performance Test II: Computer program for Windows technical guide and software manual.* North Tonwanda, NY: Multi-Health Systems.

Cook, A., Spinazzola, J., Ford, J., Lanktree, C., Blaustein, M., Cloitre, M., . . . van der Kolk, B. (2005). Complex trauma in children and adolescents. *Psychiatric Annals, 35*, 390–398.

Delis, D. C., Kaplan, E., & Kramer, J. H. (2001). *Delis–Kaplan Executive Function System (D-KEFS)*. San Antonio, TX: NCS Pearson.

Elliott, C. D. (2007). *Differential Ability Scales: Introductory and technical handbook* (2nd ed.). San Antonio, TX: NCS Pearson.

Finn, S. E. (2007). *In our clients' shoes: Theory and techniques of therapeutic assessment*. Mahwah, NJ: Erlbaum.

Gilboa, Y., Rosenblum, S., Fattal-Valevski, A., Toledano-Alhadef, H., & Josman, N. (2014). Is there a relationship between executive functions and academic success in children with neurofibromatosis type 1? *Neuropsychological Rehabilitation, 24*, 918–935.

Hachon, C., Iannuzzi, S., & Chaix, Y. (2011). Behavioral and cognitive phenotypes in children with neurofibromatosis type 1 (NF1): The link with the neurobiological level. *Brain & Development, 33*, 52–61.

Korkman, M., Kirk, U., & Kemp, S. (2007). *NEPSY-II* (2nd ed.). San Antonio, TX: NCS Pearson.

Manly, T., Robertson, I. H., Anderson, V., & Nimmo-Smith, I. (1998). *The Test of Everyday Attention for Children (TEA-Ch)*. London: Harcourt Assessment.

Meyer, G. J., Viglione, D. J., & Giromini, L. (2014). Current R-PAS transitional child and adolescent norms. Retrieved from *www.r-pas.org/CurrentChildNorms.aspx*.

Meyer, G. J., Viglione, D. J., Mihura, J. L., Erard, R. E., & Erdberg, P. (2011). *Rorschach Performance Assessment System: Administration, coding, interpretation, and technical manual*. Toledo, OH: Rorschach Performance Assessment System.

Piers, E. V., & Herzberg, D. S. (2002). *Piers–Harris Children's Self-Concept Scale (Piers–Harris 2)* (2nd ed.). Los Angeles: Western Psychological Services.

Reynolds, C. R., & Kamphaus, R. W. (2004). *Behavioral Assessment System for Children* (2nd ed.). Minneapolis, MN: NCS Pearson.

Reynolds, C. R, & Richmond, B. O. (2008). *Revised Children's Manifest Anxiety Scale (RCMAS-2)* (2nd ed.). Los Angeles: Western Psychological Services.

Schore, A. N. (2001). The effects of early relational trauma on right brain development, affect regulation, and infant mental health. *Infant Mental Health Journal, 22*(1–2), 201–269.

Smith, L. M., Diaz, S., LaGasse, L. L., Wouldes, T., Derauf, C., Newman, E., . . . Lester, B. M. (2015). Developmental and behavioral consequences of prenatal methamphetamine exposure: A review of the Infant, Development, Environment, and Lifestyle (IDEAL) study. *Neurotoxicology and Teratology, 51*, 35–44.

Wechsler, D. (2009). *Wechsler Individual Achievement Test* (3rd ed.). San Antonio, TX: NCS Pearson.

# APPENDIX 17.1. Luis's R-PAS Responses, Location Sheet, Code Sequence, and Page 1 and 2 Profiles

## Rorschach Responses "Luis"

| Respondent ID: Luis | Examiner: Jessica Lipkind, PsyD |
|---|---|
| Location: MCYAF | Date: **/**/**** |
| Start Time: 10:00 A.M. | End Time: 10:45 A.M. |

| Cd # | R # | Or | Response | Clarification | R-Opt |
|---|---|---|---|---|---|
| I | 1 | | A bat. (W) | E: (Examiner Repeats Response [ERR])<br>R: Looks like big, giant, humungous bat; wings (D2), head (Dd22).<br>[E could have queried "big, giant, humungous" for FD.] | |
| | 2 | | A woman in a dress. (W) | E: (ERR)<br>R: Woman's head (Dd22), wings (D2) on her dress, tutu shape, dress bottom (Dd24). | |
| | 3 | | Two birds. (D7) | E: (ERR)<br>R: (R yawns) Head, back. | |
| | 4 | | Three-headed dragon. (Dd99 = upper half of W)<br>[R quickly pushed card back to E, though E still should have given a reminder to give "two . . . maybe three responses."] | E: (ERR)<br>R: Head (upper protrusion of D7), head (upper protrusion of D7), tiny head (Dd22) in the middle. | |
| II | 5 | v | v That's hard . . . a drill. (D2,4) | E: (ERR)<br>R: Looks like a drill (D4), goes down into ground (D2), dirt.<br>E: Dirt?<br>R: Red dirt. | |
| | 6 | v | v A robot. (D2,3,4) | E: (ERR)<br>R: Looks like a drilling robot [drill is D4, dirt is D2], connected here this time, its head blew up.<br>E: Blew up?<br>R: Up here.<br>E: What makes it look like that?<br>R: Red brains. (D3) | |
| | 7 | v | v Erupting volcano. (W) | E: (ERR)<br>R: Lava. (D2, D3)<br>E: Lava?<br>R: Red and coming up, blasts out. | |
| III | 8 | | (R puts his head on the table) Persons (D9) took out both their hearts, connected together. (D9,3) | E: (ERR)<br>R: Ripped out hearts. (D3)<br>E: Hearts?<br>R: Pink shaped, head, hand, leg. | |
| | 9 | | People (D9) playing an instrument. (D9,2, 3) | E: (ERR)<br>R: Instrument (D3) you blow into, things coming out of instrument.<br>E: Things coming out?<br>R: Musical notes. (D2)<br>E: Notes?<br>R: Line and circle.<br>E: Instrument?<br>R: Something you blow into. | |

| Cd # | R # | Or | Response | Clarification | R-Opt |
|------|-----|----|----------|---------------|-------|
| IV | 10 | | Looks like a dragon blowing up steam. (W) | E: (ERR)<br>R: Feet (D6), hand (D4), head (D3), nose, steam (Dd30).<br>E: Steam?<br>R: Blows steam from nose.<br>E: What makes it look like steam?<br>R: Gray, exact color. | |
| | 11 | | Evil goat. (Dd99 = W – D6, D1) | E: (ERR)<br>R: Horns (D4), head (D3).<br>E: Evil?<br>R: Blowing steam; it's a shadow.<br>E: Shadow?<br>R: Same color as smoke. | |
| | 12 | | Big giant made out of shadows. (W) | E: (ERR)<br>R: Feet (D6), toe, hand (D4), head (D3).<br>E: Made of shadows?<br>R: Color as smoky shadows.<br>E: Smoky?<br>R: Color and coming out, steaming.<br>[E could have queried "big giant" for FD.] | |
| V | 13 | v | v Butterfly. (W) | E: (ERR)<br>R: Nectar (DdS27), head (D9), feet (D6).<br>E: Nectar?<br>R: Stuff that gets the nectar out. | |
| | 14 | | Bat. (W) | E: (ERR)<br>R: Ears (Dd34), wings (D4), feet (D9). | |
| | 15 | | Could be a dragon with wings that are dragon heads that has no eyes . . . my eyes are hurting. (W) | E: (ERR)<br>R: Dragon head (D6), dragon mouth (D10s), no eyes. | |
| VI | 16 | | (R makes noises with his mouth) Person throwing a smoke bomb that has a scorpion egg. (W) | E: (ERR)<br>R: Hands (Dd22), head (Dd23), throwing smoke bomb, smoke (D1) is coming out.<br>E: Smoke coming out?<br>R: It evaporates and moves into different direction.<br>E: Scorpion egg?<br>R: Coming out with big mouth. (Dd33) | |
| | 17 | | Someone throwing a crow in the air. (D3) | E: (ERR)<br>R: Reaper scarecrow.<br>E: Reaper?<br>R: Has no hands, shirt. (Dd22)<br>E: Shirt?<br>R: Cloth.<br>E: Cloth?<br>R: He's just moving around.<br>E: Crow?<br>R: No, it's a scarecrow. | |
| VII | 18 | | Two twins that are shadows looking at everyone. (D1) | E: (ERR)<br>R: Ponytail (D5), head (D9).<br>E: Shadows?<br>R: Smoky shadows, color, smoke coming out all over. | |
| | 19 | @ | Two goats. (D2) | E: (ERR)<br>R: Horns (D5), hands (Dd21) go back. | |
| VIII | 20 | | (R makes clicking noises with his mouth) Two beavers climbing up a mountain. (D1, 4)<br>I don't see anything else . . .<br>E: There's no rush: take your time and you'll probably be able to find more than one thing. | E: (ERR)<br>R: Beavers (D1), head, shape.<br>E: Mountain?<br>R: Gray up there (D4). | PR |
| | 21 | | A parachute (D5) popping, beavers popping it. (D1,5) | E: (ERR)<br>R: Beavers (D1) popping it.<br>E: Parachute?<br>R: Line hold it, shape. | |

| Cd # | R # | Or | Response | Clarification | R-Opt |
|---|---|---|---|---|---|
| IX | 22 | | Two deers howling at the moon. (D3) | E: (ERR)<br>R: Head (Dd28), ears, horns, howling because head in the air. | |
| | 23 | v | v Two deers hiding head under a tree. (D2) | E: (ERR)<br>R: Head. (Dd28)<br>E: Tree?<br>R: Stem (D5) and branches.<br>E: Under?<br>R: Head is under the tree. (D11) | |
| X | 24 | | Oh my God! Two deers wrestling. (D1,12) | E: (ERR)<br>R: Horns (upper Dd28), head (D12). | |
| | 25 | | Two lions wrestling. (D2) | E: (ERR)<br>R: Yellow mane.<br>E: Mane?<br>R: Look closely! Fur.<br>E: Fur?<br>R: (Subject rubs card.) | |
| | 26 | | Two rats fighting under a tree. It's like a wrestling match going on in here! (D11) | E: (ERR)<br>R: Fighting over a stem (D14), feet, tiny tails, hands, ears (all in D8). | |

# Rorschach Performance Assessment System (R-PAS)®

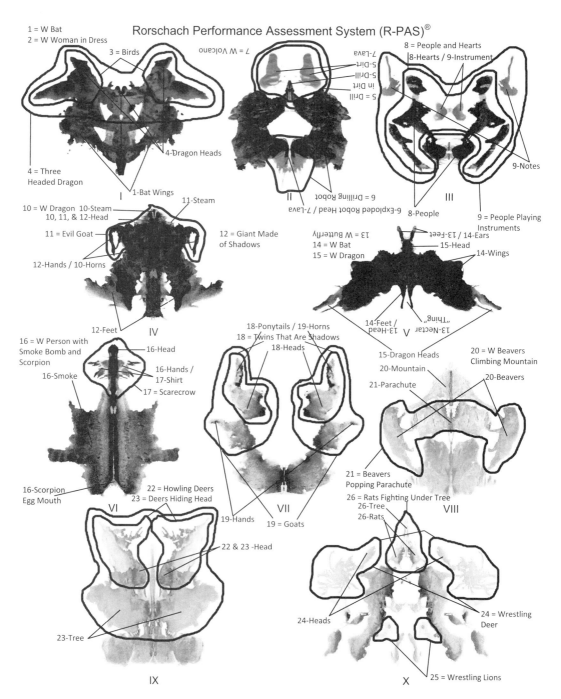

1 = W Bat
2 = W Woman in Dress
3 = Birds
4 = Three Headed Dragon
4-Dragon Heads
1-Bat Wings
I

7 = W Volcano
7-Lava
5-Dirt
5-Drill
5 = Drill in Dirt
6 = Drilling Robot
6-Exploded Robot Head / 7-Lava
II

8 = People and Hearts
8-Hearts / 9-Instrument
9-Notes
8-People
9 = People Playing Instruments
III

10 = W Dragon  10-Steam
10, 11, & 12-Head
11-Steam
11 = Evil Goat
12-Hands / 10-Horns
12-Feet
IV

12 = Giant Made of Shadows

13 = W Butterfly
14 = W Bat
15 = W Dragon
13-Feet / 14-Ears
15-Head
14-Wings
14-Feet / 13-Head
13-Nectar "Thing"
15-Dragon Heads
V

16 = W Person with Smoke Bomb and Scorpion
16-Smoke
16-Head
16-Hands / 17-Shirt
17 = Scarecrow
16-Scorpion Egg Mouth
VI

18-Ponytails / 19-Horns
18 = Twins That Are Shadows
18-Heads
19-Hands
19 = Goats
VII

20 = W Beavers Climbing Mountain
20-Mountain
21-Parachute
20-Beavers
21 = Beavers Popping Parachute
VIII

22 = Howling Deers
23 = Deers Hiding Head
22 & 23 -Head
23-Tree
IX

26 = Rats Fighting Under Tree
26-Tree
26-Rats
24-Heads
24 = Wrestling Deer
25 = Wrestling Lions
X

# R-PAS Code Sequence: "Luis"

**C-ID**: Luis    **P-ID**: 126    **Age**: 8    **Gender**: Male    **Education**: 3

| Cd | # | Or | Loc | Loc # | SR | SI | Content | Sy | Vg | 2 | FQ | P | Determinants | Cognitive | Thematic | HR | ODL (RP) | R-Opt | Text |
|----|---|----|----|------|----|----|---------|----|----|---|----|---|--------------|-----------|----------|----|------|-------|------|
| I | 1 | | W | | | | A | | | | o | P | F | | | | | | * |
| Comment: E could have queried 'big, giant, humungous' for FD. | | | | | | | | | | | | | | | | | | | |
| | 2 | | W | | | | H,Cg | Sy | | | o | | F | INC1 | | PH | | | |
| | 3 | | D | 7 | | | A | | | 2 | o | | F | | | | | | |
| | 4 | | Dd | 99 | | | (A) | | | | - | | F | INC1 | AGC | | | | |
| II | 5 | v | D | 2,4 | | | NC | Sy | | | u | | ma,CF | | | | | | |
| | 6 | v | D | 2, 4, 3 | | | (H),An,NC | Sy | | | - | | ma,CF | INC1 | MOR | PH | | | |
| | 7 | v | W | | | | Ex,NC | Sy | | | u | | ma,CF | | AGC | | | | |
| III | 8 | | D | 9,3 | | | H,An | Sy | | 2 | u | P | CF | DV1,FAB2 | AGM,MOR | PH | | | |
| | 9 | | D | 9,3,2 | | | H,NC | Sy | | 2 | u | P | Ma,mp | | COP,MAH | GH | | | |
| IV | 10 | | W | | | | (A),Fi | Sy | | | o | | FMa,C' | | AGC | | ODL | | |
| | 11 | | Dd | 99 | | | Ad,NC | Sy | | | - | | FMa,C' | INC1 | AGC | | | | |
| | 12 | | W | | | | (H) | | | | o | P | ma,C' | | AGC | GH | | | * |
| Comment: E should have queried 'big, giant' for FD. | | | | | | | | | | | | | | | | | | | |
| V | 13 | v | W | | | SI | A | | | | o | | F | DV1 | | | | | |
| | 14 | | W | | | | A | | | | o | P | F | | | | | | |
| | 15 | | W | | | | (A) | | | | u | | F | INC2 | AGC,MOR | | | | |
| VI | 16 | | W | | | | H,Ad,Fi | Sy | | | - | | Ma,mp | FAB2 | AGM,AGC | PH | ODL | | |
| | 17 | | D | 3 | | | H,Cg | Sy | | | - | | Ma,ma | | AGC,MOR | PH | | | |
| VII | 18 | | D | 1 | | | Hd,Fi | Sy | | 2 | o | P | Mp,mp,C' | DV1,INC2 | | PH | | | |
| | 19 | @ | D | 2 | | | A | | | 2 | u | | F | INC1 | | | | | |
| VIII | 20 | | D | 1,4 | | | A,NC | Sy | | 2 | o | P | FMa | | | | | Pr | |
| | 21 | | D | 1, 5 | | | A,NC | Sy | | 2 | u | P | FMa | FAB1 | MOR,MAP | | | | |
| IX | 22 | | D | 3 | | | A | | | 2 | u | | FMa | INC1 | | | ODL | | |
| | 23 | v | D | 2 | | | A,NC | Sy | | 2 | - | | FMp,FD | | | | | | |
| X | 24 | | Dd | 99 | | | A | Sy | | 2 | - | | Ma | FAB1 | AGM | PH | | | |
| | 25 | | D | 2 | | | A | Sy | | 2 | o | | FMa,CF,T | | AGM,AGC | PH | | | |
| III | 26 | | D | 8,14 | | | A,NC | Sy | | 2 | - | | FMa | | AGM | PH | | | |

©2010-2016 R-PAS

C-ID: Luis          P-ID: 126     Age: 8          Gender: Male          Education: 3

| Domain/Variables | Raw Scores | Raw A-SS | Raw C-SS | Cplx. Adj. A-SS | Cplx. Adj. C-SS | Standard Score Profile R-Optimized | Abbr. |
|---|---|---|---|---|---|---|---|
| **Admin. Behaviors and Obs.** | | | | | | | |
| Pr | 1 | 104 | 105 | | | | Pr |
| Pu | 0 | 96 | 96 | | | | Pu |
| CT (Card Turning) | 6 | 107 | 109 | | | | CT |
| **Engagement and Cog. Processing** | | | | | | | |
| Complexity | 111 | 122 | 141 | | | | Cmplx |
| R (Responses) | 26 | 107 | 109 | 91 | 90 | | R |
| F% [Lambda=0.44] (Simplicity) | 31% | 91 | 81 | 105 | 92 | | F% |
| Blend | 12 | 131 | >150 | 118 | 136 | | Bln |
| Sy | 17 | 132 | >150 | 119 | 131 | | Sy |
| MC | 10.0 | 112 | 129 | 92 | 103 | | MC |
| MC - PPD | -11.0 | 76 | 71 | 78 | 74 | | MC-PPD |
| M | 5 | 109 | 119 | 88 | 96 | | M |
| M/MC [5/10.0] | 50% | 99 | 100 | 97 | 99 | | M Prp |
| (CF+C)/SumC [5/5] | 100% | 126 | 128 | 126 | 128 | | CFC Prp |
| **Perception and Thinking Problems** | | | | | | | |
| EII-3 | 3.8 | 143 | 147 | 143 | 144 | | EII |
| TP-Comp (Thought & Percept. Com...) | 4.0 | 142 | 127 | 142 | 123 | | TP-C |
| WSumCog | 45 | 148 | >150 | 143 | 148 | | WCog |
| SevCog | 4 | 138 | 142 | 138 | 142 | | Sev |
| FQ-% | 31% | 143 | 111 | 136 | 108 | | FQ-% |
| WD-% | 22% | 127 | 101 | 119 | 96 | | WD-% |
| FQo% | 38% | 75 | 94 | 78 | 97 | | FQo% |
| P | 8 | 119 | 131 | 118 | 130 | | P |
| **Stress and Distress** | | | | | | | |
| YTVC' | 5 | 104 | 120 | 89 | 100 | | YTVC' |
| m | 8 | 143 | >150 | 131 | 147 | | m |
| Y | 0 | 85 | 92 | 85 | 77 | | Y |
| MOR | 5 | 127 | 139 | 124 | 132 | | MOR |
| SC-Comp (Suicide Concern Comp.) | NA | | | | | | SC-C |
| **Self and Other Representation** | | | | | | | |
| ODL% | 12% | 105 | 120 | 97 | 110 | | ODL% |
| SR (Space Reversal) | 0 | 87 | 90 | 87 | 90 | | SR |
| MAP/MAHP [1/2] | NA | | | | | | MAP Prp |
| PHR/GPHR [9/11] | 82% | 132 | 117 | 132 | 117 | | PHR Prp |
| M- | 3 | 129 | 146 | 129 | 146 | | M- |
| AGC | 9 | 136 | 137 | 133 | 133 | | AGC |
| H | 5 | 119 | 123 | 107 | 108 | | H |
| COP | 1 | 102 | 106 | 90 | 93 | | COP |
| MAH | 1 | 105 | 119 | 90 | 89 | | MAH |

A-SS = Adult Standard Score; C-SS = Age-Based Child or Adolescent Standard Score

© 2010-2016 R-PAS

## R-PAS Summary Scores and Profiles – Page 2

C-ID: Luis          P-ID: 126     Age: 8          Gender: Male          Education: 3

| Domain/Variables | Raw Scores | Raw A-SS | Raw C-SS | Cplx. Adj. A-SS | Cplx. Adj. C-SS | Standard Score Profile R-Optimized | Abbr. |
|---|---|---|---|---|---|---|---|
| **Engagement and Cog. Processing** | | | | | | | |
| W% | 35% | 97 | 102 | 88 | 94 | | W% |
| Dd% | 12% | 98 | 97 | 102 | 100 | | Dd% |
| SI (Space Integration) | 1 | 86 | 91 | 79 | 86 | | SI |
| IntCont | 0 | 81 | 93 | 81 | 71 | | IntC |
| Vg% | 0% | 86 | 91 | 87 | 92 | | Vg% |
| V | 0 | 92 | 95 | 92 | 65 | | V |
| FD | 1 | 104 | 104 | 96 | 97 | | FD |
| R8910% | 23% | 77 | 67 | 79 | 71 | | R8910% |
| WSumC | 5.0 | 111 | 124 | 98 | 106 | | WSC |
| C | 0 | 95 | 92 | 95 | 92 | | C |
| Mp/(Ma+Mp)  [1/5] | 20% | 85 | 87 | 85 | 87 | | Mp Prp |
| **Perception and Thinking Problems** | | | | | | | |
| FQu% | 31% | 100 | 97 | 96 | 93 | | FQu% |
| **Stress and Distress** | | | | | | | |
| PPD | 21 | 129 | 145 | 117 | 127 | | PPD |
| CBlend | 1 | 107 | 122 | 91 | 91 | | CBlnd |
| C' | 4 | 117 | 129 | 109 | 115 | | C' |
| V | 0 | 92 | 95 | 92 | 65 | | V |
| CritCont% (Critical Contents) | 62% | 135 | >150 | 133 | >150 | | CrCt |
| **Self and Other Representation** | | | | | | | |
| SumH | 8 | 109 | 113 | 96 | 98 | | SumH |
| NPH/SumH  [3/8] | 38% | 86 | 84 | 88 | 86 | | NPH Prp |
| V-Comp (Vigilance Composite) | 3.7 | 106 | 111 | 89 | 93 | | V-C |
| r (Reflections) | 0 | 95 | 96 | 95 | 96 | | r |
| p/(a+p)  [5/21] | 24% | 88 | 87 | 88 | 87 | | p Prp |
| AGM | 5 | 146 | >150 | 146 | >150 | | AGM |
| T | 1 | 107 | 123 | 107 | 123 | | T |
| PER | 0 | 92 | 92 | 92 | 92 | | PER |
| An | 2 | 108 | 114 | 108 | 114 | | An |

A-SS = Adult Standard Score; C-SS = Age-Based Child or Adolescent Standard Score

© 2010-2016 R-PAS

# CHAPTER 18

# Being in Pain

## Using R-PAS to Understand the (Non-)Dialogue of Body and Mind

Ety Berant

Human beings have an intrinsic drive toward health and recognize its importance in their lives and the lives of their loved ones. But illness creates upset and pain in life, especially when one deals with illness that has no distinct origin or clear solution on the horizon. People are most perplexed when they are told that their physical ailments may be an expression of psychological problems. For medical patients of whom this is suspected, personality assessment may clarify and deepen an understanding of their physical symptoms.

"Ms. T" is a single woman in her early 20s, born in Israel to Israeli-born parents of South American origin. She is the youngest of five children, with two brothers and two sisters. She received a BSc degree in a biological science field and now works in a laboratory. She referred herself to a public clinic due to physical pains in her abdomen and pelvis that have lasted 2 years. She cannot recall a specific event prior to the beginning of the pain. She reported that the pain limits her ability to cope and diminishes her quality of life. A series of thorough medical examinations revealed no significant findings to explain her pain.

Her doctors concluded that she suffered from fibromyalgia and recommended treatment in a pain clinic and antidepressants. These efforts gave her no relief, and she decided to stop all medications. One of her pain clinic physicians referred Ms. T to psychotherapy, concluding that her physical pain stemmed from emotional distress. The physician recommended a personality assessment in order to understand the dynamics of her pain and other symptoms, followed by a psychotherapeutic treatment that might help her. The referral questions were:

1. Is there a psychological manifestation of the patient's symptoms?
2. What are the dynamics of her symptoms?
3. What method of psychotherapy would be suitable?

## Fibromyalgia

Fibromyalgia is a medical condition characterized by chronic widespread pain and a heightened and painful response to pressure This condition is a "central sensitization syndrome" caused by biological abnormalities in the nervous system that act to produce pain and cognitive impairments, as well as psychological problems. Fibromyalgia is frequently associated with psychiatric conditions such as depression and anxiety, and with disorders such as posttraumatic stress disorder (Hawkins, 2013).

The precise cause of fibromyalgia is unknown but is thought to involve psychological, genetic, neurobiological, and environmental factors. Patients with fibromyalgia show functional and structural brain differences from those without the condition, but it is still unclear whether these anomalies cause fibromyalgia symptoms or are the product of an unknown underlying cause (Schweinhardt, Sauro, & Bushnell, 2008). In light of the fibromyalgia diagnosis, one of the aims in using the Rorschach was to determine if her symptoms were the expression of "body language" or what Joyce McDougall (1989) terms the "theatre of the body."

## Psychosomatic Psychodynamics

McDougall (1989) argues that in psychosomatic conditions the body reacts to a psychological threat as if it were a physiological threat. McDougall contends that there is a severe split between the body and mind, deriving from a disconnection of consciousness from one's emotional state. Psychoanalytic scholars claim as a basic premise that, mentally, the human body functions as a symbolic tool, as a language to communicate with others and ourselves about matters beyond corporeality. Freud stated that "The ego is first and foremost a body ego" (1923/1961, p. 26) and that the ego is ultimately derived from bodily sensations, chiefly those springing from the surface of the body. Researchers have addressed the concept of human embodiment, the role of the body in symbolization and metaphor use, and the basic assumption that the body also functions as the source area for metaphors (Duesund & Skårderud, 2003).

Metaphors are based on the perception of physical realities such as gravitation, sounds, vision, tactility, etc. For example, a depressed person "feels down" and "burdened by heavy thoughts." The essence of a metaphor is to understand and experience one phenomenon through another phenomenon. Metaphors are essential for mental representation, human understanding, fantasy, and reason.

In the case of individuals who experience somatic pain, like Ms. T, the concept of concretized metaphors enters the arena. In concretized metaphors, bodily metaphors do not function mainly as representations capable of containing an experience, but as presentations that are experienced as concrete facts in the here-and-now and are difficult to negotiate with (Skårderud, 2007). In this case there is an immediate equivalence between bodily and emotional experience. There is a problem distinguishing between the metaphor and the object or phenomenon that is metaphorized. The "as-if" quality of the more abstract meaning of the metaphor is lost and becomes an immediate concrete experience. The concretized body metaphors are viewed as a reduction of the capacity to use functioning metaphors, a collapse of the symbolic room between the body and emotion or cognition.

Within the psychoanalytic tradition of self-psychology, Atwood and Stolorow (1984) discuss "concretization" in patients with a vulnerable self-organization. Different forms of stress may threaten the integrity of the self and through concretization these individuals attempt to boost their sense of self by strengthening the experience of being grounded in their own bodies. Other scholars claim that concretized metaphors establish distance from unpleasant experiences and are signs of essential distancing defenses (Alexandrowicz, 1962; Caruth & Ekstein, 1966). Fonagy, Gergely, Jurist, and Target (2002) claim that when psychic reality is poorly integrated, the body takes on an excessively central role in the continuity of the sense of self. Mental states, unable to achieve representation as ideas or feelings, come to be represented in the bodily domain.

## Ms. T's Clinical Interview and History

Ms. T recalls that she was brought up by strict and rigid parents, an upbringing that she believes prevented her from living freely and suppressed her curiosity and self-expression. She felt that her parents were not able to contain her emotionally. Specifically, they had difficulty relating to any "negative" event in her life. She reported that when she disclosed any such difficulty, her parents made efforts to ignore it. Their attitude was painful to Ms. T, especially over the course of the last 2 years as she suffered abdominal pains. They have ignored her condition and acted as if it did not exist. Ms. T described good relationships with her siblings. One sibling, in particular, had been especially supportive but began to withdraw as Ms. T became absorbed in her medical condition and could not provide reciprocity in the relationship.

Ms. T was born and raised in a big city in southern Israel. She impressed her teachers, performed well as a student, and graduated high school with honors. She describes satisfactory relationships with classmates and added that she felt more comfortable with boys than girls. She was selected to serve in a prestigious unit in the Israeli Defense Forces (IDF) but found the teamwork required of her position difficult. After a short while, she was discharged from military service due to "social incompatibility," meaning that she did not get along with other solders or with her commanders. This was an unusual step for the IDF to take for solders in her unit. She regrets not having tried harder in her unit and feels ashamed of not completing the full mandatory service.

Ms. T claims to be unable to have intimate relations with men because of their impatience with her physical complaints; as a result, she feels emotionally alienated. Prior to her pain, she'd had no romantic relations with men. She has tried a variety of pain treatments, including acupuncture and homeopathic medicine, which did not relieve her pain. Now she is hopeful that psychotherapy will help alleviate her condition.

## Assessment Methods Used with Ms. T

For Ms. T's. assessment, a clinical interview and the Hebrew versions of the Wechsler Adult Intelligence Scale—Third Edition, Inventory of Interpersonal Problems, Beck Depression Inventory (BDI), and Experiences in Close Relationships (ECR) scale were used. The Rorschach Performance Assessment System (R-PAS) and Thematic Apperception Test were also completed in Hebrew.

## Brief Review of Other Assessment Findings

Ms. T's intelligence testing revealed high intelligence (IQ = 131) with a similar level of verbal intelligence (VIQ = 133) and performance intelligence (PIQ = 122). She endorsed a moderate level of depression (BDI = 20), which was more due to affective and self-critical items than to physical complaints. Attachment scales (ECR) revealed that she is anxiously attached (high attachment anxiety score: 4.85 out of 7; low attachment avoidance score: 2.4 out of 7).

According to attachment theory, individuals' repeated experiences of their significant others (attachment figures) result in the consolidation of working models and the formation of relatively stable patterns of expectations, needs, emotions, and behaviors in interpersonal interactions and close relationships (Hazan & Shaver, 1987). These repeated experiences have an enduring effect on an individual's intrapsychic organization and interpersonal behavior. At the intrapsychic level, such experiences can provide a resource for emotional well-being and create positive working models of self and other. Research has shown that securely attached people generally perceive themselves as valuable and lovable (Shaver & Mikulincer, 2009). Secure attachment helps a person maintain emotional balance in the face of distress and to regulate and deescalate negative emotions such as anger, anxiety, and sadness (Bowlby, 1973).

By contrast, anxiously attached individuals are concerned with the availability of their attachment figure and tend to rely on emotionally based coping mechanisms that increase their distress and reduce their ability to regulate their emotions (Mikulincer & Shaver, 2007). Attachment avoidance results in a loss of trust in others during times of need and subsequent obsessive self-reliant strategies in the face of challenging and demanding social interactions that are threatening (Bowlby, 1988). Research indicates that attachment orientation can be measured along two orthogonal dimensions: attachment anxiety and attachment avoidance (Brennan, Clark, & Shaver, 1998). Low levels on the two dimensions reflect secure attachment; a high level on attachment avoidance and a low level on attachment anxiety reflect attachment avoidance; a high score on attachment anxiety and a low score on attachment avoidance reflect attachment anxiety; high scores on both dimensions reflects fearful avoidant attachment.

## Assessment Questions for Ms. T's Rorschach

I aimed to understand the origin and dynamic of Ms. T's symptoms from the Rorschach scores and contents and to determine whether her somatic complaints interfered with her cognitive functioning or social coping. The Rorschach can provide substantive answers to these questions.

## Ms. T's Appearance and Behavior in the Assessment

Ms. T looks her chronological age. Her face is fair, she dresses simply, and her appearance would be considered plain. She was cooperative during the assessment, smiled and expressed herself openly. When she spoke about her pain and physical symptoms, she became lively but in other subjects she seemed detached, her tone monotonous and her affect flat.

I introduced the Rorschach as a segment of a battery of tests that I hoped would help us understand and treat her pain. After a short introduction of the Rorschach, I asked whether she was acquainted with the test (she was not) and then provided the standard R-Optimized instructions used in R-PAS (Meyer, Viglione, Mihura, Erard, & Erdberg, 2011). She listened attentively and appeared ready for the administration. There was no need to prompt her or to pull the card, though she did give a fourth response to Card X before handing the card back. While doing the Rorschach she worked fast and appeared impatient, even cynical at times. She noted that she enjoyed the tasks associated with the Rorschach; however, when the examiner mentioned her impatience, Ms. T said that this was due to her pain.

## Ms. T's R-PAS Results[1]

Ms. T's Rorschach scores suggested that she had cooperated with the examiner, despite giving the impression of impatience. She provided an above-average number of responses (R = 29, SS[2] = 114), indicating that she was verbally and perceptually intelligent and cooperative. Her productivity was higher than the overall complexity of her protocol (Complexity SS = 104). Furthermore, she was not prompted at all (Pr = 0, SS = 89), which suggests that she was sufficiently attentive to the task and cooperative with my instructions. These findings together may suggest that, on the one hand, she cooperated by giving an above-average number of responses without being prompted. On the other hand, she was less complexly engaged than one would expect from such an above-average-response person. Ostensibly, she was saying, "I am a cooperative person," but underneath she revealed nonverbal reservations (her impatience).

### Engagement and Cognitive Processing

Ms. T had an average capacity to detect and articulate subtleties, nuances, and personally salient aspects of her experiential world (F% = 45%, SS = 104) and an ability at the lower end of the average range to simultaneously identify and articulate multiple features of the environment (Blend = 2, SS = 91). However, given her above-average R and high intelligence, we would nevertheless expect her to have higher scores on these scales. These lower-than-expected scores perhaps reveal a tendency toward simplistic processing by neglecting or ignoring opportunities to attend to richness and complexity. This pattern might hint that there are processes that prevent her from examining her experiences in a more comprehensive and thorough manner. It seems that when she encounters situations in which she is not in full control (such as the Rorschach task), she approaches them with lower complexity, perhaps in an effort to cope more efficiently.

This tendency became more distinct when observing her low integrative cognitive activity and relational thinking. She is not very likely to engage in the synthesis and integration of ideas and different aspects of life (Sy = 3, SS = 86). Her cognitive processing focuses on common, straightforward components, along generally simple

---

[1]See Appendix 18.1 at the end of the chapter for Ms. T's R-PAS Responses, Location Sheet, Code Sequence, and Page 1 and 2 Profiles.

[2]Standard scores (SS) have a mean of 100 and an SD of 15.

lines of thinking. This is much lower than one would expect given her intelligence (Similarities = 14, Block Design = 15).

Her R-PAS results reveal another duality. On the surface, she has adequate psychological resources for adapting to developmental or life challenges and an adequate ability to mentally engage in the world with vitality, emotions, and psychological activity (MC SS = 108; MC–PPD SS = 107). Thus, her resources should be sufficient to balance her level of sensitivity to potentially distracting or discomforting internal experiences, such as needs, feelings, or concerns. She would seem to have an average internal capacity to cope effectively with daily activities, and to be stable, predictable, reliable, and resilient in handling stressful or upsetting situations. However, this was not the case because most of her coping assets rely on emotional resources versus being able to use thoughtful deliberation while making decisions and taking action (M/MC = 11%, SS = 74). That is, her responses indicate a greater tendency to react spontaneously to emotions, impulses, or circumstances rather than to reflect and to reason. Her coping is likely to be guided by trial and error, gut reaction, inspiration, and emotion, rather than thorough thought and reflection.

In addition, Ms. T displays a lower than average tendency to envision or imagine human experiences or activities. This finding suggests a struggle to mentalize and self-reflect before action (M = 1, SS = 83), perhaps indicating that she may not experience the self as the agent of her experiences, and she may have difficulty being empathic toward the experiences of others. Having only one M response is surprising given her intelligence level. It is possible that Ms. T's cognitive functioning might be better in structured situations.

The concept of mentalization—the ability "to see ourselves as others see us, and others as they see themselves" (Holmes, 2009, p. 502)—is a key to understanding Ms. T's low M score (based on one humanized animal movement, which is a less mature mentalization). Fonagy et al. (2002) define mentalization as the developed ability to "read" others' minds. Mentalization underlies the capacities for affect regulation, impulse control, self-monitoring, and the experience of self-agency—the building blocks of the organization of the self. The ability to mentalize is an achievement that develops out of a secure attachment relationship, characterized by affective attunement and accurate mirroring from caregivers who facilitate affect regulation. Anxiously attached individuals' difficulty with mentalizing stems from an inability to escape intense affects, such as fear of abandonment or loss of a loved one, as well as an inability to step back and reflect on the source of these feelings and fears, thereby impairing narrative coherence. Mentalizing involves both self-reflective and interpersonal components, which ideally provide the individual with a well-developed capacity to distinguish inner from outer reality, physical experience from mental experience, and intrapersonal mental processes from interpersonal communications.

Ms. T's history of being raised by strict, rigid, and inattentive parents contributed to her problematic affect regulation and problematic mentalization (one immature M). The determinant M manifests the deep understanding of the subjective experience of another person and the self. In a neuroscience study, Giromini and colleagues suggested that human movement on the Rorschach activates brain regions associated with social cognition, including empathy (Giromini, Porcelli, Viglione, Parolin, & Pineda, 2010).

Ms. T's R-PAS profile shows that her reactions to emotionally charged states tend to be direct, spontaneous, immediate, and absorbing. These reactions are accompanied by a relatively modest degree of cognitive control, mental filtering, intellectual processing, or restraint [(CF+C)/SumC = 78%, SS = 115], indicating that her reactions may be overly intense and encompassing, making it difficult for her to modulate negative feelings when they arise. Her difficulty with emotional regulation also appears exacerbated due to her generally high reactivity and willingness to respond to emotionally toned stimuli (WSumC SS = 126). The non-form-dominated color responses, suggesting low affect control, also appear with content suggesting body concern in general and more specifically with femininity, sexuality, and reproduction (R6: menstruation, R8: uterus, R29: placenta, R9: blood vessels and capillaries, R23: liver). It is possible that her capacity to modulate her emotions is diminished while she is preoccupied with issues regarding femininity, fertility, and sexuality. Perhaps her abdominal pain produces anxiety regarding her femininity. Or from the somatic angle, the anxiety regarding her femininity and sexuality is a trigger for the pain she is experiencing.

Anxiously attached individuals such as Ms. T are susceptible to affect regulation difficulties. Hyperactivating coping strategies used by anxiously attached people undermine the development of affect regulation. Relatedly, habitually resorting to hyperactivation may lower the threshold for triggering the sympathetic nervous system and diminish one's capacity to exert cortical control over emotional reactions (Wallin, 2007). Attachment anxiety interferes with the down-regulation of negative emotions and intense and persistent distress, which continue even after objective threats subside. As a result, anxiously attached people experience unmanageable streams of negative thoughts and feelings that contribute to cognitive disorganization and fuel distress (Ein-Dor, Mikulincer, Doron, & Shaver, 2010). The implication is that anxiously attached clients may need the therapist to help them modulate their emotional reactivity and strengthen their capacity to manage their emotions by making sense of them (Wallin, 2007).

In Ms. T's case, on the surface she demonstrates a fair ability to process her world in a holistic manner and to challenge herself by taking into account the whole situation and using all available information (W% SS = 97). But a deeper examination indicates that generally she does not provide a W to the colored cards and the only W response she provided to a colored card (R9 to Card III) is a fragmented response addressing external body parts or contours as well as internal organs such as blood vessels and capillaries with no connection to each other.

## Thought and Perception

Further examination suggests mild problems with her ego functions (EII-3 SS = 113), which appear to be largely due to crude and disturbing thought content linked with body concern, fertility, and sexuality (CritCont% = 48%, SS = 127). Ms. T does not reveal signs of thought disorder or illogical and implausible thinking (TP-Comp SS = 103), which includes no indications of significant lapses in conceptualization, reasoning, communication, or thought organization (WSumCog SS = 100; SevCog = 0, SS = 94). In addition, although there is no indication of severe reality distortion and misinterpretation (FQ-% = 14%, SS =110) that might tax her coping resources, she falls at the upper end of the average range in terms of her propensity to misperceive experiences (FQ-% SS =110; WD-% SS = 110). These mistaken perceptions generally are not at a level that would interfere with reasonable understanding of self, other, and the environment, or the ability to navigate day-to-day challenges. However, three out of her four FQ– responses occur on the chromatic cards, indicating that her reality testing may become diminished when she encounters emotionally charged situations.

In addition, Ms. T has a notable absence of conventional perceptions of the environment (FQo% = 34%, SS = 73). Although she can detect some of the most frequently seen popular responses (to Cards V and VIII), Ms. T is less likely to interpret her environment based on widely accepted interpretations, and she is less sensitive to the obvious external cues used by most people (P = 3, SS = 80). It appears that her low conventional judgment is due to very unconventional, individualistic, or personalized ways of interpreting experiences (FQu% = 48%, SS = 123). Thus, she regularly sees things from a vantage point that others would have trouble understanding without some effort, and she may behave in unconventional ways.

## Stress and Distress

The presence of just one MOR response (SS = 100) is surprising given all the Blood (SS = 141) and Anatomy (SS = 140) percepts in her protocol. This finding may point to some difficulties connecting with emotional distress or pain and draws attention to the issue of her "hiding" distress and desperation, versus expressing these emotions somatically, as her medical history reveals. It seems that she tries at times to avoid being in touch with helplessness (Y = 3, SS = 114), pain, or negative feelings (C' = 3, SS = 111). These findings converge also with some alexithymic features to her personality, with alexithymia encompassing a cluster of cognitive and affective characteristics that include difficulty identifying and communicating feelings, trouble distinguishing between feelings and somatic sensations of emotional arousal, an impoverished imaginative life, and a concrete and reality-oriented thinking style (Porcelli & Meyer, 2002; Porcelli & Mihura, 2010). Ms. T has some of the strongest alexithymic features, including impoverished mental representations (M = 1, SS = 83), difficulties modulating affect [(CF+C)/SumC, SS = 115], difficulty gaining perspective or introspecting (FD = 0, SS = 88), and low integrative skills (Sy SS = 86), but not other features, such as social conformity (P = 3, SS = 80). All of these findings are perhaps of more concern because she is at slightly elevated risk for suicide or serious self-harm (SC-Comp SS = 115).

The Rorschach results, however, indicate that these efforts to avoid pain and distress were not fully successful. Most striking is the failure to censor or inhibit problematic contents (CritCont% SS = 127). The most notable contents are Blood (SS = 141), Anatomy (An = 8, SS = 140), and Sex (Sx = 2, SS = 121). It seems that her body is "talking" for her mind and "telling" us what to focus on in therapy. Reviewing the content of these responses, it seems that she is struggling with issues of femininity, sexuality, and motherhood, as noted previously.

## Self and Other Representation

Regarding her self-concept, Ms. T does not show implicit dependency needs (ODL% SS = 101), oppositionality, or independence striving (SR = 1, SS = 102), a predominance of negative object representations (PHR/GPHR SS = 105), or a high level of aggressive thoughts and concerns (AGC SS = 100). Thus, Ms. T appears to have the potential for adequate interpersonal competence and skill in managing and understanding interactions and relationships. This does not mean that she maintains close relationships and feels empathic toward others. Indeed, her life history shows a dearth of these connections. Perhaps, her difficulties in mentalization and her deep conflicts regarding her self-value, femininity, and sexuality contribute to the latter.

Another indication of the complexity of her personality is the difficulty she showed understanding other people as complex, complete, or multifaceted individuals (H = 1, SS = 88; (NPH/SumH = 75%, SS = 111). Looking beyond the scores, however, her only H response relates to fetuses as transferred placental blood—implicating a regressive response instead of a mature human representation. In addition, she may have a tendency to view herself and others in unrealistic ways, based on part object representations. These representations may contribute to a view of herself and others in a polarized, black and white, manner. Her perceptions did not include objects in meaningful relationship, and there were no indications that relationships might be construed as supportive or cooperative (COP = 0, SS = 88; MAH = 0, SS = 90).

However, it seems that she needs mirroring and may be coping in a self-centered manner (r = 1, SS = 113), an interpretation that is bolstered by the content of the Reflection response and her demonstration of it (R15): "This is ugly; this is a parrot that is examining its image in the mirror." In the RP, while describing the parrot, she was making gestures like a woman that is examining herself in the mirror, putting her hand on her waist. In the sequence of responses to Card VI, the ugliness she perceives is intertwined with imagery of narcissistic mirroring, and the negative feelings expressed toward the object in the mirror appear resolved by the use of an omnipotence defense on the next response (R16)—commanding the examiner to "Write 'an ugly stain'" (Cooper & Arnow, 1986). It seemed troubling for her to confront her body image in the mirror, and it seems that the narcissistic defense was not working for her.

More so than others, she insecurely tries to justify her views based on private and personal knowledge, perhaps due to her need to receive external support regarding her self-esteem (PER SS = 131). Ms. T is likely to expect challenges from others and respond to insecurity with an aggrandizing and self-justifying defensive reaction. Perhaps this explains why I experienced her as defensive and irritated. This also fits with her family history of inattentive parents, an anxiously attached coping style, low self-esteem, and chronic pain, and it suggests that she feels a strong need to persuade the people in her surroundings of the value of her ideas.

As mentioned already, one of the most striking findings from the Rorschach is Ms. T's preoccupation with her body that goes hand in hand with her presenting symptoms. The high number of anatomy responses in the Rorschach (An = 8) underscores her bodily and medical concerns. She worries about physical illness and body integrity (An SS = 140). The contents of her responses reveal an intensive preoccupation with the body in general (liver, lungs, blood vessels, and capillaries) and more specifically with issues of femininity, fertility, and sexuality (menstruation, pelvis, uterus, and placenta).

Perhaps, it is "easier" for her to focus on somatic concerns than to deal with other troubling issues. Ms. T's initial responses to Card I may suggest that she wants to hide behind a mask and an apron that would hide her body and her femininity. Her final response to the card, however, points to kirigami, a decorative object that requires obsessive time to make and embodies many contortions. One could say that behind the mask of the face and the apron hides a person who feels like a decoration with no specific shape or characteristics. It also may point to the apron as a symbol of traditional femininity and that may be associated with anxiety about that role. Knowing the nature of her relationships with her mother, who is not containing and not supporting, it is perhaps not surprising. She may be looking for symbols that would protect her, contain her, and nourish her (such as fetuses in the uterus, the placenta, and the child's rocking chair that prevents falls), whereas images of powerful objects such as "rhinoceros" and "dragons" may reflect her wish for protection by symbols of power.

We still have to keep in mind that perhaps the imagery of anatomy, blood, fertility, and sexuality could be the result of trauma, particularly of a sexual or reproductive nature, or the consequence of conflicts around issues of sexuality and reproduction. The therapist should be attentive to these points.

The findings revealed in the Rorschach are clearly related to psychodynamic explanations regarding somatic preoccupation with the body. The high volume of anatomy responses, combined with the single immature M response and single immature H response (fetuses), her difficulties in affect regulation, depressed mood, high number of blood and sex contents, propensity for atypical and unconventional perceptions, and her fibromyalgia diagnosis, require an explanation of the psychodynamics of Ms. T's somatization.

## Feedback Session with Ms. T

Ms. T asked if the basis of her medical problems was mental distress. She also wondered if her mental distress was the result of her physical pain. I asked whether she thought to look for psychological help during these painful years. She answered that she did not draw any connection between her chronic pain and anything psychological. She said that she would feel guilty if her pain were due to mental reasons, and that she feels hesitant about looking inside, fears being in touch with her feelings, and has difficulties understanding subtlety. Ms. T said that until the assessment, she had avoided connecting to her need for others, especially young men her age. She behaved as if men did not interest her, but now she admitted wondering how it would feel to have a boyfriend. She also denied suicidal thoughts.

She continued, "Perhaps my physical suffering is in line with my avoidance to feel. Instead of feeling pain in my soul, I feel pain in my stomach." After a short silence, she added, "Perhaps it is better to explore my mental pains because I cannot cope any more with my physical pain." She agreed to start psychotherapy and began a mentalization-based treatment. The therapist who started to work with her reported on Ms. T's difficulties exploring mental states and reflecting on interpersonal episodes. Ms. T continued in therapy but resisted exploration and she would not understand why she was upset at times, or what caused others to withdraw from her.

## The Contribution of R-PAS to Understanding Ms. T

The R-PAS results revealed Ms. T's immature personality being disguised behind her high intelligence in specific contexts. On one hand, she gave many responses without being prompted and, on the other hand, showed a lower complexity and an inability to integrate aspects of her experience. R-PAS pointed to the fact that on the surface, it looked as if she had sufficient resources to cope with life, but these resources were dependent mostly on affect; she was unable to mentalize and organize her thinking in a productive way. She had an immature affective world that she could not regulate, which contributed to her difficulties in mentalization, as she was readily flooded by her emotions and reactions. She also was flooded by themes of bodily concern, more specifically related to femininity and sexuality. Her immaturity was demonstrated with just one pure human content (fetuses receiving placental blood), suggesting that she did not have a developmentally appropriate view of herself and her surroundings, but a one-sided way of looking at and relating to the objects in her life. The results also suggested it may be difficult to reach her because she does not have representations of cooperating human beings.

R-PAS revealed that the therapist should be as accurate as possible in his or her interpretations due to Ms. T's view of the world through private and unique lenses as well as her problems with mentalizing. Additionally, she has difficulties being in touch with unpleasant issues and her body tends to convey her mental pain, wishes, and conflicts (with alexithymic features).

The R-PAS results converged with her symptoms and further explained them, converged with her attachment orientation (anxious attachment), and clarified the link between her inability to regulate emotions and her difficulties in mentalization. R-PAS underscored the need for mentalizing-based psychotherapy that would aid in finding methods to help her self-regulate and to find words for her emotions. The R-PAS results also revealed her difficulties with trusting others and her problems in empathizing with them. The high number of anatomy responses further warns us that Ms. T will have difficulties "separating" from her somatic complaints. In short, R-PAS demonstrated that Ms. T needs careful monitoring of her therapy because of problematic mentalization, excessive investment in her bodily self that contributes to atypical and unconventional perceptions, and difficulties in affect regulation in spite of her high intelligence. Lastly, the therapist must be on guard regarding a minor chance of self-harm.

## REFERENCES

Alexandrowicz, D. (1962). The meaning of metaphor. *Bulletin of the Menninger Clinic, 26,* 92–101.

Atwood, G. E., & Stolorow, R. D. (1984). *Structures of subjectivity: Explorations in psychoanalytic phenomenology.* Hillsdale, NJ: Analytic Press.

Bowlby, J. (1973). *Attachment and loss: Vol. 2. Separation: Anxiety and anger.* New York: Basic Books.

Bowlby, J. (1988). *A secure base: Clinical implications of attachment theory.* London: Routledge.

Brennan, K. A., Clark, C. L., & Shaver, P. R. (1998). Self-report measurement of adult attachment: An integrative overview. In J. A. Simpson & W. S. Rholes (Eds.), *Attachment theory and close relationships* (pp. 46–76). New York: Guilford Press.

Caruth, E., & Ekstein, R. (1966). Interpretation within the metaphor: Further considerations. *Journal of the American Academy of Child Psychiatry, 5,* 35–45.

Cooper, S., & Arnow, D. (1986). An object relations view of borderline defenses: A review. In M.

Kissen (Ed.), *Assessing object relations phenomena* (pp. 143–171). New York: International Universities Press.

Duesund, L., & Skårderud, F. (2003). Use the body and forget the body: Treating anorexia nervosa with adapted physical activity. *Clinical Child Psychology and Psychiatry, 8,* 53–72.

Ein-Dor, T., Mikulincer, M., Doron, G., & Shaver, P. R. (2010). The attachment paradox: How can so many of us (the insecure ones) have no adaptive advantages? *Perspectives on Psychological Science, 5,* 123–141.

Fonagy, P., Gergely, G., Jurist, E. L., & Target, M. (2002). *Affect regulation, mentalization and the development of the self.* New York: Other Press.

Freud, S. (1961). The ego and the id. In J. Strachey (Ed. & Trans.), *The standard edition of the complete psychological works of Sigmund Freud* (Vol. 19, pp. 3–66). London: Hogarth Press. (Original work published 1923)

Giromini, L., Porcelli, P., Viglione, D. J., Parolin, L., & Pineda, J. A. (2010). The feeling of movement: EEG evidence for mirroring activity during the observations of static ambiguous stimuli in the Rorschach cards. *Biological Psychology, 85,* 233–241.

Hawkins, R. A. (2013). Fibromyalgia: A clinical update. *Journal of the American Osteopathic Association, 113,* 680–689.

Hazan, C., & Shaver, P. R. (1987). Romantic love conceptualized as an attachment process. *Journal of Personality and Social Psychology, 52,* 511–524.

Holmes, J. (2009). From attachment research to clinical practice: Getting it together. In J. H. Obegi & E. Berant (Eds.), *Attachment theory and research in clinical work with adults* (pp. 490–514). New York: Guilford Press.

McDougall, J. (1989). *Theatres of the body: A psychoanalytic approach to psychosomatic illness.* New York: Norton.

Meyer, G. J., Viglione, D. J., Mihura, J. L., Erard, R. E., & Erdberg, P. (2011). *Rorschach Performance Assessment System: Administration, coding, interpretation and technical manual.* Toledo, OH: Rorschach Performance Assessment System.

Mikulincer, M., & Shaver, P. R. (2007). *Attachment in adulthood: Structure, dynamics, and change.* New York: Guilford Press.

Porcelli, P., & Meyer, G. J. (2002). Construct validity of Rorschach variables for alexithymia. *Psychosomatics, 43,* 360–369.

Porcelli, P., & Mihura, J. L. (2010). Assessment of alexithymia with the Rorschach Comprehensive System: The Rorschach Alexithymia Scale (RAS). *Journal of Personality Assessment, 92,* 128–136.

Schweinhardt, P., Sauro, K. M., & Bushnell, M. C. (2008). Fibromyalgia: A disorder of the brain? *The Neuroscientist, 14,* 415–421.

Shaver, P. R., & Mikulincer, M. (2009). An overview of adult attachment theory. In J. H. Obegi & E. Berant (Eds.), *Attachment theory and research in clinical work with adults* (pp. 17–45). New York: Guilford Press.

Skårderud, F. (2007). Eating one's words: Part I. 'Concretised metaphors' and reflective function in anorexia nervosa—an interview study. *European Eating Disorders Review, 15,* 163–174.

Wallin, D. J. (2007). *Attachment in psychotherapy.* New York: Guilford Press.

**Ms. T's R-PAS Responses, Location Sheet, Code Sequence, and Page 1 and 2 Profiles**

**Rorschach Responses "Ms. T"**

| Respondent ID: Ms. T | Examiner: Ety Berant |
|---|---|
| Location: Outpatient clinic | Date: May, 201X |
| Start Time: 9.00 A.M. | End Time: 10.15 A.M. |

| Cd # | R # | Or | Response | Clarification | R-Opt |
|---|---|---|---|---|---|
| I | 1 | | A mask. (W) | E: (Examiner Repeats Response [ERR].)<br>R: Here are the eyes (DdS30), and here is the nose (Dd27). The holes of the eyes make it look like a mask. Also because it is black and the location of the white holes in the card. [E could have queried "holes" for FD or V.] | |
| | 2 | | An apron. (W) | E: (ERR)<br>R: This is the front view of the apron, and here where you tie it (Dd34), because of the things on the sides that we tie with, and the general look of an apron. | |
| | 3 | | A kirigami. (Dd99 = W – Dd34) | E: (ERR)<br>R: It reminds me that I used to once do kirigami, and to fold it in the middle, maybe because of the symmetry of the holes (DdS26). It all looks the same on both sides (she points to the whole card but takes out the edges of Dd34). | |
| II | 4 | | Devil's horns. (D2) | E: (ERR)<br>R: These two (respondent points to D2). The red color and also the way it looks. | |
| | 5 | | Lungs. (D3) | E: (ERR)<br>R: This (points to D3) looks like lungs. It has the shape of lungs and also the symmetry; it looks the same on both sides. | |
| | 6 | | Menstruation. (D3) | E: (ERR)<br>R: Because of the red spots (indicates D3); the red spots gave me the association of menstruation blood. [The Hebrew word, translated into *spots*, implies some form.] | |
| III | 7 | | An X-ray of the pelvis. (D1) | E: (ERR)<br>R: It reminds me of X-rays that I saw before; it has the structure of a pelvis. [E could have queried why it looks like an X-ray for C' or Y.] | |
| | 8 | | Uterus. (D3) | E: (ERR)<br>R: Perhaps because of the previous response. It is located near the pelvis (points to D1). Also maybe because of the red; the red reminded me of a uterus and also because of the blood of the menstruation. | |
| | 9 | | A body. (W) | E: (ERR)<br>R: It gave me a strong impression that these are parts of the body. It is not a whole body, but there are parts of a body. Here is the waistline (narrow upper part of D1), and here it is getting wider (points to Dd21). These reds (D2, D3) reminded me of parts of the body, blood vessels and capillaries. The red reminded me of blood vessels and capillaries. | |
| IV | 10 | | A rug made from an animal. (W) | E: (ERR)<br>R: I saw someone who had such a carpet made of cow's skin, and it shocked me.<br>E: What made it look like an animal's carpet?<br>C: On first sight, it looked like an animal carpet, maybe because of the symmetry. The upper part reminded me of a cat (D3). I saw that this is the way they fold these rugs in the middle (points in D5). You can see the face of the cat and the whiskers (D3). | |
| | 11 | | Puss in Boots. (W) | E: (ERR)<br>R: First I saw the shape of the boots (D6), and up here is the head of the cat (D3); that's why it gave me the association of the cat in boots. | |
| | 12 | | Geographical map of Israel. (Dd99, W – D4) | E: (ERR)<br>R: This is the way, more or less, how you draw the map of Israel (she outlined the area and specifically excluded the D4). | |

378

| Cd # | R # | Or | Response | Clarification | R-Opt |
|---|---|---|---|---|---|
| V | 13 | | A bat. (W) | E: (ERR)<br>R: Here are the wings (D4), the head (D6), and the legs (D9). It resembles a bat and also the black color made it look like a bat. | |
| | 14 | | A rabbit with wings. (W) | E: (ERR)<br>R: Here are the ears (Dd34), here are the wings (D4), and here are the legs (D9) of a rabbit that is jumping right now. | |
| VI | 15 | | This is ugly; this is a parrot that is examining its image in the mirror. (Dd31) | E: (ERR)<br>R: Here is the shape of a parrot and here is the beak and the feathers.<br>E: Feathers?<br>R: You can see the head and the lines indicate these are feathers. Because of the symmetry, I said the parrot is examining its image in the mirror. (While describing the parrot she was making gestures like a woman that is examining herself in the mirror, putting her hand on her waist.)<br>E: Ugly?<br>R: Yes, this card is ugly. | |
| | 16 | | Some sort of an ugly stain. Write "an ugly stain." (W) | E: (ERR)<br>R: Because I cannot define it; it is something ugly. It is black and ugly. | |
| VII | 17 | | Another x-ray of a pelvis. (W) | E: (ERR)<br>R: The general shape and the rounded part down here. [E could have queried why it looks like an X-ray for C' or Y.] | |
| | 18 | @ | v ^ A vase. (DS7) | E: (ERR)<br>R: Only the inner part that you can see; it is narrow up here and then getting wider. | |
| | 19 | | A chair. (W) | E: (ERR)<br>R: It reminds me of a rocking chair that is being hung by ropes (D5). This is some kind of a hammock in the shape of a chair, like a chair for a child. This is a chair in order for the child not to fall down. | |
| VIII | 20 | | Cats. (D1) | E: (ERR)<br>R: On both sides, tail, head, body. It just reminds me of a cat. | |
| | 21 | | Lungs. (Dd33) | E: (ERR)<br>R: It has the shape of lungs and also the color indicates it is an internal organ. | |
| | 22 | | A butterfly. (D7) | E: (ERR)<br>R: The shape of a butterfly, the wings, the symmetry, and the colors of a butterfly. | |
| IX | 23 | | Liver. (D6) | E: (ERR)<br>R: Because this is the color of an internal organ and also the shape resembles it a little bit. | |
| | 24 | | Two dragons. (D11) | E: (ERR)<br>R: Because of the green color and it resembles, a little bit, dragons. | |
| | 25 | | A rhinoceros. (D3) | E: (ERR)<br>R: Here is its pointy face and the horns that stick out. Why do I see only animals? Is it normal? [This sounded like a comment, so E did not respond.] | |
| X | 26 | | A pliers. (D10) | E: (ERR)<br>R: Because of its pointy shape. I use this kind of pliers. | |
| | 27 | | A grasshopper. (D14) | E: (ERR)<br>R: Because of this narrow part, and the changes in the colors, it reminds me of the shadings of the grasshopper when you draw it in black and white. | |
| | 28 | | Two crabs. (D1) | E: (ERR)<br>R: It looks like crabs, the shape of a crab. | |
| | 29 | | Two fetuses (she spontaneously hands back the card and because it was the last card, E did not give a reminder). (D9) | E: (ERR)<br>R: These two red ones look like the face of a fetus, and it looks like the placenta. The red reminds me of blood. Placenta—something in the process of being created. Placenta because of the red color. The placenta is transferring the blood. Because the changes in colors, it looks like something is happening. | |

# Rorschach Performance Assessment System (R-PAS)®

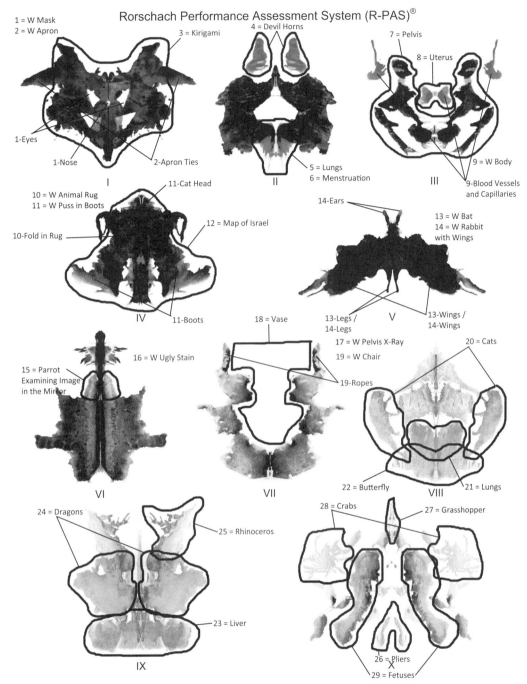

1 = W Mask
2 = W Apron
3 = Kirigami
1-Eyes
1-Nose
2-Apron Ties

I

4 = Devil Horns
5 = Lungs
6 = Menstruation

II

7 = Pelvis
8 = Uterus
9 = W Body
9-Blood Vessels and Capillaries

III

10 = W Animal Rug
11 = W Puss in Boots
11-Cat Head
10-Fold in Rug
12 = Map of Israel
11-Boots

IV

14-Ears
13 = W Bat
14 = W Rabbit with Wings
13-Legs / 14-Legs
13-Wings / 14-Wings

V

15 = Parrot Examining Image in the Mirror
16 = W Ugly Stain

VI

18 = Vase
17 = W Pelvis X-Ray
19 = W Chair
19-Ropes

VII

20 = Cats
22 = Butterfly
21 = Lungs

VIII

24 = Dragons
25 = Rhinoceros
23 = Liver

IX

28 = Crabs
27 = Grasshopper
26 = Pliers
29 = Fetuses

X

# R-PAS Code Sequence: "Ms. T"

**C-ID**: Ms. T    **P-ID**: 33    **Age**: 20s    **Gender**: Female    **Education**: 13

| Cd | # | Or | Loc | Loc # | SR | SI | Content | Sy | Vg | 2 | FQ | P | Determinants | Cognitive | Thematic | HR | ODL (RP) | R-Opt | Text |
|----|---|----|-----|-------|----|----|---------|----|----|---|----|---|--------------|-----------|----------|----|----------|-------|------|
| I | 1 | | W | | | SI | (Hd) | | | | o | | C' | | | GH | | | * |
| Comment: E could have queried 'holes' for FD or V. | | | | | | | | | | | | | | | | | | | |
| | 2 | | W | | | | Cg | | | | u | | F | | | | ODL | | |
| | 3 | | Dd | 99 | | SI | Art | | | | u | | F | | PER | | | | |
| II | 4 | | D | 2 | | | (Hd) | | | | u | | CF | | AGC | GH | | | |
| | 5 | | D | 3 | | | An | | | | u | | F | | | | | | |
| | 6 | | D | 3 | | | Bl,Sx | | Vg | | o | | CF | | | | | | |
| III | 7 | | D | 1 | | | An | | | | o | | F | | PER | | | | * |
| Comment: E could have queried why it looks like an X-ray for C' or Y. | | | | | | | | | | | | | | | | | | | |
| | 8 | | D | 3 | | | An,Bl,Sx | | | | u | | CF | | | | ODL | | |
| | 9 | | W | | | | Hd,An | | | | - | | CF | | | PH | | | |
| IV | 10 | | W | | | | Ad | | | | u | | F | | PER | | | | |
| | 11 | | W | | | | (A),Cg | Sy | | | u | | F | | | | | | |
| | 12 | | Dd | 99 | | | NC | | | | - | | F | | | | | | |
| V | 13 | | W | | | | A | | | | o | P | C' | | | | | | |
| | 14 | | W | | | | A | | | | o | | FMa | INC1 | | | | | |
| VI | 15 | | Dd | 31 | | | A | Sy | | | u | | Ma,Y,r | FAB1 | | PH | | | |
| | 16 | | W | | | | NC | | Vg | | n | | C' | | MOR | | | | |
| Comment: MOR was assigned for "stain," which implies slight damage to the object that is amplified by being an ugly stain. | | | | | | | | | | | | | | | | | | | |
| VII | 17 | | W | | | | An | | | | u | | F | | | | | | * |
| Comment: E could have queried why it looks like an X-ray for C' or Y. | | | | | | | | | | | | | | | | | | | |
| | 18 | @ | D | 7 | SR | | NC | | | | o | | F | | | | | | |
| | 19 | | W | | | | NC | Sy | | | u | | mp | | | | | | |
| VIII | 20 | | D | 1 | | | A | | | 2 | o | P | F | | | | | | |
| | 21 | | Dd | 33 | | | An | | | | o | | FC | | | | | | |
| | 22 | | D | 7 | | | A | | | | u | | FC | | | | | | |
| IX | 23 | | D | 6 | | | An | | | | u | | CF | | | | | | |
| | 24 | | D | 11 | | | (A) | | | 2 | - | | CF | | AGC | | | | |
| | 25 | | D | 3 | | | A | | | | u | | F | | AGC | | | | |
| X | 26 | | D | 10 | | | NC | | | | o | | F | | PER | | | | |
| | 27 | | D | 14 | | | A | | | | - | | Y | | | | | | |
| | 28 | | D | 1 | | | A | | | 2 | o | P | F | | | | | | |
| | 29 | | D | 9 | | | H,An,Bl | | | 2 | u | | ma,CF,Y | | | GH | ODL | | |

©2010-2016 R-PAS

# R-PAS Summary Scores and Profiles – Page 1

C-ID: Ms. T  P-ID: 33  Age: 20s  Gender: Female  Education: 13

| Domain/Variables | Raw Scores | Raw %ile | Raw SS | Cplx. Adj. %ile | Cplx. Adj. SS | Standard Score Profile R-Optimized | Abbr. |
|---|---|---|---|---|---|---|---|
| **Admin. Behaviors and Obs.** | | | | | | | |
| Pr | 0 | 24 | 89 | | | | Pr |
| Pu | 0 | 40 | 96 | | | | Pu |
| CT (Card Turning) | 1 | 38 | 95 | | | | CT |
| **Engagement and Cog. Processing** | | | | | | | |
| Complexity | 78 | 61 | 104 | | | | Cmplx |
| R (Responses) | 29 | 83 | 114 | 77 | 112 | | R |
| F% [Lambda=0.81] (Simplicity) | 45% | 61 | 104 | 63 | 105 | | F% |
| Blend | 2 | 28 | 91 | 16 | 85 | | Bln |
| Sy | 3 | 17 | 86 | 14 | 84 | | Sy |
| MC | 9.0 | 71 | 108 | 62 | 105 | | MC |
| MC - PPD | 0.0 | 68 | 107 | 71 | 108 | | MC-PPD |
| M | 1 | 13 | 83 | 3 | 72 | | M |
| M/MC [1/9.0] | 11% | 4 | 74 | 4 | 74 | | M Prp |
| (CF+C)/SumC [7/9] | 78% | 83 | 115 | 83 | 115 | | CFC Prp |
| **Perception and Thinking Problems** | | | | | | | |
| EII-3 | 0.4 | 80 | 113 | 82 | 114 | | EII |
| TP-Comp (Thought & Percept. Com...) | 0.7 | 58 | 103 | 61 | 104 | | TP-C |
| WSumCog | 6 | 50 | 100 | 48 | 99 | | WCog |
| SevCog | 0 | 35 | 94 | 35 | 94 | | Sev |
| FQ-% | 14% | 75 | 110 | 76 | 111 | | FQ-% |
| WD-% | 12% | 76 | 110 | 68 | 107 | | WD-% |
| FQo% | 34% | 4 | 73 | 3 | 72 | | FQo% |
| P | 3 | 9 | 80 | 14 | 83 | | P |
| **Stress and Distress** | | | | | | | |
| YTVC' | 6 | 70 | 108 | 65 | 106 | | YTVC' |
| m | 2 | 66 | 106 | 50 | 100 | | m |
| Y | 3 | 83 | 114 | 79 | 113 | | Y |
| MOR | 1 | 51 | 100 | 47 | 98 | | MOR |
| SC-Comp (Suicide Concern Comp.) | 6.2 | 84 | 115 | 81 | 114 | | SC-C |
| **Self and Other Representation** | | | | | | | |
| ODL% | 10% | 52 | 101 | 50 | 100 | | ODL% |
| SR (Space Reversal) | 1 | 56 | 102 | 56 | 102 | | SR |
| MAP/MAHP [0/0] | NA | | | | | | MAP Prp |
| PHR/GPHR [2/5] | 40% | 62 | 105 | 62 | 105 | | PHR Prp |
| M- | 0 | 36 | 95 | 36 | 95 | | M- |
| AGC | 3 | 49 | 100 | 46 | 99 | | AGC |
| H | 1 | 21 | 88 | 13 | 81 | | H |
| COP | 0 | 21 | 88 | 21 | 88 | | COP |
| MAH | 0 | 26 | 90 | 26 | 90 | | MAH |

© 2010-2016 R-PAS

# R-PAS Summary Scores and Profiles – Page 2

**C-ID:** Ms. T     **P-ID:** 33     **Age:** 20s     **Gender:** Female     **Education:** 13

| Domain/Variables | Raw Scores | Raw %ile | Raw SS | Cplx. Adj. %ile | Cplx. Adj. SS | Standard Score Profile R-Optimized | Abbr. |
|---|---|---|---|---|---|---|---|
| **Engagement and Cog. Processing** | | | | | | | |
| W% | 34% | 41 | 97 | 40 | 96 | | W% |
| Dd% | 14% | 52 | 101 | 55 | 102 | | Dd% |
| SI (Space Integration) | 2 | 38 | 96 | 46 | 99 | | SI |
| IntCont | 1 | 31 | 93 | 27 | 91 | | IntC |
| Vg% | 7% | 66 | 106 | 64 | 106 | | Vg% |
| V | 0 | 29 | 92 | 29 | 92 | | V |
| FD | 0 | 21 | 88 | 27 | 90 | | FD |
| R8910% | 34% | 67 | 106 | 66 | 106 | | R8910% |
| WSumC | 8.0 | 96 | 126 | 95 | 124 | | WSC |
| C | 0 | 36 | 95 | 36 | 95 | | C |
| Mp/(Ma+Mp) [0/1] | NA | | | | | | Mp Prp |
| **Perception and Thinking Problems** | | | | | | | |
| FQu% | 48% | 94 | 123 | 95 | 124 | | FQu% |
| **Stress and Distress** | | | | | | | |
| PPD | 9 | 51 | 101 | 45 | 98 | | PPD |
| CBlend | 1 | 69 | 107 | 47 | 99 | | CBlnd |
| C' | 3 | 77 | 111 | 69 | 108 | | C' |
| V | 0 | 29 | 92 | 29 | 92 | | V |
| CritCont% (Critical Contents) | 48% | 96 | 127 | 96 | 127 | | CrCt |
| **Self and Other Representation** | | | | | | | |
| SumH | 4 | 27 | 91 | 23 | 89 | | SumH |
| NPH/SumH [3/4] | 75% | 76 | 111 | 75 | 110 | | NPH Prp |
| V-Comp (Vigilance Composite) | 3.3 | 54 | 101 | 50 | 100 | | V-C |
| r (Reflections) | 1 | 81 | 113 | 81 | 113 | | r |
| p/(a+p) [1/4] | 25% | 22 | 88 | 21 | 88 | | p Prp |
| AGM | 0 | 31 | 93 | 31 | 93 | | AGM |
| T | 0 | 28 | 91 | 28 | 91 | | T |
| PER | 4 | 98 | 131 | 98 | 131 | | PER |
| An | 8 | >99 | 140 | >99 | 140 | | An |

© 2010-2016 R-PAS

# Using R-PAS in the Evaluation of an Emotional Disturbance in the School Context

Tammy L. Hughes
Kate Piselli
Cassandra Berbary

A ll children in the United States, whether emotionally disturbed, behaviorally disordered, disabled, or otherwise, must receive a free and appropriate public education (Individuals with Disability Education Act, 1997). Determining which services are provided, and where, is not only a diagnostic formulation, it is a legal matter for the school team. Psychologists working with children often find it useful to become familiar with the regulatory requirements of school psychologists so that they may better coordinate care and serve as effective advocates for their clients.

In school, children can receive mental and behavioral health services in both the general and special education setting. *Positive behavior support* is a common prevention program that is integrated into school routines and delivered to all students at the primary prevention level. These interventions promote age-appropriate social–emotional development such as teaching and supporting prosocial actions, anti-bullying behaviors, and character development. At-risk youth receive specialized services (e.g., conflict resolution, social skill training) to address problem behaviors that are not considered disabling. Students who do not benefit from these supports may be considered for special education services.

Special education eligibility is defined by the Individuals with Disabilities Education Act (IDEA), which encompasses children from birth through the age of 21. For eligible students, all services are provided free of charge by the district, or the district designee, where the children reside. At present, there are 13 categories of special education eligibility. Youth with a DSM or ICD diagnosis may or may not qualify for services under special education because the criteria also stipulate that there must be an educational need; an individualized education program (IEP) is required in order for the youth to benefit from his or her educational environment. It is possible that a child may carry a DSM or ICD diagnosis—for example, an autism spectrum disorder, obsessive–compulsive disorder, or eating disorder—and yet the disorder does not impair his or her educational performance. This group of children would not be eligible for special education services. Also, a child may exhibit a disability as defined by IDEA and not meet threshold for a DSM or ICD diagnosis. For example, a child who meets the special education criteria for Other Health Impairment due to symptoms of attention-deficit/hyperactivity disorder (ADHD) may not meet the threshold for a DSM-5 (American Psychiatric Association, 2013) ADHD diagnosis.

For behaviorally disordered youth who do not qualify for special education, treatment services *may* be individualized and either provided within the general or alternative education setting, or these students may be referred for treatment external to the school. The education program for behaviorally disordered youth who qualify for special education services *must* be individualized. One difference between the child receiving services outside the special education context (e.g., in general education) is the degree to which his or her particular school can provide interventions that are uniform and untailored. Although special education students may spend all or some of their day in the general education setting, their educational placement and support are determined solely by their individual needs.

Federal law defines protections guaranteed to all special education students, including:

- How eligibility and treatment planning is conducted (e.g., who are the required members of the multidisciplinary team).
- When evaluations and reevaluations occur, including the schedule of review of student progress.
- When and how a student may be placed in a more restrictive setting.
- Procedural safeguards (e.g., hearings for managing disputes between the school and parents).
- How discipline and sanctions (e.g., suspension) are handled.

For a child with a behavioral disruption, placement in special education directs how the school staff must conduct itself when behaviors violate the school conduct code (e.g., threatening a teacher) or become a criminal offense (e.g., assault). In short, the school may not punish, suspend, expel, or otherwise remove the child from school for a behavior that is part of the disability as defined by special education eligibility—although there are some exceptions if serious bodily injury occurs, a weapon is used, or drugs are involved (CFR §§300.530). When there are continuous or serious behavioral disruptions that would typically warrant disciplinary action, the school team must (1) demonstrate that they are adequately meeting the child's treatment needs identified in the IEP, and (2) conduct a functional behavior assessment (FBA) accompanied by a behavior intervention plan (BIP) to adjust treatment as needed. Taken together, understanding what drives the targeted behavior and not simply identifying which behaviors are present becomes an essential task for school teams treating youth with disruptive behaviors.

## Introduction to Neveah

"Neveah" was a 15-year-old African American female remanded to a residential school by juvenile court. She was adjudicated delinquent subsequent to assault, robbery, and criminal trespassing charges.

Although her charges are unrelated to her special education eligibility, the school team is concerned about eligibility, the nature of the treatments required for her success, and how to manage potential behavioral outbursts. Previous records indicate a history of aggressive and defiant behaviors; however, she does not display these behaviors at the present time. Academic problems in math, alongside angry outbursts and parental discord, have long been noted in the file history, whereas symptoms of depression and somatization were present for the first time in an evaluation conducted 1 year ago during the time of the adjudication procedures. The symptoms of depression qualified her for special education under the special education category of emotional disturbance.

There are three referral questions: Does this child qualify as a student with a disability under the special education category of emotional disturbance? If she does not qualify under the special education category of emotional disturbance, are there other diagnostic considerations? Regardless of special education eligibility, what treatment recommendations would be delivered in an alternative (general) education placement?

Quoting from IDEA, an emotional disturbance is defined as follows:

Emotional disturbance means a condition exhibiting one or more of the following characteristics over a long period of time and to a marked degree that adversely affects a child's educational performance:

(a) An inability to learn that cannot be explained by intellectual, sensory, or health factors.
(b) An inability to build or maintain satisfactory interpersonal relationships with peers and teachers.
(c) Inappropriate types of behavior or feelings under normal circumstances.
(d) A general pervasive mood of unhappiness or depression.
(e) A tendency to develop physical symptoms or fears associated with personal or school problems.

Emotional disturbance includes schizophrenia. The term does not apply to children who are socially maladjusted, unless it is determined that they have an emotional disturbance (Sec. 300.8 of the IDEA, 2004).

## Neveah's Background

Prior to the current placement, Neveah lived with her maternal grandmother, who has been her primary caregiver since her birth. Her grandmother was awarded legal custody (15 years earlier) when Neveah was 1 year old, after the courts found her to be abandoned by her biological mother. Neveah describes a chaotic and combative relationship with her mother, who has been in and out of jail throughout Neveah's life, reportedly due to drug and prostitution charges. Neveah indicates that her current assault charge occurred during a fight she and her mother were having with an aunt. Allegedly, her mother urged Neveah toward a physical confrontation and subsequently was also a participant in the assault. Although serving as Neveah's caregiver, Neveah's grandmother has had limited contact with her since her placement in the residential school. At present, the grandmother lives out of state. Neveah was relocated to a school in a state that specializes in the treatment of adolescent girls with the goal of disrupting a recent increase in aggressive actions toward others.

In school, Neveah had a history of defiance, aggression, and academic weaknesses in math, which had been consistently documented in her educational records since kindergarten. Inconsistent work effort and variable attendance were noted each year. In fifth grade she was retained. The following year she was expelled from school for "repeated violations of the student code of conduct for incidents involving insubordination, disorderly conduct, disruptive behavior, fighting, terroristic threatening, assault, and bullying." For each of her last 3 years, Neveah missed at least 30 days of school due to changing schools, suspensions, expulsions, and other unexcused absences.

Records indicate that Neveah's medical history was unremarkable aside from seasonal allergies. Results of an out-of-state psychoeducational evaluation conducted in the year before our evaluation indicated that Neveah met special education criteria for emotional disturbance due to her inability to maintain appropriate peer relationships and a general pervasive mood of unhappiness or depression.

## Assessment Methods Used with Neveah

At the current placement, where Neveah is in the ninth grade, a comprehensive psychoeducational evaluation was completed as a matter of standard practice. The ninth-grade assessment battery included cognitive, academic, and social–emotional measures, along with a record review, a clinical interview with her, and teacher interviews. Presented in this chapter are results from her eighth-grade and ninth-grade Behavior Assessment System for Children (Second Edition [BASC-2]), Self-Report of Personality (SRP), and Teacher Rating Scale (TRS), as well as results from her ninth-grade Rorschach Performance Assessment System (R-PAS; Meyer, Viglione, Mihura, Erard, & Erdberg, 2011).

## Neveah's Non-R-PAS Assessment Results

In brief, Neveah's previous eighth-grade psychoeducational evaluation results indicated that she was a student with average cognitive abilities and average academic skills in reading, writing, and oral expression. However, her math scores were below average to low average. She evidenced a poor attitude toward school, expecting and experiencing few successes. Her teachers noted poor persistence on tasks she did not like, as well as high rates of incomplete classwork and homework. Although teachers reported concerns about fighting with peers, Neveah's self-report data indicated conflict with her mother and grandmother was her concern. Results from the eighth-grade evaluation also indicated that Neveah experienced symptoms of inattention, hyperactivity, and impulsivity as well as feelings of depression. Some somatic complaints were also listed. Aggressive conduct, angry outbursts, and poor coping and adaptability were the focus of school behavioral interventions. The eighth-grade school team settled on the emotional disturbance eligibility category after reasoning that her poor school attendance made it difficult for them to determine if there was truly a learning disability in math—a required component of determining the presence of a learning disability to ensure that underachievement is not due to lack of appropriate instruction (CFR 300.304–300.306). Also, there was a statement by the eighth-grade school team that because the ADHD symptoms were not accompanied by an ADHD diagnosis from a physician, she could not be considered for the special education category of Other Health Impairment due to the requirements in her state of residence.

Upon arrival at the current placement, it became necessary to consider both the ADHD symptoms and the presence of depression to clarify Neveah's treatment needs. It is important to note that the state in which she resides for her current placement does not require a physician to diagnose ADHD, and ADHD is recognized as an area of special education eligibility as well as a DSM diagnosis.

Behavior rating scales such as the BASC-2 are routinely administered in psychoeducational evaluations. When comparing Neveah's past (eighth-grade) and current (ninth-grade) BASC-2 self-report data (see Table 19.1), there was no longer an at-risk score in Depression and Somatization, though both assessments showed problematic and clinically significant scores in the areas of Inattention and Hyperactivity.

**TABLE 19.1.  T Scores for BASC-2 Self-Report Data**

| Scale | Eighth-grade self-report | Ninth-grade self-report |
|---|---|---|
| School Problems | 60* | 55 |
|     Attitude to School | 65* | 53 |
|     Attitude to Teachers | 52 | 59 |
|     Sensation Seeking | 56 | 49 |
| Internalizing Problems | 57 | 51 |
|     Atypicality | 48 | 45 |
|     Locus of Control | 58 | 53 |
|     Social Stress | 49 | 56 |
|     Anxiety | 57 | 50 |
|     Depression | 60* | 50 |
|     Sense of Inadequacy | 56 | 55 |
|     Somatization | 62* | 48 |
| Inattention/Hyperactivity | 75** | 77** |
|     Attention Problems | 71** | 70** |
|     Hyperactivity | 73** | 77** |
| Emotional Symptoms Index | 56 | 56 |
| Personal Adjustment | 43 | 41 |
|     Relations with Parents | 30** | 35* |
|     Interpersonal Relations | 56 | 55 |
|     Self-Esteem | 48 | 40 |
|     Self-Reliance | 45 | 44 |

*Note.* $M = 50$; $SD = 10$.
*At risk; **clinically significant.

The current (ninth-grade) teachers' BASC-2 measures also indicated problematic and clinically significant Inattention and Hyperactivity scores that were previously identified in her (eighth-grade) evaluation (see Table 19.2). Current (ninth-grade) BASC-2 teacher report data also show one teacher with concern about depression, whereas the other teachers did not note depressive behaviors. Given that Neveah was found to be eligible for special education in eighth grade under the emotional disturbance category, and that decision was predicated on, in part, the presence of depressed mood, it became important to clarify the nature of Neveah's emotional status. Also, a concern to the current (ninth-grade) school team was the fact that the past (eighth-grade) BASC-2 data did not include validity scale information for either teachers or student reports. As such, the context for how those scores should be interpreted was missing.

All current (ninth-grade) teacher and self-report BASC-2 measures were considered valid and interpretable. Parent (guardian) measures were distributed but not completed for either the eighth- or ninth-grade evaluation process.

## Why R-PAS for Neveah's Case?

R-PAS was administered to help clarify (1) the drivers of Neveah's history of aggressive actions, angry outbursts, poor peer relationships, coping difficulties; and (2) the degree to which emotions influence her decision making. Given that the eighth-grade

**TABLE 19.2. T Scores for BASC-2 Teacher-Report Data**

| Scale | Eighth-grade teacher 1 | Eighth-grade teacher 2 | Ninth-grade teacher A | Ninth-grade teacher B | Ninth-grade teacher C |
|---|---|---|---|---|---|
| Externalizing Problems | 77** | 76** | 66* | 66* | 104** |
| Hyperactivity | 69* | 73** | 54 | 62* | 94** |
| Aggression | 89** | 82** | 67* | 60* | 108** |
| Conduct Problems | 69* | 69* | 74* | 71* | 97** |
| Internalizing Problems | 65* | 66* | 54 | 44 | 62* |
| Anxiety | 53 | 63* | 57 | 41 | 51 |
| Depression | 78** | 67* | 59 | 51 | 76** |
| Somatization | 55 | 59 | 43 | 43 | 55 |
| Behavioral Symptoms | 77** | 72** | 58 | 59 | 90** |
| Atypicality | 75** | 68* | 45 | 65* | 65* |
| Withdrawal | 61* | 61* | 53 | 53 | 73** |
| School Problems | 60* | 58 | 53 | 49 | 62* |
| Attention Problems | 62* | 58 | 62* | 54 | 75** |
| Learning Problems | 57 | 57 | 44 | 44 | 47 |
| Adaptive Skills | 37* | 44 | 46 | 42 | 33* |
| Adaptability | 35* | 39* | 49 | 38* | 25** |
| Social Skills | 42 | 44 | 46 | 34* | 34* |
| Leadership | 44 | 49 | 42 | 45 | 33* |
| Study Skills | 33* | 44 | 39* | 45 | 46 |
| Functional Communication | 40* | 46 | 54 | 50 | 43 |

Note. M = 50; SD = 10.
*At-risk; **clinically significant.

report provided the first indication of depression in her record, it is important to clarify if the noted depression and somatization behaviors were simply a function of situational stress—Neveah indicated poor coping due to proximity with her mother—or if her coping skills are inadequately developed. It is also important to consider the extent to which emotions contribute to her decision making and behavior. Further, because the emotional disturbance label was applied, in part, due to her inability to maintain appropriate peer relationships, it was important to consider the nature and quality of Neveah's relationships. Relatedly, the treatment team needed to consider the relationship between her actions and the ADHD symptoms. The team hypothesized that R-PAS data would add incrementally relevant information to the assessment battery.

The use of a performance-based method allows the clinician to observe and measure a person's problem solving in a way that self-report does not. R-PAS, like other performance-based measures, helps to clarify what teachers and parents observe and the child reports. Particularly when child behaviors prove to be unresponsive to straightforward evidenced-based treatment protocols, or when children present with complex treatment needs, Rorschach data can add depth toward formulating a successful treatment plan.

## Introducing R-PAS to Neveah

R-PAS was administered as part of the comprehensive psychoeducational battery used in this residential school placement to determine the treatment needs of adjudicated youth who have failed to respond to typical treatment protocols. The R-PAS task was introduced using the standard administration instructions. After the initial instructions were provided, Neveah asked the examiner to repeat them. She did not ask any additional questions regarding the task, and her approach showed that she understood the process. She reported that she had not taken the test before.

## R-PAS Administration

Testing occurred in a private room. Neveah presented as appropriately dressed, and her demeanor was calm. She was reserved when providing and elaborating on answers; however, rapport was easy to establish and maintain. Throughout the whole assessment process, Neveah was cooperative and put forth good effort. R-PAS administration was completed in 45 minutes.

## Neveah's R-PAS Results[1]

### Test Validity

Neveah provided a sufficient number of responses for an interpretable protocol, although she provided fewer responses than is typical for someone her age (R = 18, SS

---

[1] See Appendix 19.1 at the end of the chapter for Neveah's R-PAS Responses, Location Sheet, Code Sequence, and Page 1 and 2 Profiles.

= 81[2]). In addition, during the administration she had to be prompted three times to provide an adequate number of responses, which is more times than is typical for her age group (Pr SS = 131). Following two of these prompts, Neveah returned the card, stating that she did not see anything else. Neveah's refusal to follow the rule of providing "two, maybe three" responses per card is consistent with her teachers' reports that Neveah is resistant to adhering to rules, even when those rules are stated explicitly and followed by reminders. Teachers often experience and describe this type of behavior as defiant and oppositional. Neveah's need for a prompt to provide another response on the first card when the task instructions had just been given also may reflect inattention to the task directions. Inattention may also explain why right after the instructions were introduced, Neveah asked to hear the instructions repeated. Nevertheless, after two repetitions, it seems likely Neveah would have recalled the instructions on the first card—as well as the second. Her need for prompting and low R thus may suggest difficulty seeing things from multiple perspectives or difficulty responding to complex demands.

In addition to having fewer responses than expected for her age, the quality of Neveah's responses was less complex than typical for her age (Complexity SS = 83). This more simplistic approach to the task may have been due to the oppositional approach described by the teachers or representative of a limited attentional or motivational style that occurs when she is asked to perform cognitively demanding problem-solving tasks. Given that Neveah is reported as having average cognitive ability across several rounds of psychoeducational assessment, the microcosm of the R-PAS task seems to have provided an in vivo illustration of her teachers' interpretation that she "puts forth inconsistent effort in her academic work."

Taken together, the results indicated that Neveah tends to underperform when presented with tasks she finds particularly demanding or difficult. Neveah's R-PAS results were interpreted with this caution in mind. That is, for the R-PAS Engagement and Cognitive Processing variables, Neveah's results were interpreted as a typical performance task—showing how Neveah typically behaves in similar semistructured settings with an adult authority when she is asked to engage in challenging tasks that provide wide latitude for responding. Therefore, results in the Engagement and Cognitive Processing section were not adjusted for her level of Complexity, though Complexity Adjustment (CAdj) was considered for other variables.

## Engagement and Cognitive Processing

In general, Neveah evidenced adequate coping resources and cognitive flexibility. She demonstrated a developmentally appropriate ability to recognize subtleties in the environment and engage in the synthesis of information (F% SS = 107; Sy SS = 90). Neveah displayed developmentally adequate psychological resources to adapt to or contend with environmental and experiential demands (MC SS = 92; MC–PPD SS = 106). However, it is clinically important to note that although Neveah's measures of coping and psychological resources were average, her low complexity, low number of responses, and high number of prompts are indicative of her reliance on behavioral cues to complete difficult tasks. These results, considered in the context of past and

---

[2]Neveah's results were compared to same-age normative data. Results are reported in standard scores (SS) with a mean = 100 and an *SD* = 15.

current BASC-2 teacher reports noting Neveah's poor adaptability and defiant behaviors, may help to explain why, when she appears inflexible and rigid in her approach to novel situations, it is difficult to distinguish between behavioral refusal and a limited cognitive and motivational capacity to generate flexible solutions to problems.

In terms of cognitive processing style, Neveah's approach was to use the simplest solution to form her perceptions (W% SS = 112; all Ws to intact Cards I, IV, V, VI, VII). Likewise, she rarely focused her attention on small or uncommon details (Dd% SS = 80), and rarely shifted her attention to include information from various sources (SI SS = 80). This cognitive style may also contribute to the teachers' inattention concerns noted on past and present BASC-2 reports. Information from behavior rating scales indicated that Neveah displayed elevated levels of hyperactivity; however, on R-PAS, Neveah did not exhibit impulsive or reactive responses to compelling stimuli in a manner that would suggest an overinvolvement in emotional responsiveness (C SS = 92; M/MC SS = 100; R8910% SS = 91). Taken together, the results indicated that ADHD processes remain an issue of concern, although the Rorschach data did not provide evidence that impulsive emotional reactions account for these behaviors.

## Perception and Thinking

Neveah did not demonstrate evidence of significant global psychopathology or psychotic propensity (EII-3 SS = 89; TP-Comp SS = 78). She showed an average ability to organize and communicate her thoughts in a logical manner (WSumCog SS = 96). Further, she did not demonstrate any distorted or misinterpreted perceptions (FQ−% SS = 74), a result indicating that she possesses the cognitive and perceptual abilities to accurately interpret cues from the environment. In fact, Neveah had an above-average proportion of conventional perceptions (FQo% SS = 125), suggesting a sensitivity to obvious external cues. Her Popular responses were in the average range for her age (P = 3 SS = 88), and included several near Popular responses, such as a moth on Card V and a sculpture of two girls on Card VII. Given the low Complexity scores, it is possible that problems related to perception and thinking difficulties may be underestimated.

## Stress and Distress

As mentioned above, one of the goals of the evaluation was to determine whether Neveah currently experiences underlying feelings of unhappiness and depressed mood. Results suggested that Neveah does not attend to inconsistencies, nuances, and subtleties in her environment (YTVC' SS = 84). As a result, she is less likely than her peers to notice potential inconsistencies and distracting nuances that may lead to feelings of uncertainty, and less likely to recognize subtle reactions and experiences that affect her. This is probably another example of how Neveah detaches and oversimplifies as a coping method. Her low Complexity scores bring the possibility that difficulties with implicit stress and distress could be underestimated; however, of note, she did not report symptoms of depression on her most recent BASC-2.

## Self and Other Representation

Given Neveah's history of interpersonal conflict, such as family and peer fighting and bullying, it was hypothesized that she would have limited social understanding of herself and others or distorted perceptions of relationships. Two of Neveah's three current teachers rated her social skills as quite poor. However, R-PAS results suggested that Neveah has an adequate capacity to understand herself and others (PHR/GPHR SS = 95). Further, she appears to have average ability to understand others as whole people (H = 2, CAdj SS = 105). She did not evidence any difficulty related to gross misunderstandings or misperceptions of people and their actions (M– = 0, SS = 91). However, it is important to note that Neveah also did not report any perceptions of people or animals interacting with each other in clearly positive or negative ways (COP = 0, AGM = 0, MAHP = 0). Although average for her age, based on these results, it is difficult to determine the extent to which she views interpersonal relationships as healthy and benevolent or unbalanced and malevolent.

According to BASC-2 data from eighth- and ninth-grade reports, Neveah's teachers indicated that she engages in more aggressive behaviors than are typical for her age. Therefore, given her history, it was hypothesized that Neveah would demonstrate a preoccupation with thoughts or concerns about aggression, competitiveness, or power strivings. However, even considering Neveah's low number of Responses and limited engagement with the task, she was no more likely to have aggressive thoughts and images on her mind than other same-age adolescents (AGC CAdj SS = 109; AGM SS = 90). Additionally, she did not evidence a vigilant or guarded processing style characterized by sensitivity to cues indicating danger or trouble (V-Comp SS = 88), which is often noted in profiles of chronically aggressive youth. These results suggested that Neveah's aggressive interactions may be related to maladaptive patterns of behaviors that developed in the context of modeling her social environment (e.g., hostile relationship with her mother, fighting with peers), rather than with an inherent preoccupation with interpersonal aggression and suspiciousness. Instead, given her low Complexity and general lack of appreciation for subtlety and nuance, she is likely easily overwhelmed by experiences and events, resulting in her use of this modeled hostile aggression as a way to manage the environment.

## Summary of Neveah's R-PAS Results

There are many positive attributes noted in Neveah's R-PAS data, including adequate coping resources for her age, a limited preoccupation with bothersome thoughts or feelings of uncertainty, and an adequate understanding of self and others—characterized by an ability to understand others without distorted or maladaptive perceptions of relationships or a preoccupation with aggression. Nonetheless, as illustrated by her low Complexity score, when considering her skills alongside same-age peers, Neveah's behavioral repertoire is likely to be less well developed. Her scores also needed to be considered in the context of her overall approach to the task. Specifically, her fewer-than-average number of responses, low Complexity score, and a high number of prompts to follow task directions suggested that her difficulties may be underestimated in these data. For instance, the Prompt required on Card I was followed by the percept of "a sad dog," and it is possible that her lack of response to the two subsequent prompts kept similar depressive imagery at bay. Similarly, the two instances when Neveah did not comply with the Prompt occurred after her only two percepts of relational interactions, which she left ambiguous as to the positive or negative nature of the interaction (R3: "Two animals pushing their noses together";

R16: "Deer putting their antlers together"). However, the elaboration in the Response Phase for the second instance hinted at themes of loss (RP: "the green in *Bambi,* in the forest from when I saw *Bambi*").

Neveah's R-PAS performance is consistent with past and current reports from her teachers indicating that she tends to be less adaptive, resistant to adhering to rules, and puts forth inconsistent effort in completing demanding tasks. Her day-to-day functioning may be best understood in the context of a compromised ability to engage in complex problem solving along with low motivation and a limited attentional capacity. Further, it appears that her aggressive behaviors were developed and maintained in the context of maladaptive patterns of behaviors with her family members and peers, and she has found aggressive acts to be an effective method to manage her environment. Identifying and securing reliable social support remains a challenge for Neveah.

## Impact of R-PAS on Neveah

R-PAS was administered to help understand Neveah's aggressive actions, angry outbursts, problems with peer relationships, coping style, and the degree to which emotions influence her decision making. The R-PAS data, combined with other assessment data, helped to better clarify Neveah's social and emotional functioning, and resulted in the removal of a special education label of emotional disturbance.

After careful consideration of the assessment results, the school team made the decision to remove Neveah from the special education eligibility category as a student with an emotional disturbance. Foremost on the minds of these educators was that the depressive symptoms used, in part, to justify the label were transient, restricted to specific contexts, and primarily evident in times of situational stress. Neveah's R-PAS results showing low Complexity and need for Prompts helped to explain inconsistencies in her behavioral responses across contexts, as observed and reported by teachers and herself. Further, the team felt it was understandable that Neveah would resort to aggression to manage her environment, given the use of aggression in her interactions with her mother and some peer interactions. R-PAS results highlighting Neveah's need to identify appropriate sources of social support, rather than a need to acquire basic skills on how to act in a social manner, became a more specific focus of treatment. The school team felt that this type of service did not require specially designed instruction through special education services.

Special education placement decisions are not taken lightly for a variety of reasons. Foremost is the reality that placement in special education does not ensure good student academic or behavioral outcomes (Osher, 2002). Also, because there is a nationwide overrepresentation of minority students in the special education eligibility category of emotional disturbance, a minority placement in this category should receive a high level of scrutiny. R-PAS results helped to establish Neveah's problem-solving style and characterological issues in order to determine that those needs could be met in a general education setting.

When Neveah was removed from special education, she began to receive treatment within the general education setting. It is important to acknowledge, however, that her education was no longer completely individualized. Although this change may disturb those advocates who believe that all children should receive individualized treatments, the literature shows that manualized evidence-based treatments work well for a large subset of mental and behavioral health issues. Indeed, anecdotal reports from the school indicate that Neveah did not require individual modifications to her treatment in order to increase her academic or behavioral success.

Removal from special education altered the way in which the school subsequently handled Neveah's behavioral violations. Previously, as a special education student, Neveah could not be punished, suspended, or expelled for a behavior that was related to her emotional disturbance. However, when Neveah's IEP was removed, she benefited from a program that held her accountable for her behaviors as well as taught appropriate expressions of her needs. Again, reports indicate that she is participating well and shows good success.

## Summary of R-PAS Contributions to Neveah's Case

This case was selected because it highlights several ways in which R-PAS is useful in the school context. For example, this case shows that, for a child with a low Complexity score and an average IQ, her typical behavioral performance in her day-to-day life will be challenging. Although she understands how to interact in her environment, Neveah may have trouble responding effectively to environmental demands. Nevertheless, this behavioral profile is not indicative of the need for special education services.

The case also shows that any assumption that R-PAS scores will always pathologize a student's behaviors is inaccurate. Helping teachers and school personnel to appreciate Neveah's resiliency, given her personal life experiences—as noted in her average IQ, absence of thought disturbance, lack of interpersonal distortions, and absence of any preoccupation with aggression—served to reframe their approach to helping her acquire and enact prosocial behaviors. The additional information changed the course of treatment planning, which has anecdotally been reported as resulting in improved outcomes. Finally, the case shows how R-PAS information provides a check for some of the most common errors found when considering a minority child for the label of an emotional disturbance. Given that individuals with an emotional disturbance are both overidentified, especially in minority populations (Oswald, Coutinho, & Best, 2002), and underserved (Kauffman & Landrum, 2007; U.S. Department of Health and Human Services, 1999), it is important to add R-PAS to an assessment battery as these data contribute meaningful information to school-based decision making.

## REFERENCES

American Psychiatric Association. (2013). *Diagnostic and statistical manual of mental disorders* (5th ed.). Arlington, VA: Author.

Individuals with Disabilities Education Act, 20 U.S.C. § 1400 (2004). *http://idea.ed.gov/download/statute.html*

Individuals with Disability Education Act Amendments of 1997 [IDEA]. (1997). Retrieved from *http://thomas.loc.gov/home/thomas.php.*

Kauffman, J. M., & Landrum, T. J. (2007). Educational service interventions and reforms. In J. W. Jacobson, J. A. Mulick, & J. Rojahn (Eds.), *Handbook of intellectual and developmental disabilities* (pp. 173–188). New York: Springer.

Meyer, G. J., Viglione, D. J., Mihura, J. L., Erard, R. E., & Erdberg, P. (2011). *Rorschach Performance Assessment System: Administration, coding, interpretation, and technical manual.* Toledo, OH: Rorschach Performance Assessment System.

Osher, D. M. (2002). Creating comprehensive and collaborative systems. *Journal of Child and Family Studies, 11,* 91–99.

Oswald, D. P., Coutinho, M. J., & Best, A. M. (2002). Community and school predictors of overrepresentation of minority children in special education. In D. J. Losen & G. Orfield (Eds.), *Racial inequity in special education* (pp. 1–13). Cambridge, MA: Harvard Education Press.

U.S. Department of Health and Human Services. (1999). *Mental health: A report of the surgeon general.* Rockville, MD: U.S. Department of Health and Human Services, Substance Abuse and Mental Health Services Administration, Center for Mental Health Services, National Institutes of Health, National Institute of Mental Health.

# APPENDIX 19.1. Neveah's R-PAS Responses, Location Sheet, Code Sequence, and Page 1 and 2 Profiles

## Rorschach Responses "Neveah"

| Respondent ID: Neveah | Examiner: Cassandra Berbary |
|---|---|
| Location: Alternative Education School | Date: **/**/**** |
| Start Time: 10:00 A.M. | End Time: 10:45 A.M. |

| Cd # | R # | Or | Response | Clarification | R-Opt |
|---|---|---|---|---|---|
| I | 1 | | Kind of looks like a fox. I don't know, I just see a fox here. That's all. (W)<br>E: Remember, give two, maybe three responses for each card | E: (Examiner Repeats Response [ERR].)<br>R: This could be like the nose (D3) and this is the ears (D7). | Pr |
| | 2 | @ | > v < ^Maybe like a sad dog. (W) | E: (ERR)<br>R: This is the same face, but like a sad dog because the ears (D7) are pointing down [nose = D3]. | |
| II | 3 | @ | > v < ^Hmm, looks like I don't know what type of animal. I'm trying to think of the animal name, but like two animals pushing their noses together. (D6)<br>E: Remember, give two, maybe three responses for each card<br>R: Doesn't look like nothing else really, just the animals. | E: (ERR)<br>R: This looks like the animal head and the noses (D4) coming up and touching. | Pr |
| III | 4 | | Like why does everything look like a dog? Like a poodle right here and here. (D9) | E: (ERR)<br>R: The body and the hands are reaching for something (D7); this is one poodle and this is the other, heads (Dd32) here, legs (D5), hands reaching. | |
| | 5 | | Or a person or something like that, here and here. (D9) | E: (ERR)<br>R: This could just be like a lady—her body here and that is how her hair is all up like that on her head, like a do-up (upper portion of Dd34). | |
| IV | 6 | v | > v When I hold it this way, it kind of looks like water coming up. (W) | E: (ERR)<br>R: Water like shooting up out of here, this little area here like it is going up.<br>E: What makes it look like water?<br>R: All the little details sticking out made it look like it was the splashes. ["Shooting" is indicated as D1 and "splashes" is indicated as D2,4.] | |
| | 7 | @ | > v < ^ Maybe like the Abominable Snowman—is that what it's called? Or like a big monster. (W) | E: (ERR)<br>R: Yeah, because the head (D3) and face right here, and the feet (D2), and this is its arms (D4). | |
| V | 8 | v | > v Like a moth or a butterfly . . . (W) | E: (ERR)<br>R: Yeah, when you hold it like this, the wings (D4) here and the antennas (Dd34). | |
| | 9 | | or like a lady with wings. (W) | E: (ERR)<br>R: Like her wings (D4) are down and this her legs (D9) and her head (Dd30). | |
| VI | 10 | v | > v A leaf. (W) | E: (ERR)<br>R: Leaf; like the outside looks this big (respondent outlines shape) and this like the stem (D5). | |
| | 11 | | A bug. (W) | E: (ERR)<br>R: These little things sticking out here reminded me of a bug, and these on the bottom here like their little legs (Dd22) or claws (Dd33) or antenna or something; like the bug, though. | |

| Cd # | R # | Or | Response | Clarification | R-Opt |
|---|---|---|---|---|---|
| VII | 12 | | Looks like a sculpture of a girl, two of them, two sculptures. (W) | E: (ERR)<br>R: Yeah, that's their head (D9), but I can't see the face, so it's a sculpture. This is like a feather (D5) or something, and the body is turned this way facing the other: one girl here and one here. | |
| | 13 | v | > v Then this way looks kind of like an archway here. (W) | E: (ERR)<br>R: This is like the top of the arch and this is the bottom and sides like here (traces arch). | |
| VIII | 14 | | Iguanas on the sides here. (D1) | E: (ERR)<br>R: Yeah, right here, then I started looking at it and I thought something different.<br>E: What about it makes it look like iguanas?<br>R: I thought this was the iguana tail here. | |
| | 15 | | Or jaguars or mountain lions actually here. (D1) | E: (ERR)<br>R: I realized this wasn't the tail, it was the leg here of the mountain lion; there are four legs here. | |
| IX | 16 | | This looks like deer putting their antlers together. (D3,8)<br>E: Remember, give two, maybe three responses for each card.<br>R: That's it; I don't see nothing else. | E: (ERR)<br>R: Yeah, at the top.<br>E: What about it makes it look like deer?<br>R: The stick part here like antlers (Dd34) and the background (D8) here kind of reminded me of Bambi.<br>E: Reminded you of Bambi?<br>R: Yeah, the background right here, like the green in *Bambi*, in the forest from when I saw *Bambi*. [E should have queried "background" for dimensionality.] | Pr |
| X | 17 | | Some lions right here. (D2) | E: (ERR)<br>R: Yeah, right here because the yellow lion. [E could have queried for form dominance of color.] | |
| | 18 | | Some frogs or like crabs, these brown parts. (D7) | E: (ERR)<br>R: Yeah, here are the frogs or maybe it is crabs, I don't know.<br>E: What makes it look like frogs or crabs?<br>R: All the legs here; I just can't tell what animal. | |

# Rorschach Performance Assessment System (R-PAS)®

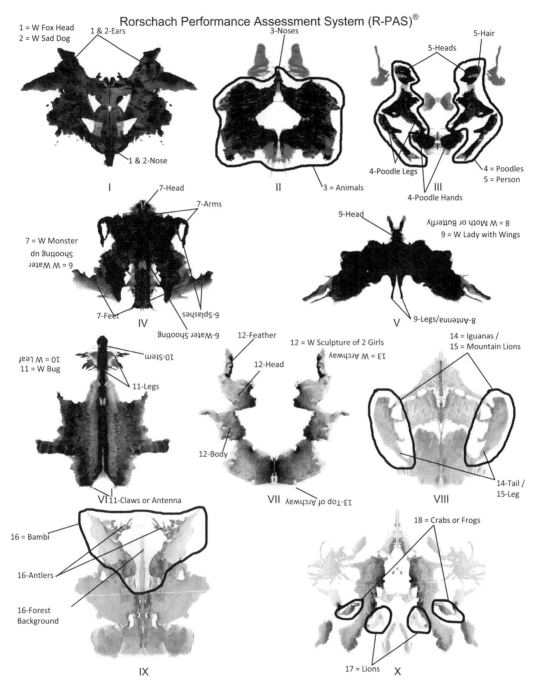

1 = W Fox Head
2 = W Sad Dog
1 & 2-Ears
1 & 2-Nose

I

3-Noses
3 = Animals

II

5-Heads
5-Hair
4-Poodle Legs
4 = Poodles
5 = Person
4-Poodle Hands

III

7-Head
7-Arms
7 = W Monster
6 = W Water Shooting up
7-Feet
6-Splashes
6-Water Shooting

IV

9-Head
8 = W Moth or Butterfly
9 = W Lady with Wings
9-Legs/Antenna
8-Antenna/6

V

10-Stem
10 = W Leaf
11 = W Bug
11-Legs
11-Claws or Antenna

VI

12-Feather
12-Head
12 = W Sculpture of 2 Girls
13 = W Archway
12-Body
13-Top of Archway

VII

14 = Iguanas /
15 = Mountain Lions
14-Tail /
15-Leg

VIII

16 = Bambi
16-Antlers
16-Forest Background

IX

18 = Crabs or Frogs
17 = Lions

X

# R-PAS Code Sequence: "Neveah"

**C-ID**: Neveah    **P-ID**: 252    **Age**: 15    **Gender**: Female    **Education**: 9

| Cd | # | Or | Loc | Loc # | SR | SI | Content | Sy | Vg | 2 | FQ | P | Determinants | Cognitive | Thematic | HR | ODL (RP) | R-Opt | Text |
|----|---|----|-----|-------|----|----|---------|----|----|---|----|---|--------------|-----------|----------|----|----------|-------|------|
| I | 1 | | W | | | | Ad | | | | o | | F | | | | | Pr | |
| | 2 | @ | W | | | | Ad | | | | o | | FMp | | MOR | | | | |
| II | 3 | @ | D | 1 | | | A | Sy | | 2 | o | | FMa | | | | | Pr | |
| III | 4 | | D | 9 | | | A | | | 2 | u | | Ma | INC1 | | PH | | | |
| | 5 | | D | 9 | | | H | | | 2 | o | P | F | DV1 | | GH | | | * |

*Comment:* Neveah appeared to be describing an "up do" hairstyle and misspoke; therefore, a DV1 was coded.

| Cd | # | Or | Loc | Loc # | SR | SI | Content | Sy | Vg | 2 | FQ | P | Determinants | Cognitive | Thematic | HR | ODL (RP) | R-Opt | Text |
|----|---|----|-----|-------|----|----|---------|----|----|---|----|---|--------------|-----------|----------|----|----------|-------|------|
| IV | 6 | v | W | | | | NC | | | | u | | ma | | | | | | * |

*Comment:* Neveah indicates a small area the water is "shooting up out of" which suggests some form over vagueness.

| Cd | # | Or | Loc | Loc # | SR | SI | Content | Sy | Vg | 2 | FQ | P | Determinants | Cognitive | Thematic | HR | ODL (RP) | R-Opt | Text |
|----|---|----|-----|-------|----|----|---------|----|----|---|----|---|--------------|-----------|----------|----|----------|-------|------|
| | 7 | @ | W | | | | (H) | | | | o | P | F | | AGC | GH | | | |
| V | 8 | v | W | | | | A | | | | o | | F | | | | | | |
| | 9 | | W | | | | H | | | | o | | F | INC1 | | PH | | | |
| VI | 10 | v | W | | | | NC | | | | o | | F | | | | | | * |

*Comment:* FQo extrapolated from upright orientation.

| Cd | # | Or | Loc | Loc # | SR | SI | Content | Sy | Vg | 2 | FQ | P | Determinants | Cognitive | Thematic | HR | ODL (RP) | R-Opt | Text |
|----|---|----|-----|-------|----|----|---------|----|----|---|----|---|--------------|-----------|----------|----|----------|-------|------|
| | 11 | | W | | | | A | | | | u | | F | | AGC | | | | |
| VII | 12 | | W | | | | (H),Art,Cg | Sy | | 2 | o | | Mp | | | GH | | | * |

*Comment:* (H) was coded because Neveah comments that she "can't see the face so it's a sculpture," suggesting they are not realistic depictions of humans. Mp was coded for "the body is turned this way."

| Cd | # | Or | Loc | Loc # | SR | SI | Content | Sy | Vg | 2 | FQ | P | Determinants | Cognitive | Thematic | HR | ODL (RP) | R-Opt | Text |
|----|---|----|-----|-------|----|----|---------|----|----|---|----|---|--------------|-----------|----------|----|----------|-------|------|
| | 13 | v | W | | | | NC | | | | u | | F | | | | | | |
| VIII | 14 | | D | 1 | | | A | | | 2 | o | | F | | | | | | |
| | 15 | | D | 1 | | | A | | | 2 | o | P | F | | AGC | | | | |
| IX | 16 | | D | 3,8 | | | A,NC | Sy | | 2 | u | | FMp,CF | | PER | | | Pr | * |

*Comment:* E should have queried "background" for dimensionality. Although aggression is implied with the deer putting their antlers together, it is not enough to establish AGM. FQu coded based on the animal (antlered or horned) at D3.

| Cd | # | Or | Loc | Loc # | SR | SI | Content | Sy | Vg | 2 | FQ | P | Determinants | Cognitive | Thematic | HR | ODL (RP) | R-Opt | Text |
|----|---|----|-----|-------|----|----|---------|----|----|---|----|---|--------------|-----------|----------|----|----------|-------|------|
| X | 17 | | D | 2 | | | A | | | 2 | o | | CF | | AGC | | | | |
| | 18 | | D | 7 | | | A | | | 2 | o | | F | | | | | | |

©2010-2016 R-PAS

C-ID: Neveah     P-ID: 252     Age: 15     Gender: Female     Education: 9

| Domain/Variables | Raw Scores | Raw A-SS | Raw C-SS | Cplx. Adj. A-SS | Cplx. Adj. C-SS | Standard Score Profile R-Optimized | Abbr. |
|---|---|---|---|---|---|---|---|
| **Admin. Behaviors and Obs.** | | | | | | | |
| Pr | 3 | 119 | 131 | | | | Pr |
| Pu | 0 | 96 | 95 | | | | Pu |
| CT (Card Turning) | 7 | 110 | 110 | | | | CT |
| **Engagement and Cog. Processing** | | | | | | | |
| Complexity | 41 | 74 | 83 | | | | Cmplx |
| R (Responses) | 18 | 77 | 81 | 93 | 92 | | R |
| F% [Lambda=1.57] (Simplicity) | 61% | 116 | 107 | 105 | 96 | | F% |
| Blend | 1 | 84 | 89 | 102 | 104 | | Bln |
| Sy | 3 | 86 | 90 | 106 | 109 | | Sy |
| MC | 4.0 | 87 | 92 | 104 | 109 | | MC |
| MC - PPD | 0.0 | 107 | 106 | 106 | 105 | | MC-PPD |
| M | 2 | 91 | 93 | 102 | 105 | | M |
| M/MC [2/4.0] | 50% | 99 | 100 | 101 | 103 | | M Prp |
| (CF+C)/SumC [2/2] | NA | | | | | | CFC Prp |
| **Perception and Thinking Problems** | | | | | | | |
| EII-3 | -0.6 | 92 | 89 | 100 | 96 | | EII |
| TP-Comp (Thought & Percept. Com...) | -0.4 | 80 | 78 | 94 | 86 | | TP-C |
| WSumCog | 5 | 98 | 96 | 105 | 102 | | WCog |
| SevCog | 0 | 94 | 94 | 94 | 94 | | Sev |
| FQ-% | 0% | 78 | 74 | 84 | 79 | | FQ-% |
| WD-% | 0% | 82 | 78 | 84 | 79 | | WD-% |
| FQo% | 72% | 112 | 125 | 105 | 116 | | FQo% |
| P | 3 | 80 | 88 | 88 | 95 | | P |
| **Stress and Distress** | | | | | | | |
| YTVC' | 0 | 73 | 84 | 89 | 95 | | YTVC' |
| m | 1 | 97 | 96 | 104 | 103 | | m |
| Y | 0 | 85 | 90 | 94 | 97 | | Y |
| MOR | 1 | 100 | 100 | 105 | 104 | | MOR |
| SC-Comp (Suicide Concern Comp.) | 3.7 | 90 | 89 | 101 | 99 | | SC-C |
| **Self and Other Representation** | | | | | | | |
| ODL% | 0% | 74 | 84 | 81 | 92 | | ODL% |
| SR (Space Reversal) | 0 | 87 | 89 | 87 | 89 | | SR |
| MAP/MAHP [0/0] | NA | | | | | | MAP Prp |
| PHR/GPHR [2/5] | 40% | 105 | 95 | 105 | 95 | | PHR Prp |
| M- | 0 | 95 | 91 | 95 | 91 | | M- |
| AGC | 4 | 108 | 106 | 111 | 109 | | AGC |
| H | 2 | 98 | 97 | 106 | 105 | | H |
| COP | 0 | 88 | 88 | 102 | 101 | | COP |
| MAH | 0 | 90 | 90 | 90 | 90 | | MAH |

A-SS = Adult Standard Score; C-SS = Age-Based Child or Adolescent Standard Score     © 2010-2016 R-PAS

# R-PAS Summary Scores and Profiles – Page 2

C-ID: Neveah    P-ID: 252    Age: 15    Gender: Female    Education: 9

| Domain/Variables | Raw Scores | Raw A-SS | Raw C-SS | Cplx. Adj. A-SS | Cplx. Adj. C-SS | Standard Score Profile R-Optimized | Abbr. |
|---|---|---|---|---|---|---|---|
| **Engagement and Cog. Processing** | | | | | | | |
| W% | 56% | 111 | 112 | 119 | 120 | | W% |
| Dd% | 0% | 75 | 80 | 75 | 78 | | Dd% |
| SI (Space Integration) | 0 | 74 | 80 | 91 | 92 | | SI |
| IntCont | 1 | 93 | 97 | 101 | 109 | | IntC |
| Vg% | 0% | 86 | 89 | 86 | 85 | | Vg% |
| V | 0 | 92 | 92 | 93 | 94 | | V |
| FD | 0 | 88 | 90 | 102 | 101 | | FD |
| R8910% | 28% | 89 | 91 | 86 | 87 | | R8910% |
| WSumC | 2.0 | 92 | 95 | 103 | 108 | | WSC |
| C | 0 | 95 | 92 | 95 | 92 | | C |
| Mp/(Ma+Mp) [1/2] | NA | | | | | | Mp Prp |
| **Perception and Thinking Problems** | | | | | | | |
| FQu% | 28% | 97 | 95 | 106 | 103 | | FQu% |
| **Stress and Distress** | | | | | | | |
| PPD | 4 | 81 | 90 | 100 | 104 | | PPD |
| CBlend | 0 | 91 | 91 | 93 | 93 | | CBlnd |
| C' | 0 | 84 | 87 | 89 | 91 | | C' |
| V | 0 | 92 | 92 | 93 | 94 | | V |
| CritCont% (Critical Contents) | 6% | 83 | 89 | 93 | 97 | | CrCt |
| **Self and Other Representation** | | | | | | | |
| SumH | 4 | 91 | 91 | 105 | 104 | | SumH |
| NPH/SumH [2/4] | 50% | 92 | 92 | 88 | 87 | | NPH Prp |
| V-Comp (Vigilance Composite) | 2.1 | 87 | 88 | 103 | 103 | | V-C |
| r (Reflections) | 0 | 95 | 93 | 95 | 93 | | r |
| p/(a+p) [3/6] | 50% | 106 | 104 | 104 | 102 | | p Prp |
| AGM | 0 | 93 | 90 | 93 | 90 | | AGM |
| T | 0 | 91 | 91 | 91 | 91 | | T |
| PER | 1 | 109 | 104 | 109 | 104 | | PER |
| An | 0 | 85 | 87 | 85 | 87 | | An |

A-SS = Adult Standard Score; C-SS = Age-Based Child or Adolescent Standard Score

© 2010-2016 R-PAS

# Index

Note. *f* or *t* following a page number indicates a figure or a table.